Metastatic Spine Disease

Rex A. W. Marco
Editor

Metastatic Spine Disease

A Guide to Diagnosis and Management

Springer

Editor
Rex A. W. Marco, MD
Department of Orthopedic Surgery
Houston Methodist Hospital
Houston, Texas, USA

ISBN 978-3-030-09443-0 ISBN 978-3-319-76252-4 (eBook)
https://doi.org/10.1007/978-3-319-76252-4

Softcover re-print of the Hardcover 1st edition 2018

Printed on acid-free paper

This Springer imprint is published by the registered company Springer International Publishing AG part of Springer Nature
The registered company address is: Gewerbestrasse 11, 6330 Cham, Switzerland

Foreword

The management of spinal metastasis is the latest horizon in musculoskeletal oncology. A new generation of clinicians brings transdisciplinary skills to catapult this field forward. With in-depth training in both oncologic and spinal surgery, surgeons can now approach these diseases in a more ambitious and sophisticated fashion. Focused collaboration between specialties is the strategy that underlies the modern approach to spinal metastases. It is captured in the chapters of this book, authored by the leading practitioners of this science and art form. Historically, the anatomic interplay of neural, vascular, and osseous elements in a three-dimensional array dissuaded investigators and surgeons from tackling cancer, especially metastases, in the spine. Medicine's aversion to treating spinal metastases is more conspicuous because this location is the most prevalent site of skeletal metastases and a principal cause of pain and morbidity in metastatic cancers. Several advances in oncology over the course of the last century have finally come together to give oncologists of all descriptions the conceptual and technical tools to handle cancers affecting these sites. Finally we have treatments that are less morbid than the disease processes, enhancing the risk-benefit analysis and favoring intelligent intervention. The approaches captured in this compendium have created successful medical, radiation, and surgical treatments that can be tailored to the individual. This is one of the most exciting advances in modern oncology and has enabled us to reduce morbidity and change the natural history of disease for many patients.

How did this progress happen? There are several specific focused advances and several macro trends that bear highlighting.

Refinement in our understanding of vascular anatomy has contributed greatly. On the arterial side of the circulation, the artery of Adamkowitz (arteria radicularis magna) has been shown to vary widely in location and importance. It may originate anywhere from the T9 to L5 vertebral levels, although it is most commonly emanating from the posterior intercostal arteries within the T9–12 levels. While it is always more satisfying to preserve this vessel, it has been recognized that it typically can be sacrificed for suitable oncologic reasons, and using appropriate technique without encountering a catastrophic neurological injury. This has emboldened more oncologically sound procedures.

There has been greater understanding of the venous circulation as well. The "grande veines rachidiennes longitudinales antéricures" described by Gilbert Breschet in 1832 were relegated to obscurity until they were rediscovered and delineated in 1940 by Oscar Batson in cadaveric and rhesus macaque experiments. Recognizing that these perivertebral valveless veins form sinuses that facilitate the characteristic pattern of metastatic spread of cancer has enabled greater understanding of the metastatic process. Such fundamental anatomic discoveries were essential to allow modern care and surgery of spinal disease.

Physiologic advances in our understanding the function of sacral neural anatomy have made sacral surgery more predictable. The role of the S3 nerve root and the value of unilateral preservation of S2 and S3 roots in the conservation of sphincter function warrant emphasis.

The indispensible role of anatomic and physiologic imaging, and magnetic resonance imaging in particular, cannot be stressed enough. Without these developments that we now take for granted, the planning of surgical and radiation procedures could never be done with accuracy or precision. High-quality imaging is the underpinning for all of the advances described in this volume. Both musculoskeletal radiologists and neuroradiologists have been essential in improving the care of patients with spinal metastases.

Surgical visionaries like Bertil Stener and Björn Gunterberg in Sweden and Katsuro Tomita in Japan have built on the anatomic, imaging, and staging advances to apply their talents to increasingly challenging problems. Their legacy is celebrated in the advances described in this book.

The management of spinal cancers has not occurred in a vacuum and the broader societal context is worth noting. President Richard Nixon, in his December 23, 1971, remarks to Congress when launching his historic War on Cancer, noted that this effort would be remembered as the most memorable act of his administration because cancer killed more Americans annually than were killed during the entirety of World War II. His vision was not to bear fruit until the early years of this new century when the overall mortality rate for cancer first declined. With the advent of personalized medicine, there is a renewed focus on enhancing cancer care with the initiation of President Barack Obama's "Cancer Moonshot." While the overall cure of cancer is not imminent, the advances from modern genomics, targeted therapies, and immunology are dramatically helping patients and converting metastatic cancer into a chronic disease. This has changed the landscape. Clinicians are no longer constrained to limited palliative surgery and radiation options, nor resignation to escalating narcotic pain management for these patients. Now the spectacular technical achievements developed for primary tumors can be offered to the patient suffering from metastatic cancer.

It is in this context that the authors of this work have brought together the latest advances in biology, surgery, and reconstruction. Practitioners of all specialties that deal with patients suffering from spinal metastatic disease will be interested in applying these new concepts clinically. Improvement of patient quality of life is the next battle in the war on cancer.

New York, NY, USA John H. Healey, MD

Preface

Few conditions are a source of greater fear and stress for both patient and practitioner than metastatic spinal cord compression (MSCC). Typically, these patients present with severe pain and impending paralysis. They are often in a deconditioned state, medically quite ill, and in great distress, so there is much pressure on the practitioner to institute rapid treatment. While MSCC is a medical emergency requiring the timely institution of treatment that will both lessen the patient's pain and preserve function, often practitioners rush into treatment without paying adequate attention to the specific features of the compression, features that are of pivotal importance to the planning of the most optimal treatment. In one's haste to "do the right thing," one may do a quick search of his or her memory for what was learned about the condition in a lecture, from an upper level resident, a book chapter, a review article, or the internet. Sometimes practitioners faced with a case of MSCC will base treatment on the findings from the most up-to-date, Level 1, prospective, randomized study reported in a national meeting or a peer-reviewed journal. Sometimes algorithms, designed to simplify the treatment decision-making process in these patients, are overly relied upon. All of these scenarios are recipes for a potentially disastrous outcome.

Occasionally, practitioners are fortunate to have trained under experienced and thoughtful mentors who teach that individualized treatment is the key to an optimal outcome in these very ill patients. Yes, MSCC is a medical emergency, but before rushing into treatment, one must first take time to consider the patient's medical and mental condition, the biology of the tumor, the responsiveness of the tumor to adjuvant treatments, the natural history of the disease, the palliative nature of the condition, the neurologic status of the patient, the degree of spinal cord compression, the physiologic stability of the spine, and the risks and benefits of operative versus nonoperative treatment options. In addition, the optimal treatment of MSCC requires the participation of a multidisciplinary team of oncologists, radiation oncologists, oncologic spinal surgeons, neuroradiologists, medical specialists, and physiatrists, all of whom play an important role in helping patients decide which treatment is best in light of the particular facets of their condition.

All of the contributors to this book have worked with such mentors, and this book is a compendium of the knowledge and experience acquired from such skilled men and women. One of the first lessons to be learned is the importance of evaluating and treating these patients with respect and compassion. All of the contributors have also had extensive experience working with cohesive multidisciplinary teams that together strive to provide optimal care to all patients with MSCC. Of perhaps the greatest importance, each contributor has had the privilege of experiencing firsthand both the joy and the anguish that always attend the treatment of patients with MSCC. The book is intended for anyone who is part of such a multidisciplinary team and desires to acquire a more in-depth understanding of the most up-to-date management techniques for MSCC. The contributing authors have not only cared for many of these patients but have also devoted much time and effort to understanding and developing better ways to achieve optimal outcomes.

Of further note, each author has made it a point to critically evaluate the existing literature and to provide up-to-date patient-centered algorithms that will help in the efficient planning of treatment that takes into consideration not only the patient but also the family, caregivers, and society in general. As an example of some of the strides made in improving the treatment of MSCC, minimally invasive surgical techniques have been developed that in combination with more effective chemotherapy and radiation therapy have enabled more patients to be treated with less invasive, and thus much less debilitating, approaches. This book contains a chapter describing a novel systematic approach for the soft tissue coverage of the surgical wounds using plastic reconstruction techniques. A unique feature of the book is chapters that describe specific approaches to the management of MSCC depending on its location along the spinal column. The unique anatomy of each location in the spine is an important focus of these chapters as well.

We, the contributors to this book, hope that it will help all those who may find themselves faced with a case of MSCC be better prepared and equipped to provide optimal, individualized care to these seriously ill patients.

Houston, TX, USA Rex A. W. Marco, MD

Acknowledgments

I would like to acknowledge everyone who has supported my professional development. My first mentor in oncologic research was Steven Rosenberg, MD, PhD, who along with Richard Alexander, MD, sparked my interest in studying cancer. John Ryan, MD, and Mark Hill, MD, taught me so much about being a doctor and surgeon. My co-residents and faculty at UC Davis became my second family and supported me throughout this wonderful time in my life and professional development. My father's battle with cancer helped me begin to understand the pain and sadness that this disease can cause. I found myself wanting to use my knowledge of orthopedics to help patients with metastatic cancer live better lives with less pain and suffering and to help save the lives of those with primary malignant bone and soft tissue tumors. John Healey, MD, taught me how to apply this knowledge with empathy and compassion. He taught me to individualize patients and care for them as if they were my loved one. Ronald L. DeWald, MD, and Howard An, MD, helped me learn the ethical application of the principles of reconstructive spine surgery to care for these patients and build spine constructs that PASS (patency, alignment, supported anteriorly, and stabilized posteriorly) the test to allow these patients to have less pain and suffering. Mark Bilsky, MD, and Ziya Gokaslan, MD, helped me learn the complex anatomy of the spine and its surrounding visceral and neurovascular structures. Jesse Dickson, MD, helped me develop proficiency in the techniques required to perform complex spine surgery. I am grateful for the friendship and support of my colleagues Darrell Hanson, MD, Vivek Kushwaha, MD, and Chris Meyer, MD, who also helped me further develop my knowledge and skills.

On a more personal level, I am extremely grateful to my mother and father who supported and encouraged me throughout my childhood, training, and career. I am grateful to Emina who supported me through the great years and remains one of my "best" teachers. I am grateful for my children who helped me understand unconditional love and through our recovery we are learning to find peace of mind and happiness. I am grateful for my PA, Jerry Buchert, PAC, and my MA, Esmeralda Salinas, who have been with me through the ups and downs of my career and life. I am grateful for the talented neurosurgeons in Istanbul, the loving staff at Columbia University, and the doctors and nurses at Mt. Sinai-St. Lukes Roosevelt Hospital for giving us the opportunity for a second chance. I am thankful for Brent Bradley, PhD, who taught me to communicate from my primary emotion from a vulnerable standpoint and for David Moore who taught me nonjudgmental self-acceptance. I will be forever grateful to Gerry and Margo Dye who taught me how to find peace by making every decision based on my sense of right. I am also grateful for Brandon and Micki Fine who introduced me to living in the present and mindfulness. I am thankful for Roger and Albina Rippy for guiding me through the 40 day personal revolution as outlined by Baron Baptiste. I am forever indebted to our recovery teams at TAFS, The Council on Recovery, Archway Academy, Elements, Academic Answers, Pure Life, Oliverian, Cornerstone, and the 12 steps. All of you have touched my life and taught me how to be a better parent and person. I am thankful for the opportunity to be reminded of the importance of kindness, compassion, humility, acceptance, honesty, accountability, commitment, forgiveness, loving kindness, and patience. I am honored to have the opportunity to apply the knowledge of my professional and life mentors to edit and contribute to this book and I am grateful to my Development Editor, Mariah Gumpert, and Springer who had the faith in me to complete this project. I am hopeful that this work will contribute to improved care for our patients with metastatic spinal cord compression.

Contents

Contributors

A. Karim Ahmed, BS Department of Neurosurgery, Johns Hopkins University School of Medicine, Baltimore, MD, USA

Syed Uzair Ahmed, MD Division of Neurosurgery, University of Saskatchewan, Saskatoon, SK, Canada

Christopher Pearson Ames, MD Department of Neurological Surgery, University of California, San Francisco, San Francisco, CA, USA

Adedayo O. Ashana, MD Department of Orthopedic Spine Surgery, OSS Health, York, PA

Mark Bilsky, MD Department of Neurosurgery, Memorial Sloan Kettering Cancer Center, New York, NY, USA

Justin Earl Bird, MD Department of Orthopedic Oncology, The University of Texas MD Anderson Cancer Center, Houston, TX, USA

Stefano Boriani, MD GSpine4 Spine Surgery Unit, IRCCS Galeazzi Orthopedic Institute, Milano, MI, Italy

Joseph Brindise, DO Department of Orthopedic and Sports Medicine, Houston Methodist Hospital, Houston, TX, USA

Jacob M. Buchowski, MD, MS Department of Orthopedic Surgery, BJC Institute of Health, Washington University in St. Louis—School of Medicine, St. Louis, MO, USA

Raphaële Charest-Morin, MD, FRCSC Department of Orthopaedic, Centre Hospitalier Universitaire de Québec, Quebec City, QC, Canada

Scott E. Dart, MD Department of Orthopedic Surgery, Carolinas Medical Center, Charlotte, NC, USA

David Dong, BS Department of Orthopedics and Sports Medicine, Houston Methodist Hospital, Houston, TX, USA

Benjamin D. Elder, MD, PhD Department of Neurosurgery, The Mayo Clinic, Rochester, MN, USA

Gisberto Evangelisti, MD Department of Oncologic and Degenerative Spine Surgery, Orthopedic Institute Rizzoli, Bologna, Italy

Charles G. Fisher, MD, MHSc, FRCSC Division of Spine, Department of Orthopaedics, The Combined Neurosurgical and Orthopaedic Spine Program at Vancouver Coastal Health, Vancouver, BC, Canada

Daryl R. Fourney, MD, FRCSC, FACS Department of Neurosurgery, University of Saskatchewan, Royal University Hospital, Saskatoon, SK, Canada

Jared Fridley, MD Department of Neurosurgery, Warren Alpert School of Medicine, Brown University, Providence, RI, USA

Steve H. Fung, MD Department of Radiology, Weill Cornell Medical College, Houston Methodist Hospital, Houston Methodist Research Institute, Houston, TX, USA

Alessandro Gasbarrini, MD Department of Oncologic and Degenerative Spine Surgery, Orthopedic Institute Rizzoli, Bologna, Italy

Riccardo Ghermandi, MD Department of Oncologic and Degenerative Spine Surgery, Orthopedic Institute Rizzoli, Bologna, Italy

Marco Girolami, MD Department of Oncologic and Degenerative Spine Surgery, Orthopedic Institute Rizzoli, Bologna, Italy

Ziya L. Gokaslan, MD, FAANS, FACS Department of Neurosurgery, The Warren Alpert Medical School of Brown University, Providence, RI, USA

Department of Neurosurgery, Rhode Island Hospital and The Miriam Hospital, Providence, RI, USA

C. Rory Goodwin, MD, PhD Department of Neurosurgery, Duke University Medical Center, Durham, NC, USA

Waqar Haque, MD CHI St. Luke's Health, Houston, TX, USA

John H. Healey, MD Department of Surgery, Memorial Sloan Kettering Cancer Center, New York, NY, USA

Charles A. Hogan, MD Department of Orthopedic Surgery, Houston Methodist Hospital, Houston, TX, USA

Wataru Ishida, MD Department of Neurosurgery, Johns Hopkins Hospital, Baltimore, MD, USA

Jack W. Jennings, MD, PhD Department of Radiology, Mallinckrodt Institute of Radiology, Washington University School of Medicine, Barnes-Jewish Hospital, St. Louis, MO, USA

Andrew B. Kay, MD Department of Orthopedic Surgery, Houston Methodist Hospital, Houston, TX, USA

Michael J. Klebuc, MD Institute for Reconstructive Surgery, Houston Methodist Hospital, Weill Cornell Medical College, Houston, TX, USA

Darryl Lau, MD Department of Neurosurgery, University of California, San Francisco, San Francisco, CA, USA

Ilya Laufer, MD Department of Neurosurgery, Memorial Sloan Kettering Cancer Center, New York, NY, USA

Daniel P. Leas, MD Department of Orthopedic Surgery, Carolinas Medical Center, Charlotte, NC, USA

Rex A. W. Marco, MD Department of Orthopedic Surgery, Houston Methodist Hospital, Houston, TX, USA

Robert F. McLain, MD Spine and Orthopedic Institute, St Vincent Charity Medical Center, Cleveland, OH, USA

Cleveland State University, Solon, OH, USA

Ehud Mendel, MD, MBA, FACS The Ohio State University-Wexner Medical Center, The James Cancer Hospital, Columbus, OH, USA

Ahmed Mohyeldin, MD, PhD Department of Neurosurgery, Ohio State University Wexner Medical Center, Columbus, OH, USA

Patrick Moody, MD Department of Orthopedics, Carolinas Medical Center, Charlotte, NC, USA

Hannah Morehouse, MD Department of Orthopedic Surgery, Houston Methodist Hospital, Houston, TX, USA

Joseph A. Osorio, MD, PhD Department of Neurosurgery, University of California, San Francisco, San Francisco, CA, USA

Adetokunbo Oyelese, MD, PhD, FAANS Department of Neurosurgery, The Warren Alpert Medical School of Brown University, Providence, RI, USA

Department of Neurosurgery, Rhode Island Hospital, Providence, RI, USA

Joshua C. Patt, MD, MPH Department of Orthopaedic Surgery, Carolinas Medical Center, Atrium Health, Charlotte, NC, USA

Levine Cancer Institute, Atrium Health, Charlotte, NC, USA

Valerio Pipola, MD Department of Oncologic and Degenerative Spine Surgery, Orthopedic Institute Rizzoli, Bologna, Italy

Joseph H. Schwab, MD, MS Harvard Medical School, Massachusetts General Hospital, Boston, MA, USA

Daniel M. Sciubba, MD Department of Neurosurgery, Johns Hopkins University School of Medicine, Baltimore, MD, USA

Sanjay K. Singh, MD Department of Radiology, Houston Methodist Hospital, Houston, TX, USA

Guiseppe Tedesco Department of Oncologic and Degenerative Spine Surgery, Orthopedic Institute Rizzoli, Bologna, Italy

Bin S. Teh, MD Radiation and Oncology Department, Houston Methodist Hospital, Houston, TX, USA

Alexander Theologis, MD Department of Orthopedic Surgery, University of California—San Francisco (UCSF), San Francisco, CA, USA

Zane Tymchak, MD Royal University Hospital, Saskatoon, SK, Canada

Max Vaynrub, MD Department of Surgery, Memorial Sloan Kettering Cancer Center, New York, NY, USA

Jean-Paul Wolinsky, MD Department of Neurosurgery, Northwestern University, Chicago, IL, USA

Dmitry Zavlin, MD Institute for Reconstructive Surgery, Houston Methodist Hospital, Houston, TX, USA

Zoe Zhang, MD Department of Neurosurgery, The Ohio State University—Wexner Medical Center, The James Cancer Hospital, Columbus, OH, USA

Scott L. Zuckerman, MD, MPH Department of Neurological Surgery, Vanderbilt University Medical Center, Nashville, TN, USA

MOSS: A Patient-Centered Approach

1

Rex A. W. Marco, Joseph Brindise, and David Dong

Background

Treating patients with spinal metastatic disease is a challenging and humbling proposition when one considers that these are patients who are often quite medically ill with life expectancies measured in months. Therefore, any treatment in these patients is primarily palliative in intent and, as such, should be aimed at ameliorating the most distressing symptoms without causing significant morbidity.

A variety of scoring systems and algorithms have been devised over time to help the spinal surgeon decide if and when surgical management is indicated. Unfortunately, however, all these systems have significant flaws that can lead the practitioner to decide on surgical intervention when non-operative treatment is really the better course of action. We currently lack more up-to-date methods of determining, first, whether surgery is called for and, second, which method of either operative or non-operative management is best for the particular patient. This is especially concerning in light of the anticipated increasing proportion of patients who will be faced with metastatic spinal disease who now can only be assessed by outdated frameworks that do not take into account newer nonsurgical treatments with a proven efficacy that makes surgery the least desirable option in most cases. For all of these urgent reasons, we have developed a framework that we believe is more up to the task of assessing patients with metastatic disease to the spine. Our framework considers several variables, the most important one, in our estimation, being the medical status of the patient. It also takes into consideration all available surgical and nonsurgical treatment options and their relative merits in a given patient. This integrated analysis has proven, in our experience, to identify the least invasive, and at the same time the most optimal, approach to the management of patients with spinal metastasis.

Historical Approaches

The treatment of patients with MSCC has changed significantly over time. Before the advent of radiotherapy, laminectomy was the only effective treatment for this problem [1]. With the advent of radiotherapy, however, there was a paradigm shift in the management of these patients, but not without a rigorous debate over the relative effectiveness of radiotherapy alone compared with the combination of laminectomy and radiotherapy. This led to the conduct of several small retrospective studies, which did indeed fail to show that the combination of laminectomy

R. A. W. Marco, MD
Department of Orthopaedic Surgery, Houston Methodist Hospital, Houston, TX, USA

J. Brindise, DO · D. Dong, BS (✉)
Department of Orthopedics and Sports Medicine, Houston Methodist Hospital, Houston, TX, USA
e-mail: jpbrindise@houstonmethodist.org

R. A. W. Marco (ed.), *Metastatic Spine Disease*, https://doi.org/10.1007/978-3-319-76252-4_1

and radiotherapy had any significant advantage over radiotherapy alone in relieving epidural metastatic compression [2, 3].

In 1980, Young et al. were the first to publish their findings from a prospective randomized study examining the relative merits of the two treatments. These authors also found that neither pain relief, ambulation, nor sphincter function was better after laminectomy plus radiotherapy than after radiotherapy alone [4]. It was still believed, however, that laminectomy alone could provide decompression and pain control. However, a further problem with this surgery not recognized at the time was that by the time of intermediate follow-up, the spinal column had collapsed in many patients because of the removal of supportive structures during the laminectomy. This therefore once again raised questions about the advisability of laminectomy. With the development of improved spinal instrumentation, some practitioners began to believe that decompression with a laminectomy or vertebrectomy, in conjunction with the implantation of the new instrumentation, could produce better functional outcomes, especially in relatively healthy patients with longer survival expectancies [5].

Then, in 2005, surgery got a boost when Patchell et al. published findings from a landmark randomized trial showing that patients with metastatic spinal cord compression who underwent surgery could expect a more favorable outcome than those treated only with radiotherapy [6]. Interestingly these investigators found that with circumferential decompression, stabilization, radiotherapy, and steroids as opposed to radiotherapy and steroids alone, significantly more patients were able to walk and maintained the ability to walk for longer duration after treatment. Additionally, those who were non-ambulatory for less than 48 h when they entered the study regained their ability to walk, and the need for corticosteroids and opioid pain medications was considerably less for the surgical treatment group. These authors therefore concluded that the best treatment for metastatic spinal cord compression is surgery followed by radiotherapy. This therefore led to a dramatic swing of the pendulum toward the use of aggressive surgical management in patients with metastatic epidural spinal cord compression.

However, this study had significant shortcomings, which raised questions about the general applicability of its findings. For example, the patients in the non-operative arm had significantly worse outcomes than those historically observed in patients treated with radiotherapy alone [7–15]. In addition, despite the participation of many high-volume centers, the enrollment of patients in the study was particularly slow, with sometimes only a single patient enrolled over the course of a decade. Understanding why so few patients being treated at these busy centers were considered eligible for inclusion in the study is key to accurately interpreting the applicability of this study's findings to one's own practice. One reason for this slow recruitment was that the inclusion criteria allowed only patients with a single area of spinal involvement and those who had not been totally paraplegic for longer than 48 h to be entered into the study. Another questionable aspect of the study was that 18/51 (35%) patients randomized to non-operative treatment presented with an unstable spine. Perhaps these patients should have undergone stabilization and not even considered as candidates for radiotherapy alone. Another criticism of the Patchell study is that tumor histology was not considered in the randomization of patients in the study. That and the relatively short median survival of 3–4 months in both the operative and non-operative groups further raise questions about the degree to which one should be influenced by the study conclusions. A final concern about the study was raised by Chi et al. [16], who conducted a sub-analysis to determine the effect of age on the outcomes. They made the troubling discovery that as patient age increased, the benefits of the combination of surgery and radiotherapy decreased. In fact, by age 65, there was no observable difference in outcomes between the two groups. Considering that over 60% of patients with cancer are over the age of 65, this may give surgery a more limited role in the care of older patients with metastatic epidural compression.

In 2008, George et al. discussed the results of a Cochrane review [17], which also questioned the generalizability of the findings in the Patchell study. This study was designed with the overall purpose of determining definitively the effectiveness of radiotherapy, surgery, and corticosteroids in the treatment of patients with metastatic epidural spinal cord compression. Specifically, the authors assessed the quality of six randomized controlled trials of radiotherapy, surgery, and corticosteroids and calculated the relative risk ratios and numbers of patients needed to enable treatment with 95% confidence intervals. Among their conclusions, they found that high-dose steroids are associated with more serious side effects than moderate-dose steroids. They also concluded that patients with stable spines can be treated with radiation therapy only and still retain their ability to walk. Surgery was deemed beneficial for ambulatory patients with a relatively radioresistant tumor, as well as for non-ambulatory patients with a single area of involvement who had been paraplegic for less than 48 h, had a relatively radioresistant tumor, and had a more than 3-month life expectancy.

Now, with improvements in technology and refinements in treatment options, an effort has been made to develop comprehensive, multidisciplinary decision frameworks for determining the most optimal treatment in patients with metastatic epidural spinal compression. The most popular of these has been the neurologic, oncological, mechanical, and systemic (NOMS) framework, developed at Memorial Sloan-Kettering Cancer Center over 15 years ago [18, 19].

The goal of NOMS is to provide a dynamic framework that will identify the optimal treatment for these patients. It does so by integrating the four sentinel decision points (i.e., neurological, oncological, mechanical, and systemic), which guides the type and extent of radiation therapy, surgery, and/or systemic therapy. Although this framework has been useful in accomplishing these goals, it is not without significant drawbacks.

For example, the neurological component of the NOMS framework focuses on the degree of spinal cord compression shown by MRI [19], which is then classified as high or low grade. The treatment algorithm then directs the clinician to the oncologic diagnosis, which involves classifying the tumors as radioresistant or radiosensitive. The algorithm is most suitable, however, for directing non-operative treatment in patients with low-grade spinal cord compression and radiosensitive or radioresistant tumors. However, the way the algorithm is designed, it favors surgery for the treatment of high-grade spinal cord compression caused by radioresistant tumors even though the clinical significance of this compression is not yet entirely clear.

In addition, the framework generally regards renal cell carcinoma (RCC), lung carcinoma, and sarcoma as radioresistant tumors. Thus, according to the NOMS framework, a patient with RCC and high-grade epidural compression should undergo surgical intervention. We believe, however, that such patients could benefit more from antiangiogenic chemotherapeutic agents (e.g., sunitinib, sorafenib, and pazopanib) that can provide sufficient local control, increase time to tumor progression, and potentially sensitize the tumor to radiation therapy; at the same time, these patients would be spared the risks and morbidity associated with surgery [20, 21]. Similarly, despite the presence of high-grade spinal cord compression, some patients with non-small cell lung carcinoma and small cell lung carcinoma are amenable to treatment with chemotherapy, such as erlotinib, combined with decompressive stereotactic radiotherapy. A final criticism of the NOMS framework is that sarcoma is generally considered a radioresistant tumor in this treatment algorithm, when in fact sarcomas such as Ewing's sarcoma, leiomyosarcoma, alveolar soft-parts sarcoma, myxoid liposarcoma, and synovial sarcoma are relatively radiosensitive tumors compared to many other sarcomas and carcinomas.

Regardless, since the NOMS framework was first adopted into clinical use, the picture in patients with metastasis to the spine has been changed dramatically by the increasing availability of very effective noninvasive treatments. Recent advances in the image-guided delivery of high-dose radiation therapy have further changed the nature of therapy in these patients. These advances have already translated into great improvements in the outcome of treatment.

One of these new radiotherapies is stereotactic radiosurgery (SRS), which can deliver high doses of radiation close to the spinal cord without exposing the cord and other adjacent vital structures to unsafe levels of radiation. In many cases now, SRS can achieve durable local tumor control regardless of tumor pathology, degree of spinal cord compression, and its past response to conventional radiotherapy. As proof of this, clinical response rates of greater than 85% and partial or complete pain response rates of 85–92% have been reported for patients treated with this technique [22–26].

Despite these significant advances, Bilsky et al. [19] have relegated the use of SRS to patients with radioresistant tumors who do not have high-grade epidural compression. They advocate surgical intervention in those patients with radioresistant tumors who have high-grade compression. This decided overemphasis on the MRI findings to determine whether the patient requires surgery unfortunately ignores other less invasive treatment options with proven efficacy that should be considered before surgery.

Of further concern, Bilsky et al. justified their recommendation for surgery in patients with high-grade epidural compression on the basis of the Patchell study, which showed a more favorable outcome in such patients compared with those who underwent radiotherapy alone. However, the surgery these authors advocate for such patients is separation surgery, not the decompression and debulking procedure Patchell et al. performed. In separation surgery, the intent is to do only minimal tumor resection to separate the tumor margin from the spinal cord, usually by as little as 2 mm, thereby leaving the bulk of the tumor to be treated with radiation, not the more extensive surgical debulking procedure Patchell et al. described. Furthermore, only conventional radiotherapy was available at the time of the Patchell study, which differs considerably in scope and intent from the SRS used by Bilsky et al. Therefore, one must question the appropriateness of using data from one study of somewhat outmoded treatments, or at least the only available treatments at the time, to support the adoption of new ones that, albeit, fall into the same categories as the earlier treatments but are far different in nature and effectiveness.

There are additional important drawbacks to the NOMS framework that in the light of current knowledge further make its reliability questionable. One of these has to do with the fact that it relies on the Spine Oncology Study Group (SOSG) proposed system for the mechanical assessment of the spine. The Spine Instability Neoplastic Score (SINS) yielded by the assessment evaluates spinal instability on the basis of clinical and radiographic information [27]. The SINS uses six variables: location, type of pain, radiographic spinal alignment, nature of the lesion (lytic, mixed, or blastic), vertebral body collapse, and involvement of the posterior elements. In this assessment, each variable is given a numerical score and these are totaled to arrive at an overall score. A low score (0–6) indicates a stable lesion that does not require surgical intervention. A high score (13–18) indicates spinal instability that does call for surgical intervention. Intermediate scores (7–12) are considered to indicate potential, but not definite, instability. Although SINS helps the clinician decide whether to consider surgical intervention for spinal instability in a patient with metastatic spinal disease, it does not offer much help in identifying the best surgical intervention in a particular patient. Furthermore, curiously, the SOSG also gave higher scores to metastases in the junctional regions of the spine such as the occipitocervical junction. This would suggest to practitioners that surgery is the preferable treatment option in these patients. In our experience, however, tumors at the occipito-cervical and lumbosacral junctions can frequently be treated non-operatively and rarely become unstable. For example, because odontoid tumors often spread in a cephalocaudal direction, they rarely cause spinal cord compression or instability. The SOSG also gave a high score for vertebral body collapse of more than 50%. Our experience has shown, however, that, even in cases where there is 100% vertebral body collapse or vertebra plana, the spine can often remain very stable.

The systemic, final, component of the NOMS framework assesses the ability of patients to tolerate the proposed intervention on the basis of the extent of systemic comorbidities and tumor burden. Bilsky et al. named several scoring systems for predicting the survival of patients with metastases, but they favored an individualistic approach that involves the oncologist in the discussion concerning life expectancy [27]. These authors noted that oncologists tend to overestimate a patient's life expectancy and therefore they are more inclined to recommend surgery as long as patients are likely to adequately recover from the indicated surgery and/or radiation therapy in order to continue systemic treatment. Once again, therefore, surgical interventions are ultimately favored over nonsurgical options that may actually be of greater benefit to the patient and also spare him or her the risks and morbidities associated with any kind of surgery.

Regardless, this systemic component of the NOMS framework has significant shortcomings. In sharp contrast to the approach taken in the NOMS framework, we believe the systemic assessment should be the primary consideration in all patients with metastatic disease. Yet in the NOMS system, this component is considered last, and the least amount of space is devoted to its discussion. The consequence of this, in effect, is the downplaying of the systemic aspect of a patient's medical status. Of greatest concern, is the strong bias for surgical intervention whenever NOMS is used. For instance, the framework will call for surgery in patients with metastatic lung cancer on the basis of neurological compression and oncological (radioresistance) and mechanical (e.g., greater than 50% tumor vertebral involvement) considerations before the systemic status of the patient is considered. If systemic considerations were considered first, then surgery maybe deemed of limited benefit regardless of neurological compression and spinal instability because of the typically short life-expectancy and high burden of disease in many of these patients.

Fortunately, an improved understanding of tumor biology has led to the discovery of a host of newer agents that is changing the landscape of non-operative treatment. For example, antiangiogenic, tyrosine kinase inhibitors such as sutinitib, sorafenib, and pasopanib can shrink renal cell carcinomas and thereby increase the median time until tumor progression into the spinal canal. These agents may also sensitize these tumors to radiotherapy. Tumor shrinkage, slower progression and radiosensitization makes such patients better candidates for non-operative treatment [20, 21]. Similarly, other tyrosine kinase inhibitors such as erlotinib that act on mutated EGFRs may improve local control in patients with non-small cell lung carcinoma [28–30]. These agents also appear to increase the likelihood that stereotactic radiation therapy will provide local control without the need for surgery.

Even in those patients who need surgery, an emphasis on their systemic status would encourage the search for the least invasive intervention possible for addressing any given problem. For example, combining limited separation surgery (described above) with SRS has in many cases supplanted the need for traditional excisional surgery. Similarly, percutaneous cement augmentation has been shown to be excellent for reducing pain secondary to spinal metastases. Balloon kyphoplasty has also proven to be very safe and effective in the short term. This was shown in the Cancer Patient Fracture Evaluation [31] study, in which 134 patients were randomized to receive either balloon kyphoplasty or usual care. Outcomes were assessed with the Roland Morris Disability Questionnaire (RMDQ), which showed that patients treated with kyphoplasty had an 8.4 point change in their RMDQ results at 1 month versus 0.1 in those who received usual care.

MOSS, A Patient-Centered Approach to Metastatic Disease of the Spine

As the foregoing discussion suggests, there is now a great need for a framework that is more adapted to the needs of patients with spinal metastases based on the greater understanding of the underlying disease processes and that also takes into consideration the new and improved surgical and nonsurgical treatments for spinal metastases. To meet this need, we have developed a novel framework (MOSS: medical/mental, oncological, stenosis, stability) for evaluating patients with MSCC. There are several aspects of this framework that are important for practitioners to understand. First, it applies to the palliative (not curative) care of these patients. Second, it reestablishes a patient's systemic status as the dominant consideration. Third, it encourages the evaluation of all treatment modalities (including newer adjuvant therapies) to determine the least invasive treatment strategy.

In our experience, use of this framework has significantly reduced the proportion of patients treated with surgical interventions. For us this is an important objective, because we believe that most patients are best served when treated with less invasive strategies, including radiotherapy, chemotherapy, newer biological agents, and hospice care in certain cases.

Medical/Mental Component

Because metastatic disease is a systemic problem, conceptually it should be treated as such. Thus, in keeping with the concerns we expressed earlier, the patient's medical and mental status and life expectancy take precedence in our approach. When first dealing with new patients with metastatic spine disease, we immediately attempt to obtain information about the patient's functional status, disease burden, medical history, and overall well-being. The patient is closely observed for any clinical findings that may indicate deteriorating or poor health. A frail, cachectic, and non-ambulatory patient with metastatic spinal disease, for example, is likely to have a short life expectancy and is unlikely to benefit from aggressive surgical management. The same goes for a patient with lung and liver lesions who appears close to death. In such cases the onus is on the surgeon to show that surgery will not improve such a patient's remaining life. Similarly, the surgeon must question the benefit of surgery in patients with multiple medical comorbidities. It may also be unwise to consider a major operation in a smoker with critical aortic stenosis, chronic obstructive pulmonary disease, or uncontrolled diabetes, as the risks of surgery may be unacceptably high and outweigh any benefits.

Patient performance status is quantified using simple, practical and intuitive systems. It should be an integral part of the management of cancer patients because it is highly correlated with survival and the identification of a need for other care. It should also help predict a patient's ability to tolerate treatment. We have found the Eastern Cooperative Oncology Group (ECOG)/Zubrod score to be a useful and simple way of determining functional status [32, 33]. The ECOG scores range from 0 to 5 and these scores correlate with the Karnofsky Scale. The ECOG score has the further advantage of identifying the full range of patient performance status, from asymptomatic and fully able to perform all pre-disease activities without restriction to bedbound and incapable of any self-care (Table 1.1).

A patient's mental status and preferences for treatment must also be considered at this stage. Someone who has, for example, already been through many rounds of aggressive therapy may not have the mental stamina to undergo a grueling perioperative and postoperative recovery. Surgical intervention is also best avoided in patients with an altered mental status or other conditions that interfere with their ability to fully comprehend the risks associated with an invasive intervention. We personally advocate terminal or supportive care (as an alternative to surgery) for very ill patients with poor functional status.

Table 1.1 ECOG performance status

ECOG performance status	Definition
0	No symptoms; normal activity level
1	Symptomatic, but able to carry out normal daily activities
2	Symptomatic; in bed <50% of the day; needs some assistance with daily activities
3	Symptomatic; in bed >50% of the day
4	Bedridden 100% of the day

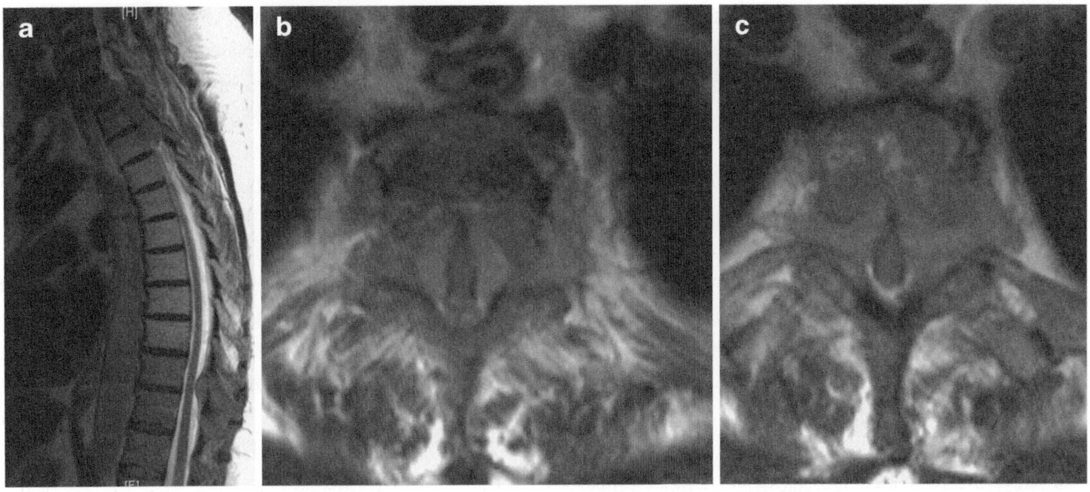

Fig. 1.1 (**a–c**) Sagittal T2-weighted MRI (**a**) of a 73-year-old male with multilevel, high-grade spinal cord compression associated with metastatic lung carcinoma who presented with <24 h of complete paraplegia, multiple medical problems, and newly developed brain metastases. Axial T2-weighted MRI images show high-grade spinal cord compression (**b**) and bilobed epidural compression consistent with metastatic tumor protruding posteriorly to the dense midline fibers of the posterior longitudinal ligament (**c**). Reproduced with permission from: Marco R, Ashana D, Kay A: Modern Techniques in the Treatment of Patients with Metastatic Spine Disease, in Parvizi J, Huddleston JI III (eds): Instructional Course Lectures 67. Rosemont, IL, American Academy of Orthopaedic Surgeons, 2018

For the reasons we give above, systemic evaluation takes precedence over other considerations in the MOSS framework. The advantage of this is that sick patients with multiple comorbidities, poor functional status, and an overall poor prognosis, regardless of the degree of spinal compression or instability, are almost always treated with non-operative measures. We have increasingly favored this conservative approach for the treatment of these very sick patients because, in our experience, they derive very limited benefit from surgical intervention. Instead, the emphasis of such end-of-life treatment should be on noninvasive strategies that optimize the quality of these patients' remaining lifetimes (Fig. 1.1).

Oncologic Component

Oncologic considerations in the MOSS framework focus primarily on tumor histology, stage, and prognosis. A complete workup includes making a diagnosis on the basis of tissue biopsy findings and complete staging of the disease with imaging studies. One thing that we have noted in particular is that visceral metastases almost certainly indicate a poor prognosis, and these patients are therefore unlikely to live long enough to benefit from surgery. Other tumors that carry a poor clinical prognosis include non-small cell lung carcinoma without the epidermal growth factor receptor (EGFR) mutation, colon carcinoma, and hepatocellular carcinoma.

A patient's tumor response to conventional radiotherapy plays an important role in guiding the non-operative management of patients with metastatic spinal disease. It is particularly important to bear in mind that those with radiosensitive spinal metastases can often be managed with radiotherapy alone even in the presence of high-grade epidural spinal cord compression. For instance, patients with spinal compression from a lymphoma or myeloma can almost always be treated successfully with chemotherapy and radiation therapy. Table 1.2 lists the most common tumors in the order of their radiosensitivity, starting with those that are most radiosensitive and ending with those that are least radiosensitive [34]. Unlike the other frameworks discussed, MOSS also considers all currently available

Table 1.2 Relative radiosensitivity from radiosensitive to relatively radioresistant

• Myeloma
• Lymphoma
• Germ cell tumor
• Ewing's sarcoma
• Rhabdomyosarcoma
• Small cell lung carcinoma
• Naïve follicular thyroid carcinoma
• Prostate carcinoma
• Breast carcinoma
• Untreated medullary thyroid carcinoma
• Myxoid liposarcoma
• Synovial sarcoma
• Leiomyosarcoma
• Non-small cell lung carcinoma with the EGFR mutation and sensitive to targeted chemotherapy
• Renal cell carcinoma treated with antiangiogenic agents and stereotactic radiosurgery
• Colon carcinoma
• Non-small cell lung carcinoma
• Carcinoma of unknown origin
• Radioactive iodine–resistant thyroid carcinoma
• Malignant fibrous histiocytoma
• Renal cell carcinoma untreated with antiangiogenic agents
• Melanoma
• Radio- and chemoresistant renal cell carcinoma
• Chordoma
• Osteosarcoma
• Chondrosarcoma

adjuvant treatments in determining the relative radiosensitivity of a tumor compressing the spinal cord. For instance, a distinction is made between patients with renal cell carcinomas that are responsive to antiangiogenic agents and those that are not. The particular strength of this approach is that it allows a comprehensive surveillance of all available treatment options before aggressive surgical management is considered.

The responsiveness to radiation therapy and the overall prognosis help guide treatment recommendations. Practitioners must stay the course with regard to favoring nonsurgical treatment in patients with radioresistant tumors and a poor life expectancy. Indeed, surgery has virtually no place in these patients. Underscoring this point is the observation that the life expectancy in a patient with a non-small cell lung carcinoma that is chemoresistant is likely to be less than 3 months. Similarly, metastatic thyroid cancer may be relatively radioresistant as many of these patients have received radioactive iodine by the time spinal metastases are discovered. Unlike patients with chemoresistant non-small cell lung carcinoma, patients with previously treated thyroid carcinoma usually have a long life expectancy. Stereotactic radiosurgery or surgery is often considered in these patients. In contrast, naïve follicular thyroid cancer and medullary thyroid carcinoma are usually radiosensitive before any medical treatments have been initiated and can be treated with radioactive iodine with or without conventional radiation therapy or stereotactic radiotherapy.

The prognosis regarding life expectancy and disease burden is paramount in decision-making and is most ideally determined by a multidisciplinary team consisting of medical, medical oncology, surgical oncology, radiation oncology, and palliative care staff. However, when a situation necessitates rapid clinical decision-making and it is unfeasible to assemble the entire multidisciplinary team for this purpose, we have found the revised Tokuhashi score to be a practical point-of-service tool for estimating prognosis and helping guide treatment [35]. This scoring system is especially useful for determining prognosis in patients irrespective of treatment modality. The scoring system consists of six parameters: the assessment of each parameter yields a numeric score, and the individual scores are then added together to get a total score. The six parameters include the general condition of the patient, the number of extraspinal bone metastases, the number of vertebral body metastases, metastases to major internal organs, the primary cancer site, and the severity of spinal neurologic compromise. Total scores of 0–8 predict a life expectancy of less than 6 months. Total scores of 9–11 predict a life expectancy of 6 months or more. And total scores of 12–15 predict a life expectancy of 1 year or more. In both a prospective and retrospective evaluation of the score, the authors found the score was, respectively, 86.4% and 82.5% consistent in predicting prognosis. We find this scoring system practical because of its ease of use, its consistency, and its usefulness for both surgical and nonsurgical management. The Tomita scoring system, which examines histology in conjunction with the number of bony metastases and the location of visceral metastases, has been found to also yield useful prognostic information [36]. It has proved to be particularly useful when an en bloc spondylectomy is being considered in the very rare patient with a solitary metastasis, prolonged life expectancy, and possibility for cure.

Stenosis (Ambulatory/Neurologic) Component

The next component assessed in our MOSS framework is the status of stenosis or neurologic function. Historical studies prior to Patchell's demonstrated that 90% of patients with MSCC who were ambulatory upon presentation would remain ambulatory even though treated with only conventional radiation therapy and steroids [7–15]. The Cochrane review of randomized controlled trials comparing the effectiveness of radiotherapy, surgery, and steroids yielded similar findings that patients with stable spines can be treated with radiation therapy only and still retain their ability to walk. This review also found surgery to be beneficial only for ambulatory patients with a relatively radioresistant tumor and for non-ambulatory patients with a single area of involvement who had been paraplegic for less than 48 h, had a relatively radioresistant tumor, and had more than a 3-month life expectancy [17]. Generally speaking, all these authors found surgery to be useful in very limited and specific circumstances and not necessarily contingent on the degree of stenosis. As an example, regardless of the degree of spinal cord compression, patients with myeloma or other chemosensitive or radio-responsive tumors should routinely first be treated with non-operative measures. This should also apply to patients with conventionally radioresistant tumors that, nonetheless, are responsive to decompressive stereotactic radiosurgery and, further, could be radiosensitized by more modern chemotherapy. It should also be borne in mind that the separation surgery for high-grade spinal cord compression described earlier is still an invasive intervention that is not without risks even despite its minimalist design. Therefore, its routine use in every patient with radioresistant pathology and high-grade compression, as Bilsky et al. suggest and as discussed previously, is probably not necessary given that there is data to support the use of decompressive stereotactic radiotherapy alone in these patients. Nonetheless, research to delineate those patients with high-grade spinal cord compression from relatively radioresistant tumors who may benefit from the combination of separation surgery and SRS is important. For patients who are ambulatory, we evaluate the degree of spinal cord compression based on Bilsky's grading system and then discuss the treatment options with the patient. We would explain to a patient with high-grade stenosis associated with chemoresistant non-small cell lung carcinoma that Bilsky et al. might recommend surgery, whereas some radiation oncologists would recommend decompressive stereotactic radiosurgery. We further explain to the patient the respective risks and benefits of their treatment options. Armed with what we consider to be a comprehensive understanding of the treatment options in light of their particular clinical state, the patients are then given time to decide whether to proceed with a non-operative or operative intervention. It is important, however, that healthy, non-ambulatory patients know that they are generally considered surgical candidates if they have a life expectancy of greater than 3 months and have a radioresistant tumor or unstable spine.

Rapid deterioration of neurologic function with complete loss of motor and sensory function except for maintenance of deep touch and proprioception may indicate that the spinal cord compression has led to thrombosis of the anterior spinal artery with anterior spinal cord infarction. These patients are not likely to regain neurologic function after surgical decompression. Non-operative management is thus considered unless the patient has a life expectancy greater than 3 months, a radioresistant tumor, and an unstable spine.

Stability Component

The final variable assessed in the MOSS framework is spinal stability. In this regard, we, and others, believe the White-Panjabi definition of physiologic instability is preferable to the Spine Instability Neoplastic Score (SINS) [27, 37]. As discussed previously, the SINS score gives higher scores for tumors in junctional sites and for vertebral collapse which thus potentially increases the frequency with which surgery is performed. In our experience, however, tumors in junctional sites (i.e., occipitocervical and lumbosacral junctions) and tumors causing 100% vertebral collapse can frequently be treated non-operatively and can remain very stable. In the White-Panjabi definition, a spine is physiologically unstable if it cannot maintain its patterns of displacement under physiologic loads. Conditions that qualify as physiologically unstable include progressive neurologic dysfunction, progressive deformity, and uncontrolled pain. Nevertheless, patients with a physiologically unstable spine may benefit from surgery if they are medically well, have a life expectancy of greater than 3 months, and have a type of tumor that is relatively resistant to available adjuvant therapies. Using the MOSS criteria, we have been able to avoid surgical interventions, and most importantly its risks and resultant morbidity, in many patients who, if assessed using other frameworks such as the NOMS or SINS, would be treated more aggressively with surgical options.

Summary

Metastatic disease to the spine poses a difficult challenge for most practitioners because of the need to carefully weigh the well-being of the patient against the potential efficacy of treatment, be it aggressive or otherwise. In most instances, non-operative treatment is more appropriate. This is not just because of the significant risks associated with surgery. Of greater importance, it is because of the limited life expectancies of many of these patients who cannot expect to fully recover from their surgery before succumbing to their cancer. It is important to understand that the more aggressive surgical options advocated in the past were based on studies that may have misinterpreted or overemphasized the advantages of surgical management. The significant advances in chemotherapy, radiotherapy, and newer biological agents have dramatically improved local tumor control without surgery for many patients with tumors that were previously not responsive to conventional radiation or chemotherapy, which is a further reason to favor non operative or less invasive treatment.

In conclusion, the MOSS framework was developed to eliminate the shortcomings of other frameworks. For example, in the MOSS assessment, the patient's medical and mental status is examined first and given the highest priority. After this, the patient's tumor histology, neurologic status, and, finally, spinal stability are assessed. At each step of the way, every attempt is made to determine whether a non-operative or less invasive method can be employed instead of surgery. When there is no less invasive approach that can adequately serve the patient's needs, it is up to the surgeon to clearly define the benefits of surgery and identify those who are likely to benefit from it.

Application of MOSS: Three Case Reports

The following case reports illustrate how MOSS has been applied in three different patients with MSCC and how this approach has proved successful in both meeting patient preferences and managing discomfort stemming from the MSCC.

Case 1

A 73-year-old male with spinal cord compression and progressive neurologic dysfunction presented with 0/5 strength and no sensation in the lower extremities (Fig. 1.1a–c). He had been ambulatory the day before. **M**edically, the patient was elderly and had a history of atrial fibrillation, Parkinson's disease, and polio. **M**entally, the patient was alert and oriented and conveyed that he had a desire to live. His ECOG score was 4 as he was in bed 100% of the time. **O**ncologically, the patient had recently been diagnosed with lung carcinoma, and staging studies showed new metastases to the brain and spine (Fig. 1.2a–d). His tumor did not have the epidermal growth factor receptor (EGFR) mutation, so he was not a candidate for treatment with ertonolib, currently

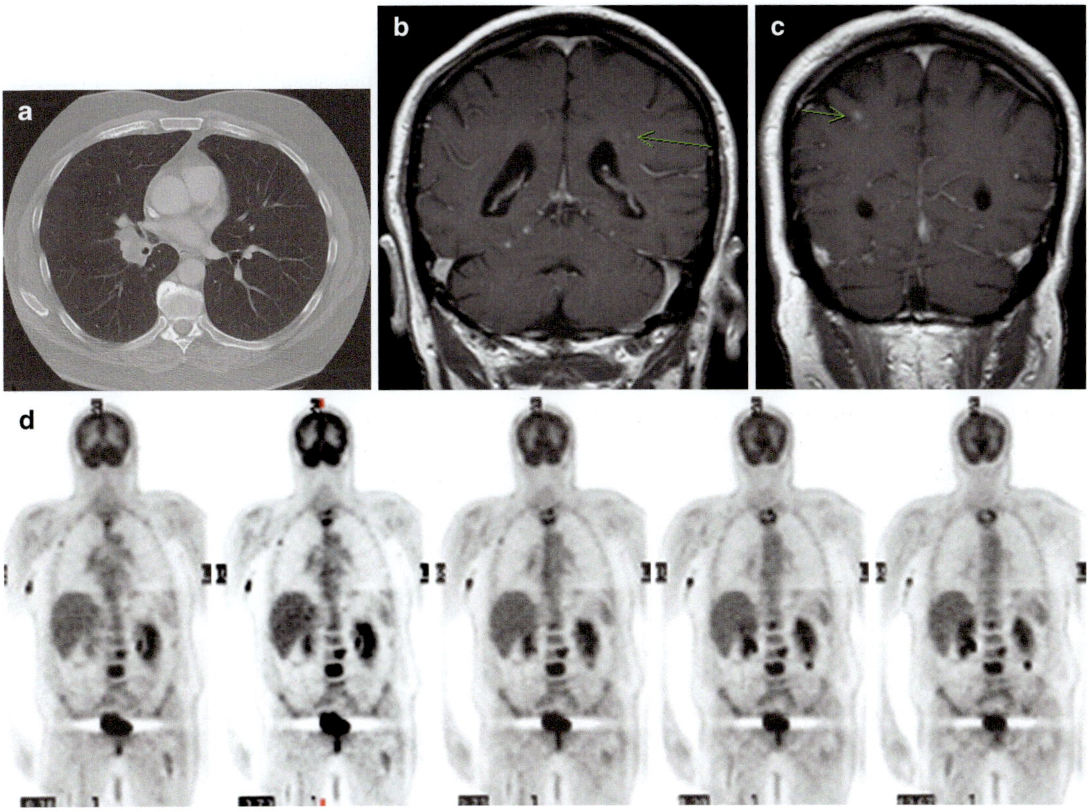

Fig. 1.2 (**a**–**d**) Staging studies revealed the primary right hilar lung lesion on the chest CT scan (**a**), multiple brain metastases on the brain CT scan (**b**, **c**), and multiple spine metastases on the bone scan (**d**)

one of the only nonsurgical options that might otherwise have increased progression-free survival in this patient. Our multidisciplinary team estimated that survival in this patient would unlikely exceed 3 months. His Tokuhashi score (Fig. 1.3) [38] was 0, which indicated that "conservative treatment" was the more advisable option. In addition, his Tomita score (Fig. 1.4) [39] was 10, which indicated that "supportive care" was more advisable than surgery.

The use of the MOSS assessment tool allowed the team to give the patient's medical and oncologic condition priority over the degree of stenosis, neurologic status, or spinal column stability. Before decisive treatment was undertaken, only corticosteroids were administered. Up-front radiation therapy was recommended to provide some local control but it was not instituted.

Evaluation of the stenosis/neurologic status confirmed the patient had high-grade spinal cord compression (Fig. 1.5) [40] and that he was non-ambulatory. Evaluation of spinal stability according to White and Panjabi's definition showed that he had progressive neurologic dysfunction, which indicated physiologic instability.

Some might contend that the patient was physiologically stable at this point because no further progressive neurological deficit was possible, thus suggesting, to their way of thinking, that the patient was physiologically stable from a neurologic standpoint. In addition, since his pain was controlled, some would take this to indicate physiologic stability. The patient's SINS score (Tables 1.3 and 1.4) [41, 42] was 12, which suggests potential instability.

Our team recommended non-operative management based on the patient's fragile medical and oncologic condition. We believed this would also ensure a better quality of life during the end stage of the patient's disease. However, the patient asked

Characteristic	***Score***
General condition (performance status)	0
Poor (PS 10 ~ 40%)	0
Moderate (PS 50 ~ 70%)	1
Good (PS 80 ~ 100%)	2
No. of extraspinal bone metastases foci	
≥3	0
1 – 2	1
0	2
No. of metastases in the vertebral body	
≥3	0
2	1
1	2
Metastases to the major internal organs	
Unremovable	0
Removable	1
No metastases	2
Primary site of the cancer	
Lung, osteosarcoma, stomach, bladder, esophagus, pancreas	0
Liver, gallbladder, unidentified	1
Others	2
Kidney, uterus	3
Rectum	4
Thyroid, breast, prostate, carcinoid tumor	5
Palsy	
Complete (Frankel A, B)	0
Incomplete (Frankel C, D)	1
None (Frankel E)	2

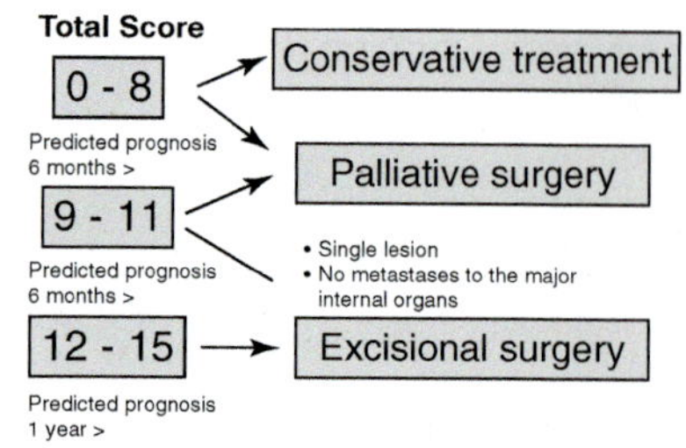

Criteria of predicted prognosis: Total Score (TS)0 ~ 8=>6 months: TS 9 ~ 11= ≤ 6 months: TS 12 ~ 15= ≤ 1year

Fig. 1.3 Prognosis and treatment recommendation based on Tokuhashi score. From Tokuhashi Y, Matsuzaki H, Oda H, Oshima M, Ryu J. A Revised Scoring System for Preoperative Evaluation of Metastatic Spine Tumor Prognosis. Spine. 2005 Oct 1;30(19)

Scoring system			
	Prognostic factors		
Point	Primary tumor	Visceral mets.[a)]	Bone mets.[b)]
1	Slow growth (breast, thyroid, etc.)		Solitary or isolated
2	Moderate growth (Kidney, uterus, etc.)	Treatable	Multiple
4	Rapid growth (lung, stomach, etc.)	Un-treatable	

Prognostic score	Treatment goal	Surgical strategy
2, 3	Long-term local control	Wide or marginal excision
4, 5	Middle-term local control	Marginal or intralesional excision
6, 7	Short-term local control	Palliative surgery
8, 9, 10	Terminal care	Supportive care

Fig. 1.4 Prognostic score, treatment goal, and surgical strategy based on Tomita score. From Tomita K, Kawahara N, Kobayashi T, Yoshida A, Murakami H, Akamaru T. Surgical Strategy for Spinal Metastases. Spine. 2001 Feb 1;26(3)

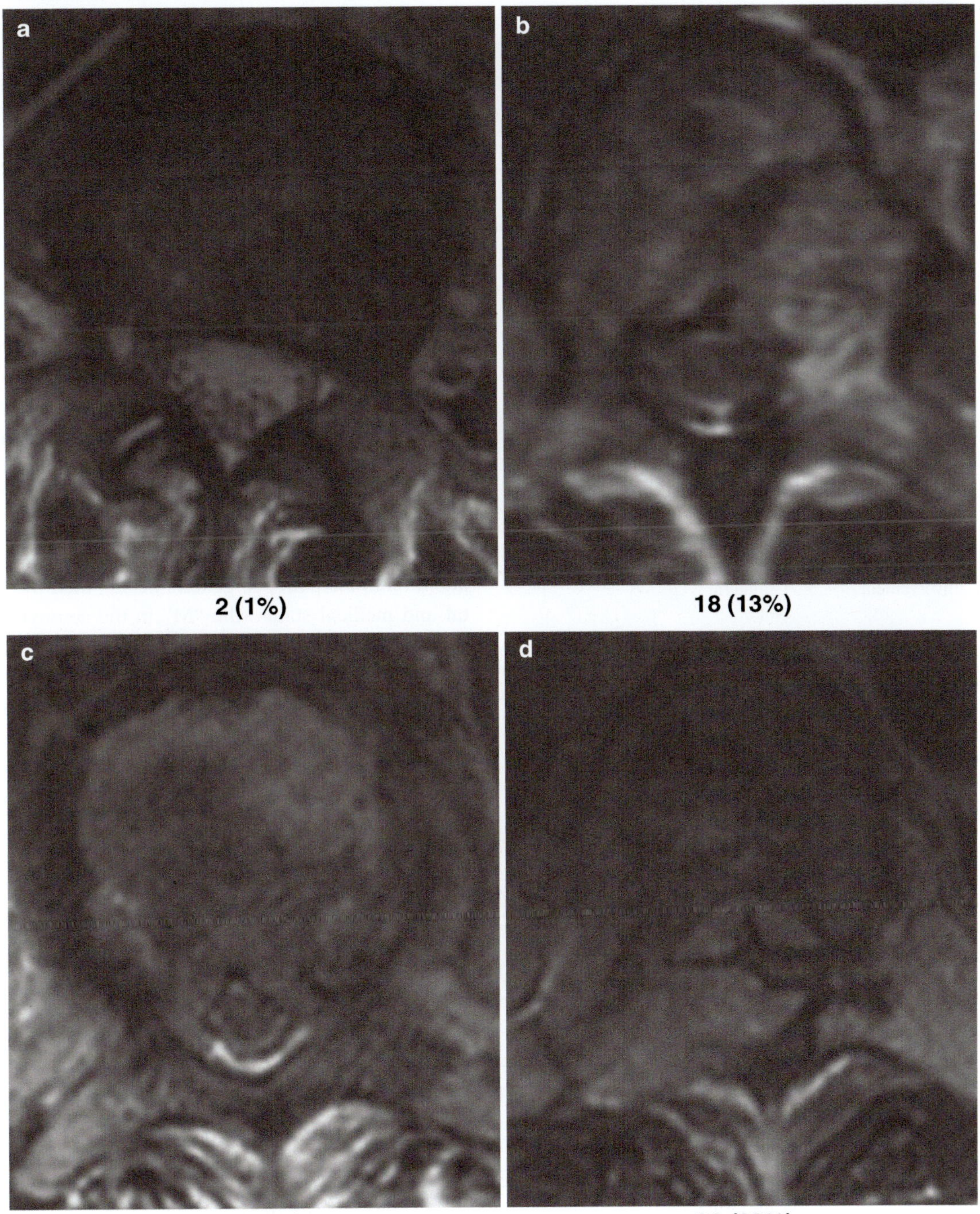

Fig. 1.5 Stenosis based on degree of spinal cord compression as defined by Wang et al. A: Grade 0. B: Grade 1. C: Grade 2. D: Grade 3. Degree of ESCC. Axial T_2-weighted MR images obtained to assess the degree of ESCC and the extent of SSO. The number and percentage of patients with each grade of ESCC are also shown. A: ESCC Grade 0. B: ESCC Grade 1. C: ESCC Grade 2. D: ESCC Grade 3. Grades 2 and 3 are considered high-grade spinal cord compression. From Wang JC et al. Single-stage posterolateral transpedicular approach for resection of epidural metastatic spine tumors involving the vertebral body with circumferential reconstruction: results in 140 patients. J Neurosurg Spine. 2004 October;1(3): 287–298

Table 1.3 Spinal Instability Neoplastic Score (SINS)

SINS component	Description	Score
Location	Junctional (Occ-C2, C7-T2, T11-L1, L5-S) Mobile (C3-6, L2-4) Semirigid (T3-10) Rigid (S2-5)	3 2 1 0
Pain	Yes* Occasional nonmechanical pain No	3 1 0
Bone lesion	Lytic Mixed Blastic	2 1 0
Alignment	Subluxation/translation De novo deformity Normal	4 2 0
Vertebral body	>50% collapse <50% collapse No collapse with >50% VB involved None of above	3 2 1 0
Posterolateral involvement	Bilateral Unilateral None	3 1 0

From Fisher C, et al. Reliability of the Spinal Instability Neoplastic Score (SINS) among radiation oncologists: an assessment of instability secondary to spinal metastases. *Radiation Oncology*. 2014; 9:69

Table 1.4 Likelihood of instability based on SINS

Stable	Potentially unstable	Unstable
0–6	7–12	13–18

From Fisher C, et al. Reliability of the Spinal Instability Neoplastic Score (SINS) among radiation oncologists: an assessment of instability secondary to spinal metastases. *Radiation Oncology*. 2014; 9:69

for a second opinion and decided to undergo a decompressive laminectomy without instrumentation. Interestingly, a decompressive laminectomy as performed by the other team has not been shown to have improved outcomes over conventional radiation therapy plus steroids. Moreover, this procedure probably increased the instability of the spine and predisposed the patient to progressive kyphosis. The patient was discharged to hospice care and he did not regain any neurologic function.

Of note, the use of NOMS (neurologic, oncologic, mechanical stability, and systemic) might have also caused some practitioners to favor surgical intervention with a laminectomy, separation surgery, and spinal stabilization combined with stereotactic radiosurgery because this treatment algorithm starts with evaluation of the **n**eurology, which in this patient was high-grade stenosis, followed by evaluation of the **o**ncology, which in this patient was NSCLC (Fig. 1.6) [43].

It is also important to note that total reliance on the SINS score might have guided the treatment team to recommend surgical stabilization, as the score in this patient indicated potential spinal instability. However, in making such a call, we are in full agreement with the Spine Oncology Study Group's conclusions on the application of the SINS score [27] that: "Most importantly, we must emphasize that in making surgical treatment decisions, stability is only 1 component of the process. Patient general health, tumor histology, prognosis, neurology and patient choice must also be considered." The MOSS assessment tool that we have devised is in keeping with this stance, in that it gives priority attention to the patients' general health, their mental and medical status (the "M" in the acronym), followed by the tumor histology status and prognosis ("O") and patients' neurologic status ("S"). Only lastly is spinal stability ("S") considered in determining whether operative or non-operative intervention is better for the patient. In this case, the patient was given the choice of either option, and he chose the operative intervention, although we had advised against this. Regardless, this case shows how a systematic, patient-centered approach to treatment planning in patients with MSCC can be relied upon to help the practitioner know whether surgery and/or conservative treatment can be confidently offered to the patient.

Case 2

A 57-year-old female with T5 spinal cord compression presented with bilateral lower extremity weakness (4-/5 strength) and urinary retention (Fig. 1.7a, b). **M**edically, she had type II diabetes mellitus and hypertension. **M**entally, she was alert and oriented and she had a desire to live. Her ECOG performance score was a 3 as she was in bed more than 50% of the time. **O**ncologically, her laboratory values and biopsy confirmed a diagnosis of multiple myeloma. Staging studies revealed bone marrow involvement but no other bone lesions. On the basis of these findings, her

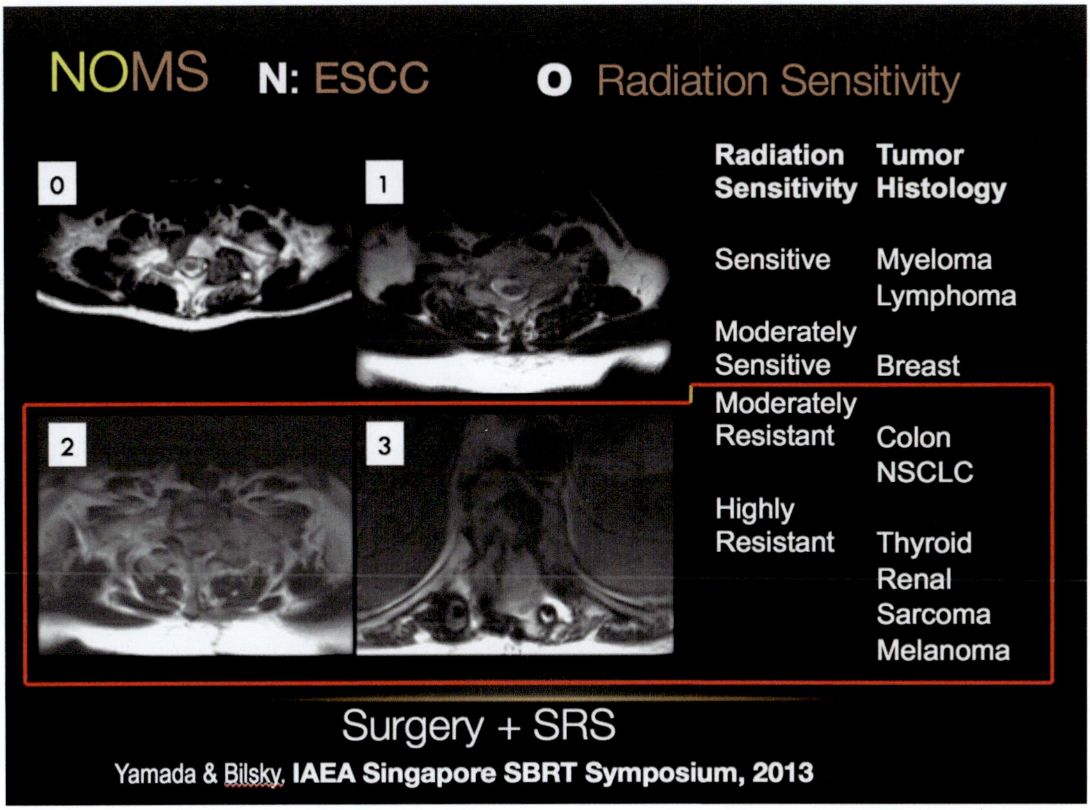

Fig. 1.6 Recommendations for surgery plus stereotactic radiation therapy for a high-grade spinal cord compression associated with a radioresistant tumor based on NOMS as presented by Yamada and Bilsky at IAEA Singapore SBRT Symposium in 2013. With permission from Yoshiya (Josh) Yamada, MD

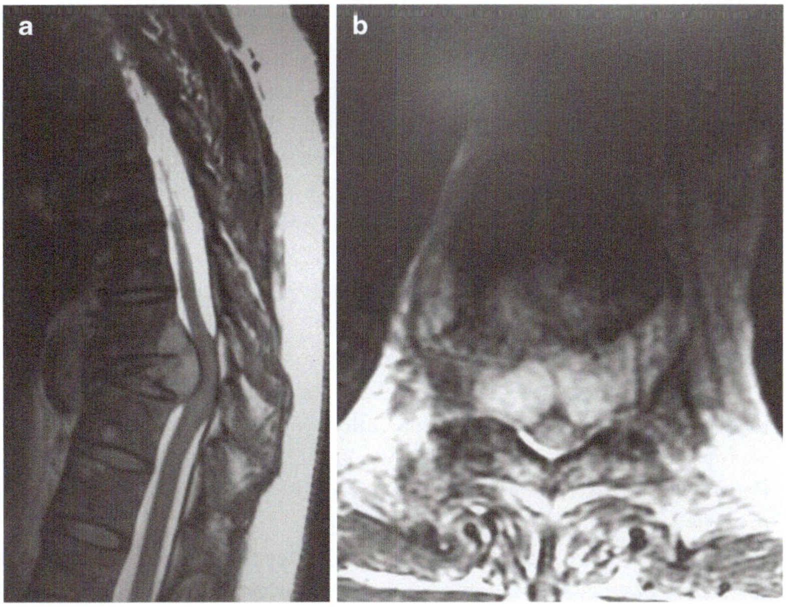

Fig. 1.7 (**a**, **b**) Sagittal T2-weighted MRI (**a**) demonstrating spinal cord compression and 100% vertebral body collapse associated with multiple myeloma. Axial T1-weighted MRI (**b**) with contrast demonstrating bilobed, high-grade spinal cord compression

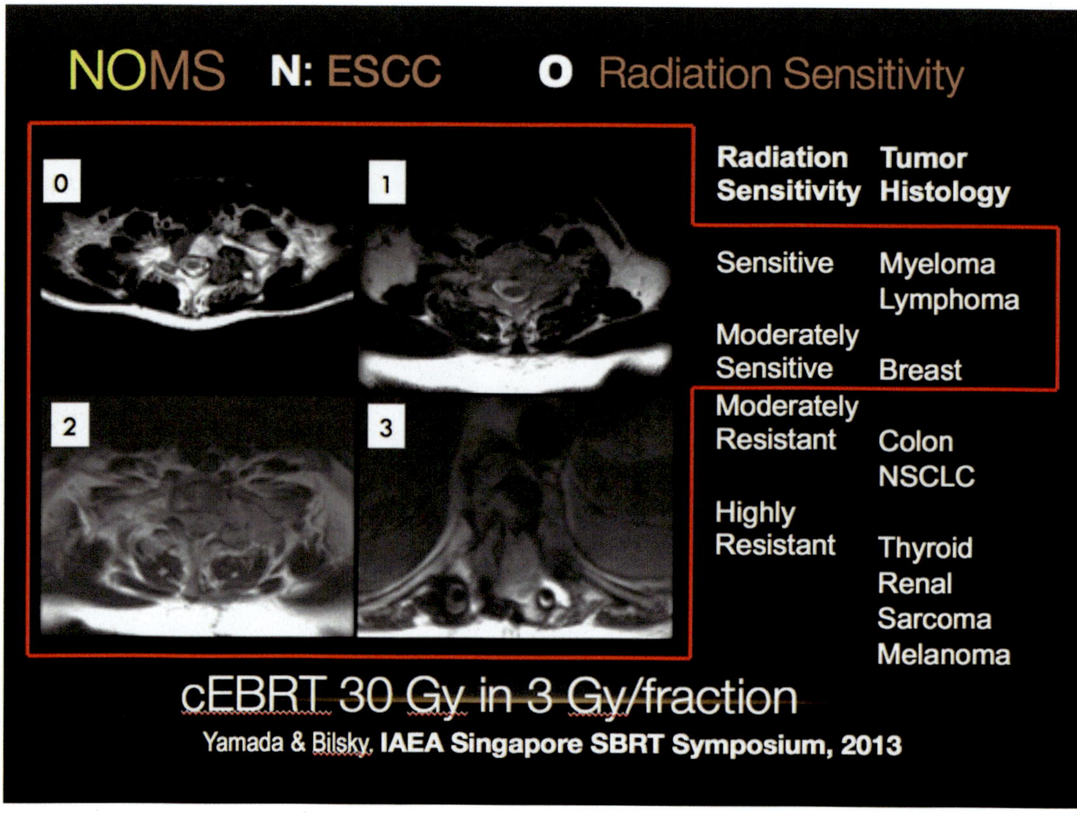

Fig. 1.8 Recommendations for conventional external beam radiation therapy for high-grade spinal cord compression associated with a radiation sensitive tumor based on NOMS as presented by Yamada and Bilsky at IAEA Singapore SBRT Symposium in 2013. With permission from Yoshiya (Josh) Yamada, MD

median survival time was estimated to be 5 years. Stenosis evaluation revealed high-grade spinal cord compression. Despite this, the patient was still ambulatory. Stability evaluation, done using White and Panjabi's criteria, further showed her to be physiologically stable, in that there were no signs of progressive deformity, progressive neurologic dysfunction, or persistent pain under physiologic loading.

Because multiple myeloma is exquisitely sensitive to radiation therapy, steroids and chemotherapy, these were at the top of the list of treatment options in this patient. In fact, because invasive surgery is generally not called for in such patients, Tokuhashi et al., Tomita et al., and Patchell et al. excluded patients with multiple myeloma from their studies [6, 35, 36]. If the NOMS assessment had been done in this patient, it too may have guided the practitioner to recommend external beam radiation therapy (Fig. 1.8) [43]. A further concern in this patient was that, although physiologic stability had been indicated by White and Panjabi's assessment criteria, the patient's SINS score of 11 indicated that her spine was potentially unstable. However, in our experience with vertebral plana (100% vertebral body collapse), we have found that the spine is usually physiologically stable unless there is facet incongruity, diastasis, or subluxation seen on MRI or CT scans.

On the basis of all these collective findings and our personal experience, our team recommended non-operative treatment consisting of corticosteroids and radiation therapy followed by systemic chemotherapy. The patient agreed to this approach. She remained physiologically stable (Fig. 1.9a, b) and went on to regain full lower extremity strength.

Case 3

A 67-year-old male presented with T11 spinal cord compression associated with previously radiated prostate carcinoma (Fig. 1.10a, b). **M**edically, he had hypertension. **M**entally he was alert and oriented and had a desire to live. His ECOG performance status was 3 as he was in bed greater than 50% of the time. **O**ncologically, his tumor was resistant to hormonal treatment and radiation therapy. His Tokuhashi score was 12, indicating that he could expect to survive for more than 1 year. Thus palliative surgery was considered reasonable in this patient. His Tomita score of 3 indicated that "wide or marginal excision" was a reasonable. Stenosis evaluation revealed high-grade spinal cord compression. Of further note, **s**tenosis evaluation revealed high-grade spinal cord compression. Despite this, the patient

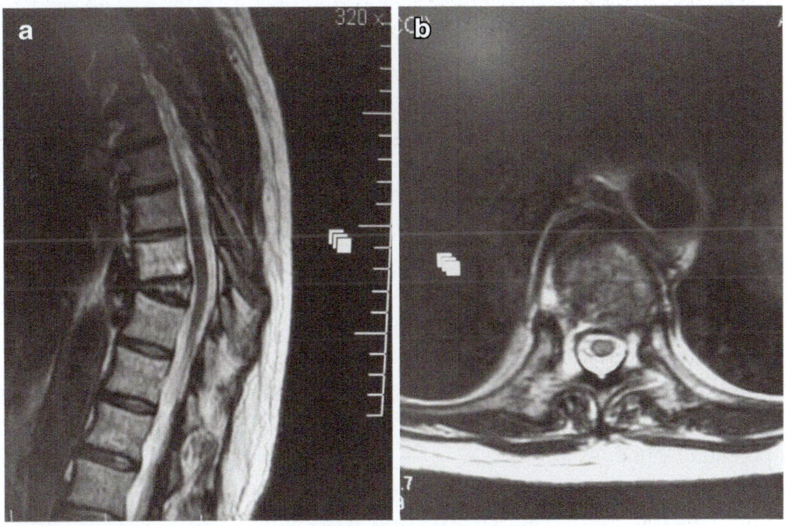

Fig. 1.9 (**a**, **b**) Sagittal (**a**) and axial (**b**) T2-weighted MRI 2 years after radiation therapy demonstrates elimination of spinal cord compression and maintenance of spinal alignment. Reproduced with permission from: Marco R, Ashana D, Kay A: Modern Techniques in the Treatment of Patients with Metastatic Spine Disease, in Parvizi J, Huddleston JI III (eds): Instructional Course Lectures 67. Rosemont, IL, American Academy of Orthopaedic Surgeons, 2018

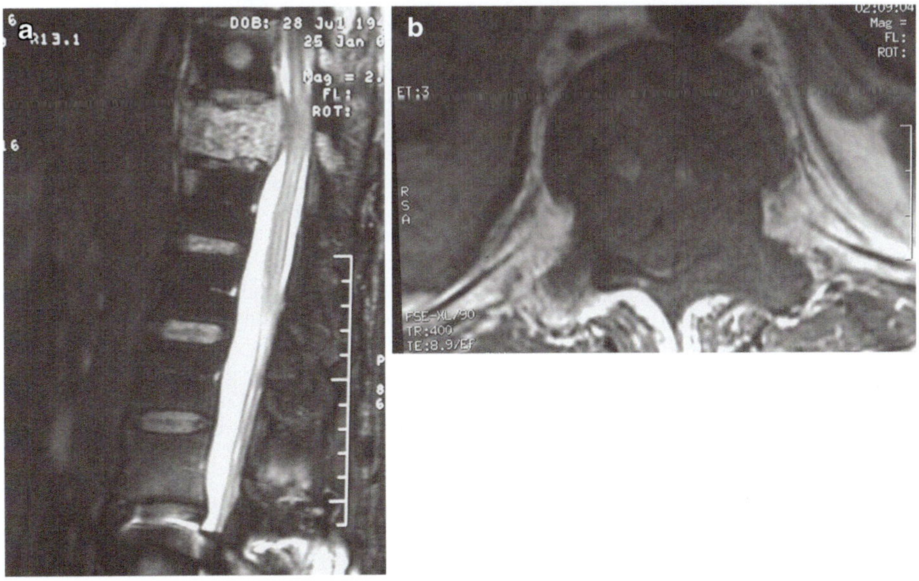

Fig. 1.10 (**a**, **b**) Sagittal T2-weighted MRI (**a**) demonstrating recurrent spinal cord compression associated with previously irradiated and hormonally treated prostate carcinoma. Axial T1-weighted MRI (**b**) demonstrates high-grade, bilobed spinal cord compression with pedicle, lamina, and transverse process involvement

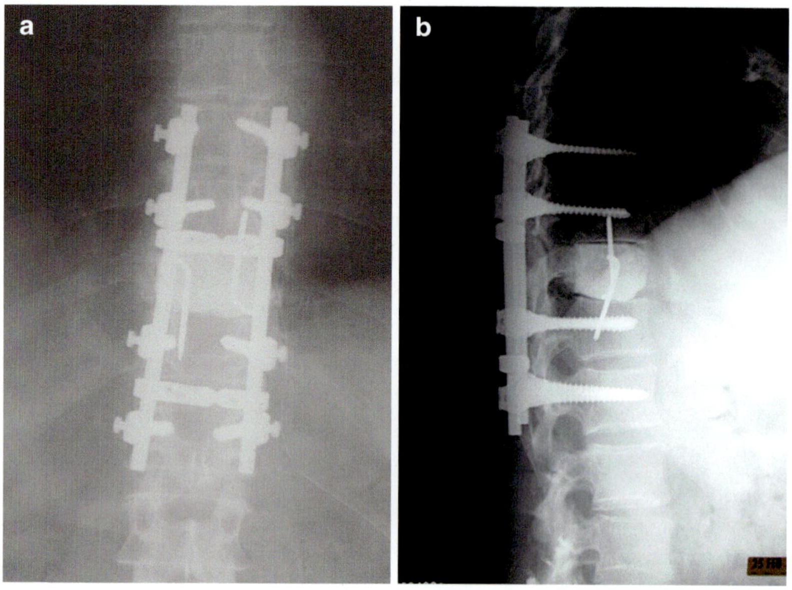

Fig. 1.11 (**a**, **b**) AP and lateral radiograph of the thoracic spine following transpedicular excision of tumor with anterior column reconstruction with polymethylmethacrylate cement and Steinman pins and posterior stabilization with spinal instrumentation

remained ambulatory. Stability evaluation done using White and Panjabi's criteria showed this patient to be physiologically unstable as his associated pain was recalcitrant to medical management. His SINS score of 8 likewise suggested potential spinal instability.

On the basis of these findings, our team recommended a transpedicular excision with anterior cement and pin reconstruction and posterior spinal instrumentation (Fig. 1.11a, b). The patient regained full strength and was alive and well at his last follow-up.

References

1. Dunn RC, Kelly WA, Wohns RNW, Howe JF. Spinal epidural neoplasia. J Neurosurg. 1980;52(1):47–51. https://doi.org/10.3171/jns.1980.52.1.0047.
2. Gilbert RW, Kim J-H, Posner JB. Epidural spinal cord compression from metastatic tumor: diagnosis and treatment. Ann Neurol. 1978;3(1):40–51. https://doi.org/10.1002/ana.410030107.
3. Livingston KE, Perrin RG. The neurosurgical management of spinal metastases causing cord and cauda equina compression. J Neurosurg. 1978;49(6):839–43. https://doi.org/10.3171/jns.1978.49.6.0839.
4. Young RF, Post EM, King GA. Treatment of spinal epidural metastases. J Neurosurg. 1980;53(6):741–8. https://doi.org/10.3171/jns.1980.53.6.0741.
5. Rompe JD, Hopf CG, Eysel P. Outcome after palliative posterior surgery for metastatic disease of the spine—evaluation of 106 consecutive patients after decompression and stabilisation with the Cotrel-Dubousset instrumentation. Arch Orthop Trauma Surg. 1999;119(7–8):394–400.
6. Patchell RA, Tibbs PA, Regine WF, Payne R, Saris S, Kryscio RJ, et al. Direct decompressive surgical resection in the treatment of spinal cord compression caused by metastatic cancer: a randomised trial. Lancet. 2005;366(9486):643–8. https://doi.org/10.1016/s0140-6736(05)66954-1.
7. Cassady JR, Sagerman RH, Chang CH. Radiation therapy for lymphoma of the spinal canal. Radiology. 1967;89(2):313–5. https://doi.org/10.1148/89.2.313.
8. Friedman M, Kim TH, Panahon AM. Spinal cord compression in malignant lymphoma—treatment and results. Cancer. 1976;37(3):1485–91. https://doi.org/10.1002/1097-0142(197603)37:3<1485::aid-cncr2820370334>3.0.co;2-l.
9. Khan FR, Glicksman AS, Chu FCH, Nickson JJ. Treatment by radiotherapy of spinal cord compression due to extradural metastases. Radiology. 1967;89(3):495–500. https://doi.org/10.1148/89.3.495.
10. Martin WE. Radiation therapy for paraplegia due to multiple myeloma. JAMA. 1965;191(3):247. https://doi.org/10.1001/jama.1965.03080030091020.
11. Mones RJ, Dozier D, Berrett A. Analysis of medical treatment of malignant extradural spinal cord tumors. Cancer. 1966;19(12):1842–53. https://doi.org/10.1002/1097-0142(196612)19:12<1842::aid-cncr2820191212>3.0.co;2-v.
12. Murphy WT, Bilge N. Compression of the spinal cord in patients with malignant lymphoma. Radiology. 1964;82(3):495–501. https://doi.org/10.1148/82.3.495.
13. Raichle ME, Posner JB. The treatment of extradural spinal cord compression. Neurology. 1970;20(4):391.
14. Rubin P, Miller G. Extradural spinal cord compression by tumor. Radiology. 1969;93(6):1243–8. https://doi.org/10.1148/93.6.1243.

15. Rubin P, Mayer E, Poulter C. Part II: high daily dose experience without laminectomy. Radiology. 1969;93(6):1248–60. https://doi.org/10.1148/93.6.1248.
16. Chi JH, Gokaslan Z, McCormick P, Tibbs PA, Kryscio RJ, Patchell RA. Selecting treatment for patients with malignant epidural spinal cord compression—does age matter? Spine. 2009;34(5):431–5. https://doi.org/10.1097/brs.0b013e318193a25b.
17. George R, Jeba J, Ramkumar G, Chacko AG, Leng M, Tharyan P. Interventions for the treatment of metastatic extradural spinal cord compression in adults. Cochrane Database Syst Rev. Wiley; 2008.
18. Laufer I, Rubin DG, Lis E, Cox BW, Stubblefield MD, Yamada Y, et al. The NOMS framework: approach to the treatment of spinal metastatic tumors. Oncologist. 2013;18(6):744–51. https://doi.org/10.1634/theoncologist.2012-0293.
19. Bilsky MH, Laufer I, Fourney DR, Groff M, Schmidt MH, Varga PP, et al. Reliability analysis of the epidural spinal cord compression scale. J Neurosurg Spine. 2010;13(3):324–8. https://doi.org/10.3171/2010.3.spine09459.
20. Lim ZD, Mahajan A, Weinberg J, Tannir NM. Outcome of patients with renal cell carcinoma metastatic to the brain treated with sunitinib without local therapy. Am J Clin Oncol. 2013;36(3):258–60. https://doi.org/10.1097/coc.0b013e3182467b9a.
21. Rousseau B, Kempf E, Desamericq G, Boissier E, Chaubet-Houdu M, Joly C, et al. First-line antiangiogenics for metastatic renal cell carcinoma: a systematic review and network meta-analysis. Crit Rev Oncol Hematol. 2016;107:44–53. https://doi.org/10.1016/j.critrevonc.2016.08.012.
22. Gerszten PC, Mendel E, Yamada Y. Radiotherapy and radiosurgery for metastatic spine disease. Spine. 2009;34(22 Suppl):S78–92. https://doi.org/10.1097/brs.0b013e3181b8b6f5.
23. Gerszten PC, Burton SA, Ozhasoglu C, Welch WC. Radiosurgery for spinal metastases. Spine. 2007;32(2):193–9. https://doi.org/10.1097/01.brs.0000251863.76595.a2.
24. Ryu S, Rock J, Jain R, Lu M, Anderson J, Jin J-Y, et al. Radiosurgical decompression of metastatic epidural compression. Cancer. 2010;116(9):2250–7. https://doi.org/10.1002/cncr.24993.
25. Ryu S, Rock J, Rosenblum M, Kim JH. Patterns of failure after single-dose radiosurgery for spinal metastasis. J Neurosurg. 2004;101(Suppl 3):402–5. https://doi.org/10.3171/jns.2004.101.supplement3.0402.
26. Gerszten PC, Burton SA, Ozhasoglu C, Vogel WJ, Welch WC, Baar J, et al. Stereotactic radiosurgery for spinal metastases from renal cell carcinoma. J Neurosurg Spine. 2005;3(4):288–95. https://doi.org/10.3171/spi.2005.3.4.0288.
27. Fisher CG, DiPaola CP, Ryken TC, Bilsky MH, Shaffrey CI, Berven SH, et al. A novel classification system for spinal instability in neoplastic disease. Spine. 2010;35(22):E1221–E9. https://doi.org/10.1097/brs.0b013e3181e16ae2.
28. Kris MG, Natale RB, Herbst RS, Lynch JTJ, Prager D, Belani CP, et al. Efficacy of gefitinib, an inhibitor of the epidermal growth factor receptor tyrosine kinase, in symptomatic patients with non–small cell lung cancer. JAMA. 2003;290(16):2149. https://doi.org/10.1001/jama.290.16.2149.
29. Rosell R, Carcereny E, Gervais R, Vergnenegre A, Massuti B, Felip E, et al. Erlotinib versus standard chemotherapy as first-line treatment for European patients with advanced EGFR mutation-positive non-small-cell lung cancer (EURTAC): a multicentre, open-label, randomised phase 3 trial. Lancet Oncol. 2012;13(3):239–46. https://doi.org/10.1016/s1470-2045(11)70393-x.
30. Paez JG. EGFR mutations in lung cancer: correlation with clinical response to gefitinib therapy. Science. 2004;304(5676):1497–500. https://doi.org/10.1126/science.1099314.
31. Berenson J, Pflugmacher R, Jarzem P, Zonder J, Schechtman K, Tillman JB, et al. Balloon kyphoplasty versus non-surgical fracture management for treatment of painful vertebral body compression fractures in patients with cancer: a multicentre, randomised controlled trial. Lancet Oncol. 2011;12(3):225–35. https://doi.org/10.1016/s1470-2045(11)70008-0.
32. Oken MM, Creech RH, Tormey DC, Horton J, Davis TE, McFadden ET, et al. Toxicity and response criteria of the Eastern Cooperative Oncology Group. Am J Clin Oncol. 1982;5(6):649–56. https://doi.org/10.1097/00000421-198212000-00014.
33. Conill C, Verger E, Salamero M. Performance status assessment in cancer patients. Cancer. 1990;65(8):1864–6. https://doi.org/10.1002/1097-0142(19900415)65:8<1864::aid-cncr2820650832>3.0.co;2-u.
34. Maranzano E, Latini P. Effectiveness of radiation therapy without surgery in metastatic spinal cord compression: final results from a prospective trial. Int J Radiat Oncol Biol Phys. 1995;32(4):959–67. https://doi.org/10.1016/0360-3016(95)00572-g.
35. Tokuhashi Y, Matsuzaki H, Oda H, Oshima M, Ryu J. A revised scoring system for preoperative evaluation of metastatic spine tumor prognosis. Spine. 2005;30(19):2186–91. https://doi.org/10.1097/01.brs.0000180401.06919.a5.
36. Tomita K, Kawahara N, Kobayashi T, Yoshida A, Murakami H, Akamaru T. Surgical strategy for spinal metastases. Spine. 2001;26(3):298–306. https://doi.org/10.1097/00007632-200102010-00016.
37. Panjabi MM. Clinical spinal instability and low back pain. J Electromyogr Kinesiol. 2003;13(4):371–9. https://doi.org/10.1016/s1050-6411(03)00044-0.
38. Tokuhashi Y, Matsuzaki H, Oda H, Oshima M, Ryu J. A revised scoring system for preoperative evaluation of metastatic spine tumor prognosis. In: Tumors TRESftPoMS, editor. Spine (Phila Pa 1976): Ovid Technologies (Wolters Kluwer Health); 2005. p. Table 2. Revised Evaluation System for the Prognosis of Metastatic Spine Tumors.

39. Tomita K, Kawahara N, Kobayashi T, Yoshida A, Murakami H, Akamaru T. Surgical strategy for spinal metastases. In: metastases FSsfs, editor. Spine: Ovid Technologies (Wolters Kluwer Health); 2001. p. Figure 1. Surgical strategy for spinal metastases.
40. Wang JC, Boland P, Mitra N, Yamada Y, Lis E, Stubblefield M, et al. Single-stage posterolateral transpedicular approach for resection of epidural metastatic spine tumors involving the vertebral body with circumferential reconstruction: results in 140 patients. J Neurosurg Spine. 2004;1(3):287–98. Figure 1.
41. Fisher CG, DiPaola CP, Ryken TC, Bilsky MH, Shaffrey CI, Berven SH, et al. A novel classification system for spinal instability in neoplastic disease. Spine: Ovid Technologies (Wolters Kluwer Health); 2010. p. Table 1 The SINS classification according to Fisher et al.
42. Fisher CG, DiPaola CP, Ryken TC, Bilsky MH, Shaffrey CI, Berven SH et al. A novel classification system for spinal instability in neoplastic disease. Spine: Ovid Technologies (Wolters Kluwer Health); 2010. p. Table 2 SINS scores organized as a total score, three-clinical categories, and binary scale with their corresponding levels of stability where surgical consultation is recommended for a total score >7.
43. Yamada Y, Bilsky MH. IAEA Singapore SBRT Symposium. 2013.

2 Relative Radiosensitivity of Metastatic Spine Disease

Waqar Haque and Bin S. Teh

Cancer metastasizing to the spine is a common clinical condition seen in approximately 10% of all patients with cancer and up to 40% of patients with metastatic disease [1–3]. Spinal metastases often initially present as back pain, though other symptoms include sensory deficit, radicular pain, weakness, bowel/bladder dysfunction, and paralysis. The goals of treatment with radiation therapy are to provide palliation, tumor control, improvement or recovery of neurologic function, spine stability, and improvement of quality of life [4]. There is substantial heterogeneity of response to EBRT among patients, different tumor histologies, different metastatic nodules within the same patient, and even different regions of the same tumor. The present report will describe radiosensitivity of metastatic disease within the spine and the implications this has in guiding treatment for this disease process.

Before describing radiosensitivity, it may be beneficial to provide a brief summary of the mechanism of action of EBRT delivered with the use of photons. Please note that the mechanism of action of radiation therapy delivered by charged particles is different than the process described herein. Typically, a linear accelerator shoots high-energy photons into tissue, ejecting orbital electrons from atoms in a process called ionization [5]. Radiation can damage DNA directly, in which the electron ejected from the atom damages DNA, or indirectly, in which the electron ejected from the atom interacts with a water molecule to create a hydroxyl free radical which then causes DNA damage. Types of DNA damage induced by ionizing radiation include single-strand breaks, double-strand breaks (DSBs), base damage, and DNA-protein cross-links, with DSBs thought to be the primary method of radiation-induced cell kill [6, 7]. The predominant pathway of cell killing caused by radiation is mitotic cell death, a process in which cells attempting to undergo mitosis will be unable to replicate and will die due to chromosome damage [7]. Radiation can also induce apoptosis within tumor cells, though this is more prominent in lymphoid and hemopoietic cells and is not seen in some solid tumors [8]. Cells are most radiosensitive in the M and G_2 phases of the cell cycle and least sensitive in the later part of the S phase, possibly due to the greater ability of DNA to repair double-strand breaks by homologous recombination when an undamaged sister chromatid is present [9, 10].

The radiosensitivity of a cancer cell is further influenced by the following four factors. The first is the number of clonogenic cells, that is, a cell that has retained reproductive integrity and is able to proliferate indefinitely to produce a colony, within the tumor [11]. A greater number of

W. Haque, MD • B. S. Teh, MD (✉)
Radiation Oncology Department, Houston Methodist Hospital, Houston, TX, USA
e-mail: bteh@houstonmethodist.org

R. A. W. Marco (ed.), *Metastatic Spine Disease*, https://doi.org/10.1007/978-3-319-76252-4_2

clonogens increased the likelihood that it will be able to withstand treatment with radiation. Secondly, the number of cells that are proliferating and the tumor growth kinetics within the tumor can have an impact on response to EBRT. Rapidly dividing cells are typically more radiosensitive because they are less likely to be able to repair DNA damage, are more likely to be in a radiosensitive portion of the cell cycle when receiving radiation, and are more likely to reassort into a radiosensitive portion of the cell cycle with fractionation of treatment [11, 12]. Additionally, increasing levels of hypoxia adversely impact the effect of EBRT. Since most of the radiation damage delivered by photons is mediated by oxygenated free radicals, the absence of oxygen limits the potency of radiation therapy, and tumors with poor circulation display increased radioresistance [13, 14]. Fourth, different tumor cells have a varying degree of ability to repair DNA damage, and this intrinsic ability to repair the DNA has a significant impact on radiosensitivity. In one study, investigators transfected the double-strand break repair gene DNA-PKcs into a cloned tumor cell line from severe combined immunodeficient mice and then transplanted this tumor in the same strain of mice and were able to show an increase in tumor cell radioresistance by the introduction of DNA-PKcs, leading the authors to conclude that the intrinsic radiosensitivity of tumor cells is a major factor in determining radiosensitivity [15].

Multiple methods have been proposed as ways to measure radiosensitivity. One such method has been to record the fraction of tumor cells that survives after being exposed to 2 Gray (Gy), though clinically this did not demonstrate a relevant predictive parameter for patients with head and neck squamous cell cancer [16]. Investigators have attempted to measure the potential doubling time from tumor cells obtained in vitro from patients with head and neck cancer, though this also failed to have a correlation with oncologic outcome [17]. Measurement of pretreatment tumor oxygenation can predict radiosensitivity. In patients receiving definitive radiation therapy for cervical cancer and head and neck cancer, pretreatment tumor hypoxia was predictive of worse overall survival, disease-free survival, and local control [18, 19]. Functional positron emission tomography-computerized tomography (PET/CT) imaging conducted twice during the early course of EBRT after the initiation of treatment can also quantify the responsiveness of the tumor to therapy, potentially allowing for adjustment of treatment based on the radiosensitivity displayed by the tumor [20]. Proteomic methods have revealed the presence of specific protein biomarkers that can predict for radiosensitivity prior to the initiation of treatment in breast, colon, rectal, and prostate cancers [21–24]. Bioinformatical analysis has demonstrated that the overexpression of certain plasma miRNAs was associated with a greater response to EBRT in patients with non-small cell lung cancer [25].

Unfortunately, none of the abovementioned methods have to date gained widespread clinical application. The primary method of determining radiation sensitivity in clinical practice has been based on tumor histology, despite the known heterogeneity of radiation response within the tumors [4, 26]. The tumors that have been demonstrated to have relative radiosensitive histologies include lymphoma, seminoma, and myeloma; tumors with relative radioresistant histologies include melanoma, renal cell carcinoma, some sarcomas, and gastrointestinal cancers; and tumors with an intermediate degree of radiosensitivity include prostate cancer and breast cancer [4, 27]. It is necessary to keep in mind that this is a broad overview, and while this classification does have treatment applications, there are certain subgroups of patients within these disease sites that can have different responses to radiation. For example, it has been demonstrated that there are tumor markers within patients with breast cancer that can predict for treatment response, and patients with triple-negative disease may have decreased radiosensitivity than those with estrogen receptor (ER)-positive, progesterone receptor (PR)-positive disease [28, 29].

The radiosensitivity of the cancer can be used to guide management of patients with spinal metastatic disease. Conventional radiation therapy (CRT) alone can improve neurologic function in select patients with radiosensitive tumors, and in one study 67% of patients with radiosensitive tumor histologies regained ambulation following CRT alone [30]. A retrospective review from Japan demonstrated a difference in response for patients with spinal metastases treated with CRT alone based on the radiosensitivity of the tumor, with 87% of patients with radiosensitive tumors responding to radiation, compared to a response rate of just 49% for patients with radioresistant histologies [31]. Other studies have confirmed that the histology of the tumor is associated with response to radiation treatment for metastatic spinal cord compression [32, 33]. The optimal radiation dose and fractionation for treatment of radiosensitive tumors with CRT are controversial. While there is data showing equivalent palliation with single-fraction (SF) or multi-fraction (MF) treatments, MF treatments are associated with better longer-term local control and decreased re-treatment, suggesting that MF treatment may be preferable for patients with spinal metastases [33–35]. The most typical MF fractionation scheme is 30 Gy in 10 fractions. Due to the superior outcomes associated with CRT or radiosensitive tumors, some authors advocate for CRT alone in patients with spinal metastatic disease with or without cord compression in this patient population, though the American Society for Radiation Oncology (ASTRO) guidelines recommend surgical intervention for most patients with a good performance status and life expectancy >3 months, regardless of histology with postoperative CRT [4, 36] (Fig. 2.1).

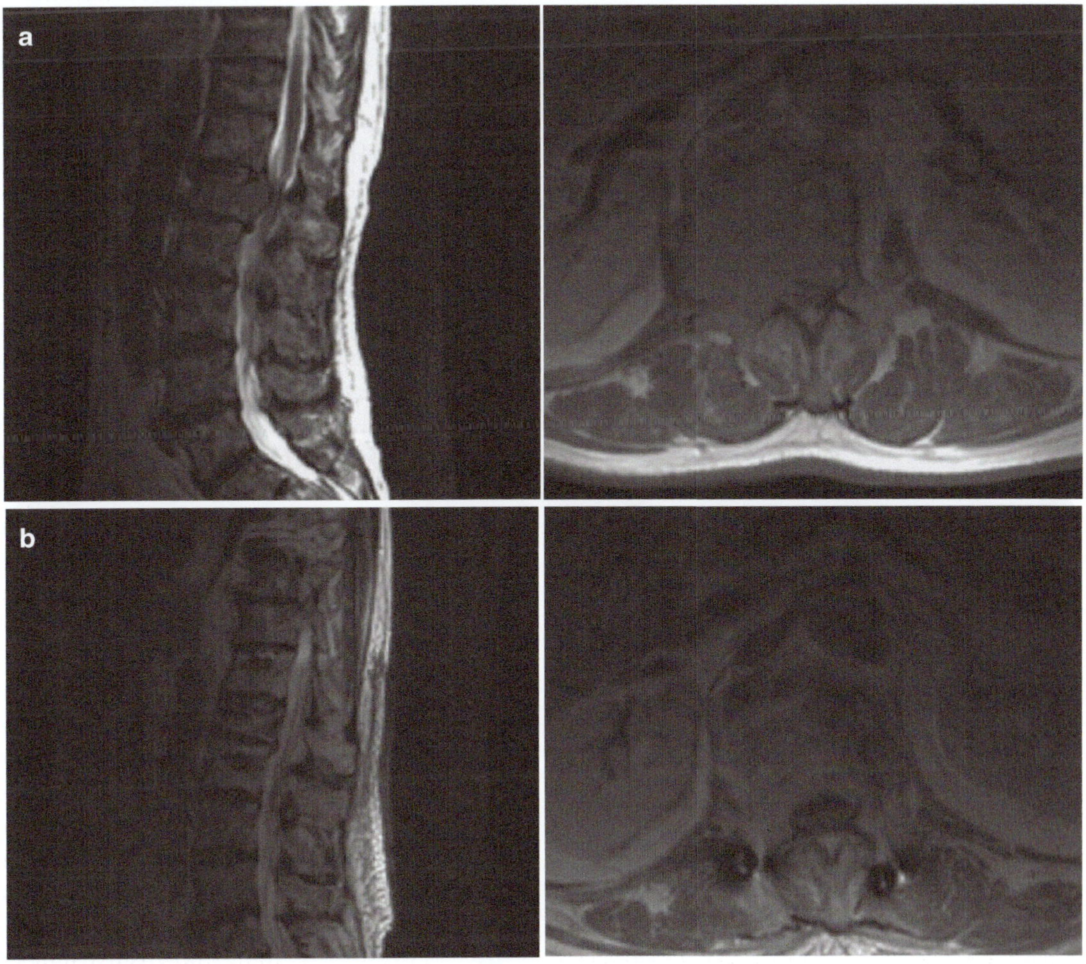

Fig. 2.1 Images displaying a patient with cord compression at L1 due to multiple myeloma and complete resolution of the compression 11 weeks after completion of conventionally fractionated radiation (from [4])

Radioresistant tumors do not respond well to CRT, with studies reporting only a 20–33% response rate with CRT alone in this patient population, with a time to progression of 1–3 months in patients who respond [30, 31]. This is partially because of the inability to achieve a tumoricidal dose with conventional techniques, as in CRT the dose delivered to the tumor within the spine is the same dose received by the spinal cord. Consequently, the radiation dose is limited by the radiation tolerance dose of the spinal cord. One solution to overcome radioresistance is to deliver higher, ablative doses to the tumor while sparing the dose delivered to the spinal cord using a technique called stereotactic body radiation therapy (SBRT). Advances in radiation therapy technology including the use of image fusion, development of more rigid immobilization devices, computerized treatment planning, image-guided radiation treatment (IGRT), and intensity-modulated radiation therapy (IMRT) have allowed the delivery of this conformal treatment [37] (Fig. 2.2).

Intracranial, single-fraction SBRT has been demonstrated to overcome radioresistance for intracranial metastatic disease and demonstrated equivalent local control for both radioresistant and radiosensitive tumor histologies [38–40]. The success of treatment of radioresistant intracranial disease with SBRT leads to experimentation of radioresistant extracranial disease with SBRT, with similarly successful outcomes. In the largest series of patients treated with single-fraction spine SBRT, 500 patients with metastases in the spine were treated to a mean dose of 20 Gy and achieved a 90% local control rate, with 84% of patients displaying neurologic improvement [41]. There was no difference in outcome based on tumor histology. In a review of 103 patients with radioresistant oligometastatic disease treated with spine SBRT to a dose of 18–24 Gy, Yamada et al. demonstrated a local control rate of 92% [42]. In a later review of this cohort, a higher dose was associated with superior local control, with a 97% local control rate at 3 years reported for patients receiving a dose of 24 Gy [43]. Due to the excellent outcomes achieved with SBRT for spinal metastatic disease, patients with radioresistant tumors without cord compression are recommended to receive treatment with SBRT alone [4].

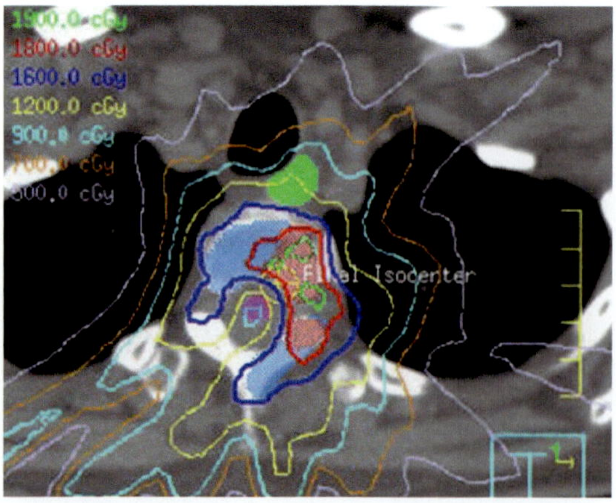

Fig. 2.2 Image demonstrating the ability to sculpt dose around the spinal cord with SBRT. Red color indicates the tumor (from [55])

Patients with radioresistant tumors with cord compression, however, are considered for upfront decompressive surgery followed by postoperative SBRT [44]. In a retrospective review from Memorial Sloan-Kettering, 186 patients with epidural spinal cord compression were treated with surgical decompression followed by postoperative single-fraction SBRT to 24 Gy, high-dose hypofractionated SBRT to 24–30 Gy in 3 fractions, or low-dose hypofractionated SBRT to 18–36 Gy in 5–6 fractions. Local progression was 4.1% for the high-dose SBRT arm, while it was 22.6% for the low-dose SBRT arm, with equivalent outcomes seen for patients with radiosensitive and radioresistant histologies [45]. A second retrospective review reporting on outcomes for patients with spinal metastases treated postoperatively with SBRT from the University of Toronto showed a 1-year local control rate of 84%, with equivalent outcomes for patients regardless of histology, though superior local control was observed for patients treated with high-dose SBRT (18–26 Gy in 1 or 2 fractions) when compared to patients treated with low-dose SBRT (18–40 Gy in 3–5 fractions) [46] (Table 2.1).

Table 2.1 Consensus guidelines for patients eligible for postoperative SBRT (adapted from [44])

Indications	Contraindications
Radioresistant primary	Involvement of more than three contiguous vertebral bodies
1–2 levels of adjacent disease	Complete spinal cord injury without preservation of motor or sensory function
Prior overlapping radiation therapy	Spinal cord compression without any CSF around the spinal cord

Table 2.2 Suggested treatment recommendations for spinal metastatic disease based on radiosensitivity (adapted from [4])

Spinal cord compression	Tumor histology	Treatment decision
No	Radioresistant	SBRT
No	Radiosensitive	CRT
Yes	Radioresistant	Surgery followed by SBRT
Yes	Radiosensitive	Surgery followed by CRT

The effectiveness of SBRT in radioresistant histologies has changed the goals of surgical intervention in the setting of spinal cord compression. Prior to the advent of SBRT, the surgical goal was to aggressively resect the tumor, a procedure associated with prolonged anesthesia time, increased length of hospital stay, and trend of lower survival rates [47]. The minimum tumor-spinal cord distance that allows radiation oncologists to deliver adequate, tumoricidal dose to the tumor while maintaining the ability to keep the spinal cord within the tolerated dose is 3 mm [48]. The advent of SBRT has allowed surgeons to perform a "separation surgery," with the goal of providing an adequate margin of separation between the tumor and the spinal cord such that an adequate SBRT dose can be delivered to the tumor while respecting the spinal cord dose tolerance, with studies suggesting equivalent oncologic outcomes along with decreased morbidity [49] (Table 2.2).

Additionally, there is data to suggest single-fraction spinal SBRT may be effective in management of epidural cord compression in patients with symptomatic epidural cord compression. Ryu et al. investigated the use of single-fraction spinal SBRT for management of patients with high-grade spinal cord compression and motor strength 4/5 or higher [50]. Of note, patients with radioresistant histologies, such as melanoma and chordoma, were included in the study, while patients with radiosensitive histologies, such as lymphoma or myeloma, were not included. The rate of neurologic improvement or preservation was 84% after SBRT, leading the authors to conclude that the epidural space would potentially be decompressed with the use of single-fraction SBRT. Importantly, there have been no trials comparing SBRT or surgery for management of spinal cord compression, and surgery remains the standard of care. However, due to high rate of neurologic preservation in patients managed with SRS alone in the aforementioned trial, some authors advocate that patients with minimal neurologic symptoms may be adequately treated by SBRT alone [51].

In the above paragraphs, we have demonstrated that advances in radiation physics have allowed physicians to overcome the limited radiosensitivity of certain tumor histologies to provide adequate local control. A numerical example may further illustrate the radiobiological principle behind the increased efficacy of SBRT over CRT in controlling radioresistant tumors. As stated previously, a limitation of conventional radiation techniques is that the dose delivered to the tumor is constrained by the tolerance dose of the spinal cord, since in CRT, the dose delivered to the tumor is the same as that delivered to the cord. However, SBRT allows physicians to sculpt the dose distribution to create a conformal treatment plan that maximizes dose to the tumor while simultaneously minimizing the dose delivered to the spinal cord. Therefore, using the equation for the biologically effective dose (BED), BED = $n * d\ x\ (1 + d/[\alpha/\beta])$, we can compare the BED delivered using SBRT to BED delivered using CRT, where n is number of fractions, d is dose per fraction, and the α/β ratio is the dose at which the linear and quadratic components of cell killing are equal [52]. Using an α/β ratio of 7 for melanoma [53], we find that a CRT dose of 30 Gy in 10 fractions yields a BED of 42.9 Gy_7, whereas a SBRT dose of 18 Gy in a single fraction yields a BED of

64.3 Gy_7. It is likely that this increase in BED to the tumor is the radiobiological explanation for the improvement in oncologic outcome for radioresistant tumors that is observed with SBRT treatment; that is to say, the increased BED offered by SBRT allows physicians to overcome unfavorable tumor radiobiology. Additionally, there is data to suggest that the high dose per fraction of SBRT may produce enhanced antitumor immunity, which can further potentiate tumor kill, a process not seen in CRT [54].

We have illustrated that radiosensitivity of the tumor can guide treatment management for patients with spinal metastatic disease. Currently, the most widely clinically used method to determine radiosensitivity is tumor histology. However, this is not ideal, as significant heterogeneity can exist in terms of radiation response within the same tumor histology [28, 29]. It is likely that more sophisticated techniques, such as proteomic analysis or analysis of plasma miRNA, may have increased clinical application in order to provide a more accurate measure of radiosensitivity [21–25]. Additionally, the use of systemic agents may be used concurrently with SBRT to further improve tumor control. The use of tyrosine kinase inhibitors concurrently with spine SBRT has been demonstrated to improve outcomes for patients with metastatic renal cell carcinoma [55, 56]. The development of newer targeted agents may provide additional opportunities for use in combination with SBRT. Future improvements in technology, in both methods of determination of radiosensitivity and treatment delivery, will allow physicians to offer a greater degree of personalized medicine, tailoring treatments for patients based on the unique radiobiological characteristics of their tumor, while also taking advantage of possible synergy between systemic agents and radiation therapy to optimize treatment and improve outcomes for patients.

References

1. Fornasier VL, Horne JG. Metastases to the vertebral column. Cancer. 1975;36:590–4.
2. Grant R, Papadopoulos SM, Greenberg HS. Metastatic epidural spinal cord compression. Neurol Clin. 1991;9:825–41.
3. Hatrick NC, Lucas JD, Timothy AR, et al. The surgical treatment of metastatic disease of the spine. Radiother Oncol. 2000;56:335–9.
4. Laufer I, Rubin DG, Lis E, et al. The NOMS framework: approach to the treatment of spinal metastatic tumors. Oncologist. 2013;18:744–51.
5. Johns HE, Cunningham JR. The physics of radiology. Springfield: Charles C Thomas; 1969.
6. Carrano AV. Chromosome aberrations and radiation-induced cell death: II. Predicted and observed cell survival. Mutat Res. 1973;17:355–66.
7. Cornforth MN, Bedford JS. A quantitative comparison of potentially lethal damage repair and the rejoining of interphase chromosome breaks in low passage normal human fibroblasts. Radiat Res. 1987;111:385–405.
8. Williams GT. Programmed cell death: apoptosis and oncogenesis. Cell. 1991;65:1097–8.
9. Sinclair WK, Morton RA. X-ray sensitivity during the cell generation cycle of cultured Chinese hamster cells. Radiat Res. 1966;29:450–74.
10. Hammond EM, Pires I, Giacca AJ. Chapter 2: DNA damage and repair. In: Libel S, Phillips TL, Hoppe RT, Roach M, editors. Textbook of radiation oncology. Philadelphia: Elsevier; 2010.
11. Hall EJ, Giaccia AJ. Radiobiology for the radiobiologist. 7th ed. Philadelphia: Lippincott Williams and Wilkins; 2012.
12. Tubiana M. Repopulation in human tumors. A biological background for fractionation in radiotherapy. Acta Oncol. 1988;27:83–8.
13. Gray LH, Conger AD, Ebert M, Hornsey S, Scott OC. The concentration of oxygen dissolved in tissues at the time of irradiation as a factor in radiotherapy. Br J Radiol. 1953;26:638–48.
14. Thomlinson RH, Gray LH. The histological structure of some human lung cancers and the possible implications for radiotherapy. Br J Cancer. 1955;9:539–49.
15. Gerweck LE, Vijayappa S, Kurimasa A, Ogawa K, Chen DJ. Tumor cell radiosensitivity is a major determinant of tumor response to radiation. Cancer Res. 2006;66:8352–5.
16. Eschwege F, Bourhis J, Girinski T, et al. Predictive assays of radiation response in patients with head and neck squamous cell carcinoma: a review of the Institute Gustave Roussy experience. Int J Radiat Oncol Biol Phys. 1997;39:849–53.
17. Bourhis J, Dendale R, Hill C, et al. Potential doubling time and clinical outcome in head and neck squamous cell carcinoma treated with 70 Gy in 7 weeks. Int J Radiat Oncol Biol Phys. 1996;35:471–6.
18. Höckel M, Vorndran B, Schlenger K, Baussmann E, Knapstein PG. Tumor oxygenation: a new predictive parameter in locally advanced cancer of the uterine cervix. Gynecol Oncol. 1993;51:141–9.
19. Brizel DM, Dodge RK, Clough RW, Dewhirst MW. Oxygenation of head and neck cancer: changes

during radiotherapy and impact on treatment outcome. Radiother Oncol. 1999;53:113–7.
20. Brahme A. Biologically optimized 3-dimensional *in vivo* predictive assay-based radiation therapy using positron emission tomography–computerized tomography imaging. Acta Oncol. 2003;42:123–36.
21. Smith L, Qutob O, Watson MB, et al. Proteomic identification of putative biomarkers of radiotherapy resistance: a possible role for the 26S proteasome? Neoplasia. 2009;11(11):1194–207.
22. Allal AS, Kähne T, Reverdin AK, et al. Radioresistance-related proteins in rectal cancer. Proteomics. 2004;4:2261–9.
23. Skvortsova I, Skvortsov S, Stasyk T, et al. Intracellular signaling pathways regulating radioresistance of human prostate carcinoma cells. Proteomics. 2008;8:4521–33.
24. Ramsamooj P, Kasid U, Dritschilo A. Differential expression of proteins in radioresistant and radiosensitive human squamous carcinoma cells. J Natl Cancer Inst. 1992;84:622–8.
25. Chen X, Xu Y, Liao X, et al. Plasma miRNAs in predicting radiosensitivity in non-small cell lung cancer. Tumour Biol. 2016;37:11927–36.
26. Rofstad EK. Radiation sensitivity in vitro of primary tumors and metastatic lesions of malignant melanoma. Cancer Res. 1992;52:4453–7.
27. Gerszten PC, Mendel E, Yamada Y. Radiotherapy and radiosurgery for metastatic spine disease: what are the options, indications, and outcomes? Spine. 2009;34:S78–92.
28. Kyndi M, Sørensen FB, Knudsen H, et al. Estrogen receptor, progesterone receptor, HER-2, and response to postmastectomy radiotherapy in high-risk breast cancer: the Danish Breast Cancer Cooperative Group. J Clin Oncol. 2008;26:1419–26.
29. Nguyen PL, Taghian AG, Katz MS, et al. Breast cancer subtype approximated by estrogen receptor, progesterone receptor, and HER-2 is associated with local and distant recurrence after breast-conserving therapy. J Clin Oncol. 2008;26:2373–8.
30. Maranzano E, Latini P. Effectiveness of radiation therapy without surgery in metastatic spinal cord compression: final results from a prospective trial. Int J Radiat Oncol Biol Phys. 1995;32:959–67.
31. Katagiri H, Takahashi M, Inagaki J, et al. Clinical results of nonsurgical treatment for spinal metastases. Int J Radiat Oncol Biol Phys. 1998;42:1127–32.
32. Gilbert RW, Kim JH, Posner JB. Epidural spinal cord compression from metastatic tumor: diagnosis and treatment. Ann Neurol. 1978;3:40–51.
33. Rades D, Fehlauer F, Schulte R, et al. Prognostic factors for local control and survival after radiotherapy of metastatic spinal cord compression. J Clin Oncol. 2006;24:3388–93.
34. Steenland E, Leer JW, van Houwelingen H, et al. The effect of a single fraction compared to multiple fractions on painful bone metastases: a global analysis of the Dutch Bone Metastasis Study. Radiother Oncol. 1999;52:101–9.
35. Hartsell WF, Scott CB, Bruner DW, et al. Randomized trial of short- versus long-course radiotherapy for palliation of painful bone metastases. J Natl Cancer Inst. 2005;97:798–804.
36. Lutz S, Berk L, Chang E, et al. Palliative radiotherapy for bone metastases: an ASTRO evidence-based guideline. Int J Radiat Oncol Biol Phys. 2011;79:965–76.
37. Sahgal A, Roberge D, Schellenberg D, et al. The Canadian Association of Radiation Oncology scope of practice guidelines for lung, liver and spine stereotactic body radiotherapy. Clin Oncol (R Coll Radiol). 2012;24:629–39.
38. Brown PD, Brown CA, Pollock BE, Gorman DA, Foote RL. Stereotactic radiosurgery for patients with "radioresistant" brain metastases. Neurosurgery. 2002;51:656–65.
39. Yaeh A, Nanda T, Jani A, et al. Control of brain metastases from radioresistant tumors treated by stereotactic radiosurgery. J Neurooncol. 2015;124:507–14.
40. Teh BS, Bloch C, Paulino AC, et al. Pathologic complete response in renal cell carcinoma brain metastases treated with stereotactic radiosurgery. Clin Genitourin Cancer. 2007;5:334–7.
41. Gerszten PC, Burton SA, Ozhasoglu C, et al. Radiosurgery for spinal metastases: clinical experience in 500 cases from a single institution. Spine. 2007;32:193–9.
42. Yamada Y, Bilsky MH, Lovelock DM, et al. High-dose, single-fraction image-guided intensity-modulated radiotherapy for metastatic spinal lesions. Int J Radiat Oncol Biol Phys. 2008;71:484–90.
43. Yamada Y, Cox B, Zelefsky MJ, et al. An analysis of prognostic factors for local control of malignant spine tumors treated with spine radiosurgery. Int J Radiat Oncol Biol Phys. 2011;81:S132–3.
44. Redmond KJ, Lo SS, Soltys SG, et al. Consensus guidelines for postoperative stereotactic body radiation therapy for spinal metastases: results of an international survey. J Neurosurg Spine. 2017;26(3):299–306.
45. Laufer I, Iorgulescu JB, Chapman T, et al. Local disease control for spinal metastases following "separation surgery" and adjuvant hypofractionated or high-dose single-fraction stereotactic radiosurgery: outcome analysis in 186 patients. J Neurosurg Spine. 2014;18:207–14.
46. Al-Omair A, Masucci L, Masson-Cote L, et al. Surgical resection of epidural disease improves local control following postoperative spine stereotactic body radiotherapy. Neuro Oncol. 2013;15:1413–9.
47. Yang Z, Yang Y, Zhang Y, et al. Minimal access versus open spinal surgery in treating painful spine metastasis: a systematic review. World J Surg Oncol. 2015;13:68.
48. Ryu S, Pugh SL, Gerszten PC, et al. RTOG 0631 phase 2/3 study of image guided stereotactic radiosurgery for localized (1-3) spinal metastases: phase 2 results. Pract Radiat Oncol. 2014;4:76–81.

49. Zuckerman SL, Laufer I, Sahgal A, et al. When less is more: the indications for MIS techniques and separation surgery in metastatic spine disease. Spine (Phila Pa 1976). 2016;41:S246–53.
50. Ryu S, Rock J, Jain R, et al. Radiosurgical decompression of metastatic epidural compression. Cancer. 2010;116:2250–7.
51. Ryu S, Yoon H, Stessin A, et al. Contemporary treatment with radiosurgery for spinal metastasis and spinal cord compression in 2015. Radiat Oncol J. 2015;33:1–11.
52. Fowler JF. A review: the linear quadratic formula and progress in fractionated radiotherapy. Br J Radiol. 1989;62:679–5.
53. Rofstad EK. Radiation biology of malignant melanoma. Review article. Acta Radiol Oncol. 1986;25:1–10.
54. Brown JM, Carlson DJ, Brenner DJ. The tumor radiobiology of SRS and SBRT: are more than the 5 R's involved? Int J Radiat Oncol Biol Phys. 2014;88:254–62.
55. Miller JA, Balagamwala EH, Angelov L, et al. Spine stereotactic radiosurgery with concurrent tyrosine kinase inhibitors for metastatic renal cell carcinoma. J Neurosurg Spine. 2016;25:766–74.
56. Kroeze SGC, Fritz C, Hoyer M, et al. Toxicity of concurrent stereotactic radiotherapy and targeted therapy or immunotherapy: a systematic review. Cancer Treat Rev. 2017;53:25–37.

Relative Chemo-, Hormonal, and Immunosensitivity

3

Max Vaynrub and John H. Healey

Introduction

The decision regarding the best approach to treating a spinal metastasis depends on two factors: (1) the current state of the lesion and (2) the projected course of the lesion. The first factor requires an evaluation of the damage already done by the lesion. Any existing mechanical instability warrants surgical intervention regardless of tumor sensitivity to adjuvant therapy for patients who are medically able to undergo surgical intervention. Similarly, aside from cases of relatively radiosensitive tumors (as can be seen with some neoplasms such as lymphoma, myeloma, and breast carcinoma), most instances of severe epidural spinal cord compression will require timely decompression surgery. The second factor is more difficult to analyze and depends on the known chemo-, hormonal, or immunosensitivity of the tumor histology as well as the patient's past response to the adjuvant therapy. Although the spine surgeon may not necessarily dictate the specifics of adjuvant treatment, it is imperative that he/she understands the anticipated caliber, timeframe, and durability of response, as well as the patient's projected survival, in order to make an informed decision regarding management of the patient's spinal lesions.

M. Vaynrub, MD · J. H. Healey, MD (✉)
Department of Surgery, Memorial Sloan Kettering Cancer Center, New York, NY, USA
e-mail: healeyj@mskcc.org

Assessing Response to Treatment

A discussion of the relative response of malignant lesions to systemic therapy necessitates precise definitions and measurements of response. Trending laboratory biomarkers may provide information about overall disease activity but cannot directly quantify lesion size. Response Evaluation Criteria in Solid Tumors (RECIST) version 1.1 [1] is a widely accepted system for radiographically quantifying size and objective response of known metastatic lesions. It standardizes the anatomical measurement of disease burden by dictating that up to five lesions (maximum of two per organ) be measured in the single greatest dimension on CT or MRI. A subsequent increase of 20% or decrease of 30% of the sum of measured lesions defines progressive disease (PD) or partial response (PR), respectively. Resolution of all lesions defines complete response (CR). Of note, blastic bone lesions are considered nonmeasurable, and lytic bone lesions are included only if the soft tissue component is sufficiently measurable.

Limitations of RECIST 1.1 are its reliance on a unidimensional anatomical measurement, which is an imperfect representation of three-dimensional tumor size, and the lack of information on tumor activity. An additional useful assessment of response on CT is the observation of sclerotic change in a lytic osseous lesion in response to therapy, whereas progression of lytic change indicates progressive disease. MRI is

R. A. W. Marco (ed.), *Metastatic Spine Disease*, https://doi.org/10.1007/978-3-319-76252-4_3

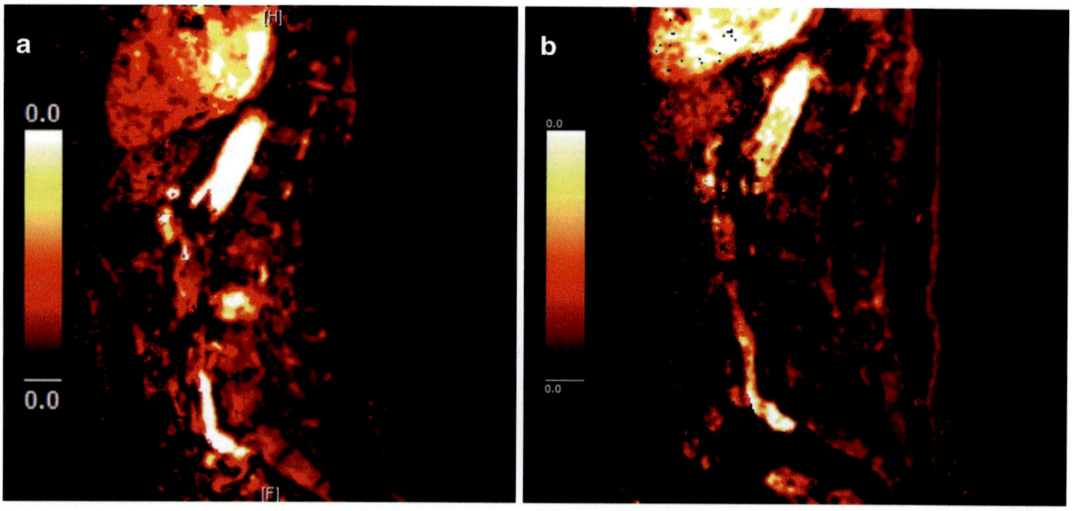

Fig. 3.1 The images illustrate the use of MRI to evaluate lesion perfusion. A 64-year-old male with metastatic renal cell carcinoma with a lesion at L4 imaged with dynamic contrast-enhanced perfusion MRI prior to (**a**) and 10 weeks following (**b**) treatment with hypofractionated radiation therapy. The lack of perfusion in the posttreatment image demonstrates inactive lesion status

excellent at depicting bone marrow involvement and soft tissue response but is not well-suited to differentiating osteolytic and blastic changes [2]. Bone scintigraphy may also be informative but when used alone in the first 6 months of therapy has a high false-positive rate due to the flare phenomenon, an osteoblastic reaction following response to treatment [3, 4]. The MD Anderson (MDA) classification combines plain radiograph, CT, MRI, and bone scintigraphy evaluations of bone metastasis treatment response and has been shown to correlate with progression-free survival (PFS) [5–7].

Cytostatic agents may decrease tumor activity without a change in tumor size on anatomical imaging [8]. Furthermore, changes in tumor activity may offer an earlier indication of response than changes in the size or radiographic character of a lesion on CT [2, 9]. The integration of metabolic imaging technologies has led to the development of PET Response Criteria in Solid Tumors (PERCIST) [10]. Treatment evaluation with PERCIST shows substantial agreement with RECIST 1.1 (κ = 0.689) with PERCIST showing an overall better treatment response [10]. Further validation studies are required to demonstrate that PERCIST can reliably show treatment response and time to progression. Additionally, functional imaging using dynamic contrast-enhanced MRI can be used to assess vascular perfusion of a target lesion following treatment with systemic therapy or radiotherapy [11–13] (Fig. 3.1).

Tissue Procurement

Several indications for biopsy exist in metastatic disease of the spine. Biopsy of a vertebral metastasis may be used as a planned procedure to establish a primary cancer diagnosis, though initial staging imaging will usually reveal a more accessible location to biopsy [14]. In situations where the presenting symptom is spinal instability or epidural compression, urgent operative intervention may precede diagnosis, and an intraoperative biopsy will be required. In patients with a known primary neoplasm without proven metastatic disease, biopsy can serve to confirm metastatic status of the known primary or to establish a new diagnosis. Patients with previously biopsy-proven osseous metastases may, in specific instances, benefit from additional biopsy of a specific vertebral lesion for genetic or immunohistochemical testing, as therapeutic sensitivity patterns can vary among lesions. Patients presenting with a compression fracture that is radiographically ambiguous may require biopsy to differentiate a fragility fracture from a pathologic fracture, which will guide treatment [15].

Biopsy technique can be either open or percutaneous. The lower morbidity of percutaneous image-guided biopsy has made this the preferred initial approach. A large-bore core biopsy needle is used and inserted via a transpedicular, transcostovertebral, paraspinal, anterolateral, or transoral approach [16] (Fig. 3.2). Transpedicular biopsy can be performed in conjunction with vertebroplasty/kyphoplasty in order to reduce the morbidity of a separate procedure [15].

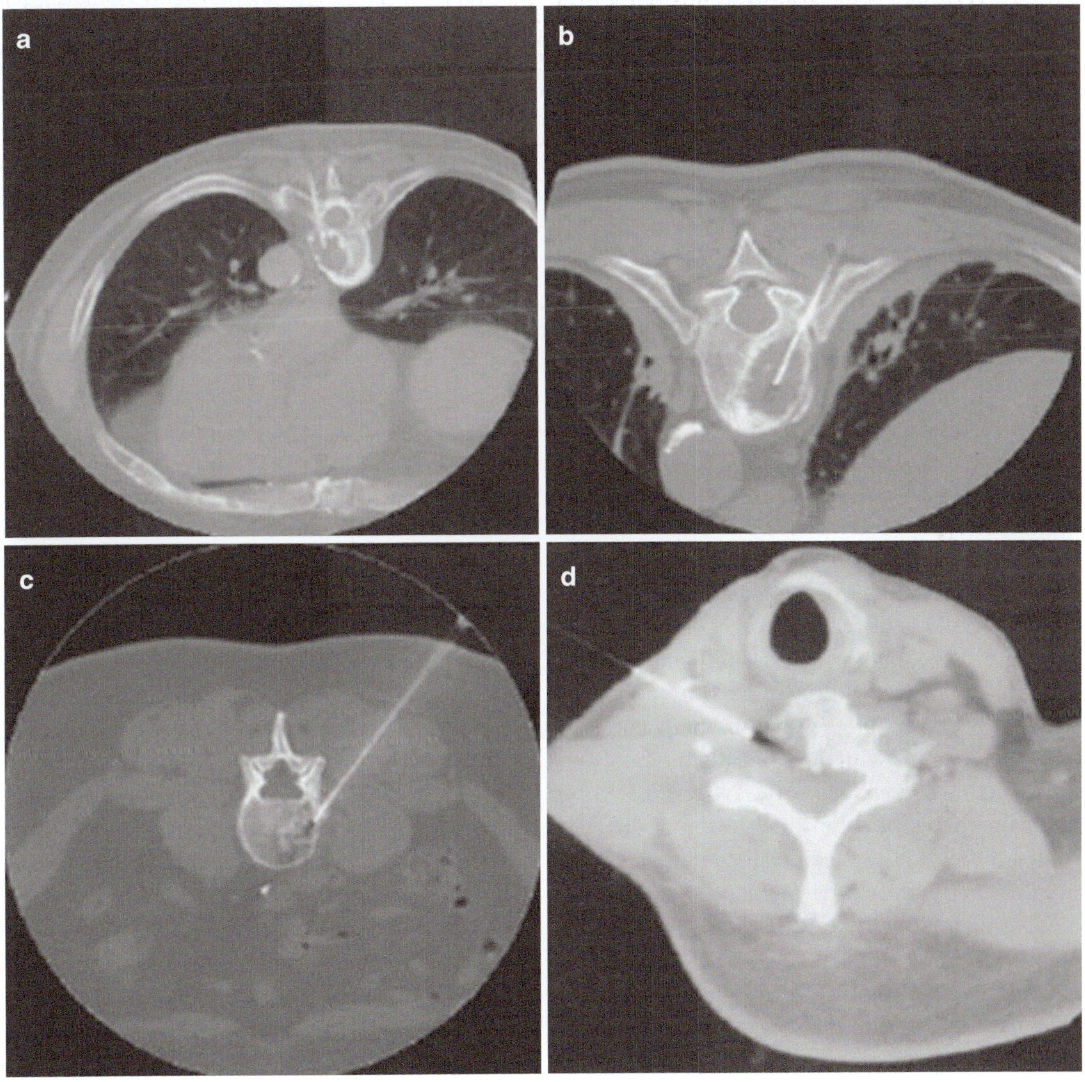

Fig. 3.2 Axial CT images. (**a**) Transpedicular approach to a T6 lytic lesion in a patient without a prior cancer history. Cytologic and histologic findings revealed numerous plasma cells compatible with plasma cell neoplasm-plasmacytoma. (**b**) Transcostovertebral approach to a T8 lytic lesion in a patient with a history of papillary thyroid cancer. Biopsy confirmed metastatic thyroid cancer. (**c**) Paraspinal approach to a mixed L3 lytic-sclerotic lesion in a patient with breast cancer. Biopsy showed adenocarcinoma consistent with a mammary origin. (**d**) Anterolateral approach to a C5 lytic lesion in a patient with a history of gastric cancer. Cytology was compatible with metastatic gastric carcinoma. Images from Lis E, Bilsky MH, Pisinski L, Boland P, Healey JH, O'Malley B, et al. Percutaneous CT-guided biopsy of osseous lesion of the spine in patients with known or suspected malignancy. *Am J Neuroradiol.* 2004;25(9):1586. © 2004 American Society of Neuroradiology. Reproduced with permission

It is essential to procure sufficient amounts of tissue for histologic and genetic examination, which can be crucial in determining systemic therapy. Equally crucial is obtaining the appropriate tissue. Thus, prior to biopsy, imaging should be carefully reviewed to determine the location that is expected to have the highest yield. Central necrotic portions of tumor may be avoided in favor of more active tissue at the periphery. Metabolic imaging such as positron emission tomography (PET) may be useful in this regard. It is also important to note the sclerotic and lytic characteristics of the lesion, in terms of ease of procurement and diagnostic yield. Overall accuracy with percutaneous biopsy is 89%, though it is lower in sclerotic lesions, which have shown a 24% false-negative rate [16]. Lesions that are sclerotic may require decalcification as part of pathological analysis; it is vital in these cases to request EDTA decalcification (as opposed to hydrochloric or nitric acid), as this will minimize degradation of genetic material [17].

Variability of Sensitivity

The relative sensitivity to systemic treatment varies widely, not just between broad categories (e.g., sarcoma vs. carcinoma) and different organs of primary origin (e.g., lung adenocarcinoma vs. breast adenocarcinoma), but also between patients with the same histological subtypes and even between different lesions within the same patient or the same lesion at different time points. Additional variables that can determine sensitivity include mutational status, time course of treatment, and the anatomic location of the lesion of interest.

Approximately 50% of all spinal metastases originate from primary breast, lung, or prostate cancers, with spinal metastasis rates of 74.3%, 44.9%, and 90.5%, respectively, among those patients with metastatic disease [18]. The remaining burden of spinal metastatic disease originates largely from renal cell carcinoma, gastrointestinal neoplasms, thyroid cancer, lymphoma, multiple myeloma, or sarcoma. While lymphoma is often exquisitely chemosensitive, with frequent complete responses, the benefits of chemotherapy in metastatic sarcoma and carcinoma are variable and often temporary, even in the face of an encouraging initial response.

The timeline of disease and treatment are important factors when considering sensitivity. As neoplasms exhibit genomic instability and a certain spontaneous mutation rate, the natural history is that of advancing aggressiveness and resistance [19]. In addition, clonal heterogeneity and the selective pressure applied by the presence of chemotherapeutics (assuming a certain amount of surviving tumor cells) further drive the abatement of sensitivity to systemic therapy over time [20, 21]. Thus, a tumor that was sensitive to certain classes of therapy initially cannot be assumed to respond to the same agents at a different time point.

Sensitivity to various therapies can differ between the primary tumor and its spinal metastases, as well as between various spinal metastases in the same patient. Clonal differences in genetic profiles and shorter doubling times in metastatic lesions contribute to this difference in response [22]. The tumor microenvironment also plays a crucial role. The anatomic location assumes certain mutations as a prerequisite for its migration to and survival in that foreign environment. Additionally, the size, vascularity, and activity of a given lesion will affect its metabolic and hypoxic gradient and, in turn, the effective drug concentrations delivered to its cells [23, 24]. These factors create differences in sensitivity in the metastatic lesions, and one cannot assume that a treatment that is effective on the primary tumor will have an equal effect on the spinal metastases of interest. As an example the discordance in hormonal receptor status between primary and metastatic breast cancer lesions and, consequently, primary and metastatic sensitivity to hormonal therapy, can range from 10 to 50% [25]. For this reason, it is sometimes prudent to biopsy a spine lesion in a patient with proven metastases, as it may provide additional therapeutic guidance.

The response rates and relative sensitivities mentioned below are current as of the publication of this text but are bound to change in the coming years. The field of medical oncology is a rapidly evolving one, and patients with cancers that have previously been deemed chemoresistant to conventional antiproliferative drugs now benefit from major advances in the form of novel therapies. One area that holds great promise is immunotherapy—the concept of harnessing and augmenting the patient's immune system to invoke a directed and durable attack on tumor cells. This is accomplished with exogenous monoclonal antibodies, cancer vaccines, and immune checkpoint inhibitors (ICIs), which target inhibitory receptor proteins to disinhibit the T-cell response to cancer antigens. While many of the treatments in this category are still investigational, several are already in clinical use and have demonstrated promising results [26].

Breast Cancer

The expression of estrogen receptor (ER), progesterone receptor (PR), and human epidermal growth factor receptor 2 (HER2) is key to determining sensitivity to hormonal and targeted therapies in breast cancer. ER expression confers tumor susceptibility to endocrine therapy and often allows initial treatment without conventional chemotherapy. Endocrine therapy may include ovarian chemical suppression or surgical ablation, selective estrogen receptor modulators (SERMs) such as tamoxifen, aromatase inhibitors such as anastrozole, ER antagonists such as fulvestrant, and other agents [27]. The choice of agent depends on menopause status and prior response to specific endocrine therapies. Progression to multiline endocrine therapy resistance prompts the initiation of conventional chemotherapy. Overexpression of HER2 confers sensitivity to targeted treatment with monoclonal antibodies against the receptor, including trastuzumab and pertuzumab [28, 29].

Receptor status not only predicts response to hormonal therapy but also predicts sensitivity to conventional chemotherapy (such as doxorubicin and cyclophosphamide) [30]. Of note, the genetic subtypes with the most favorable prognosis and response to hormonal therapy (so-called luminal A or ER+, HER2−, low proliferation) are the least sensitive to chemotherapy. These subtypes are less likely to metastasize or recur, but when such patients do develop metastasis or recurrence, they are likely to have the poorest responses to chemotherapy. Conversely, in what has come to be known as the "triple-negative paradox," tumors lacking hormone receptor expression (ER−, PR−, HER2−) demonstrate the most robust response to chemotherapy, but patients who do not achieve a complete response have the shortest survival [31, 32].

The genetic profile of breast cancer is known to predict survival and sensitivity to hormonal or chemotherapy [30, 33, 34]. Gene expression profiles of breast cancer tissue, and more specifically of migratory cells, can be predictive of the clinical course [35]. BRCA1 and BRCA2 mutations can be prognostic of survival and response to various classes of chemotherapy, including platinum agents, anthracyclines, taxanes, and PARP inhibitors [36–39]. BRCA1 and BRCA2 carriers demonstrate increased sensitivity to anthracycline-based regimens, while the CHEK2 mutation confers a poor response to this therapy [36, 40]. However, the improved response is not uniform; among breast cancers that are hormone receptor negative, the BRCA1 mutation portends a poorer response to taxanes [37].

Lung Cancer

Lung cancer has long been considered a relentlessly progressive disease with uniformly dismal outcome. More recently, however, patients with lung cancer have benefitted from advances in genetic analysis and targeted therapy, which have prolonged survival times, although 5-year survival remains about 15%. Heavy smoking is associated with squamous cell, small cell, and large cell subtypes with high rates of TP53 mutation and no targetable oncogene mutations. However, lung adenocarcinoma may display mutations in epidermal growth factor receptor (EGFR), anaplastic lymphoma kinase (ALK), and several other oncogenes that present options for targeted therapy [41].

EGFR mutations are seen in 15–40% of lung adenocarcinomas, more frequently in Asians and never-smokers [42, 43]. When compared with conventional platinum-based chemotherapy, tyrosine kinase inhibitors (TKIs) such as gefitinib, erlotinib, and afatinib result in better objective response rates (ORR) and, in certain EGFR mutations, improved overall survival [43, 44]. ALK rearrangement is present in 3–6% of lung adenocarcinoma and is also more prevalent in never-smokers. First-line targeted therapy with crizotinib (a small-molecule TKI) in these patients has shown an ORR of 74% and a PFS of 10.9 months [45]. Though EGFR and ALK have proven to be the most effective targets thus far, they appear in a small subset of lung cancer patients; ongoing trials involving other potential targets, including MET, ROS-1, and KRA, may yield greater rates of therapeutic response in the future.

Prostate Cancer

The cornerstone of prostate cancer treatment is androgen deprivation therapy (ADT), entailing medical or surgical castration. One method of pharmacologic ADT is continuous administration of luteinizing hormone-releasing hormone (LHRH), which causes a paradoxical cessation of androgen production due to pituitary desensitization. Of particular importance to the spine surgeon is the potential for tumor flare in the first 7–10 days after initiation of treatment, as testosterone release is stimulated prior to hormonal desensitization [46]. For this reason, antiandrogen therapy is co-administered during this period—an especially vital detail in patients with lesions that confer risk of epidural spinal cord compression. Additionally, corticosteroids, associated with both androgen-lowering and anti-inflammatory effects, are routinely used to treat tumor-related symptoms [47].

Sensitivity to ADT is initially high, with response in 80–90% of patients with advanced prostate cancer, though progression to castration-resistant prostate cancer (CRPC) usually occurs 1–3 years after initiation of treatment [48]. Docetaxel can be incorporated into the treatment regimen before or after the development of castration resistance and has been shown to prolong survival. With further progression, there are options for immunotherapy, including the dendritic cell vaccine sipuleucel-T and the ICI ipilimumab, though clinical studies to demonstrate their efficacy are still ongoing [49].

Renal Cell Carcinoma

There has been substantial recent progress in the systemic treatment of metastatic renal cell carcinoma. TKIs targeting vascular endothelial growth factor receptor (sunitinib and pazopanib) have an ORR of 25–31% and PFS of 10.2–10.5 months [50]. Cytokine therapy with interferon or interleukin has shown an ORR up to 25% and PFS of 4.2 months but is associated with high levels of toxicity [51]. Following progression on antiangiogenic therapy, ICIs, such as nivolumab, have demonstrated an ORR of 25% and PFS of 4.6 months, an improvement over the accepted second-line therapy with mTOR inhibitors (everolimus) [52]. Higher rates of durable response have been seen when ICIs have been used in combination with another agent [49].

Lymphoma

Lymphomatous spinal lesions are predominantly of diffuse large B-cell lymphoma (DLBCL) histology. The etiology of a single spinal lesion (without visceral lesions) may be primary lymphoma of bone (Stage IE or IIE), whereas multiple bony lesions may either be multifocal osseous lymphoma (Stage IVE) or, more commonly, disseminated systemic lymphoma with secondary bone involvement (Stage IV). The initial systemic treatment for all three categories is similar, though the response rates and overall prognoses differ significantly [53]. Of note, response to therapy may be difficult to judge on imaging, as plain radiographs may show persistent alterations in bony structure and PET imaging may continue to demonstrate increased activity secondary to bone remodeling after therapy.

First-line therapy consists of R-CHOP (cyclophosphamide, doxorubicin, vincristine, prednisone followed by the monoclonal antibody rituximab) [54]. Response rates vary from 65% complete response (CR) in secondary lymphoma of bone (Stage IV) to 95% CR in primary lymphoma of bone (Stage IE or IIE) [55]. Given the substantial sensitivity of DLBCL of bone to chemotherapy, immunotherapy, steroids, and radiation, surgical management is rarely indicated outside of biopsy or stabilization of an acutely unstable bony lesion. An additional surgical indication is decompression of high-grade epidural compression; however, in contrast to the results in metastatic carcinoma, it is not clear that the functional outcomes in lymphoma are superior with decompression surgery versus chemotherapy and radiation [56].

Myeloma

The present discussion will focus on active multiple myeloma, exclusive of solitary plasmacytoma, smoldering multiple myeloma, and monoclonal gammopathy of undetermined significance—disease entities for which systemic treatment is not routinely indicated. The mainstay of systemic therapy for active myeloma consists of induction chemotherapy with agents such as bortezomib, thalidomide/lenalidomide, and corticosteroids, followed by hematopoietic cell transplantation (HCT) in eligible candidates. Patients who are ineligible for HCT receive maintenance chemotherapy [57].

The choice of therapy and anticipated sensitivity or time to progression are influenced by risk stratification models that are based on FISH analysis of known translocations, gene expression profiles, serum lactate dehydrogenase levels, and response to prior therapy [58]. Patients typically demonstrate good sensitivity to the above therapy regimens initially, but those with high-risk profiles can experience disease progression in 8–18 months, as compared with 25–36 months for standard-risk myeloma patients [59, 60]. Other predictors of early disease progression on therapy (and, by association, shorter overall survival) include age >65 years, albumin <3 g/dL, serum β_2 microglobulin >4 mg/dL, hemoglobin <10 g/dL, platelets <150/mm^3, and involvement of more than three bones [61].

Sarcoma

Metastatic sarcomatous lesions of the spine are relatively infrequent, and their systemic and local management is controversial. However, myxoid liposarcoma does show a predilection for metastasis to the spine and, therefore, warrants a discussion in this context. Spine metastases are present in 8–14% of patients with myxoid liposarcoma and in 82–83% of those with bone metastases [62, 63]. Screening is most appropriately performed with MRI [64]. Treatment is usually palliative, though reports of long-term control with en bloc excision exist [65]. Compared to other liposarcoma subtypes, myxoid liposarcoma is relatively chemosensitive to conventional regimens, including doxorubicin with or without ifosfamide, with a partial response rate of 48%. The PFS is short, though, at a median of 4 months [66]. A promising second line of therapy has been reported with trabectedin, which demonstrates specific efficacy against translocation-associated sarcomas and has been shown to produce a PFS of 7.3 months in myxoid liposarcomas that were unresponsive to doxorubicin therapy [67].

Bone Antiresorptive Therapy

A discussion of metastatic disease of the spine would not be complete without inclusion of bone antiresorptive therapy, namely, bisphosphonates and denosumab. The relevant indications for initiating these medications include (1) minimizing vertebral fragility fracture risk due to treatment-related decline in bone mineral density (BMD), (2) lowering the rate of skeletal-related events (SRE) from metastatic spine lesions, and (3) potentially reducing disease recurrence.

Antineoplastic therapy can contribute to bone loss via alterations of hormonal balance (e.g., aromatase inhibitors in breast cancer or LHRH in prostate cancer) [68, 69], administration of

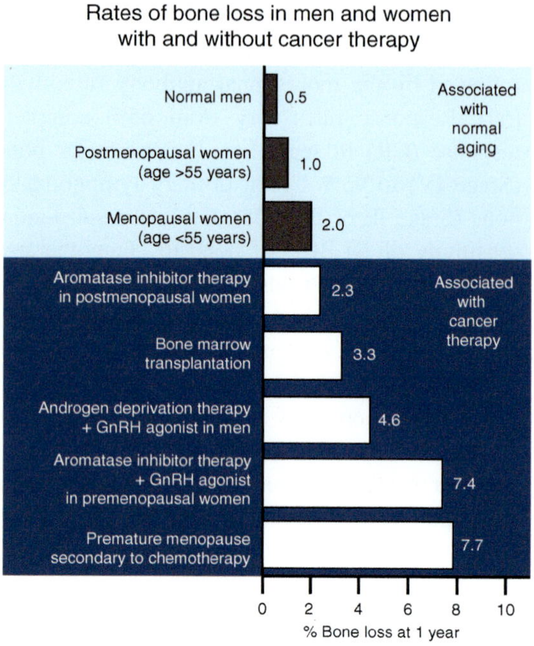

Fig. 3.3 One-year rates of bone loss in men and women are shown. Bone loss while receiving cancer therapy [68–72] tends to occur at a higher rate than bone loss associated with normal aging [74]. *GnRH*, gonadotropin-releasing hormone

exogenous corticosteroids (e.g., prednisone in lymphoma), bone marrow transplantation [70], and/or chemotherapy-induced ovarian failure (common to many chemotherapy regimens) [71, 72]. The effect of chemotherapy-induced premature menopause may be the most potent, resulting in a 7.7% reduction in vertebral BMD after 1 year compared to a 2.0% decline with normal menopause [71, 73, 74] (Fig. 3.3). Interestingly, tamoxifen can have a protective effect on BMD in postmenopausal patients but a paradoxical deleterious effect on BMD in patients who remain premenopausal [75]. Denosumab 60 mg subcutaneously every 6 months carries FDA approval for treatment-related bone loss [76], and bisphosphonates also have proven efficacy for this indication [77, 78]. In contrast, teriparatide is generally avoided in patients with bone malignancy or a history of radiation to the bone, due to a theoretical increased risk of secondary osteosarcoma [79].

Antiresorptive therapy is fundamental to decreasing pain, improving quality of life, and preventing or delaying the time to skeletal-related events (SRE) in patients with established metastatic disease of the spine [80, 81]. SRE in this context includes pain requiring surgical or radiotherapy intervention, vertebral pathologic compression fracture, or spinal cord compression. Denosumab 120 mg subcutaneously every 4 weeks and zoledronic acid 4 mg intravenous infusion every 3–4 weeks are both FDA-approved for prevention of SRE in bone metastases from solid tumors (and myeloma in the case of zoledronic acid) [82, 83]. Denosumab has shown superiority to bisphosphonates in this regard in breast cancer and prostate cancer [84, 85]. Noninferiority of denosumab compared with zoledronic acid was demonstrated for bony metastases from other solid tumors as well as multiple myeloma [86].

In addition to their beneficial effects on BMD and SRE, there is evidence that antiresorptive medications have antitumor antimetastatic activity. In vitro and animal studies have shown a pro-apoptotic effect as well as alteration of the interaction of disseminated tumor cells with the bone microenvironment [73]. The most compelling evidence is in breast cancer studies, as a recent meta-analysis has indicated that postmenopausal breast cancer patients taking bisphosphonates seem to demonstrate improved overall survival and disease-free survival as compared with controls [87].

Conclusion

Systemic management options factor heavily into surgical decision-making for metastatic disease of the spine. A systematic approach starts with selection of appropriate biopsy timing, anatomic location, method, and approach. A comprehensive histologic and molecular analysis will allow an informed consultation with the medical oncologist regarding anticipated response rate, timeline, and durability, as well as expected patient survival. Malignancies with poor responses to systemic therapy may require more aggressive surgical or radiation intervention, while those with reliable and rapid responses may not require any invasive intervention. Patients with longer life expectancies may require more durable reconstruction, while the emphasis may shift to minimizing surgical morbidity and the postoperative recovery timeline in those with limited remaining life expectancy. The implications of proposed systemic therapy on bone mineral density require consideration of bone-reinforcing medications to minimize the risk of insufficiency fractures. Once equipped with this knowledge, the spine surgeon can truly develop the best palliative decisions with the patient.

References

1. Eisenhauer EA, Therasse P, Bogaerts J, Schwartz LH, Sargent D, Ford R, et al. New response evaluation criteria in solid tumours: revised RECIST guideline (version 1.1). Eur J Cancer. 2009;45(2):228–47.
2. Vassiliou V, Andreopoulos D, Frangos S, Tselis N, Giannopoulou E, Lutz S. Bone metastases: assessment of therapeutic response through radiological and nuclear medicine imaging modalities. Clin Oncol (R Coll Radiol). 2011;23(9):632–45.
3. Vogel CL, Schoenfelder J, Shemano I, Hayes DF, Gams RA. Worsening bone scan in the evaluation of antitumor response during hormonal therapy of breast cancer. J Clin Oncol. 1995;13(5):1123–8.
4. Coleman RE, Mashiter G, Whitaker KB, Moss DW, Rubens RD, Fogelman I. Bone scan flare predicts successful systemic therapy for bone metastases. J Nucl Med. 1988;29(8):1354–9.
5. Hamaoka T, Costelloe CM, Madewell JE, Liu P, Berry DA, Islam R, et al. Tumour response interpretation with new tumour response criteria vs the World Health Organisation criteria in patients with bone-only metastatic breast cancer. Br J Cancer. 2010;102(4):651–7.
6. Hayashi N, Costelloe CM, Hamaoka T, Wei C, Niikura N, Theriault RL, et al. A prospective study of bone tumor response assessment in metastatic breast cancer. Clin Breast Cancer. 2013;13(1):24–30.
7. Woolf DK, Padhani AR, Makris A. Assessing response to treatment of bone metastases from breast cancer: what should be the standard of care? Ann Oncol. 2015;26(6):1048–57.
8. Costelloe CM, Chuang HH, Madewell JE, Ueno NT. Cancer response criteria and bone metastases: RECIST 1.1, MDA and PERCIST. J Cancer. 2010;1:80–92.
9. Du Y, Cullum I, Illidge TM, Ell PJ. Fusion of metabolic function and morphology: sequential [18F] fluorodeoxyglucose positron-emission tomography/computed tomography studies yield new insights into the natural history of bone metastases in breast cancer. J Clin Oncol. 2007;25(23):3440–7.
10. Min SJ, Jang HJ, Kim JH. Comparison of the RECIST and PERCIST criteria in solid tumors: a pooled analysis and review. Oncotarget. 2016;7(19):27848–54.
11. Bauerle T, Merz M, Komljenovic D, Zwick S, Semmler W. Drug-induced vessel remodeling in bone metastases as assessed by dynamic contrast enhanced magnetic resonance imaging and vessel size imaging: a longitudinal in vivo study. Clin Cancer Res. 2010;16(12):3215–25.
12. Lecouvet FE, Larbi A, Pasoglou V, Omoumi P, Tombal B, Michoux N, et al. MRI for response assessment in metastatic bone disease. Eur Radiol. 2013;23(7):1986–97.
13. Chu S, Karimi S, Peck KK, Yamada Y, Lis E, Lyo J, et al. Measurement of blood perfusion in spinal metastases with dynamic contrast-enhanced magnetic resonance imaging: evaluation of tumor response to radiation therapy. Spine (Phila Pa 1976). 2013;38(22):E1418–24.
14. Rose PS, Buchowski JM. Metastatic disease in the thoracic and lumbar spine: evaluation and management. J Am Acad Orthop Surg. 2011;19(1):37–48.
15. Mukherjee S, Thakur B, Bhagawati D, Bhagawati D, Akmal S, Arzoglou V, et al. Utility of routine biopsy at vertebroplasty in the management of vertebral compression fractures: a tertiary center experience. J Neurosurg Spine. 2014;21(5):687–97.
16. Lis E, Bilsky MH, Pisinski L, Boland P, Healey JH, O'Malley B, et al. Percutaneous CT-guided biopsy of osseous lesion of the spine in patients with known or suspected malignancy. Am J Neuroradiol. 2004;25(9):1583–8.
17. Singh VM, Salunga RC, Huang VJ, Tran Y, Erlander M, Plumlee P, et al. Analysis of the effect of various decalcification agents on the quantity and quality of nucleic acid (DNA and RNA) recovered from bone biopsies. Ann Diagn Pathol. 2013;17(4):322–6.

18. Klimo P Jr, Schmidt MH. Surgical management of spinal metastases. Oncologist. 2004;9(2):188–96.
19. Goldie JH, Coldman AJ. A mathematic model for relating the drug sensitivity of tumors to their spontaneous mutation rate. Cancer Treat Rep. 1979;63(11–12):1727–33.
20. Foo J, Michor F. Evolution of acquired resistance to anti-cancer therapy. J Theor Biol. 2014;355:10–20.
21. Gerlinger M, Swanton C. How Darwinian models inform therapeutic failure initiated by clonal heterogeneity in cancer medicine. Br J Cancer. 2010;103(8):1139–43.
22. Dexter DL, Leith JT. Tumor heterogeneity and drug resistance. J Clin Oncol. 1986;4(2):244–57.
23. Hanahan D, Weinberg RA. Hallmarks of cancer: the next generation. Cell. 2011;144(5):646–74.
24. Mumenthaler SM, Foo J, Choi NC, Heise N, Leder K, Agus DB, et al. The impact of microenvironmental heterogeneity on the evolution of drug resistance in cancer cells. Cancer Inform. 2015;14(Suppl 4):19–31.
25. Rossi S, Basso M, Strippoli A, Dadduzio V, Cerchiaro E, Barile R, et al. Hormone receptor status and HER2 expression in primary breast cancer compared with synchronous axillary metastases or recurrent metastatic disease. Clin Breast Cancer. 2015;15(5):307–12.
26. Martin-Liberal J, Ochoa de Olza M, Hierro C, Gros A, Rodon J, Tabernero J. The expanding role of immunotherapy. Cancer Treat Rev. 2017;54:74–86.
27. Barrios C, Forbes JF, Jonat W, Conte P, Gradishar W, Buzdar A, et al. The sequential use of endocrine treatment for advanced breast cancer: where are we? Ann Oncol. 2012;23(6):1378–86.
28. National Comprehensive Cancer Network. NCCN Clinical Practice Guidelines in Oncology (NCCN Guidelines(R)): breast cancer. Version 2.2016 (5/6/2016). Fort Washington: National Comprehensive Cancer Network; 2016. https://www.nccn.org/professionals/physician_gls/pdf/breast.pdf.
29. Taghian A, El-Ghamry MN, Merajver SD. Overview of the treatment of newly diagnosed, non-metastatic breast cancer. UpToDate. New York: Wolters Kluwer; 10 Aug 2016. https://www.uptodate.com/contents/overview-of-the-treatment-of-newly-diagnosed-non-metastatic-breast-cancer. Accessed 5 Apr 2017.
30. Kim SR, Paik S. Genomics of adjuvant therapy for breast cancer. Cancer J. 2011;17(6):500–4.
31. Bhargava R, Beriwal S, Dabbs DJ, Ozbek U, Soran A, Johnson RR, et al. Immunohistochemical surrogate markers of breast cancer molecular classes predicts response to neoadjuvant chemotherapy: a single institutional experience with 359 cases. Cancer. 2010;116(6):1431–9.
32. Carey LA, Dees EC, Sawyer L, Gatti L, Moore DT, Collichio F, et al. The triple negative paradox: primary tumor chemosensitivity of breast cancer subtypes. Clin Cancer Res. 2007;13(8):2329–34.
33. van de Vijver MJ, He YD, van't Veer LJ, Dai H, Hart AA, Voskuil DW, et al. A gene-expression signature as a predictor of survival in breast cancer. N Engl J Med. 2002;347(25):1999–2009.
34. Gupta A, Mutebi M, Bardia A. Gene-expression-based predictors for breast cancer. Ann Surg Oncol. 2015;22(11):3418–32.
35. Patsialou A, Wang Y, Lin J, Whitney K, Goswami S, Kenny PA, et al. Selective gene-expression profiling of migratory tumor cells in vivo predicts clinical outcome in breast cancer patients. Breast Cancer Res. 2012;14(5):R139.
36. Kriege M, Seynaeve C, Meijers-Heijboer H, Collee JM, Menke-Pluymers MB, Bartels CC, et al. Sensitivity to first-line chemotherapy for metastatic breast cancer in BRCA1 and BRCA2 mutation carriers. J Clin Oncol. 2009;27(23):3764–71.
37. Kriege M, Jager A, Hooning MJ, Huijskens E, Blom J, van Deurzen CH, et al. The efficacy of taxane chemotherapy for metastatic breast cancer in BRCA1 and BRCA2 mutation carriers. Cancer. 2012;118(4):899–907.
38. Smith KL, Isaacs C. BRCA mutation testing in determining breast cancer therapy. Cancer J. 2011;17(6):492–9.
39. Bayraktar S, Gluck S. Systemic therapy options in BRCA mutation-associated breast cancer. Breast Cancer Res Treat. 2012;135(2):355–66.
40. Pfeifer W, Sokolenko AP, Potapova ON, Bessonov AA, Ivantsov AO, Laptiev SA, et al. Breast cancer sensitivity to neoadjuvant therapy in BRCA1 and CHEK2 mutation carriers and non-carriers. Breast Cancer Res Treat. 2014;148(3):675–83.
41. Sholl LM. The molecular pathology of lung cancer. Surg Pathol Clin. 2016;9(3):353–78.
42. Paez JG, Janne PA, Lee JC, Tracy S, Greulich H, Gabriel S, et al. EGFR mutations in lung cancer: correlation with clinical response to gefitinib therapy. Science. 2004;304(5676):1497–500.
43. Korpanty GJ, Graham DM, Vincent MD, Leighl NB. Biomarkers that currently affect clinical practice in lung cancer: EGFR, ALK, MET, ROS-1, and KRAS. Front Oncol. 2014;4:204.
44. Greenhalgh J, Dwan K, Boland A, Bates V, Vecchio F, Dundar Y, et al. First-line treatment of advanced epidermal growth factor receptor (EGFR) mutation positive non-squamous non-small cell lung cancer. Cochrane Database Syst Rev. 2016;(5):CD010383.
45. Solomon BJ, Mok T, Kim DW, Wu YL, Nakagawa K, Mekhail T, et al. First-line crizotinib versus chemotherapy in ALK-positive lung cancer. N Engl J Med. 2014;371(23):2167–77.
46. National Comprehensive Cancer Network. NCCN Clinical Practice Guidelines in Oncology (NCCN Guidelines(R)): prostate cancer. Version 2.2017 (02/21/17). Fort Washington: National Comprehensive Cancer Network; 2017. https://www.nccn.org/professionals/physician_gls/pdf/prostate.pdf. Accessed 20 Mar 2017.
47. Dorff TB, Crawford ED. Management and challenges of corticosteroid therapy in men with metastatic castrate-resistant prostate cancer. Ann Oncol. 2013;24(1):31–8.
48. Hellerstedt BA, Pienta KJ. The current state of hormonal therapy for prostate cancer. CA Cancer J Clin. 2002;52(3):154–79.

49. Hurwitz ME, Sokhn J, Petrylak DP. Cancer immunotherapy: new applications in urologic oncology. Curr Opin Urol. 2016;26(6):535–42.
50. Motzer RJ, Hutson TE, Cella D, Reeves J, Hawkins R, Guo J, et al. Pazopanib versus sunitinib in metastatic renal-cell carcinoma. N Engl J Med. 2013;369(8):722–31.
51. McDermott DF, Cheng SC, Signoretti S, Margolin KA, Clark JI, Sosman JA, et al. The high-dose aldesleukin "select" trial: a trial to prospectively validate predictive models of response to treatment in patients with metastatic renal cell carcinoma. Clin Cancer Res. 2015;21(3):561–8.
52. Motzer RJ, Escudier B, McDermott DF, George S, Hammers HJ, Srinivas S, et al. Nivolumab versus everolimus in advanced renal-cell carcinoma. N Engl J Med. 2015;373(19):1803–13.
53. Messina C, Christie D, Zucca E, Gospodarowicz M, Ferreri AJ. Primary and secondary bone lymphomas. Cancer Treat Rev. 2015;41(3):235–46.
54. National Comprehensive Cancer Network. NCCN Clinical Practice Guidelines in Oncology (NCCN Guidelines (R)): B-cell lymphomas. Version 2.2017 (02/21/17). Fort Washington: National Comprehensive Cancer Network; 2017. https://www.nccn.org/professionals/physician_gls/pdf/b-cell.pdf. Accessed 20 Mar 2017.
55. Pellegrini C, Gandolfi L, Quirini F, Ruggieri P, Stefoni V, Derenzini E, et al. Primary bone lymphoma: evaluation of chemoimmunotherapy as front-line treatment in 21 patients. Clin Lymphoma Myeloma Leuk. 2011;11(4):321–5.
56. McDonald AC, Nicoll JA, Rampling RP. Non-Hodgkin's lymphoma presenting with spinal cord compression; a clinicopathological review of 25 cases. Eur J Cancer. 2000;36(2):207–13.
57. National Comprehensive Cancer Network. NCCN Clinical Practice Guidelines in Oncology (NCCN Guidelines(R)): multiple myeloma. Version 3.2017 (11/28/16). Fort Washington: National Comprehensive Cancer Network; 2017. https://www.nccn.org/professionals/physician_gls/pdf/myeloma.pdf. Accessed 20 Mar 2017.
58. Ooi MG, de Mel S, Chng WJ. Risk stratification in multiple myeloma. Curr Hematol Malig Rep. 2016;11(2):137–47.
59. Gertz MA, Lacy MQ, Dispenzieri A, Greipp PR, Litzow MR, Henderson KJ, et al. Clinical implications of t(11;14)(q13;q32), t(4;14)(p16.3;q32), and -17p13 in myeloma patients treated with high-dose therapy. Blood. 2005;106(8):2837–40.
60. Kapoor P, Kumar S, Fonseca R, Lacy MQ, Witzig TE, Hayman SR, et al. Impact of risk stratification on outcome among patients with multiple myeloma receiving initial therapy with lenalidomide and dexamethasone. Blood. 2009;114(3):518–21.
61. Durie BG, Jacobson J, Barlogie B, Crowley J. Magnitude of response with myeloma frontline therapy does not predict outcome: importance of time to progression in southwest oncology group chemotherapy trials. J Clin Oncol. 2004;22(10):1857–63.
62. Schwab JH, Boland P, Guo T, Brennan MF, Singer S, Healey JH, et al. Skeletal metastases in myxoid liposarcoma: an unusual pattern of distant spread. Ann Surg Oncol. 2007;14(4):1507–14.
63. Moreau LC, Turcotte R, Ferguson P, Wunder J, Clarkson P, Masri B, et al. Myxoid\round cell liposarcoma (MRCLS) revisited: an analysis of 418 primarily managed cases. Ann Surg Oncol. 2012;19(4): 1081–8.
64. Schwab JH, Boland PJ, Antonescu C, Bilsky MH, Healey JH. Spinal metastases from myxoid liposarcoma warrant screening with magnetic resonance imaging. Cancer. 2007;110(8):1815–22.
65. Kato S, Kawahara N, Murakami H, Demura S, Shirai T, Tsuchiya H, et al. Multi-level total en bloc spondylectomy for solitary lumbar metastasis of myxoid liposarcoma. Orthopedics. 2010;33(6):446.
66. Jones RL, Fisher C, Al-Muderis O, Judson IR. Differential sensitivity of liposarcoma subtypes to chemotherapy. Eur J Cancer. 2005;41(18):2853–60.
67. Kawai A, Araki N, Sugiura H, Ueda T, Yonemoto T, Takahashi M, et al. Trabectedin monotherapy after standard chemotherapy versus best supportive care in patients with advanced, translocation-related sarcoma: a randomised, open-label, phase 2 study. Lancet Oncol. 2015;16(4):406–16.
68. Eastell R, Hannon RA, Cuzick J, Dowsett M, Clack G, Adams JE, et al. Effect of an aromatase inhibitor on bmd and bone turnover markers: 2-year results of the Anastrozole, Tamoxifen, Alone or in Combination (ATAC) trial (18233230). J Bone Miner Res. 2006;21(8):1215–23.
69. Maillefert JF, Sibilia J, Michel F, Saussine C, Javier RM, Tavernier C. Bone mineral density in men treated with synthetic gonadotropin-releasing hormone agonists for prostatic carcinoma. J Urol. 1999;161(4):1219–22.
70. Lee WY, Cho SW, Oh ES, Oh KW, Lee JM, Yoon KH, et al. The effect of bone marrow transplantation on the osteoblastic differentiation of human bone marrow stromal cells. J Clin Endocrinol Metab. 2002;87(1):329–35.
71. Shapiro CL, Manola J, Leboff M. Ovarian failure after adjuvant chemotherapy is associated with rapid bone loss in women with early-stage breast cancer. J Clin Oncol. 2001;19(14):3306–11.
72. Gnant M, Mlineritsch B, Luschin-Ebengreuth G, Kainberger F, Kassmann H, Piswanger-Solkner JC, et al. Adjuvant endocrine therapy plus zoledronic acid in premenopausal women with early-stage breast cancer: 5-year follow-up of the ABCSG-12 bone-mineral density substudy. Lancet Oncol. 2008;9(9): 840–9.
73. Gralow JR, Biermann JS, Farooki A, Fornier MN, Gagel RF, Kumar R, et al. NCCN Task Force Report: bone health in cancer care. J Natl Compr Canc Netw. 2013;11(Suppl 3):S1–50; quiz S1.

74. Kanis JA. Determinants of skeletal mass and strength [chapter 4]; causes of osteoporosis [chapter 5]. In: Kanis JA, editor. Textbook of osteoporosis. Oxford and Cambridge: Blackwell Science; 1996. p. 106–99.
75. Vehmanen L, Elomaa I, Blomqvist C, Saarto T. Tamoxifen treatment after adjuvant chemotherapy has opposite effects on bone mineral density in premenopausal patients depending on menstrual status. J Clin Oncol. 2006;24(4):675–80.
76. Prolia(R) (denosumab) Injection [package insert]. Thousand Oaks: Amgen Inc.; 2011. https://www.accessdata.fda.gov/drugsatfda_docs/label/2011/125320s5s6lbl.pdf.
77. Ellis GK, Bone HG, Chlebowski R, Paul D, Spadafora S, Smith J, et al. Randomized trial of denosumab in patients receiving adjuvant aromatase inhibitors for nonmetastatic breast cancer. J Clin Oncol. 2008;26(30):4875–82.
78. Van Poznak C, Hannon RA, Mackey JR, Campone M, Apffelstaedt JP, Clack G, et al. Prevention of aromatase inhibitor-induced bone loss using risedronate: the SABRE trial. J Clin Oncol. 2010;28(6):967–75.
79. Canalis E, Giustina A, Bilezikian JP. Mechanisms of anabolic therapies for osteoporosis. N Engl J Med. 2007;357(9):905–16.
80. Wong MH, Stockler MR, Pavlakis N. Bisphosphonates and other bone agents for breast cancer. Cochrane Database Syst Rev. 2012;(2):CD003474.
81. Lipton A. Efficacy and safety of intravenous bisphosphonates in patients with bone metastases caused by metastatic breast cancer. Clin Breast Cancer. 2007;7(Suppl 1):S14–20.
82. ZOMETA(R) (zoledronic acid) Injection [package insert]. East Hanover: Novartis Pharmaceuticals Corporation; 2014. https://www.accessdata.fda.gov/drugsatfda_docs/label/2014/021223s028lbl.pdf.
83. XGEVA(R) (denosumab) Injection [package insert]. Thousand Oaks: Amgen Inc.; 2013. https://www.accessdata.fda.gov/drugsatfda_docs/label/2013/125320s094lbl.pdf.
84. Fizazi K, Carducci M, Smith M, Damiao R, Brown J, Karsh L, et al. Denosumab versus zoledronic acid for treatment of bone metastases in men with castration-resistant prostate cancer: a randomised, double-blind study. Lancet. 2011;377(9768):813–22.
85. Martin M, Bell R, Bourgeois H, Brufsky A, Diel I, Eniu A, et al. Bone-related complications and quality of life in advanced breast cancer: results from a randomized phase III trial of denosumab versus zoledronic acid. Clin Cancer Res. 2012;18(17):4841–9.
86. Henry DH, Costa L, Goldwasser F, Hirsh V, Hungria V, Prausova J, et al. Randomized, double-blind study of denosumab versus zoledronic acid in the treatment of bone metastases in patients with advanced cancer (excluding breast and prostate cancer) or multiple myeloma. J Clin Oncol. 2011;29(9):1125–32.
87. Ben-Aharon I, Vidal L, Rizel S, Yerushalmi R, Shpilberg O, Sulkes A, et al. Bisphosphonates in the adjuvant setting of breast cancer therapy—effect on survival: a systematic review and meta-analysis. PLoS One. 2013;8(8):e70044.

4 NOMS

Scott L. Zuckerman, Ilya Laufer, and Mark Bilsky

The spine is the most common site of bony metastases in patients with cancer [1, 2]. Spinal metastases occur in 30–50% of patients, and common primary cancers known to metastasize to the spine include breast, prostate, renal, and lung [3, 4]. Through tumor spread from the arterial system, epidural venous plexus, cerebrospinal fluid (CSF), or direct extension, symptoms develop secondary to painful vertebral body involvement or neurologic compromise from metastatic epidural spinal cord compression (ESCC) [5]. Improved treatment has led to an increase in the incidence and prevalence of patients both living with metastatic spine disease and undergoing therapy for these tumors [6–8].

Patients with spinal metastases are medically complex. Deconditioned and malnourished, they have often undergone or are actively receiving chemotherapy and/or radiation. These factors require consideration when pursuing surgical intervention. Major treatment decisions are often made in conjunction with a team of oncologic providers. As cancer treatments rapidly evolve, so does the role of the spine surgeon. Operative treatments have progressed from simple stabilization [9] to invasive resections [10] to separation surgery [11, 12]. The spine surgeon must now be aware of both minimally invasive surgical (MIS) techniques in addition to novel radiosurgical options.

The NOMS framework consists of four sentinel considerations used to guide choice of therapy for patients with spinal metastases. The NOMS decision points include neurologic, oncologic, mechanical, and systemic considerations and provide a dynamic framework that may incorporate novel therapies. Herein we describe the NOMS framework with a special emphasis on the role of the surgeon. Notable concepts are subsequently discussed in addition to challenging case presentations.

NOMS Framework

The NOMS algorithm utilizes four decision points of assessment in order to determine the optimal combination of systemic therapy, radiation and surgery (Fig. 4.1).

Neurologic

The neurologic assessment includes a neurologic examination and determination of ESCC severity. ESCC is a radiologic evaluation and dichotomized to low or high grade, whereas myelopathy is determined through physical exam and also

S. L. Zuckerman, MD, MPH
Department of Neurological Surgery, Vanderbilt University Medical Center, Nashville, TN, USA
e-mail: scott.zuckerman@vanderbilt.edu

I. Laufer, MD · M. Bilsky, MD (✉)
Department of Neurosurgery, Memorial Sloan Kettering Cancer Center, New York, NY, USA
e-mail: lauferi@mskcc.org; bilskym@mskcc.org

R. A. W. Marco (ed.), *Metastatic Spine Disease*, https://doi.org/10.1007/978-3-319-76252-4_4

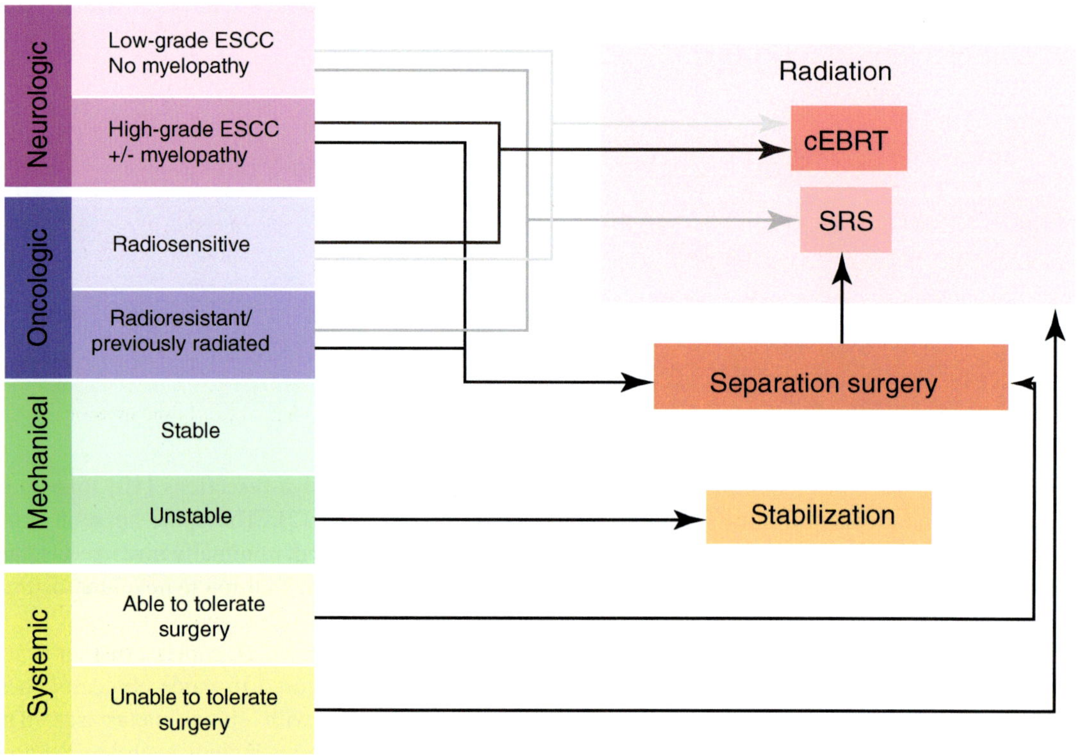

Fig. 4.1 NOMS framework. From Laufer et al., The NOMS Framework: Approach to the Treatment of Spinal Metastatic Tumors. Oncologist. 2013 Jun;18(6):744–51. doi: 10.1634/theoncologist.2012-0293. Epub 2013 May 24

dichotomized into presence or absence of neurologic deficit (myelopathy or radiculopathy). It is of paramount importance that the neurologic evaluation is standardized; care becomes fractured if medical and surgical teams cannot communicate, and meaningful treatment decisions cannot be made. We cannot overemphasize the importance of the neurologic exam.

The examining physician should first take a thorough history, taking note of specific symptoms (dropping things, trouble buttoning shirt, difficulty with utensils or counting change, gait imbalance, or bowel/bladder dysfunction) and signs (hyperreflexia, clonus, decreased rectal tone, or a positive Hoffman, Babinski, Romberg, Spurling's, or Lhermitte's sign). Motor or sensory deficits can be determined by one of the several commonly used grading scales. The American Spinal Injury Association (ASIA) classification is commonly used, ranging from neurologically intact (E) to a complete injury (A) [13], which is a modification of the Frankel scale. The Nurick and Ranawat scales are older and slightly more complex but can still be used to quantify the level of dysfunction. Myelopathy-specific scales include the McCormick scale [14] that assesses motor, sensory, and gait, originally developed for intradural tumors, or the Aminoff-Logue scale [15] for gait and micturition, originally developed for spinal arteriovenous malformations.

Radiologic ESCC is best evaluated by a six-point grading scale [16] that was developed from a previous four-point grading scale [17]. The six-point grading scale describes bone-only disease (0), epidural impingement without deformation of the thecal sac (1a), deformation of the thecal sac without spinal cord abutment (1b), deformation of the thecal sac with spinal cord abutment (1c), spinal cord compression with CSF visible (2), and spinal cord compression without CSF visible (3) (Fig. 4.2). In a study of seven spine surgeons, 25 MRI scans of

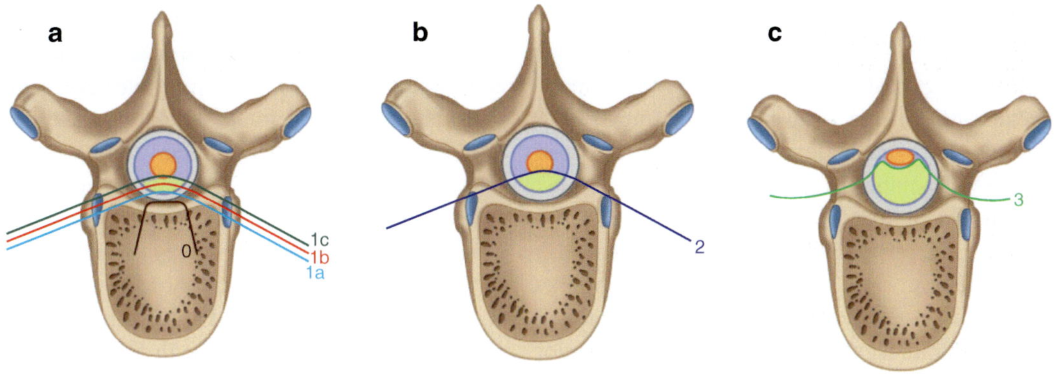

Fig. 4.2 (**a–c**) ESCC scale. From Bilsky et al., Reliability Analysis of the Epidural Spinal Cord Compression Scale. Journal of Neurosurgery: Spine. 2010 Sep; 13(3):324–328

cervical and thoracic tumors were shown three times at 2-week intervals, and the T2-weighted images produced good to excellent inter-rater (ICC 0.701–0.782) and intra-rater (ICC 0.619–0.819) reliability, which was significantly superior to T1-weighted images [16]. The NOMS framework considers Grades 0 and 1a–c low grade and Grades 2 and 3 high grade.

Armed with a reliable neurologic and ESCC assessment, low-grade ESCC is universally considered for radiation treatment in the absence of any mechanical instability, regardless of radiosensitivity. For high-grade ESCC with or without neurologic deficit (Grades 2 and 3), separation surgery is offered unless the tumor is radiosensitive, in which case radiation is pursued. As previously stated, the role of 1c ESCC remains ill defined and depends on the patient's neurologic status. If there is a significant neurologic deficit due to tumor abutment and/or inflammation, surgery may be more suitable. However, if the patient is neurologically intact, a hypofractionated radiation regimen may provide desired response while avoiding surgery.

Within the scope of the neurologic assessment, the time and severity of a neurologic deficit are of paramount importance. Most often in the emergency department, but sometimes encountered during a clinic visit, the acuity and severity of neurologic deficit deterioration must be determined quickly. In the setting of spinal cord compression by solid tumor resulting in neurologic deficit, surgery provides the most rapid and reliable decompression of the spinal cord. Laufer et al. [18] conducted a systematic review to outline what preoperative indicators were associated with neurologic improvement after surgery, and both duration of symptoms and severity of deficit were consistently found to predict outcome. Five articles endorsed an association between duration of symptom onset and severity of symptoms that was discussed in two studies. These two factors were the most powerful influences of neurologic recovery.

The same authors administered a survey to 32 members of the AOSpine Knowledge Forum Tumor group (94% surgeons, 6% radiation oncologists) with a median practice duration of 8 years (range 1–38) [18]. A satisfactory surgical outcome was defined as motor improvement (69%) or preservation of bowel/bladder function without ambulation (90%). Agreement was unanimous that duration of ambulation loss should be considered when deciding on surgery. Forty-one percent responded that surgery could be pursued in the case of prolonged duration of ambulation loss. In terms of specific timing, 13% excluded surgery at >24 h of ambulation loss, and 69% stated patients were less likely to recover at 48 h of ambulation loss. In terms of severity of weakness, 94% believed this was an important variable. Forty percent stated 0/5 lower extremity strength excluded patients from surgery, and 23% used their surgical cut-off at 1/5 strength.

Oncologic

The oncologic assessment considers the responsiveness of a tumor to available treatments. For the most part, this is determined by the effect of radiation. Radiation is the least invasive and most successful option for local tumor control. However, increasing success is being seen with chemotherapy and immunotherapy options. Thus, the oncologic perspective is determined mostly by radiosensitivity of the primary tumor but can be further modified by effective chemotherapy and/or immunotherapy options.

Radiation

Currently the main methods of radiation delivery include cEBRT and SRS. cEBRT delivers two opposing radiation beams to a fairly large region using additive low-dose fractions. Ten fractions of 3 Gy to a total dose of 30 Gy represent the most commonly utilized cEBRT dosing in the spine. Advances in radiation technology have allowed delivery of radiation in highly focused and conformal manner using image guidance. This form of radiation therapy, known as stereotactic radiosurgery (SRS), allows delivery of high-dose radiation to tumors while sparing the surrounding organs at risk (OAR).

Radiosensitive. A recent review of the literature shows that different tumor histology dictates responsiveness to cEBRT (Table 4.1). Universally, lymphoma, seminoma, and myeloma are radiosensitive. It makes intuitive sense that the nonsolid tumors rarely require surgery and have an excellent response to radiation. Among solid tumors, breast and prostate are also categorized as radiosensitive. In 1995, Maranzano and Latini [20] conducted a prospective trial and reported that when diagnosed early or late, radiosensitive histologies (myeloma, breast, prostate) were associated with higher median response times and improved survival. The more recent literature agrees with these early results. Rades and colleagues [21] retrospectively analyzed 238 patients with ESCC secondary to myeloma and found that cEBRT alone led to a positive response in 97%—motor improvement in 53% and stable motor deficit in 44%. The same group treated 29 patients with lymphoma causing ESCC and found that 72% improved motor function and 28% were stable with cEBRT alone [22]. Similarly favorable results were reported in four young men with seminomas [23]. Tumors with radiosensitive histology also respond significantly better to increased doses of radiation, even when doses extend beyond 30 Gy [24]. Breast and prostate cancers are also radiosensitive but less so than the nonsolid tumors. The NOMS framework states that for radiosensitive tumors, even with high-grade ESCC, cEBRT can be used for local tumor control [25]. However, in cases of symptomatic spinal cord compression, especially by solid radiosensitive malignancies, surgery still plays an important role.

Radioresistant. Many solid tumors on the other hand are quite radioresistant. Renal cell carcinoma (RCC), gastrointestinal (GI), and non-small cell lung cancer (NSCLC) are encountered often and less responsive to cEBRT. SRS employs tumor kill pathways that are different from cEBRT and therefore overcomes radioresistance to cEBRT. Radioresistant

Table 4.1 Response to radiation based on histology [19]

	Lymphoma Seminoma Myeloma	Breast	Prostate	Sarcoma	Melanoma	GI	NSCLC	Renal
Gilbert	F	F	U	U	U	U	U	U
Maranzano	F	F	F	U	U	U	U	U
Rades	F	I	I	I	U	I	U	I
Rades	F	F	F	U	U	U	U	U
Katagiri	F	F	F	U	U	U	U	U
Maranzano	F	F	F	U	U	U	U	U
Rades	F	I	I	I	U	I	U	I

Responses: *F* favorable, *I* intermediate, *U* unfavorable

tumors with low-grade ESCC and no neurologic deficits can be treated with SRS and do not require surgery. A recent large, single-institution study from MSKCC evaluated 657 patients receiving SRS as first-line therapy, which was decided using the NOMS criteria and a multidisciplinary team [26]. Of 811 total lesions, 665 (82%) were radioresistant histologies, most commonly RCC (170), sarcoma (113), and NSCLC (102). A total of 28 cases progressed with mean time to failure of 26 months, and interestingly the dose of radiation given, rather than histology, was the most predictive factor of local failure. The authors concluded that high-dose, single-session SRS provided durable long-term control for radioresistant tumors and that lesions irradiated to higher doses had improved local control. Tumor control through SRS can be effectively achieved without the need to reduce tumor volume [27–29]. Based on the excellent local control provided by SRS, the Spine Oncology Study Group (SOSG) recommended for radioresistant tumors to undergo radiosurgery in the absence of ESCC with neurologic deficit [30].

However, in the case of high-grade ESCC, by radioresistant tumors, surgical decompression and stabilization followed by radiation often lead to a better functional outcome. Treatment is dictated by a landmark prospective randomized controlled study by Patchell and co-authors [9], where 101 patients with metastatic spine disease were randomized to surgery and radiotherapy versus radiotherapy alone. The study was ended early due to the superior outcomes in the surgery group, where those patients had over six times the odds of ambulating after treatment compared to the radiation alone group. The surgery group also saw improved outcomes in days of ambulation and opioid/corticosteroid use. The conclusion of the seminal article was that surgery, in the form of decompression and stabilization, improved neurologic outcomes in patients with spinal metastases. The current recommendations for patients with high-grade MESCC by the Spine Oncology Study Group (SOSG) are to undergo surgical decompression followed by radiation [30].

Furthermore, while SRS provides outstanding local tumor control, it must be delivered without injuring the critical structures surrounding the tumor, such as the spinal cord. Initial experience with single-fraction SRS showed that a minimal dose of 15 Gy must be delivered to the entire tumor volume in order to avoid local recurrences. However, this cannot be safely done when the tumor abuts the spinal cord without risking spinal cord toxicity. Due to the high spatial precision of SRS, a separation of 2–3 mm between the tumor and the spinal cord is adequate in order to provide the necessary safety margin for spinal SRS. Therefore, in the era of spinal SRS, decompressive surgery is required for patients with high-grade ESCC in order to provide a separation between the tumor and the spinal cord and to provide favorable conditions for SRS.

Chemotherapy and Immunotherapy

Novel chemotherapy and immunotherapy options have significantly altered the landscape of all cancer treatment. From the perspective of the NOMS framework and the treatment of spinal metastases, immunotherapy plays an important role in conjunction with radiation when considering the oncologic assessment. Here, we briefly mention common examples. For melanoma, cells with BRAF mutations have a worse prognosis, and targeted antibody therapy has been developed to inhibit the proliferation of BRAF-mutated cells. Cytokine-based therapies such as interferon and IL-2 and checkpoint blockade therapies that blunt the immune response have had good success. Common agents include ipilimumab, vemurafenib, dabrafenib, and trametinib, as seen in melanoma spine metastasis treatment algorithm [31]. Thyroid cancer has been treated with lenvatinib, an antibody that induces a multi-targeted tyrosine kinase inhibition, and its broad antitumor activity has led to promising results [32]. NSCLC has seen improved outcomes with epidermal growth factor receptor (EGFR)-targeted agents, such as erlotinib, gefitinib, and afatinib. These targeted agents have shown superior results to cytotoxic chemotherapy alone [33]. Lastly, cabozantinib is an oral tyrosine kinase inhibitor used in renal cell carcinoma and has shown improved survival benefits compared to mTOR inhibitor everolimus [34]. Historically the response of osseous metastases to systemic therapy has been very limited, requiring local therapy with surgery and/or radiation. However, the new systemic therapies are showing remarkable responses even in bone, emphasizing the importance of close collaboration between the surgeons, radiation oncologists, and medical oncologists when deciding the need for surgery or radiotherapy.

Mechanical

Mechanical instability is an independent indication for surgical stabilization. Though radiation is a powerful means of tumor control, it provides no structural integrity—unstable fractures cannot be made stable with radiation. No matter the tumor histology or radiosensitivity, an unstable spine requires surgical intervention to provide stability. Determination of mechanical integrity is a clinical and radiographic decision.

The mainstay of mechanical determination is the spinal instability neoplastic score (SINS) developed by the Spinal Oncology Study Group (SOSG) (Table 4.2) [36]. The grading scheme uses a combination of clinical and radiographic parameters, each with varying degrees of severity, to determine the ultimate stability of the spine. The final score allocates the patient into a stable (0–6), unstable (13–18), or intermediate (7–12) group. More points are given to junctional lesions compared to rigid or semirigid areas, as are those with mechanical pain. The quality of the bony lesion—whether it is lytic, mixed, or blastic—is also weighed and is best determined by x-ray or CT. The involvement of the posterolateral elements is also factored. Perhaps the greatest value in the SINS is that it can be interpreted by many different specialties and not just surgeons. Where previously the oncologist may have had to rely on a radiology report alone to determine stability, the SINS fosters improved multidisciplinary understanding of spinal stability.

Table 4.2 SINS [35]

SINS component		Score
Location	Junctional (occiput–C2, C7–T2, T11–L1, L5–S1)	3
	Mobile spine (C3–C6, L2–L4)	2
	Semirigid (T3–T10)	1
	Rigid (S2–S5)	0
Pain	Yes	3
	Occasional pain but not mechanical	1
	Pain-free lesion	0
Bone lesion	Lytic	2
	Mixed (lytic/blastic)	1
	Blastic	0
Radiographic spinal alignment	Subluxation/translation present	4
	De novo deformity (kyphosis/scoliosis)	2
	Normal alignment	0
Vertebral body collapse	>50% collapse	3
	<50% collapse	2
	No collapse with >50% body involved	1
	None of the above	0
Posterolateral involvement of spinal elements	Bilateral	3
	Unilateral	1
	None of the above	0
Total score	Stable	0–6
	Indeterminate	7–12
	Unstable	13–18

The role of pain in determining spinal stability warrants further discussion. Three different categories of pain represent distinct clinical processes—biologic, neurologic, and mechanical pain. Biologic pain is unrelated to movement or axial loading, often constant or worse at night, and responds to steroids and radiation [25]. The pathophysiology of biologic pain is secondary to inflammatory mediators secreted by the tumor that becomes manifest at night or early morning due to reduced endogenous, nocturnal steroids levels and can typically be treated with exogenous steroids and radiation therapy. Neurologic pain is the result of spinal cord, cauda equina, or nerve root compression and can present with numbness or weakness. Mechanical pain is a sign of instability and occurs with axial loading or movement. One important clinical encounter is the evaluation of the inpatient with painful spinal metastases. When taking a history, the patient has been lying in bed for several days, and it should be no surprise they deny pain at the time of interview. However, it is imperative to walk each patient and to observe transitions from sitting to supine and standing, especially hospital inpatients, and ask them about their pain when they were at home or when ambulating; otherwise, an unstable lesion requiring stabilization may be missed.

Stabilization is principally achieved through cement augmentation or lateral mass/pedicle screw fixation. While a review of stabilization techniques is outside the scope of this chapter, a brief discussion of percutaneous fixation is mentioned later. However, it is worth noting which lesions can be treated with simple cement augmentation, as considerable evidence reports decreased mechanical pain, improved mobility, and restoration of anterior column height [37–41]. Kyphoplasty is a percutaneous technique in which a balloon is inflated within the vertebral body, creating space for radiopaque polymethyl methacrylate (PMMA) to be injected into the vertebral body [37, 42]. Vertebroplasty is a similar percutaneous procedure without balloon inflation, in which PMMA is injected into the vertebral body under fluoroscopy [43]. The only study to provide Class I evidence of balloon kyphoplasty compared to non-operative management for treatment of painful metastatic fractures was the Cancer Patient Fracture Evaluation (CAFE) study [39]. The randomized, multicenter trial evaluated 65 patients treated with kyphoplasty compared to 52 treated non-operatively and found a statistically significant improvement in pain, activity, analgesic requirement, and quality of life in the kyphoplasty group. No significant changes were found in the nonsurgical group.

Radiation therapy in patients at risk of mechanical instability generally fails to provide symptom relief and leads to adverse events. Huisman and co-authors [44] investigated how mechanical back pain due to instability responded to radiation by matching 38 patients who failed RT and required re-treatment to 76 control patients without failure. Their results showed that the SINS was independently associated with RT failure (OR 1.3, 95% CI 1.1–1.5 $p = 0.01$), concluding that significant spinal instability increases the risk of RT failure independent of related variables. Lam et al. [45] studied 299 spinal metastasis patients without ESCC who received cEBRT. Spinal adverse events were the primary outcome and included vertebral fracture, hospitalization for pain, neurologic compromise, or surgery. Multivariable analysis revealed that adverse events were significantly higher in SINS ≥11 (HR 2.5, 95% CI 1.3–4.9, $p = 0.007$).

Systemic

Surgical decision-making must take into consideration overall patient health and prognosis. If a comprehensive assessment is overlooked, unanticipated morbidity can ensue that could have otherwise been avoided. The NOMS framework is predicated on the patient's ability to tolerate surgery, a decision based on two components: (1) acute preoperative assessment and (2) expected survival.

The acute preoperative assessment is made in conjunction with the treating oncologists and anesthesiologist. While survival may be promising, an acute deterioration due to side effects from chemotherapy can defer surgical intervention. In cachectic and malnourished patient, nutritional status should also be evaluated. In a study of 4310 non-cancer patients undergoing lumbar spinal fusion, hypoalbuminemia was an independent predictor of wound dehiscence, infection, and readmission [46]. This same trend was seen in a study of 161 patients undergoing surgery for spinal metastases [47]. After multivariable logistic regression, albumin <3.5 g/dL was an independent predictor of death at 1-year post surgery.

The expected survival is predicated on tumor histology, extent of metastatic tumor burden, medical comorbidities, and overall response to systemic therapy. Several prognostic scoring systems have been developed including the Tokuhashi [48] or Tomita [49] scores. However, in an era of rapidly evolving systemic therapy and continually changing survival expectations for cancer patients, their heavy reliance on primary tumor histology to predict survival challenges their relevance. More recently, Pereira et al. [50] developed and validated a survival algorithm that placed less weight on primary tumor histology. Creating a model and scoring system from 649 patients from two tertiary centers, multivariate cox regression revealed the following factors to be predictive of survival: older age, poor performance status, primary cancer type, more than one spine metastasis, lung/liver metastasis, brain metastasis, systemic therapy, higher white blood cell count, and lower hemoglobin. Surgery for spinal metastases provides palliation of local symptoms and may play a role even in the setting of expected short survival if the symptoms are severe.

Surgical Considerations

Separation Surgery

In the era of SRS, the goals of surgery for MESCC have changed. Since SRS provides reliable tumor control regardless of tumor volume and histology, extensive cytoreductive surgery is no longer necessary. As discussed above, the primary goal of surgery is to provide adequate separation between the tumor and the spinal cord in order to safely undergo SRS and to provide spinal column stability. Separation surgery is a procedure that separates tumor from the spinal cord to allow delivery of radiation to the tumor site [12]. The spinal fluid space is reconstituted so that an adequate distance (2–3 mm) is created between tumor and the spinal cord, and SRS can be initiated safely without fear of periprocedural cord compression progression or overdosing the spinal cord [51]. Adequate circumferential spinal cord decompression is vital to the success of the operation [11, 52]. The decompression is generally achieved with laminectomy, bilateral facetectomy, and pedicle removal, providing access to the ventral epidural space. Since the majority of epidural metastatic tumors originate in the vertebral body, sectioning of the posterior longitudinal ligament (PLL) is of paramount importance in order to access the epidural tumor and to ensure adequate decompression of the spinal cord and reconstitution of the thecal sac.

While corpectomies may be performed for the purpose of anterior column stabilization, standalone posterior constructs have been shown to provide reliable stabilization with low risk of instrumentation failure. Amankulor and colleagues [53] reported symptomatic instrumentation failure, defined as reoperation, in a very low percentage (2.8%) of patients undergoing separation surgery with posterior segmental instrumentation only. Anterior column instrumentation was utilized in a small subset of patients (17.4%) with the most severe forms of anterior column compromise. In a recent review of MIS and separation surgery, three studies reported their experience with separation surgery using an open approach. The mean local failure rate was 17.1% with a mean time to local recurrence of 13.6 months. The single study that investigated OS rates found a 78% 1-year survival rate in patients with systemic therapy post-SRS compared to 56% in patients without systemic therapy ($p = 0.02$). Several factors were found to offer improved control and survival, including a higher dose of hypofractionated SRS, concomitant systemic treatment, and lower epidural disease grade [11, 53].

However, newer techniques are evolving. Perhaps the most notable is the use of laser interstitial thermal therapy (LITT) to provide adequate separation of tumor from the dura. Tatsui et al. [54] published an exploratory analysis in 11 patients undergoing LITT followed by SRS. Intraoperative MRI guidance was used to place a laser probe into the involved epidural space, and laser thermal therapy ablates the offending tumor. MRI changes are seen as a thermal map to allow real-time monitoring of intensity and spread of heat within the involved tissue [54]. A second study of 19 patients with long-term follow-up (range 10–64 weeks) showed excellent results [55]. Systemic therapy was continued for all patients with statistically significant improvement in pain and function at 3 months. LITT can also be done in conjunction with percutaneous fixation, as seen in a second report of eight patients requiring decompression and stabilization [56].

Surgical Stabilization

Within the mechanical assessment, the primary decision point is deciding whether the patient needs to be stabilized or not. In fact, many forms of stabilization exist, ranging from cement augmentation to open instrumented stabilization. Patients with vertebral compression fractures benefit from vertebroplasty or kyphoplasty as evidenced by the previously cited CAFÉ study. In instances of fracture extension into the posterior elements, percutaneous pedicle instrumentation is required in order to restore stability. In cases of more extensive fractures, open surgical stabilization may be required. Open and percutaneous instrumented stabilization provides comparable pain relief, and stabilization and selection technique is predicated on the preference of the surgeon. However, the risk of wound complications may be lower after percutaneous stabilization. Wound complications after open surgery for MESCC have been reported to range from 12 to 26% of cases [57–59], and prior conventional radiation is perhaps the strongest risk factor for wound breakdown [59, 60]. On the other hand, decreased invasiveness can facilitate earlier return to radiation or systemic therapy, and even conventionally fractionated radiation can be started within 1 week of surgery and sometimes 2–3 days [61].

It has been our practice to utilize cement augmentation of the screws when performing short-segment stabilization. Adjuvant therapy, comorbidities, and malnourishment prevent a biologically favorable environment for a bony fusion, and the hardware is heavily relied upon for the remaining years of life. Cement augmentation along the pedicle screw tract can increase pullout strength [62] and has also been shown to decrease rates of pseudoarthroses in osteoporotic patients [63]. Screw pullout or pedicle fracture can be catastrophic, especially in a short-segment fusion with adjacent sites of tumor infiltration. From 2011 to 2014, we reported 44 patients who underwent short-segment cement-augmented percutaneous spinal fixation for unstable tumors. Pain was markedly decreased without perioperative morbidity, and only two patients required subsequent decompression [64]. Three other large studies reported similar positive results [65–67]. One study also reported percutaneous placement of iliac screws for lumbopelvic instability [68]. Percutaneous screws can also be used in mini-open decompressions or corpectomies [69, 70].

Case Illustrations

Case #1 Fig. 4.3

A 62-year-old woman with esophageal adenocarcinoma presented with lower back pain exacerbated by movement. Imaging showed an L3 lytic metastasis with <50% loss of vertebral body

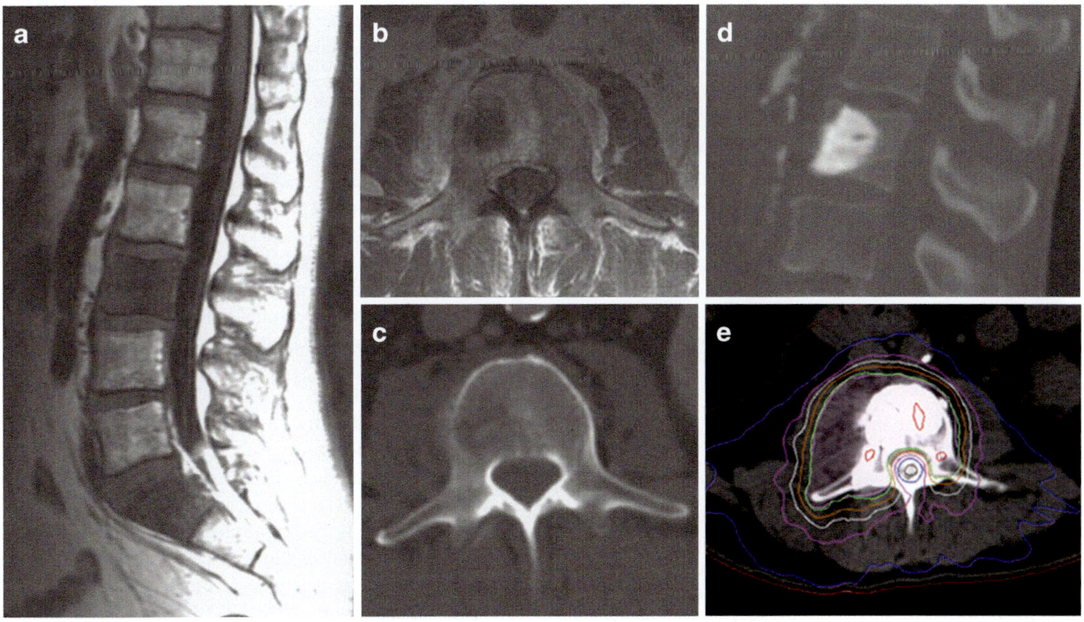

Fig. 4.3 (**a–e**) Case 1: L3 metastasis treated with kyphoplasty and radiosurgery

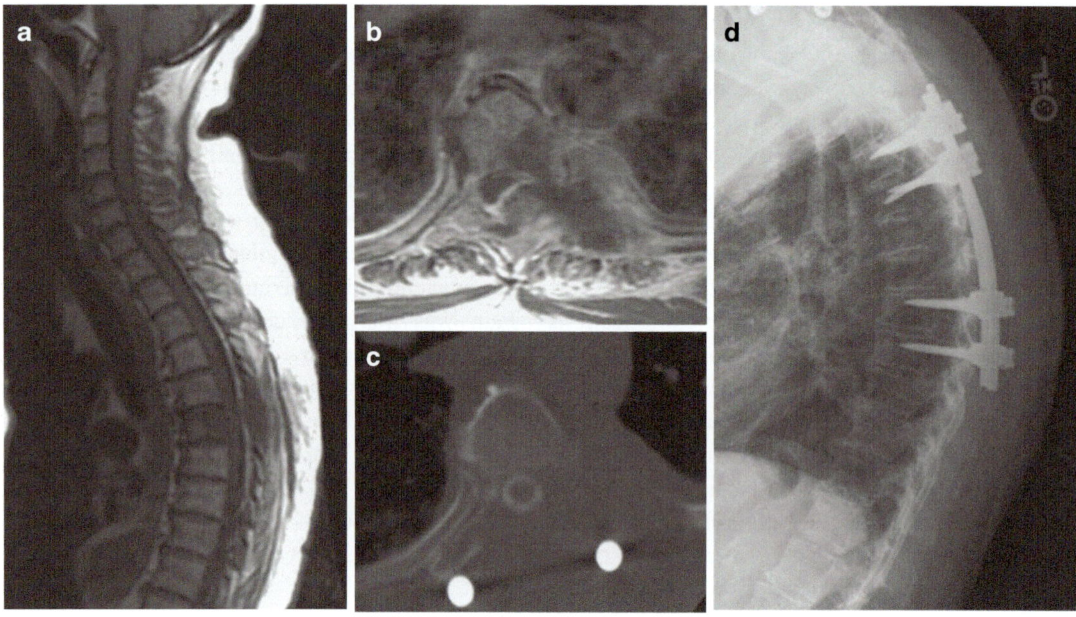

Fig. 4.4 (**a–d**) Case 2: T6 metastasis treated with separation surgery and radiosurgery

height (SINS 11) and low-grade epidural tumor extension (a, b, c). Patient underwent kyphoplasty for stabilization (d) and 24 Gy single-fraction stereotactic radiosurgery treatment (e).

Case #2 Fig. 4.4

A 76-year-old woman with squamous cell carcinoma of the lung presented with thoracic back pain, with an intact neurologic examination. Imaging showed a T6 metastasis with high-grade compression of the spinal cord (ESCC 3) (a, b). Patient underwent separation surgery for decompression of the spinal cord (c) and spinal stabilization (d). She subsequently underwent hypofractionated radiotherapy to T5 and T6.

References

1. Hatrick NC, Lucas JD, Timothy AR, Smith MA. The surgical treatment of metastatic disease of the spine. Radiother Oncol. 2000;56(3):335–9.
2. Ortiz Gomez JA. The incidence of vertebral body metastases. Int Orthop. 1995;19(5):309–11.
3. Jacobs WB, Perrin RG. Evaluation and treatment of spinal metastases: an overview. Neurosurg Focus. 2001;11(6):e10.
4. Steinmetz MP, Mekhail A, Benzel EC. Management of metastatic tumors of the spine: strategies and operative indications. Neurosurg Focus. 2001;11(6):e2.
5. Harel R, Angelov L. Spine metastases: current treatments and future directions. Eur J Cancer. 2010;46(15):2696–707.
6. Choi D, Crockard A, Bunger C, Harms J, Kawahara N, Mazel C, et al. Review of metastatic spine tumour classification and indications for surgery: the consensus statement of the Global Spine Tumour Study Group. Eur Spine J. 2010;19(2):215–22.
7. Fehlings MG, Nater A, Holmer H. Cost-effectiveness of surgery in the management of metastatic epidural spinal cord compression: a systematic review. Spine (Phila Pa 1976). 2014;39(22 Suppl 1):S99–S105.
8. Yoshihara H, Yoneoka D. Trends in the surgical treatment for spinal metastasis and the in-hospital patient outcomes in the United States from 2000 to 2009. Spine J. 2014;14(9):1844–9.
9. Patchell RA, Tibbs PA, Regine WF, Payne R, Saris S, Kryscio RJ, et al. Direct decompressive surgical resection in the treatment of spinal cord compression caused by metastatic cancer: a randomised trial. Lancet. 2005;366(9486):643–8.
10. Yao KC, Boriani S, Gokaslan ZL, Sundaresan N. En bloc spondylectomy for spinal metastases: a review of techniques. Neurosurg Focus. 2003;15(5):E6.
11. Laufer I, Iorgulescu JB, Chapman T, Lis E, Shi W, Zhang Z, et al. Local disease control for spinal metastases following "separation surgery" and adjuvant hypofractionated or high-dose single-fraction stereotactic radiosurgery: outcome analysis in 186 patients. J Neurosurg Spine. 2013;18(3):207–14.

12. Moussazadeh N, Laufer I, Yamada Y, Bilsky MH. Separation surgery for spinal metastases: effect of spinal radiosurgery on surgical treatment goals. Cancer Control. 2014;21(2):168–74.
13. American Spinal Injury Association. International standards for neurological classification of spinal cord injury (ISNCSCI). 2016. http://asia-spinalinjury.org/wp-content/uploads/2016/02/International_Stds_Diagram_Worksheet.pdf.
14. McCormick PC, Torres R, Post KD, Stein BM. Intramedullary ependymoma of the spinal cord. J Neurosurg. 1990;72(4):523–32.
15. Aminoff MJ, Logue V. Clinical features of spinal vascular malformations. Brain. 1974;97(1):197–210.
16. Bilsky MH, Laufer I, Fourney DR, Groff M, Schmidt MH, Varga PP, et al. Reliability analysis of the epidural spinal cord compression scale. J Neurosurg Spine. 2010;13(3):324–8.
17. Bilsky MH, Boland PJ, Panageas KS, Woodruff JM, Brennan MF, Healey JH. Intralesional resection of primary and metastatic sarcoma involving the spine: outcome analysis of 59 patients. Neurosurgery. 2001;49(6):1277–86.
18. Laufer I, Zuckerman SL, Bird JE, Bilsky MH, Lazary A, Quraishi NA, et al. Predicting neurologic recovery after surgery in patients with deficits secondary to MESCC: systematic review. Spine (Phila Pa 1976). 2016;41(Suppl 20):S224–S30.
19. Gerszten PC, Mendel E, Yamada Y. Radiotherapy and radiosurgery for metastatic spine disease: what are the options, indications, and outcomes. Spine (Phila Pa 1976). 2009;34(22S):S78–92.
20. Maranzano E, Latini P. Effectiveness of radiation therapy without surgery in metastatic spinal cord compression: final results from a prospective trial. Int J Radiat Oncol Biol Phys. 1995;32(4):959–67.
21. Rades D, Conde-Moreno AJ, Cacicedo J, Segedin B, Rudat V, Schild SE. Excellent outcomes after radiotherapy alone for malignant spinal cord compression from myeloma. Radiol Oncol. 2016;50(3):337–40.
22. Rades D, Conde-Moreno AJ, Cacicedo J, Segedin B, Rudat V, Schild SE. Radiation therapy alone provides excellent outcomes for spinal cord compression from vertebral lymphoma. Anticancer Res. 2016;36(6):3081–3.
23. Bolm L, Janssen S, Bartscht T, Rades D. Radiotherapy alone for malignant spinal cord compression in young men with seminoma. Anticancer Res. 2016;36(4):2033–4.
24. Rades D, Panzner A, Rudat V, Karstens JH, Schild SE. Dose escalation of radiotherapy for metastatic spinal cord compression (MSCC) in patients with relatively favorable survival prognosis. Strahlenther Onkol. 2011;187(11):729–35.
25. Laufer I, Rubin DG, Lis E, Cox BW, Stubblefield MD, Yamada Y, et al. The NOMS framework: approach to the treatment of spinal metastatic tumors. Oncologist. 2013;18(6):744–51.
26. Yamada Y, Katsoulakis E, Laufer I, Lovelock M, Barzilai O, McLaughlin LA, et al. The impact of histology and delivered dose on local control of spinal metastases treated with stereotactic radiosurgery. Neurosurg Focus. 2017;42(1):E6.
27. Chang EL, Shiu AS, Mendel E, Mathews LA, Mahajan A, Allen PK, et al. Phase I/II study of stereotactic body radiotherapy for spinal metastasis and its pattern of failure. J Neurosurg Spine. 2007;7(2):151–60.
28. Moussazadeh N, Lis E, Katsoulakis E, Kahn S, Svoboda M, DiStefano NM, et al. Five-year outcomes of high-dose single-fraction spinal stereotactic radiosurgery. Int J Radiat Oncol Biol Phys. 2015;93(2):361–7.
29. Ghia AJ, Chang EL, Bishop AJ, Pan HY, Boehling NS, Amini B, et al. Single-fraction versus multifraction spinal stereotactic radiosurgery for spinal metastases from renal cell carcinoma: secondary analysis of Phase I/II trials. J Neurosurg Spine. 2016;24(5):829–36.
30. Bilsky MH, Laufer I, Burch S. Shifting paradigms in the treatment of metastatic spine disease. Spine (Phila Pa 1976). 2009;34(22 Suppl):S101–7.
31. Caruso JP, Cohen-Inbar O, Bilsky MH, Gerszten PC, Sheehan JP. Stereotactic radiosurgery and immunotherapy for metastatic spinal melanoma. Neurosurg Focus. 2015;38(3):E6.
32. Wang E, Karedan T, Perez CA. New insights in the treatment of radioiodine refractory differentiated thyroid carcinomas: to lenvatinib and beyond. Anticancer Drugs. 2015;26(7):689–97.
33. Greenhalgh J, Dwan K, Boland A, Bates V, Vecchio F, Dundar Y, et al. First-line treatment of advanced epidermal growth factor receptor (EGFR) mutation positive non-squamous non-small cell lung cancer. Cochrane Database Syst Rev. 2016;(5):CD010383.
34. Choueiri TK, Escudier B, Powles T, Tannir NM, Mainwaring PN, Rini BI, et al. Cabozantinib versus everolimus in advanced renal cell carcinoma (METEOR): final results from a randomised, open-label, phase 3 trial. Lancet Oncol. 2016;17(7):917–27.
35. Fisher CG, DiPaola CP, Ryken TC, Bilsky MH, Shaffrey CI, Berven SH, et al. A novel classification system for spinal instability in neoplastic disease: an evidence-based approach and expert consensus from the Spine Oncology Study Group. Spine (Phila Pa 1976). 2010;35:E1221–9.
36. Fourney DR, Frangou EM, Ryken TC, Dipaola CP, Shaffrey CI, Berven SH, et al. Spinal instability neoplastic score: an analysis of reliability and validity from the spine oncology study group. J Clin Oncol. 2011;29(22):3072–7.
37. Burton AW, Mendoza T, Gebhardt R, Hamid B, Nouri K, Perez-Toro M, et al. Vertebral compression fracture treatment with vertebroplasty and kyphoplasty: experience in 407 patients with 1,156 fractures in a tertiary cancer center. Pain Med. 2011;12(12):1750–7.
38. Dalbayrak S, Onen MR, Yilmaz M, Naderi S. Clinical and radiographic results of balloon kyphoplasty for treatment of vertebral body metastases and multiple myelomas. J Clin Neurosci. 2010;17(2):219–24.
39. Berenson J, Pflugmacher R, Jarzem P, Zonder J, Schechtman K, Tillman JB, et al. Balloon kyphoplasty

versus non-surgical fracture management for treatment of painful vertebral body compression fractures in patients with cancer: a multicentre, randomised controlled trial. Lancet Oncol. 2011;12(3):225–35.
40. Tseng YY, Lo YL, Chen LH, Lai PL, Yang ST. Percutaneous polymethylmethacrylate vertebroplasty in the treatment of pain induced by metastatic spine tumor. Surg Neurol. 2008;70 Suppl 1:S1:78–83; discussion S1:83–4.
41. Mendel E, Bourekas E, Gerszten P, Golan JD. Percutaneous techniques in the treatment of spine tumors: what are the diagnostic and therapeutic indications and outcomes? Spine. 2009;34(22 Suppl):S93–100.
42. Gerszten PC. Spine metastases: from radiotherapy, surgery, to radiosurgery. Neurosurgery. 2014;61(Suppl 1):16–25.
43. Jensen ME, Kallmes DE. Percutaneous vertebroplasty in the treatment of malignant spine disease. Cancer J. 2002;8(2):194–206.
44. Huisman M, van der Velden JM, van Vulpen M, van den Bosch MA, Chow E, Oner FC, et al. Spinal instability as defined by the spinal instability neoplastic score is associated with radiotherapy failure in metastatic spinal disease. Spine J. 2014;14(12):2835–40.
45. Lam TC, Uno H, Krishnan M, Lutz S, Groff M, Cheney M, et al. Adverse outcomes after palliative radiation therapy for uncomplicated spine metastases: role of spinal instability and single-fraction radiation therapy. Int J Radiat Oncol Biol Phys. 2015;93(2):373–81.
46. Bohl DD, Shen MR, Mayo BC, Massel DH, Long WW, Modi KD, et al. Malnutrition predicts infectious and wound complications following posterior lumbar spinal fusion. Spine (Phila Pa 1976). 2016;41(21):1693–9.
47. Goodwin CR, Schoenfeld AJ, Abu-Bonsrah NA, Garzon-Muvdi T, Sankey EW, Harris MB, et al. Reliability of a spinal metastasis prognostic score to model 1-year survival. Spine J. 2016;16(9):1102–8.
48. Tokuhashi Y, Matsuzaki H, Oda H, Oshima M, Ryu J. A revised scoring system for preoperative evaluation of metastatic spine tumor prognosis. Spine. 2005;30(19):2186–91.
49. Tomita K, Kawahara N, Kobayashi T, Yoshida A, Murakami H, Akamaru T. Surgical strategy for spinal metastases. Spine. 2001;26(3):298–306.
50. Paulino Pereira NR, Janssen SJ, van Dijk E, Harris MB, Hornicek FJ, Ferrone ML, et al. Development of a prognostic survival algorithm for patients with metastatic spine disease. J Bone Joint Surg Am. 2016;98(21):1767–76.
51. Bilsky MH, Laufer I, Matros E, Yamada J, Rusch VW. Advanced lung cancer: aggressive surgical therapy vertebral body involvement. Thorac Surg Clin. 2014;24(4):423–31.
52. Bate BG, Khan NR, Kimball BY, Gabrick K, Weaver J. Stereotactic radiosurgery for spinal metastases with or without separation surgery. J Neurosurg Spine. 2015;22(4):409–15.
53. Amankulor NM, Xu R, Iorgulescu JB, Chapman T, Reiner AS, Riedel E, et al. The incidence and patterns of hardware failure after separation surgery in patients with spinal metastatic tumors. Spine J. 2014;14(9):1850–9.
54. Tatsui CE, Stafford RJ, Li J. Utilizaiton of laser interstitial thermotherapy guided by real-time thermal MRI as an alternative to separation surgery in the management of spinal metastases. J Neurosurg Spine. 2015;23(4):400–11.
55. Tatsui CE, Lee SH, Amini B, Rao G, Suki D, Oro M, et al. Spinal laser interstitial thermal therapy: a novel alternative to surgery for metastatic epidural spinal cord compression. Neurosurgery. 2016;79(Suppl 1):S73–82.
56. Tatsui CE, Belsuzarri TA, Oro M, Rhines LD, Li J, Ghia AJ, et al. Percutaneous surgery for treatment of epidural spinal cord compression and spinal instability: technical note. Neurosurg Focus. 2016;41(4):E2.
57. Jansson KA, Bauer HC. Survival, complications and outcome in 282 patients operated for neurological deficit due to thoracic or lumbar spinal metastases. Eur Spine J. 2006;15(2):196–202.
58. Itshayek E, Yamada J, Bilsky M, Schmidt M, Shaffrey C, Gerszten P, et al. Timing of surgery and radiotherapy in the management of metastatic spine disease: a systematic review. Int J Oncol. 2010;36(3):533–44.
59. Ghogawala Z, Mansfield FL, Borges LF. Spinal radiation before surgical decompression adversely affects outcomes of surgery for symptomatic metastatic spinal cord compression. Spine (Phila Pa 1976). 2001;26(7):818–24.
60. Sundaresan N, Rothman A, Manhart K, Kelliher K. Surgery for solitary metastases of the spine: rationale and results of treatment. Spine. 2002; 27(16):1802–6.
61. Disa JJ, Smith AW, Bilsky MH. Management of radiated reoperative wounds of the cervicothoracic spine: the role of the trapezius turnover flap. Ann Plast Surg. 2001;47(4):394–7.
62. Burval DJ, McLain RF, Milks R, Inceoglu S. Primary pedicle screw augmentation in osteoporotic lumbar vertebrae: biomechanical analysis of pedicle fixation strength. Spine (Phila Pa 1976). 2007;32(10):1077–83.
63. Sawakami K, Yamazaki A, Ishikawa S, Ito T, Watanabe K, Endo N. Polymethylmethacrylate augmentation of pedicle screws increases the initial fixation in osteoporotic spine patients. J Spinal Disord Tech. 2012;25(2):E28–35.
64. Moussazadeh N, Rubin DG, McLaughlin L, Lis E, Bilsky MH, Laufer I. Short-segment percutaneous pedicle screw fixation with cement augmentation for tumor-induced spinal instability. Spine J. 2015;15(7):1609–17.
65. Versteeg AL, Verlaan JJ, de Baat P, Jiya TU, Stadhouder A, Diekerhof CH, et al. Complications after percutaneous pedicle screw fixation for the treatment of unstable spinal metastases. Ann Surg Oncol. 2016;23(7):2343–9.
66. Kwan MK, Lee CK, Chan CY. Minimally invasive spinal stabilization using fluoroscopic-guided

percutaneous screws as a form of palliative surgery in patients with spinal metastasis. Asian Spine J. 2016;10(1):99–110.

67. Zairi F, Vielliard MH, Bouras A, Karnoub MA, Marinho P, Assaker R. Long-segment percutaneous screw fixation for thoracolumbar spine metastases: a single centre experience. J Neurosurg Sci. 2017;61(4):365–70.
68. Liu G, Hasan MY, Wong HK. Minimally invasive iliac screw fixation in treating painful metastatic lumbosacral deformity: a technique description and clinical results. Eur Spine J. 2016;25(12):4043–51.
69. Lau D, Chou D. Posterior thoracic corpectomy with cage reconstruction for metastatic spinal tumors: comparing the mini-open approach to the open approach. J Neurosurg Spine. 2015;23(2):217–27.
70. Miscusi M, Polli FM, Forcato S, Ricciardi L, Frati A, Cimatti M, et al. Comparison of minimally invasive surgery with standard open surgery for vertebral thoracic metastases causing acute myelopathy in patients with short- or mid-term life expectancy: surgical technique and early clinical results. J Neurosurg Spine. 2015;22(5):518–25.

Spinal Instability in Metastatic Disease

5

Joshua C. Patt and Daniel P. Leas

Introduction

The vast majority of patients presenting with metastatic disease of the spine will not require any intervention. The overall prognosis for these patients is uniformly poor, and every effort must be made to understand their burden of disease, performance status, and life expectancy before considering intervention. If after a thorough multidisciplinary discussion, it seems reasonable to consider intervention, the treating physician must determine if surgery is indicated or not.

The most quoted and evidence-based indication for surgery is based on the Patchell et al. study which demonstrated a statistically significant advantage for surgical intervention for patients with acute loss of ambulatory ability or impending loss of ambulatory status with epidural spinal cord compression from non-highly radiosensitive tumors [1]. With a careful understanding of this article, one will notice that this study was specifically looking at cord compression. With the average cord terminus at approximately L1, this study cannot routinely be used to justify intervention in the lumbar spine. Acute neurologic deficit in lumbar spine metastatic disease is less common, and intervention should be considered on an individual basis. Moreover, this study has several limitations that are discussed in the chapter entitled "Critical evaluation of the current literature."

A second major category for intervention in spinal metastatic disease is instability. Spinal instability was classically defined by Panjabi and White [2] in their landmark study. Their work is helpful in understanding the basic elements required for spinal stability, particularly in iatrogenic instability and trauma. A variety of systems have been developed to better understand stability, and these will be discussed below. The most recent advance in understanding neoplastic instability comes from the Spinal instability neoplastic score (SINS) developed by a multi-institutional working group. We will highlight a number of historical classification systems and end on this comprehensive system and its ability to guide management, particularly in the lumbar spine.

Initial Evaluation

Clinical Evaluation

Clinical instability is classically considered with one or more of the three key domains: the spinal column (intrinsic), the paraspinal musculature and tendinous attachments (dynamic), and the central neuromotor control. Dysfunction in any of these three categories can cause pain and

J. C. Patt, MD, MPH (✉)
Levine Cancer Institute, Atrium Health, Charlotte, NC, USA
e-mail: Joshua.Patt@carolinashealthcare.org

D. P. Leas, MD
Department of Orthopaedic Surgery, Carolinas Medical Center, Atrium Health, Charlotte, NC, USA
e-mail: Daniel.Leas@carolinashealthcare.org

R. A. W. Marco (ed.), *Metastatic Spine Disease*, https://doi.org/10.1007/978-3-319-76252-4_5

failure of stability, but the passive structure of the spinal column is most commonly the region affected by metastatic disease [3–5].

Pain continues to be a significant clinical finding and the most common presenting symptom in patients with metastatic spine disease [6]. This pain is an indicator of the failure of the spinal column to maintain anatomic relationships under physiologic stresses [2, 7].

As with any initial patient encounter, time must be dedicated toward a thorough patient interview and physical exam. It is important to consider that some patients will already have a preexisting oncologic diagnosis or are in the process of a formal workup, while others may have been sent from a primary care provider or an emergency room for evaluation of pain or neurologic deficit. Taking the time to recognize what the patient understands about their symptoms at baseline will help in establishing a rapport and improve the flow of information between parties throughout the visit.

Careful questioning regarding the length and character of symptoms should elicit enough information to start down a differential path, as well as help determine whether this patient is at risk for more rapid progression of symptoms. Classic descriptors of pain, such as pain with activity, nighttime pain, or progression of symptoms (both pain and neurologic) over longer periods of time, can be hints that the patient may suffer from a spine that is not capable of resisting physiologic stresses and at risk of mechanical failure. Questions should also highlight symptoms of neurologic dysfunction, such as trouble with fine motor skills or balance, indicative of a myelopathic process, radicular pain (a very common scenario in the lumbar spine), or even bowel/bladder changes in a more urgent presentation such as a frank cauda equina syndrome.

Radiographic Evaluation

Before discussing the evidence surrounding imaging of suspected metastatic disease, it is important to understand the translation of bone loss to actual instability. Cadaveric studies perfumed by Abumi et al. provided significant insight into progressive instability from the loss of posterior elements. Two-level lumbar specimens were sequentially released in stepwise fashion and subjected to vectored stresses to determine the loss of intrinsic stability, starting with division of the posterior ligamentous complex and working through unilateral medial facetectomy, bilateral medial facetectomy, unilateral complete with contralateral medial facetectomy, and finally bilateral total facetectomy [8]. Their findings correlated with a progressive increase in relative range of motion that has been critical for interpreting findings of bone loss in axial and sagittal imaging studies. Relative increases in flexion, lateral bending, and axial rotation were significantly different, implying a translation to in vivo loss of these structures.

Plain Radiographs

Standing radiographs are of foremost importance when initiating a workup of pain in the setting of potential metastatic disease. Standing anterior-posterior and lateral films allow an outlined look at existing bony anatomy, providing contrast between adjacent levels of normal and abnormal bony structure [9]. An upright film or gravity stress view is the simplest form of a stress radiograph of the spine. An interesting direct translation of the work done evaluating the contribution of the posterior facet structure to spinal stability is the "winking owl" sign. In this case, the A/P film shows an absence of a clinically involved pedicle, causing the absence of its circular cortical rim (Fig. 5.1).

Functional radiographs continue to be a core component of imaging in the office, both at initial encounter and following progressive disease over time. Dynamic instability can occasionally be visualized with flexion and extension views either in an upright or lateral decubitus position. Some authors advocate for a lateral position as it relaxes the paraspinal musculature and will allow for a purely passive exam of structural instability. In a study by Wood et al., they found that 31 of 50 patients demonstrated instability with flexion/extension, and of the 31, 18 were only unstable on lateral decubitus imaging [10]. This indicated a potential increase in sensitivity but also a potential increase in false-positive test results.

Nizard and colleagues highlighted, however, that there are multiple limitations to dynamic radiography: First, functionally dynamic studies are difficult to reproduce in patient populations.

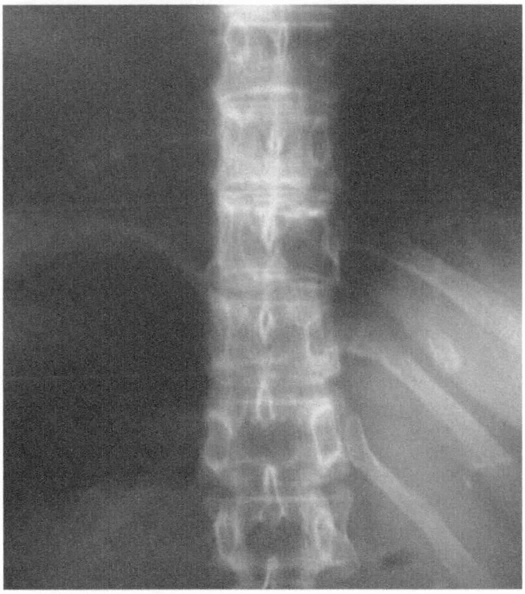

Fig. 5.1 A/P radiograph of the thoracolumbar spine. This patient was diagnosed with metastatic disease erosion of the left T10 pedicle, as demonstrated by the "winking owl" sign with the absence of the cortical rim at this level on the left side compared to adjacent segments

Even small variations in imaging directionality and patient positioning between studies can result in up to 10–15% difference in the amount of perceived translation. Second, while radiographic landmarks have been described, there is no fundamentally standard technique to image these patients. And finally, a lack of "gold standard" for the diagnosis of instability means that any study obtained with conventional radiography will provide only part of the whole picture [11].

Unfortunately, disease processes can advance silently even with dedicated serial radiographs obtained. In an early study by Edelstyn et al., a cadaveric lumbar spine was sectioned in the sagittal plane, and the cancellous bone of the vertebral body was sequentially removed with interval radiographs [12]. They found that 60% of the bone had to be removed before any changes were detected on lateral imaging, and the entire body had to be decorticated before it was detectable on an A/P view. Because of this important limitation, other advanced imaging modalities serve an important role in characterizing spinal disease.

Despite these limitations, changes in alignment seen as both coronal and sagittal collapse as compared to supine imaging (x-rays, CT scans, and MRIs) remain a mainstay in the identification of spinal instability, especially when accompanied by position-dependent pain.

Nuclear Medicine Scans

Nuclear imaging studies are an important tool in the identification of metastatic disease, but do not provide any clinical benefit with respect to determining stability or potential need for future fixation. It is routinely utilized as a supplemental method of detecting skeletal metastases with a new diagnosis of many soft tissue cancer including breast, lung, prostate, thyroid, renal, and many others. In some cases, a positive bone scan can be present 3–18 months before any other radiographic abnormality appears [13].

Computed Tomography

Computed tomography (CT) continues to be the gold standard with respect to evaluating bony anatomy. Sagittal and coronal reformats, in addition to the standard axial sections, provide nearly all bony parameters needed when defining lesion size and quality.

Axial cuts provide an excellent look at facet orientation, most importantly in the lumbar spine. As these facets become more sagittally aligned, experience with degenerative spondylolisthesis has demonstrated a reduced mechanical resistance to listhesis under physiologic loads. These facets may be at an increased risk for early instability as a disease process progresses (Fig. 5.2).

Sagittal and coronal reformats provide measurable information with respect to single-level translation in a supine position. Asymmetric disc space collapse can represent early signs of facet failure and unilateral subsidence. Finally, sagittal images can also show disproportional interspinous spacing that may indicate mass effect or compromise of the posterior ligamentous complex.

Magnetic Resonance

Utilization of magnetic resonance imaging (MRI) in the setting of segmental instability is still in its early stages. One well-understood benefit of MRI in the setting of spine pathology is its exceptional soft tissue and fluid characterization providing insight into both specific tumor characteristics

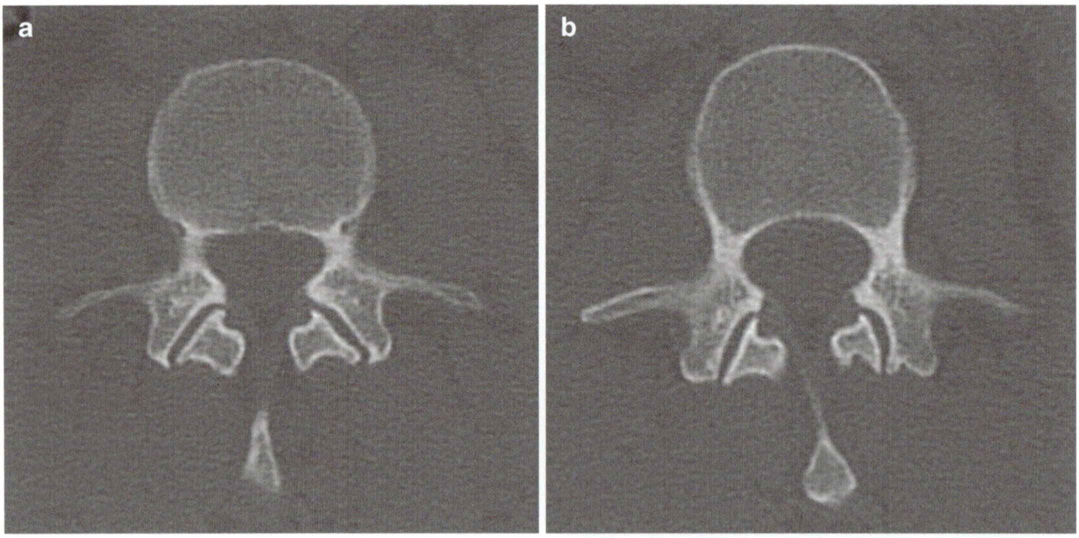

Fig. 5.2 Figure (**a**, **b**) demonstrates two adjacent levels in a patient with back pain and clinical symptoms of instability. Figure (**a**) demonstrates a more typical alignment of the lumbar facet orientation. Figure (**b**) demonstrates facet articulations in a near completely sagittal plane where the patient also demonstrated radiographic signs of instability. This patient went on to instrumented fusion at this level

and evaluation of potential spinal cord compression/involvement. The increasing prevalence of upright MRI capabilities and the option for flexion and extension imaging would theoretically provide some information about stability in neoplastic disease; however to date it has only been described in degenerative disease [14].

Classically, identification of increased fluid signal within the facet capsule is used as an indication of hypermobility at that level. Data in this realm exclusively centers on degenerative cervical and lumbar disease processes. Axial T2 imaging allows for a strong contrast between the darker bone structures and bright fluid within the facet capsule (Fig. 5.3). Increases in fluid appear to correlate in a linear fashion with instability, and fluid space measuring over 1.5 mm can suggest early instability in the absence of translation on a supine MRI in degerative disease [15–19].

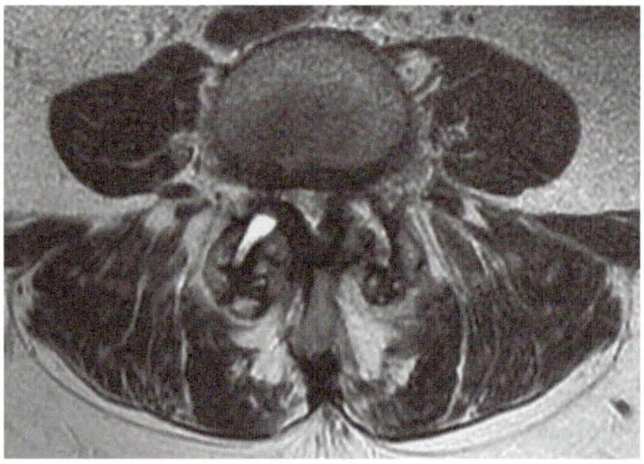

Fig. 5.3 Figure is an axial cut of the lumbar spine with T2-weighted enhancement. Most notable is the high intensity of the fluid in the right facet complex, particularly compared to the less affected left facet complex

Classification Systems

A number of authors have worked to quantify and qualify the risk for instability based on clinical and radiographic characteristics. This section will outline several of these systems and finish with a discussion of the Spinal Instability Neoplastic Disease Score (SINS).

Denis

The work done by Francis Denis is well quoted in the spinal trauma, and with good reason. His three-column model provides a fundamental understanding of the different anatomic sections moving from anterior to posterior, as well as providing analysis should one or more of these columns show deficiency [20, 21].

In an evaluation of over 400 injuries, Denis highlighted three separate zones of injury in the spine. This was a departure at the time from the previous two-column model. These three areas consisted of the anterior, middle, and posterior columns. The anterior column includes the anterior longitudinal ligament, the anterior vertebral body cortex, and the anterior aspect of the annulus and ends in the midpoint of the end plate. The middle column starts at the midportion of the end plate and includes the posterior annulus, the posterior cortex of the vertebral body, and the posterior longitudinal ligament. Finally, the posterior column includes the ligamentum flavum, the posterior bony elements (pedicle, lamina, spinous process, facet articulations), and the inter-/supraspinous ligaments (Fig. 5.4).

His retrospective review of injury patterns in trauma provided insight into the modes of

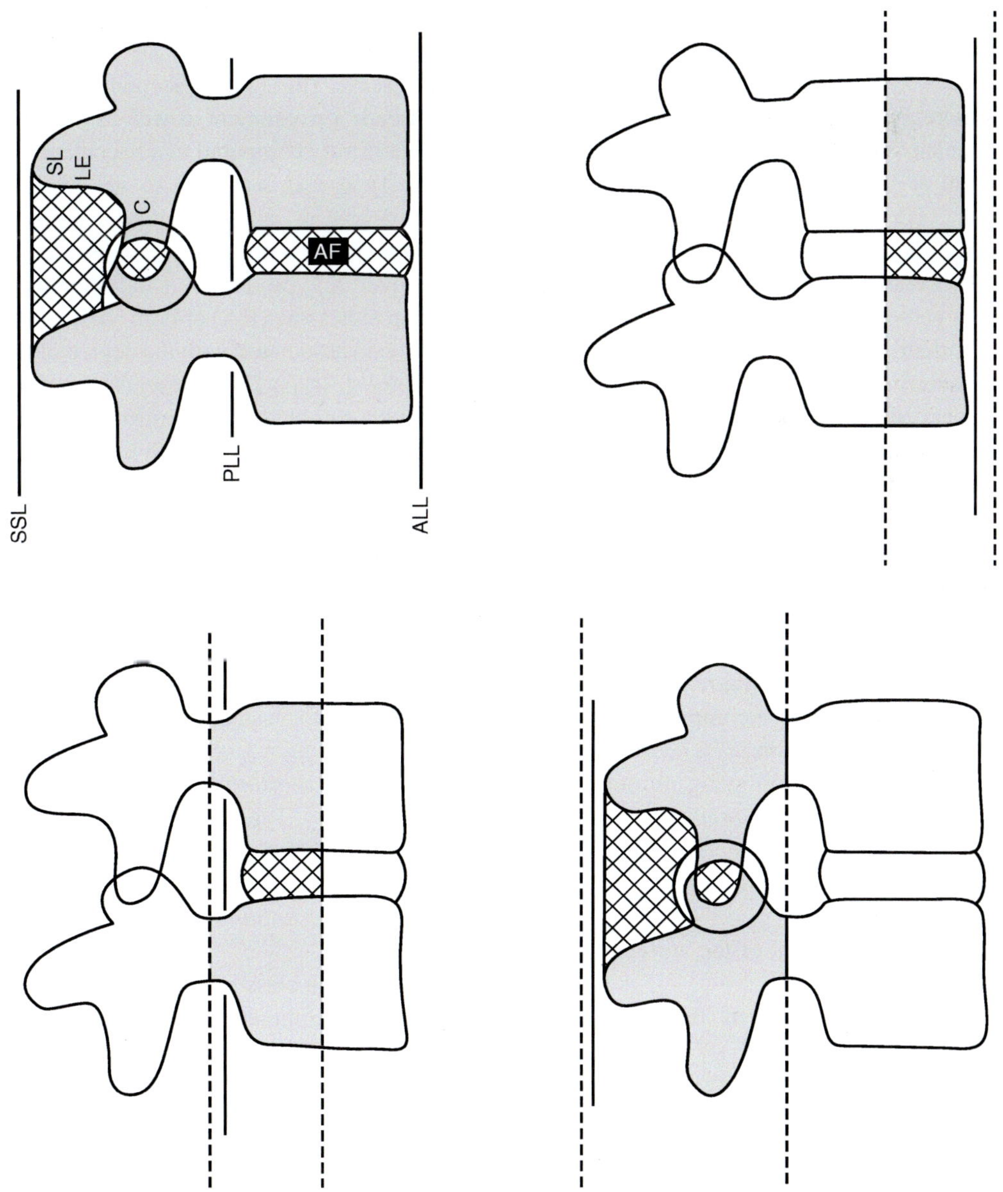

Fig. 5.4 Three-column model demonstrated by Denis. From Francis Denis, The Three Column Spine and Its Significance in the Classification of Acute Thoracolumbar Spinal Injuries, Spine, 1983 Jan 1;8(8)

failure with specific column incompetence. For example, a spine with an insufficient posterior column could be at risk for instability in both flexion and rotation. Disruption of the anterior column would in theory fail in extension due to the absence of a competent anterior longitudinal ligament. This foundation allowed future research to incorporate his work into additional classification systems as we will see moving forward.

Taneichi

In a thorough assessment of risk factors for thoracolumbar collapse with metastatic disease, Taneichi et al. took a series of 100 thoracic and lumbar vertebrae with osteolytic lesions and captured data points from radiographic studies. Particular data points of interest were tumor size (in percentage of vertebral body occupancy), pedicle destruction, posterior element destruction, and costovertebral destruction. The last three data points are again well demonstrated to have an association with clinical instability based on the cadaveric biomechanical studies done by Abumi in 1990 [8].

A multivariate logistic regression model demonstrated that costovertebral joint destruction and tumor size were predictors in the thoracic spine, while size and pedicle destruction were the leading factors in the thoracolumbar region. These data points were based on computed tomography for better bony evaluation.

Ultimately, the following criteria were selected by the authors as predictive of impending collapse [22]:

Thoracic spine:
- 50–60% involvement of the vertebral body in isolation
- 25–30% involvement of the costovertebral joint

Thoracolumbar/lumbar spine:
- 35–40% involvement of the vertebral body in isolation
- 20–25% involvement of the posterior elements

Asdourian

Using a series of patients with metastatic breast cancer in the vertebral body, Asdourian and colleagues worked to define a set of criteria for instability and thus a protocol for treatment of metastatic spinal disease [23, 24]. They took a series of 31 magnetic resonance imaging studies across 27 patients to define these patterns prior to suggesting the said criteria and subsequent protocol.

Observationally, they identified four stages of vertebral body deformity in the setting of metastatic disease. These stages accounted for percentage of body involvement as well as the degree of body deformity compared to adjacent, unaffected levels. Type I is assigned to vertebral bodies with a degree of involvement or complete body involvement but without any collapse (IA and IB, respectively). Type II demonstrates endplate collapse on either one (IIA) or both (IIB) ends of the body, again associated with the degree of marrow replacement. Type III represents end-stage collapse with complete bony destruction. These are subcategorized into those with kyphotic collapse (IIIA) and symmetric collapse (IIIB). Finally, Type IV is described to represent those with translational deformity due to collapse. In each of the five patients studied with this deformity, there was associated posterior element involvement of the disease process (Fig. 5.5).

These stages were then grouped into a classification system for instability as follows:

Impending axial instability: Type IA or IB
Axial instability: Type II or III
Impending translational instability: Type II or III with posterior element involvement
Translational instability: Type IV

Finally, each class in the system was assigned a treatment recommendation by the authors:

Impending axial instability without canal compromise: Radiation/chemotherapy
Impending axial instability with canal compromise: Radiation/chemotherapy and surgical decompression if radioresistant

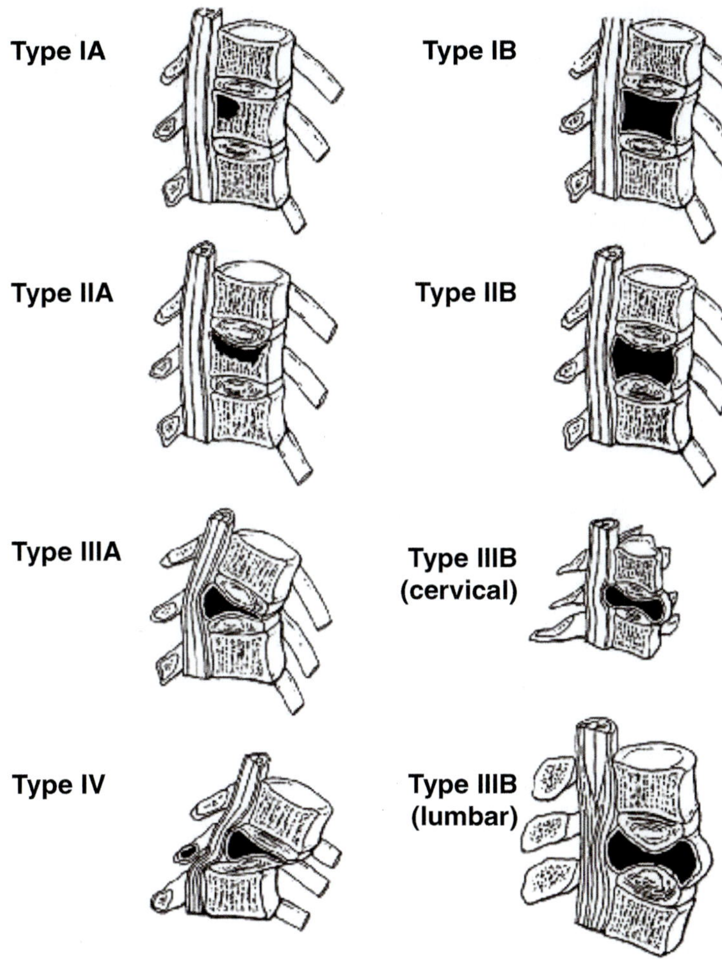

Fig. 5.5 Four stages of vertebral body collapse as defined by Asdourian et al. From Asdourian PL, Mardjetko S, Rauschning W, Jónsson H Jr, Hammerberg KW, Dewald RL, An Evaluation of Spinal Deformity in Metastatic Breast Cancer, Clin Spine Surg, 1990, Jan 1;3(2)

Axial instability: Anterior surgical stabilization if single level, posterior if multilevel

Impending translational instability: Anterior versus anterior/posterior stabilization

Translational instability: Posterior stabilization with posterolateral or anterior decompression

White and Panjabi

The conclusive definition of spinal instability was provided by White and Panjabi in 1990 as they outlined a series of evaluation criteria as a "checklist" for instability. They stated that clinical instability was the loss of the spine's ability to maintain normal patterns of displacement under physiologic loads, protecting against initial or additional neurologic deficits, major deformity, and incapacitating pain [2].

Initially, their work exploring the biomechanical properties of cadaveric cervical spine models provided great insight into the passive restraints to supraphysiologic motion [25–27]. They sequentially sectioned specimens in a controlled fashion, first in an anterior to posterior method followed by independent specimens from posterior to anterior. These sections were then subjected to deforming forces and the displacement was measured. Their suggestion after the review of their own results was that stability was an entity defined solely by osseous and ligamentous restraints and did not rely on active management by cervical musculature [28].

Additionally, they were able to cement the concept that anterior structures restrained extension forces, while posterior structures were tethers to flexion.

In total, the understanding offered by this detailed look at the passive biomechanics in spinal stability paved the way for creating the lower cervical and lumbar spine checklists [2, 29]. In each case, a cumulative score of five points is enough to have a high clinical suspicion of segmental instability of the spine (Tables 5.1 and 5.2).

Table 5.1 Lumbar spine checklist

Element	
Anterior elements destroyed or unable to function	2
Posterior elements destroyed or unable to function	2
Radiographic criteria	4
Flexion-extension radiographs	
Sagittal plane translation > 4.5mm or 15%	2
Sagittal plane rotation	
15 at L1-2, L2-3, and L3-4	2
20 at L4-5	2
25 at L5-S1	2
Resting radiographs	
Sagittal plane displacement >4.5mm or 15%	2
Relative sagittal plane angulation >22°	2
Cauda equina damage	3
Dangerous loading anticipated	1

From White A, Panjabi, M, Clinical Biomechanics of the Spine, 2nd ed., Wolters Kluwer, 1990

Table 5.2 Cervical spine checklist

Element	
Anterior elements destroyed or unable to function	2
Posterior elements destroyed or unable to function	2
Positive stretch test	2
Radiographic criteria	4
Flexion-extension radiographs	
Sagittal plane translation > 3.5mm or 20%	2
Sagittal plane rotation > 20°	2
Resting radiographs	
Sagittal plane displacement >3.5mm or 20%	2
Relative sagittal plane angulation >11°	2
Abnormal disc narrowing	1
Developmentally narrow spinal canal	
Sagittal diameter < 13mm	1
Pavlov's ratio > 0.8	1
Spinal cord damage	2
Nerve root damage	1
Dangerous loading anticipated	1

Reproduced with permission from: White AA III, Panjabi MM: Update on the Evaluation of Instability of the Lower Cervical Spine, in: Griffin PP (ed): Instructional Course Lectures 36. Rosemont, IL, American Academy of Orthopaedic Surgeons, 1987, pp 513–520

The editor applies White and Panjabi's definition of physiologic instability to help determine whether a patient has spinal instability that may warrant stabilization. A clinical example of the utility of this definition compared to Asdourian and SINS is the example of symmetric, end stage vertebral body collapse. Asdourian and SINS would consider this an unstable spine. However, the editor has treated many patients with this presentation who did not demonstrate physiologic instability with progressive deformity, progressive neurologic dysfunction, or pain recalcitrant to medical management. These patients remained stable after radiation therapy and corticosteroids. We have seen a couple patients with complete vertebral body collapse and facet incongruity or diastasis who did demonstrate physiologic instability. The editor believes that the White and Panjabi definition of physiologic instability is helpful to determine spinal instability.

SINS

In 2010, the Spine Oncology Study Group released a comprehensive review of the available literature, combined with their own professional experience, using the Delphi technique of assessing member's opinions on the relevant factors associated with instability in the setting of an oncologic process. These serial opinions were then adapted in tandem with the existing literature base to create the Spinal Instability Neoplastic Score (SINS) [30].

Variables including character of pain, disease location, and descriptors of bony involvement were presented before the study group, and a relative scoring system was then adapted as follows in Table 5.3.

Table 5.3 Spinal Instability Neoplastic Score (SINS)

Element		Score
Location		
	Junctional (occiput–C1, C7–T2, T11–L1, L5–S1	3
	Mobile spine (C3–C6, L2–L4)	2
	Semirigid (T3–T10)	1
	Rigid (S2–S5)	0
Pain relief with recumbency and/or pain with movement/loading of the spine		
	Yes	3
	No (occasional pain but not mechanical)	1
	Pain-free lesion	0
Bone lesion		
	Lytic	2
	Mixed (lytic/blastic)	1
	Blastic	0
Radiographic spinal alignment		
	Subluxation/translation present	4
	De novo deformity (kyphosis/scoliosis)	2
	Normal alignment	0
Vertebral body collapse		
	>50% collapse	3
	<50% collapse	2
	No collapse with >50% body involved	1
	None of the above	0
Posterolateral involvement of the spinal elements		
	(Facet, pedicle, or CV joint fracture or replacement with tumor)	
	Bilateral	3
	Unilateral	1
	None of the above	0

The SINS system notably includes many characteristics from previous classification systems covered and assigned relative scores to each category to help weight associated symptoms appropriately. As patients progressed with higher and higher scores, the increased risk of instability is immediately understood.

As a conclusion to their outlined scoring system, the authors provided insight into what numerical score denoted concern for instability in the hope that oncologists and surgeons alike would have guidance on the next step of treatment. For patients with a score from 0 to 6, the authors suggested that these were likely "stable" spines and could be managed nonoperatively from the perspective of stability. Consultation with a spine surgeon was not necessary, and systemic and/or radiation therapy could be considered. With a score of 7–12, patients were categorized as indeterminate instability, and any score greater than 7 merited surgical consultation. Finally, scores of 13–18 denoted instability, and intervention was likely necessary if the patient was deemed a reasonable surgical candidate.

When considering the SINS scoring system, it is important to note at this point that while patients may start at one end numerically, progressive disease processes may move their score up with time and they should be monitored for these changes. Additionally, this scoring system is one defined around stability at a single level and does not account for discontinuous lesions nor does it account for neurologic symptoms.

The study group went on to provide a clinical validation in 2011 where 30 patients were presented to the members of the study group individually [31]. Scoring of each subcategory and the final categorization of stable, potentially unstable, and unstable were analyzed and inter- and intra-observer reliability calculated. There was near-perfect correlation of the total SINS score with an inter- and intra-observer reliability of 0.846 and 0.886, respectively. The sensitivity and specificity of the SINS scoring system were demonstrated to be 95.7 and 79.5%, respectively. Additionally, and perhaps most importantly, no "unstable" were grouped into the "stable" category.

Separate evaluations and validations were performed using the SINS system. A validation was performed in radiation oncologists where they found substantial interobserver and excellent intra-observer reliability between providers. And again, most importantly, there were no cases of an unstable spine being categorized as "stable" by the providers [32]. A separate evaluation by oncologists noted the gradual decrease in the mean SINS score for patients, positing that an increased awareness of relevant clinical criteria provided an earlier diagnosis of risk factors for instability and appropriate referral [33]. Galasko et al. highlighted a significant need for education of potential referring providers after identifying that many patients present to their clinic in a delayed fashion despite symptoms of instability [34].

Conclusions

Instability of the spine from metastatic disease is difficult to quantify, but there are a number of systems that have been designed to assist the clinician to appropriately stratify their patient's risks and direct them toward the most appropriate treatment pathway.

Fundamental components of patient care, such as a thorough history and physical examination, remain at the foundation of diagnosis and treatment. Decision-making can be supported by routine and advanced imaging studies, confirming the clinical impression. Baseline imaging studies with plain radiographs should always be obtained to allow for longitudinal evaluation of disease processes and progression, particularly as more advance imaging modalities are both costly and less convenient for routine follow-up. However, the advanced studies of CT and MR imaging should be part of the initial workup to help better understand the disease process that each patient faces.

The Cancer Center at Memorial Sloan Kettering uses a combination of clinical and pathologic criteria to assist with determining the treatment pathway for spinal neoplastic processes. One of their most important contributions is the neurologic, oncologic, mechanical, and systemic (NOMS) decision framework. This framework importantly includes the mechanical impact of spinal neoplasms when determining treatment pathways, and a thorough understanding of instability is a critical step in providing excellent care for our patients [35] (Fig. 5.6).

There are many systems which can assist the clinician with clinical decision-making and help us to provide our patients with an understanding of their individual risk of instability and potential morbidity from intrinsic spinal instability due to neoplastic disease (both benign and malignant). Depending on the clinical scenario, components of multiple systems may need to be employed, so a thorough understanding of these concepts is essential for the clinician. This understanding of risk can be translated to the bedside to help determine the potential surgical and nonsurgical treatment options best suited to the individual patient's stage of disease.

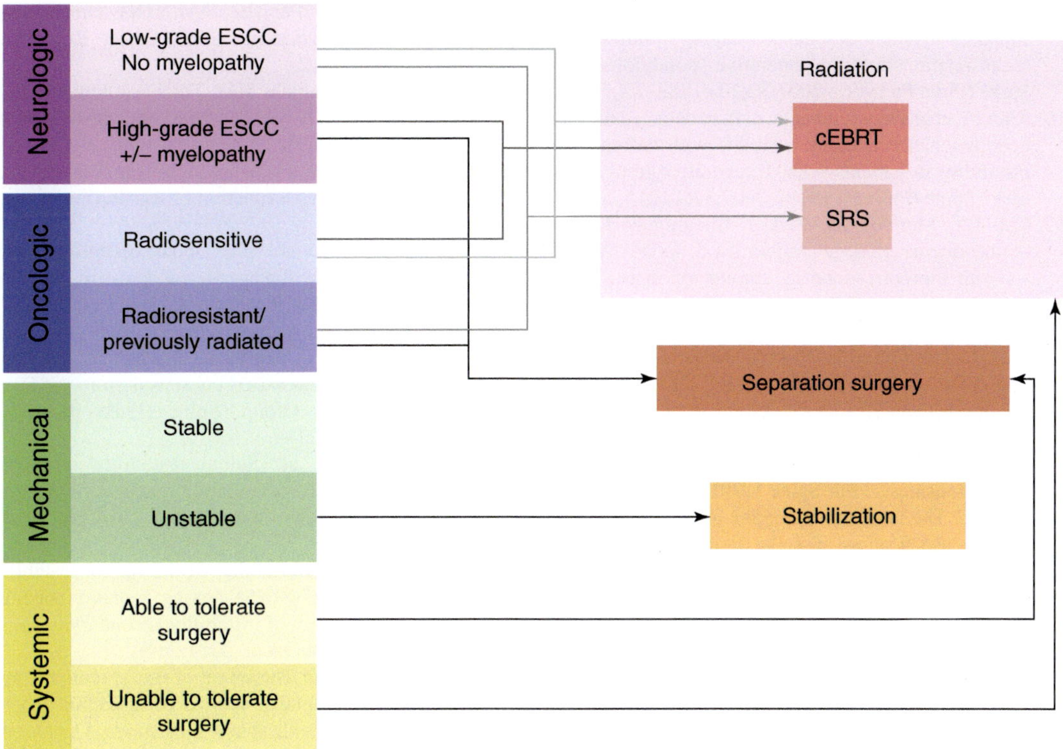

Fig. 5.6 Neurologic, oncologic, mechanical, and systemic decision framework by Memorial Sloan Kettering (2013). Republished with permission from John Wiley and Sons, from Laufer I, Rubin DG, Lis E, Cox BW, Stubblefield MD, Yamada Y, Bilsky MH, The NOMS framework: approach to the treatment of spinal metastatic tumors, Oncologist, 2013 Jun;18(6):744–51, doi: 10.1634/theoncologist.2012-0293, epub 2013 May 24, permission conveyed through Copyright Clearance Center, Inc.

References

1. Patchell RA, et al. Direct decompressive surgical resection in the treatment of spinal cord compression caused by metastatic cancer: a randomised trial. Lancet. 2005;366(9486):643–8.
2. White AA, Panjabi MM. Clinical biomechanics of the spine. 2nd ed. Philadelphia: Lippincott; 1990. xxiii, 722 p.
3. Demoulin C, et al. Lumbar functional instability: a critical appraisal of the literature. Ann Readapt Med Phys. 2007;50(8):677–84, 669–76.
4. Posner I, et al. A biomechanical analysis of the clinical stability of the lumbar and lumbosacral spine. Spine (Phila Pa 1976). 1982;7(4):374–89.
5. Panjabi MM. The stabilizing system of the spine. Part I. Function, dysfunction, adaptation, and enhancement. J Spinal Disord. 1992;5(4):383–9; discussion 397.
6. Fourney DR, et al. Use of pedicle screw fixation in the management of malignant spinal disease: experience in 100 consecutive procedures. J Neurosurg. 2001;94(1 Suppl):25–37.
7. Panjabi MM. Clinical spinal instability and low back pain. J Electromyogr Kinesiol. 2003;13(4):371–9.
8. Abumi K, et al. Biomechanical evaluation of lumbar spinal stability after graded facetectomies. Spine (Phila Pa 1976). 1990;15(11):1142–7.
9. Salvo N, et al. The role of plain radiographs in management of bone metastases. J Palliat Med. 2009;12(2):195–8.
10. Wood KB, et al. Radiographic evaluation of instability in spondylolisthesis. Spine (Phila Pa 1976). 1994;19(15):1697–703.
11. Nizard RS, Wybier M, Laredo JD. Radiologic assessment of lumbar intervertebral instability and degenerative spondylolisthesis. Radiol Clin North Am. 2001;39(1):55–71, v–vi.
12. Edelstyn GA, Gillespie PJ, Grebbell FS. The radiological demonstration of osseous metastases. Experimental observations. Clin Radiol. 1967;18(2):158–62.
13. Tatsui H, et al. Survival rates of patients with metastatic spinal cancer after scintigraphic detection of abnormal radioactive accumulation. Spine (Phila Pa 1976). 1996;21(18):2143–8.
14. Alyas F, Connell D, Saifuddin A. Upright positional MRI of the lumbar spine. Clin Radiol. 2008;63(9):1035–48.

15. Chaput C, et al. The significance of increased fluid signal on magnetic resonance imaging in lumbar facets in relationship to degenerative spondylolisthesis. Spine (Phila Pa 1976). 2007;32(17):1883–7.
16. Rihn JA, et al. Does lumbar facet fluid detected on magnetic resonance imaging correlate with radiographic instability in patients with degenerative lumbar disease? Spine (Phila Pa 1976). 2007;32(14):1555–60.
17. Cho BY, Murovic JA, Park J. Imaging correlation of the degree of degenerative L4-5 spondylolisthesis with the corresponding amount of facet fluid. J Neurosurg Spine. 2009;11(5):614–9.
18. Schinnerer KA, Katz LD, Grauer JN. MR findings of exaggerated fluid in facet joints predicts instability. J Spinal Disord Tech. 2008;21(7):468–72.
19. Snoddy MC, et al. Can facet joint fluid on MRI and dynamic instability be a predictor of improvement in back pain following lumbar fusion for degenerative spondylolisthesis? Eur Spine J. 2016;25(8):2408–15.
20. Denis F. The three column spine and its significance in the classification of acute thoracolumbar spinal injuries. Spine (Phila Pa 1976). 1983;8(8):817–31.
21. Denis F. Spinal instability as defined by the three-column spine concept in acute spinal trauma. Clin Orthop Relat Res. 1984;(189):65–76.
22. Taneichi H, et al. Risk factors and probability of vertebral body collapse in metastases of the thoracic and lumbar spine. Spine (Phila Pa 1976). 1997;22(3):239–45.
23. Asdourian PL, et al. An evaluation of spinal deformity in metastatic breast cancer. J Spinal Disord. 1990;3(2):119–34.
24. Asdourian PL, et al. The pattern of vertebral involvement in metastatic vertebral breast cancer. Clin Orthop Relat Res. 1990;(250):164–70.
25. White AA 3rd, et al. Biomechanical analysis of clinical stability in the cervical spine. Clin Orthop Relat Res. 1975;(109):85–96.
26. White AA 3rd, Panjabi MM. The clinical biomechanics of scoliosis. Clin Orthop Relat Res. 1976;(118):100–12.
27. White AA 3rd, Panjabi MM. The basic kinematics of the human spine. A review of past and current knowledge. Spine (Phila Pa 1976). 1978;3(1):12–20.
28. Panjabi MM, White AA 3rd, Johnson RM. Cervical spine mechanics as a function of transection of components. J Biomech. 1975;8(5):327–36.
29. White AA 3rd, Panjabi MM. Update on the evaluation of instability of the lower cervical spine. Instr Course Lect. 1987;36:513–20.
30. Fisher CG, et al. A novel classification system for spinal instability in neoplastic disease: an evidence-based approach and expert consensus from the Spine Oncology Study Group. Spine (Phila Pa 1976). 2010;35(22):E1221–9.
31. Fourney DR, et al. Spinal instability neoplastic score: an analysis of reliability and validity from the spine oncology study group. J Clin Oncol. 2011;29(22):3072–7.
32. Fisher CG, et al. Reliability of the Spinal Instability Neoplastic Score (SINS) among radiation oncologists: an assessment of instability secondary to spinal metastases. Radiat Oncol. 2014;9:69.
33. Versteeg AL, et al. The effect of introducing the spinal instability neoplastic score in routine clinical practice for patients with spinal metastases. Oncologist. 2016;21(1):95–101.
34. Galasko CS, Norris HE, Crank S. Spinal instability secondary to metastatic cancer. J Bone Joint Surg Am. 2000;82(4):570–94.
35. Laufer I, et al. The NOMS framework: approach to the treatment of spinal metastatic tumors. Oncologist. 2013;18(6):744–51.

Imaging Metastatic Spinal Disease

6

Sanjay K. Singh and Steve H. Fung

Background

Classically, the spine is divided into anterior and posterior elements, with the *anterior element* composed of the vertebral body/intervertebral disc and the *posterior element* composed of the neural arch including pedicles, facet joints, laminae, and transverse and spinous processes. Surgeons prefer to divide the spine into three columns [1] with the *anterior column* composed of the anterior half of vertebral body/intervertebral disc and anterior longitudinal ligament, the *middle column* composed of the posterior half of vertebral body/intervertebral disc and posterior longitudinal ligament, and the *posterior column* composed of posterior elements, ligamentum flavum, and interspinous and supraspinous ligaments.

Pathologies involving the spine, including metastases from primary cancers elsewhere, are classified by location (Tables 6.1 and 6.2) [2].

Approximately 90–95% of spinal metastases are extradural in location, mostly as osseous metastases that can extend into the epidural space or result in pathologic fracture with mass effect on the thecal sac [3, 4]. Pure extraosseous epidural, intradural extramedullary (leptomeningeal), and intramedullary metastases are less frequently encountered. Indeed, the most common location for osseous metastases is the spine with vertebral bodies most often involved, presumably from hematogenous spread via highly vascular Batson's venous plexus connecting deep pelvic and thoracic veins to internal vertebral venous plexus [5] and modulated by molecular characteristics of tumor cells [6, 7]. Approximately 80% of all osseous metastases originate from breast, prostate, thyroid, kidney, and lung cancers with 70–90% of patients with breast or prostate cancer and 30–40% of patients with thyroid, kidney, or lung cancer having osseous metastases on postmortem examination [8–10]. Spinal involvement can also be extensive in patients with multiple myeloma and Hodgkin and non-Hodgkin lymphomas [11]. When spinal metastases are present, 60–80% involve the thoracic spine, 15–30% involve the lumbar spine, and <10% involve the cervical spine [4].

Osseous metastases are generally classified as *osteolytic* or *osteoblastic*, depending on if dysregulated bone resorption (from increased osteoclast activity) or bone formation (from increased osteoblast activity) is the dominant mechanism, respectively [12, 13]. Despite this dichotomous classification, most cancer types display a range of dysregulated bone resorption and bone formation activity, so that patients can have a varying

S. K. Singh, MD (✉)
Department of Radiology, Houston Methodist Hospital, Houston, TX, USA
e-mail: ssingh@houstonmethodist.org

S. H. Fung, MD
Department of Radiology, Weill Cornell Medical College, Houston Methodist Hospital, Houston Methodist Research Institute, Houston, TX, USA
e-mail: shfung@houstonmethodist.org

R. A. W. Marco (ed.), *Metastatic Spine Disease*, https://doi.org/10.1007/978-3-319-76252-4_6

Table 6.1 Differential diagnosis of spinal pathologies by location

Extradural	Intradural extramedullary	Intramedullary
Spondylosis	*Tumors*	*Tumors*
Disc bulge/herniation	Peripheral nerve sheath tumor	Astrocytoma
Osteophyte	Schwannoma	Intramedullary ependymoma
Facet hypertrophy	Neurofibroma	Ganglioglioma
Synovial/ganglion cyst	Meningioma	Hemangioblastoma
Ligamentous hypertrophy	Leptomeningeal metastasis	Intramedullary metastasis
Tumors	Lipoma, dermoid/epidermoid	Lymphoma
Osseous and epidural metastasis	Extramedullary ependymoma	*Demyelinating disease/myelitis*
Primary spinal/paraspinal tumor extension	Lymphoma	Multiple sclerosis
See Table 6.2	*Other*	Neuromyelitis optica
Multiple myeloma/plasmacytoma	Guillain-Barré syndrome	Acute disseminated
Lymphoma	Chronic inflammatory	encephalomyelitis
Other	demyelinating	Systemic lupus erythematosus
Inflammatory arthritis	polyneuropathy	Sjögren's syndrome
Rheumatoid arthritis/odontoid pannus	Arachnoid cyst	Infectious/postinfectious
Seronegative spondyloarthropathies	Arachnoiditis/meningitis	myelitis
Metabolic disease	Sarcoidosis	Viral infection
Paget's disease	Arteriovenous fistula/	Bacterial infection
Renal osteodystrophy/brown tumor	malformation	Postvaccination myelitis
Vertebral fracture		Paraneoplastic syndrome
Pathologic fracture from malignancy		Sarcoidosis
Osteoporosis		Idiopathic transverse myelitis
Trauma		*Other*
Epidural abscess		Syringohydromyelia
Pyogenic infection		Subacute combined
Tuberculous infection		degeneration
Epidural hematoma		Spinal cord contusion
Epidural lipomatosis		Spinal cord infarction
Sarcoidosis		Arteriovenous malformation

degree of mixed lesions containing both osteolytic and osteoblastic elements (Table 6.3). Osteolytic metastases are more common than osteoblastic metastases, including metastases from breast, lung, kidney, and thyroid cancers and multiple myeloma, whereas osteoblastic metastases occur most often in patients with prostate cancer, 15–20% of breast cancer, and osteosclerotic myeloma/POEMS syndrome [12–14].

Although most patients with spinal metastasis present with no or few symptoms, the most common initial symptoms include local pain and radicular pain that may be associated with anesthesia, hyperesthesia, paresthesia, muscle weakness, and loss of reflexes [15]. A serious complication that can occur with spinal metastasis is *malignant spinal cord compression* (MSCC), which is defined as compression of the spinal cord and/or cauda equina by extradural mass effect from epidural extension of tumor or pathologic vertebral fracture. In addition to pain, symptoms of MSCC can include muscle weakness and sensory deficits in distributions distal to the point of compression, progressive myelopathy, autonomic dysfunction manifesting as urinary retention, incontinence, and impotence [10, 15]. MSCC is an oncologic emergency that requires immediate treatment with corticosteroids, radiotherapy, and/or surgery to prevent irreversible loss of neurological function [11, 16].

Table 6.2 Differential diagnosis of spinal tumors by tissue of origin and location

Tissue of origin	Vertebral body	Posterior element
Osteogenic	*Malignant*	*Benign*
Bone island/enostosis	Metastasis[b]	Osteoid osteoma
Osteoid osteoma	Multiple myeloma/plasmacytoma[b]	Osteoblastoma[c]
Osteoblastoma	Lymphoma[b]	Osteochondroma
Osteosarcoma	Chordoma	Aneurysmal bone cyst[c]
Chrondogenic	*Benign*	*Malignant*
Osteochondroma	Hemangioma	Sarcoma
Chondroblastoma	Langerhans cell histiocytosis	Chondrosarcoma[c]
Chondrosarcoma	Giant cell tumor[b]	Osteosarcoma[c]
Fibrogenic		Ewing's sarcoma[c]
Fibrous dysplasia		
Benign fibrous histiocytoma[a]		
Malignant fibrous histiocytoma[a]		
Vascular		
Hemangioma		
Paraganglioma[a]		
Hemangioendothelioma/hemangiosarcoma[a]		
Hemangiopericytoma[a]		
Hematopoietic		
Multiple myeloma/plasmacytoma		
Lymphoma		
Leukemia		
Langerhans cell histiocytosis		
Ewing's sarcoma		
Notochordal		
Chordoma		
Other		
Aneurysmal bone cyst		
Giant cell tumor		

Modified from Rodallec et al. 2008
[a]Rare in spine
[b]Can extend to posterior element
[c]Can extend to vertebral body

Table 6.3 Typical radiographic appearance of osseous metastases

Predominantly osteolytic	Predominantly osteoblastic	Mixed osteolytic/osteoblastic
Breast cancer (can be mixed or osteoblastic)	Prostate cancer (most common)	Breast cancer (often mixed or osteolytic)
Non-small cell lung cancer (can be mixed)	Breast cancer (15–20% osteoblastic)	Lung cancer (often osteolytic)
Renal cell carcinoma	Small cell lung cancer	Prostate cancer (often osteoblastic)
Thyroid cancer	Transitional cell carcinoma	Cervical cancer
Melanoma	Carcinoid tumor	Testicular cancer
Hepatocellular carcinoma	Medulloblastoma	Gastrointestinal cancers
Ewing's sarcoma	Neuroblastoma	Squamous cell carcinoma
Multiple myeloma	Hodgkin lymphoma	
Non-Hodgkin lymphoma	Osteosclerotic myeloma/POEMS syndrome	

Imaging Considerations

Imaging plays an essential role in the diagnosis and staging of cancer patients, differentiating malignant from benign spinal lesions such as spondylosis and infection, evaluating involved sites for pathologic fracture and MSCC, and follow-up of treatment response and complications. Although a wide range of imaging modalities are available, the oncologist should be mindful of which imaging study is the most accurate and economical in addressing a given clinical indication and have a well-designed imaging strategy in approaching the cancer patient.

In patients with known or suspected cancer and significant back pain, contrast-enhanced spinal magnetic resonance imaging (MRI) should be obtained as early as possible and is the imaging modality of choice for determining if symptoms are from spinal metastasis, acute fracture, spondylosis, or other causes. If spinal metastasis is present, MRI provides information on the extent of metastatic disease and any complications including pathologic fracture, epidural extension of tumor, MSCC, and spinal instability. A T1- and T2-weighted MRI without contrast usually provides sufficient information to treat the patient with less cost, time, and risk to the patient.

X-ray computed tomography (CT) scans offer complimentary information on the structural integrity of bone including better delineation of fractures, spinal alignment, posterior element involvement, and characterization of osseous metastasis as osteolytic, osteoblastic, or mixed. In patients who are unable to have MRI because of implanted medical devices or metallic foreign bodies, CT scan with or without myelography should be obtained.

Other imaging modalities potentially helpful in the evaluation of spinal metastasis are reviewed in the following sections.

Radiography

Plain radiography is commonly used for the initial evaluation of patients with new symptoms related to the spine because of the imaging technique's low cost, widespread availability, and ease of use. A radiograph is a projectional image of the patient's body created by an x-ray beam that is attenuated variably by different structures of the body depending on its density as it casts a shadow of the patient's anatomy onto a planar detector [17]. Anatomical structures are described by their density with a dense structure like bone (which appears bright on the image) attenuating more of the x-ray beam than a lower-density structure like soft tissue (which appears gray on the image), and air (which appears dark on the image) has the least density and attenuation of the x-ray beam. At least two orthogonal projectional images usually in anteroposterior (AP) and lateral orientations are necessary to adequately evaluate spinal anatomy. A systematic approach should be used to evaluate spinal alignment, bone integrity, spacing, and surrounding soft tissue.

Although patients presenting with spinal symptoms are commonly initially evaluated with radiography, plain radiographs should not be generally used for screening osseous metastases because of their poor sensitivity (44–50%) in detecting metastatic lesions [18] due to overlapping of structures and poor contrast resolution.

Osteolytic metastases often present as regions of decreased density or loss of normal trabecular pattern in cancellous bone (also called spongy or trabecular bone), which has limited contrast compared to lesions affecting cortical bone. Therefore, osteolytic metastases can be missed on plain radiographs until up to 50% of the vertebral body is affected and 30–75% of bone density is lost [18]. Osteoblastic lesions often present as regions with increased density or can have mixed osteolytic elements with sclerotic rims.

Despite this limitation for detecting osseous metastases, radiographs are still useful for screening vertebral fractures, spinal deformities, malalignment, spondylosis, gross osteolytic or osteoblastic lesions, and large soft tissue masses. Any suspicion for vertebral fracture or mechanical instability of the spine should be followed by MRI and/or CT scans.

Computed Tomography

Computed tomography (CT) scanning uses an array of detectors and an x-ray beam to form a reconstructed picture of the body. CT allows rapid assessment of patients because it is readily available and has few contraindications. It is still the primary method for detection of calcification [19] and of the bony matrix of a spinal mass. The reconstructed image of CT scanning does not suffer from the overlapping of different structures that plagues plain film radiographs. In addition CT scanning has higher spatial resolution but lower contrast resolution compared with MRI [20]. Similar to plain film radiographs, CT scanning is most sensitive to lytic change in cortical bone and less sensitive to changes in cancellous/spongy bone. Overall sensitivity of CT for detection of bone metastatic disease is around 73% [21].

Placing contrast into the subarachnoid space helps evaluate compromise of nerve root sleeves, the thecal sac and the spinal cord. CT myelography also helps to differentiate the cause of MSCC from tumor extension into the epidural space or from retropulsion of osseous fragments from pathological fracture.

Magnetic Resonance Imaging

Magnetic resonance imaging (MRI) utilizes the interaction of hydrogen nuclei (protons) in tissue with radiofrequency waves and magnetic fields. Various MRI sequences allow one to visualize different qualities of tissue based on their chemical environment. One sequence ("T1-weighted" or T1W) shows normal fatty tissue (such as in yellow bone marrow) as high signal (bright or hyperintense) and water (such as cerebrospinal fluid [CSF] and edema) as low signal (dark or hypointense). Another sequence ("T2-weighted" or T2W) shows regions with high water content (CSF and edema) as high signal. Proteinaceous fluid and blood can have a range of low to high T1W and T2W signal depending on protein concentration and age of blood product (methemoglobin produces high T1W signal). This range of T1W and T2W signal in tissue on MRI allows for higher sensitivity and specificity in characterizing tissue than that possible based on density differences in tissue using radiographic techniques such as CT scanning.

A drawback of MRI is that a typical MRI scan of the spine takes much longer to perform (20–30 min) than a CT scan (1–2 min). Modern MRI sequences utilize fast spin-echo (FSE) technique to shorten scan time, which results in higher signal in normal fat on T2W FSE images. Therefore, normal fat-containing yellow bone marrow appears bright on both T1W and T2W FSE images. The STIR ("short tau inversion recovery") sequence produces a fat-suppressed T2W image that is useful for evaluating bone marrow edema (such as in acute fracture and marrow-replacing tumor) that appears bright on STIR, whereas normal yellow bone marrow appears dark on STIR.

Intravascular contrast in MRI studies generally has relied on the T1-shortening effect of paramagnetic contrast agents containing gadolinium. This leads to higher signal ("enhancement") on T1W images where gadolinium contrast agents concentrate (such as in areas of neovascularity and increased capillary permeability). Because normal fat appears bright on conventional T1W images, fat-suppressed post-contrast T1W images are usually used to evaluate for enhancement on spinal MRI.

In evaluating a spinal mass, MRI possesses multiple advantages over radiographic techniques. The normal adult bone marrow (yellow marrow) has high intrinsic signal on T1W images making a neoplasm easy to identify because the vast majority of neoplasms have low T1 signal and (if lytic) high T2 signal. Marrow-replacing lesions with high T2 signal are best seen on STIR, and enhancement can be determined using fat-suppressed T1W images as described above. The subarachnoid space is well seen as bright signal on T2W images, and the spinal cord can be delineated because of its lower signal within the bright CSF.

In the setting of the oncology patient, MRI provides high sensitivity (up to 90.6%) and specificity (up to 96.0%) [21] for detecting skeletal metastatic disease.

Bone Scintigraphy

Skeletal scintigraphy (bone scan) is low risk, widely available, and easy to perform. The compounds are ^{99m}Tc(technetium-99m)-labeled diphosphonates. The accumulation in bone is related to blood flow and the rate of new bone formation [22]. The new bone formation in metastatic disease is predominantly osteoblastic activity in response to neoplastic osteolysis. Bone scintigraphy is less sensitive in aggressive neoplasms such as multiple myeloma where there is little osteoblastic activity compared to the osteoclastic activity. These patients can thus have minimal uptake of the radionuclide despite large amounts of lytic activity within the bone [23].

In the setting of the oncology patient, bone scintigraphy has the advantage of routinely imaging the entire body and having high sensitivity for skeletal metastases of about 78% [24]. False-positive activity can occur in bone scintigraphy from benign bone tumors, degenerative disease, or fractures. Treatment of bone metastases can result in transiently increased bone reparative activity ("flare phenomenon") which can be falsely interpreted as worsening metastatic disease on bone scintigraphy.

Routine bone scintigraphy is acquired with a planar detector in which there is overlap of anatomic structures. Single-photon emission computed tomography (SPECT) acquires bone scintigraphy images in a cross-sectional manner allowing better delineation of anatomical distribution of the radiotracer. This increases the sensitivity of bone scintigraphy for skeletal metastases to 87% [24].

Positron-Emission Tomography

PET, or positron-emission tomography, generates high-resolution tomographic images from the detection of pairs of photons emitted during the annihilation of positrons with electrons. The positrons are the result of decay of specific radioisotopes which are in certain compounds. ^{18}F-fluorodeoxyglucose (FDG) and ^{18}F-NaF are the radiopharmaceuticals used in bone evaluation. Similar to conventional bone scintigraphy, ^{18}F-NaF PET shows activity where osteoblastic activity occurs. FDG is an analogue of glucose and will accumulate where metabolism of glucose is high. ^{18}F-FDG PET is commonly used in oncology imaging due to the high glucose metabolism of many cancers. Unlike technetium and ^{18}F-NaF bone scanning, FDG scanning directly images the cancer cells in the bone. The sensitivity of ^{18}F-FDG PET for detecting bone metastases is high (89.7%) [21]. The tomographic images from PET scanning can be fused with routine CT images. The resulting ^{18}F-FDG PET/CT allows analysis of the radiographic anatomy and appearance of areas of abnormal metabolic activity. The sensitivity for detecting skeletal metastatic disease of ^{18}F-FDG PET/CT has been reported to be as high as 97% [25].

Approach to Evaluating the Spine

The diagnostic imaging approach to a spinal lesion begins with determining its exact location. The differential diagnosis of spinal cord masses will differ from that of intradural but extramedullary tumors. Extradural (epidural) masses are the most common abnormalities seen in spine imaging. Extradural pathologies are located outside the thecal sac and can involve the bone (e.g., osseous metastasis), intervertebral disc (e.g., herniated disc), or epidural space (e.g., epidural abscess). Extradural lesions can compress the thecal sac and its contents, i.e., spinal cord and nerve roots. Intradural extramedullary pathologies are located outside the spinal cord but inside the thecal sac, which can include tumors (e.g., peripheral nerve sheath tumor, meningioma, and leptomeningeal metastasis) and non-tumors (e.g., arachnoid cyst, arachnoiditis, and arteriovenous fistula). Intradural extramedullary lesions tend to expand the subarachnoid space on the lesion side and displace the spinal cord and nerve roots away from the lesion. Intramedullary pathologies involve the spinal cord and include tumors (e.g., astrocytoma, ependymoma, and rarely spinal cord metastasis) and non-tumors (e.g., demyelinating disease/myelitis, syringohydromyelia, spinal cord contusion and infarction). Intramedullary lesions with mass effect tend to expand the spinal cord and narrow the surrounding subarachnoid space.

After localizing a lesion, the imaging characteristics of a tumor need to be evaluated. A mass involving bone or adjacent to bone may have an internal bony matrix identifiable on CT scan or plain films. If the matrix is calcified, it may offer a clue to the histology of the underlying mass. For example, cartilaginous neoplasms can have ringlike or arc-like calcifications. In addition the bony edge or margin of a lesion should be examined. A sharp, well-defined edge usually indicates a slow-growing process. Irregular, poorly defined margins often indicate an aggressive process. Finally some tumors (such as giant cell tumor, osteoblastoma, and aneurysmal bone cyst) can expand the bones they involve, and this can be detected with CT scan and plain radiographs [26]. CT scan evaluation of soft tissues can be augmented with intravenous contrast material. In patients with suspected malignant spinal cord compression (MSCC), subarachnoid (intrathecal or myelographic) contrast can help detect the level of spinal cord compromise due to epidural mass effect from metastatic disease. CT myelography also helps discern intramedullary tumors from intradural-extramedullary tumors.

The MRI characteristics of a mass can help better define its extent and histology. Internal lesion hemorrhage, melanin, fat, or cyst-like features can be evident on MRI. Enhancement within a mass is easier to detect with MRI compared to CT scan and is most conspicuous when fat suppression is used in T1W images. Bone neoplasms can be seen on T2W images especially if fat suppression is utilized. Short tau/T1 inversion recovery (STIR) images are commonly used in spine imaging to provide T2-like images with fat suppression. Some tumors (chordomas and chondrosarcomas) tend to be very bright on T2W images [27]. A soft tissue component of a lesion can easily be detected on MRI. Compromise of the spinal canal by bone (displaced fracture) or epidural soft tissue mass is an important imaging finding. A limitation of MRI is the setting of the postoperative spine with metal implants which distort the local magnetic field and render MRI nondiagnostic. In such patients, CT scan with myelographic contrast can provide better anatomic information than MRI.

The imaging of spinal metastasis provides basic information important to assessing stability [28]. The information should include the location/level of mass in the spinal column. What is the quality of the mass (lytic or not)? Does the tumor involve posterior elements and/or the vertebral body? If the vertebral body is involved, is greater than 50% of the body affected? If there is a pathologic fracture, is the deformity greater or less than 50% of the height of the vertebral body? Is there subluxation or acquired deformity in either the sagittal or coronal plane? [28]

Illustrative Cases in Diagnostic Imaging

Case 1

This case of a 79-year-old male with neck pain shows typical appearance of tumors in bone. The normal, bright bone marrow on T1W images is replaced by focal areas of dark signal (Fig. 6.1a). Most neoplasms are higher signal on T2W images, and unfortunately typical fatty bone marrow is also higher signal on T2W images. Therefore T2-weighted images with fat suppression/saturation (such as STIR) are needed to clearly identify neoplastic masses (Fig. 6.1b).

The MR (Fig. 6.1c) and CT images show tumor in pedicles and pars (arrowheads in Fig. 6.2a, b) and areas of cortical bone loss (anterior aspect of right C1, white arrow in Fig. 6.2b). The lesions have no internal matrix. The margins varied: poorly defined in most areas and well-defined in a few other places.

Many features important in assessing spinal stability are present [28]. The quality of the bone lesions is that they are lytic. The pathologic fracture of C4 is greater than 50% of the height of

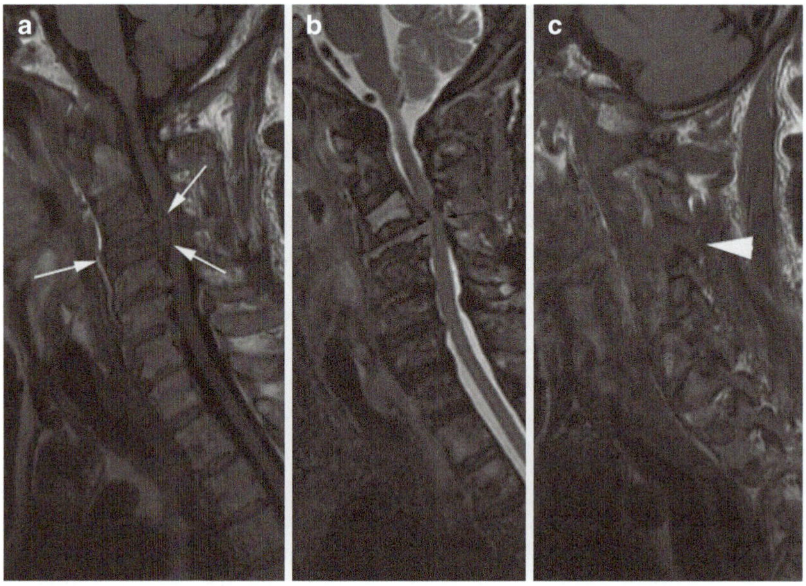

Fig. 6.1 Case 1: MRI in 79-year-old male with neck pain. (a) Sagittal T1W image shows pathologic fracture of C4 vertebral body with loss of greater than 50% of the height of the vertebral body and epidural tumor compromising the spinal canal (white arrows). Metastatic disease is also present in C3 vertebral body. (**b**) Sagittal STIR image shows the deformity and compression of the spinal cord (short black arrows). (**c**) Sagittal T1W image to the right of midline shows tumor involvement of the C4 pars interarticularis (white arrowhead) and pedicle. Metastatic disease is also present in right C1 vertebral arch

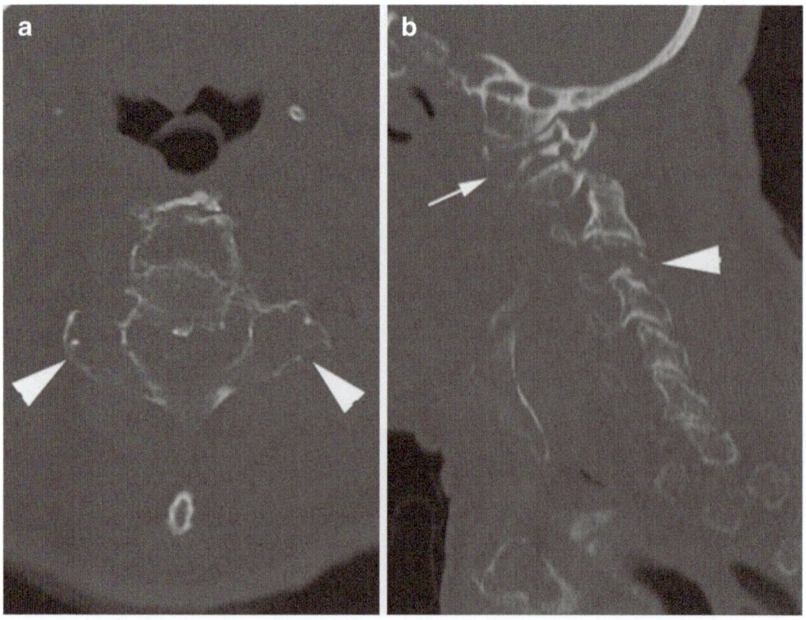

Fig. 6.2 Case 1: CT scan images in 79-year-old male with neck pain. (**a**) Axial CT bone technique image shows lytic disease in C4 pars interarticularis bilaterally (white arrowheads). (**b**) Sagittal CT bone technique image to the right of midline shows tumor involvement of the C4 pars interarticularis (white arrowhead). Tumor and pathologic fracture are seen in the right C1 vertebral arch (white arrow)

the vertebral body. There is involvement of the posterior elements. Multiple lesions are noted. Taken together the imaging suggests multiple aggressive neoplasms such as metastases or multiple myeloma (or lymphoma) in this patient's age group. The final histopathologic diagnosis was multiple myeloma.

Case 2

This case of a 73-year-old female with mild back pain illustrates a spinal lesion that should not be confused with a metastasis. The benign hemangioma of the spine is most often bright on T1W images (Fig. 6.3a) but can enhance on contrast-enhanced T1W images with fat saturation (Fig. 6.3c) [29]. It is often high signal on T2W images (Fig. 6.3b). CT scan shows the characteristic thickened vertical trabeculae (Fig. 6.3d) [2]. Bone scan typically shows no abnormal activity especially in smaller (less than 3 cm) hemangiomas [29].

Case 3

An 84-year-old male with primary lung cancer and back pain had CT scan for metastatic evaluation because cardiac pacemaker precluded MRI. Previous MRI obtained 12 years before was unremarkable (Fig. 6.4a). Suspicious new lytic areas were identified in the L1 and T11 vertebral bodies (Fig. 6.4b, c, arrows). The density of these abnormalities was higher than fat and there was no significant internal matrix. The margins were fairly well-defined. Overall metastatic disease remained a possibility. However, careful examination shows subtle endplate defects (Fig. 6.4c, arrowheads) indicating that the disc has herniated through the endplate into the vertebral body (Schmorl's node). A subsequent bone

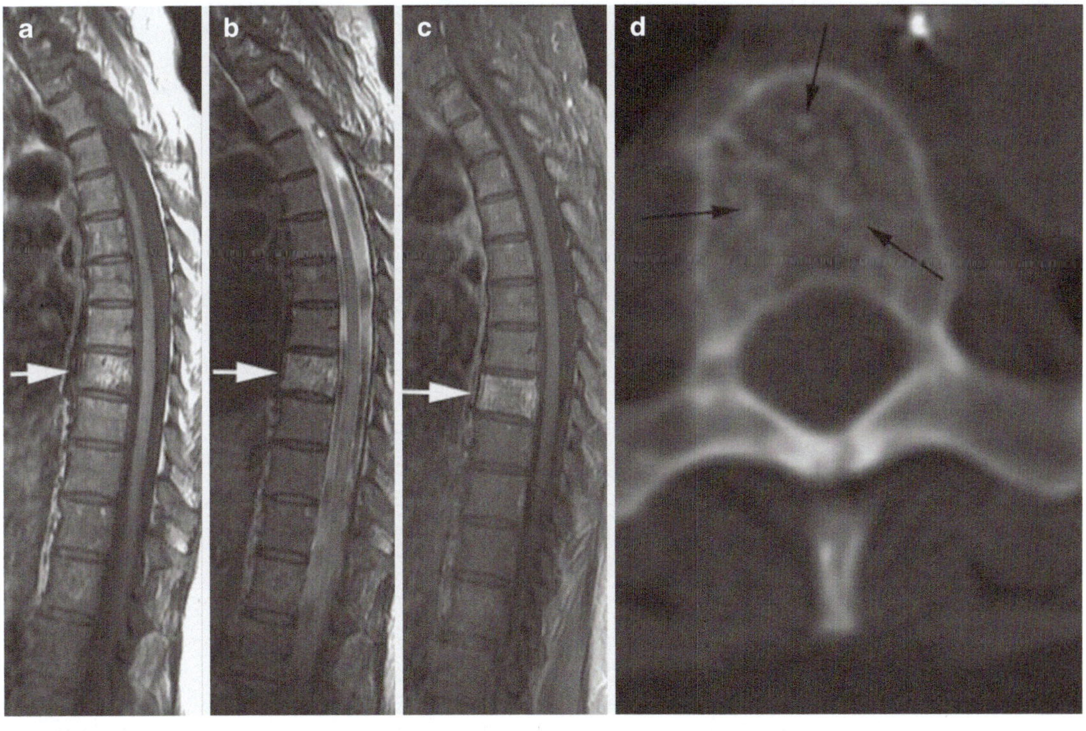

Fig. 6.3 Case 2: MRI and CT scan images in 73-year-old female with typical hemangioma. (**a**) Sagittal T1W image shows areas of bright signal in T8 vertebral body (white arrow). (**b**) Sagittal T2W image shows mostly areas of bright signal in T8 vertebral body (white arrow). (**c**) Sagittal T1W image with fat saturation and after intravenous contrast shows enhancement in the T8 vertebral body (white arrow). (**d**) Axial CT scan image from chest study shows typical thickened vertical trabeculae within the T8 hemangioma (black arrows)

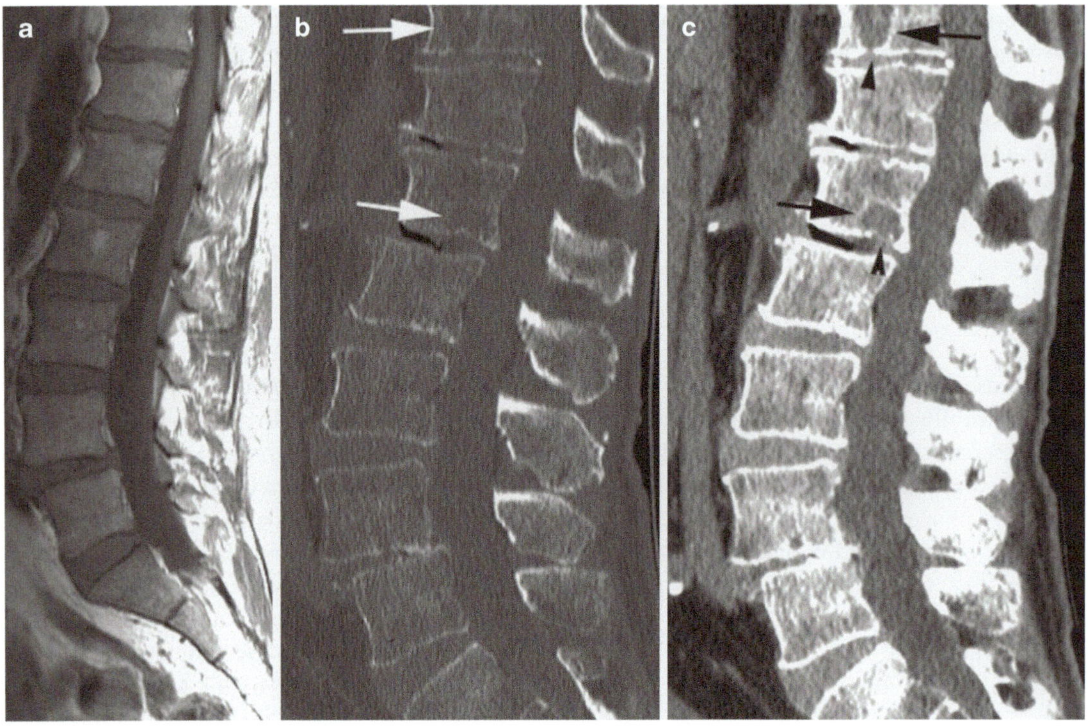

Fig. 6.4 Case 3: 84-year-old male with cardiac pacemaker was imaged with CT scan to evaluate for metastatic disease. (**a**) Previous MRI obtained 12 years ago showing normal bone marrow at L1 and T11. (**b**) CT Sagittal bone technique reconstruction. (**c**) CT Sagittal soft tissue technique. Suspicious new lucent areas were identified in the L1 and T11 vertebral bodies (arrows). Subtle endplate defects (arrowheads) indicating that the disc has herniated through the endplate into the vertebral body (Schmorl's node)

scan did not reveal any metastatic disease activity. An intraosseous disc herniation can mimic a neoplasm in the bone marrow [2]. Often on MRI, disc fragments can be dark on T1W images and intermediate to bright on T2W. They can even show enhancement, typically marginal.

Case 4

This 73-year-old female presents with an unusual abnormality. The T7 vertebral body lesion has a predominantly sclerotic matrix that is nonspecific (Fig. 6.5a). The anterior bony margin on axial CT image is fairly well-defined, but not a sharp sclerotic line (Fig. 6.5b). MRI shows extension across the disc into the upper T8 vertebral body (Fig. 6.6). A process that involves the disc always should bring to mind the possibility of infection. However the bulk of the abnormality is in the vertebral body, is well-defined, and does not enhance (Fig. 6.6). There is no soft tissue mass outside of the spine and adjacent to the abnormality; the endplates around the disc are sharp and well-defined. All of these features argue against infection. A neoplasm that can involve the disc and is high signal on T2W images is chordoma [27], but chordomas usually have some internal enhancement [2]. The final histopathologic diagnosis was benign notochordal neoplasm.

Case 5

The imaging evaluation of a 57-year-old female with back pain relies on MRI scans. Abnormalities (dark on T1W images and mostly bright on T2W images) involve multiple vertebral bodies and in the lower thoracic spine extend across disc spaces

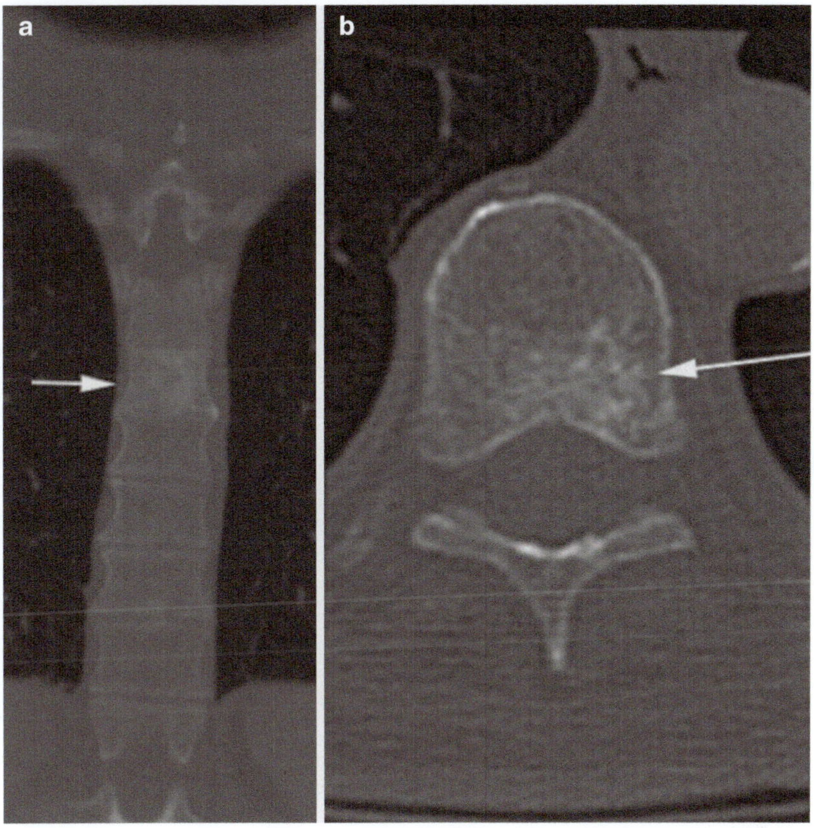

Fig. 6.5 Case 4: CT scan in 73-year-old female with unknown spine lesion. (**a**) Coronal CT scan reconstruction in bone window shows mostly sclerotic change in T7 lesion with small lytic component (white arrow). (**b**) Axial CT scan in bone window shows mainly sclerotic change (white arrow)

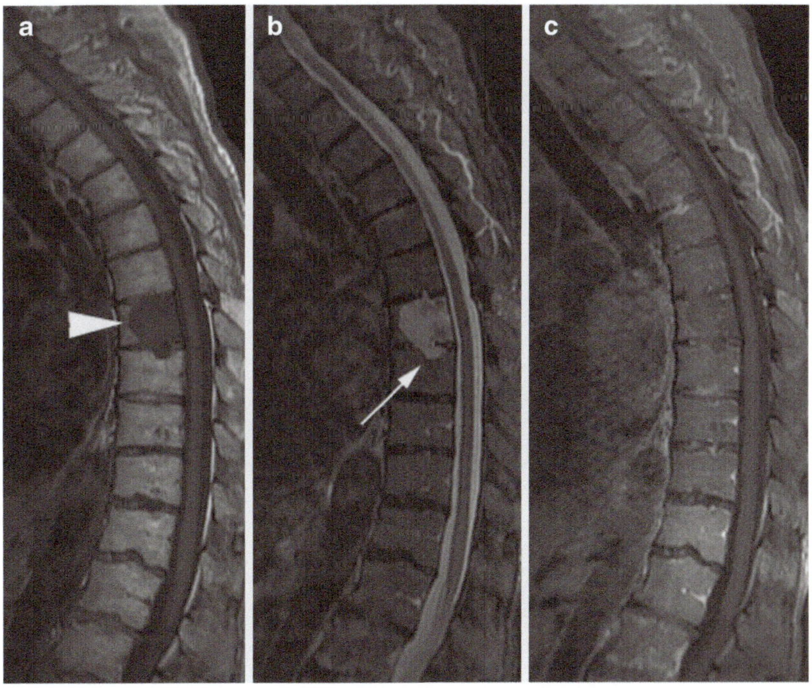

Fig. 6.6 Case 4: MRI in 73-year-old female with unknown spine lesion. (**a**) Sagittal T1W image shows areas of low signal in T7 vertebral body (white arrowhead). (**b**) Sagittal T2 STIR image very bright signal in T7 vertebral body which extends across disc into superior T8 vertebral body (white arrow). (**c**) Sagittal T1W image with fat saturation and after intravenous contrast shows no enhancement

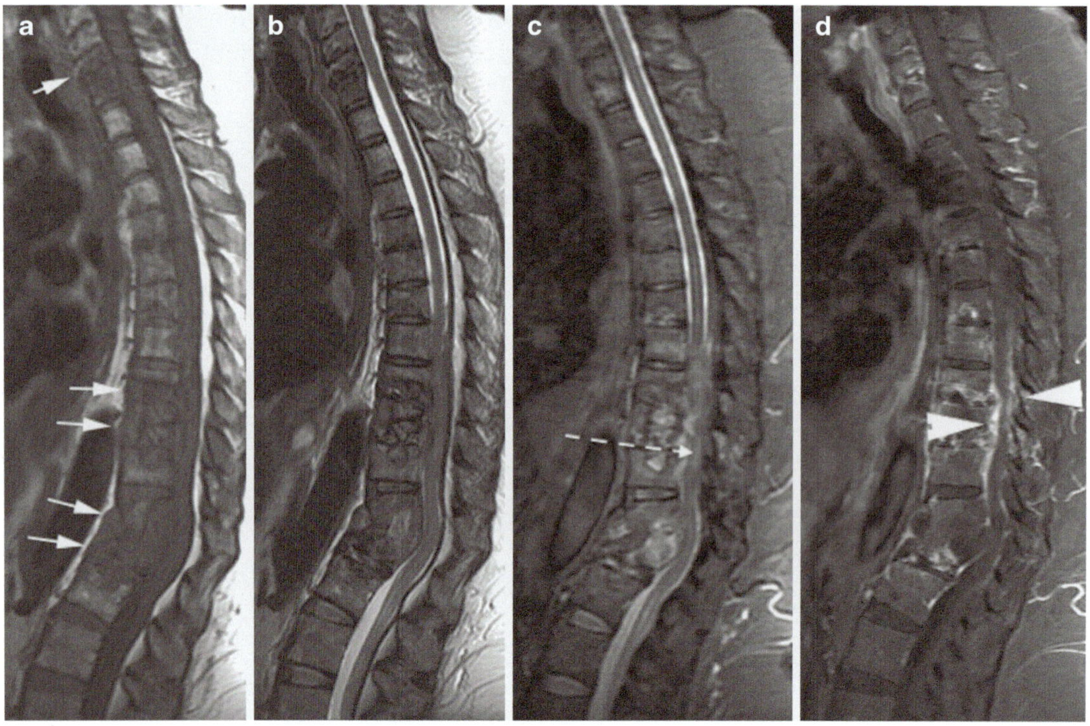

Fig. 6.7 Case 5: MRI in 57-year-old female with multiple spine lesions. (**a**) Sagittal T1W image shows areas of low signal in multiple thoracic vertebral bodies (white arrows). Compression deformity at the lowest arrow. (**b**) Sagittal T2W image demonstrates involvement across multiple intervertebral discs. (**c**) Sagittal T2 STIR image shows many of the lesions are bright/high signal. The epidural involvement results in signal change in the cord (dashed white arrow). (**d**) Sagittal T1W image with fat saturation and after intravenous contrast shows epidural extension, both ventrally and dorsally (arrowheads)

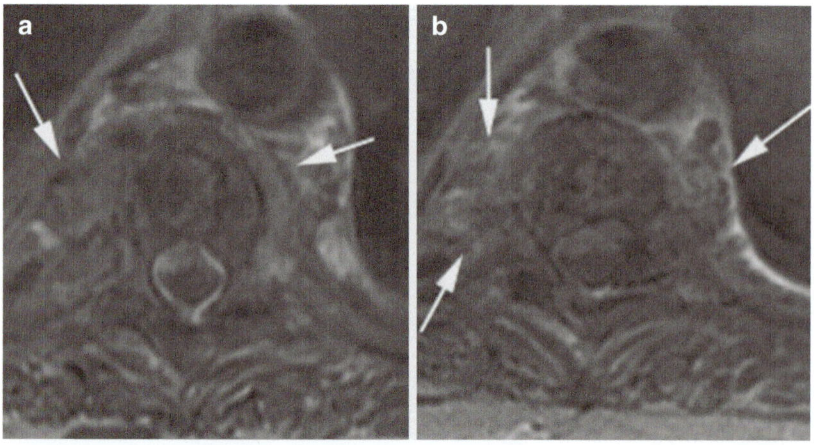

Fig. 6.8 Case 5: MRI in 57-year-old female with multiple spine lesions. (**a**, **b**) Axial T1W images after intravenous contrast show extensive paravertebral enhancing tissue (white arrows) in addition to epidural disease

(Fig. 6.7). The multiple disc space involvement argues against typical metastatic disease or multiple myeloma. The typical T2W very high signal of chordoma is not present. There is prominent paravertebral enhancing material as well as epidural involvement (Fig. 6.8). One of the lower thoracic vertebral bodies shows considerable deformity. Unusually for neoplasms, different areas show different enhancement characteristics: considerable enhancement of epidural and paravertebral disease (Fig. 6.8a), but little enhancement in many of the vertebral body lesions (Fig. 6.7d).

The disc involvement again raises the concern for infection. However, in contrast to bacterial spinal infection, the amount of disc disease (Fig. 6.7d) is small (little contrast-enhanced disease) in relation to the degree of vertebral body or paravertebral disease. This pattern suggests fungus or tuberculosis as the cause [30]. Indeed, the final diagnosis was tuberculosis.

Case 6

The case illustrates the analysis of the imaging of an unknown spinal mass in a 42-year-old male. The enhancing mass involves the spinal canal, right neural foramen, and paravertebral soft tissues (Figs. 6.9 and 6.10). The flow void of the right vertebral artery is displaced anteriorly (Fig. 6.10b). There is involvement of the C4 vertebral body with a mild pathologic fracture (Figs. 6.10 and 6.11) as well as the right pedicle and pars (Figs. 6.9d and 6.11c). In some areas the bone cortex is completely gone (Fig. 6.11c). The margins of the mass in the bone are slightly sclerotic in places (Fig. 6.11) and have a narrow margin or transition zone. CT scan does not identify an internal matrix of the mass either in the bone or outside bone. The lack of disc involvement and the large, fairly solidly enhancing appearance argue against infection and in favor of neoplasm. A neoplasm that involves both bone and adjacent soft tissues suggests an aggressive process such as metastases, multiple myeloma, or lymphoma [2]. The complete loss of cortical bone in areas also hints at a more aggressive process. However, the areas of sclerotic margins that seem well-defined or narrow favor a slow-growing neoplasm [2]. The final imaging diagnosis favored an aggressive neoplasm.

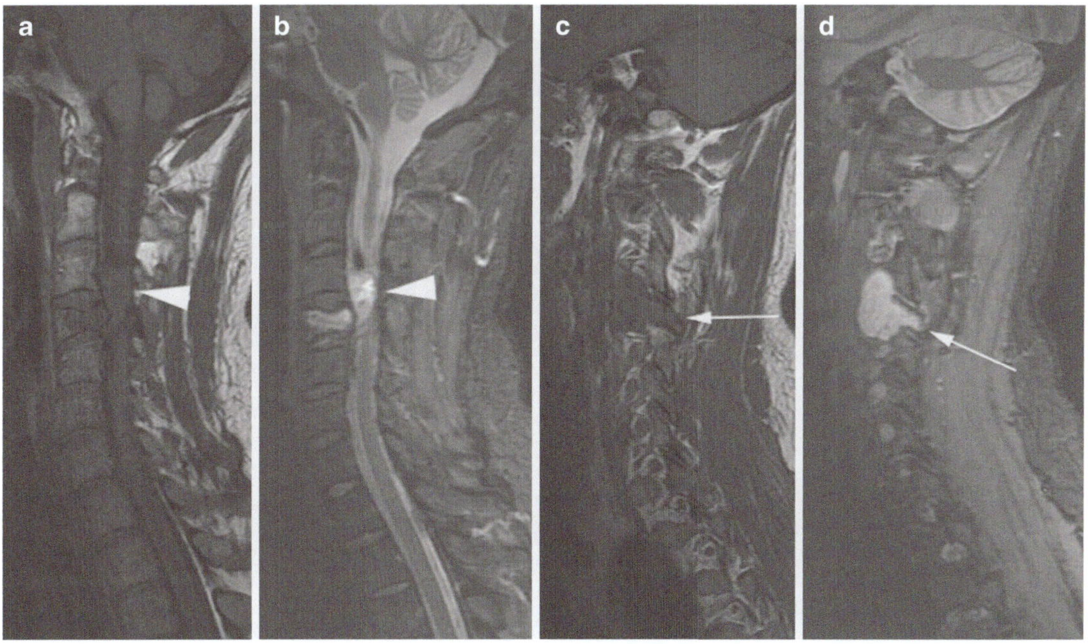

Fig. 6.9 Case 6: MRI in 42-year-old male with large spine mass. (**a**) Sagittal midline T1W image shows area of low signal in C4 vertebral body with epidural extension into spinal canal (arrowhead). (**b**) Sagittal midline T2 STIR image shows the lesion has bright/high signal including epidural component (arrowhead) and mild deformity of C4 vertebral body. (**c**) Sagittal right-sided T1W image shows lateral extension and involvement of the pars interarticularis (arrow). (**d**) Sagittal right-sided T2 STIR image shows lateral extension and involvement of the pars interarticularis (arrow)

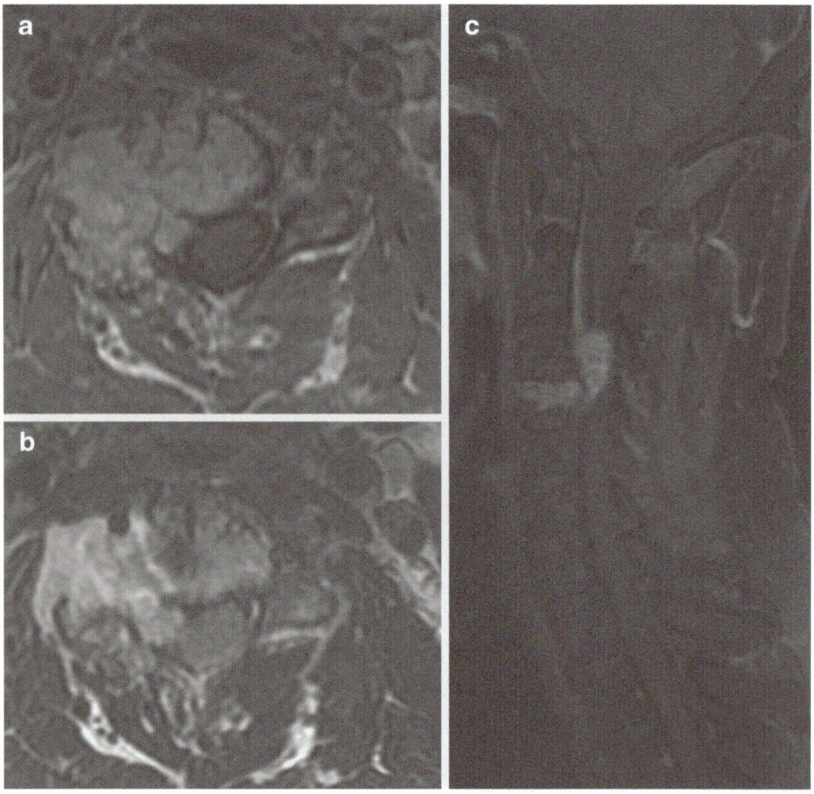

Fig. 6.10 Case 6: MRI in 42-year-old male with large spine mass. (**a**) Axial T1W image after intravenous contrast shows extensive right spinal and paravertebral enhancing tissue in addition to vertebral body and epidural disease. (**b**) Axial T2W image shows high signal in mass with anterior round dark flow void of right vertebral artery. (**c**) Sagittal T1W image after intravenous contrast shows enhancement in the mass

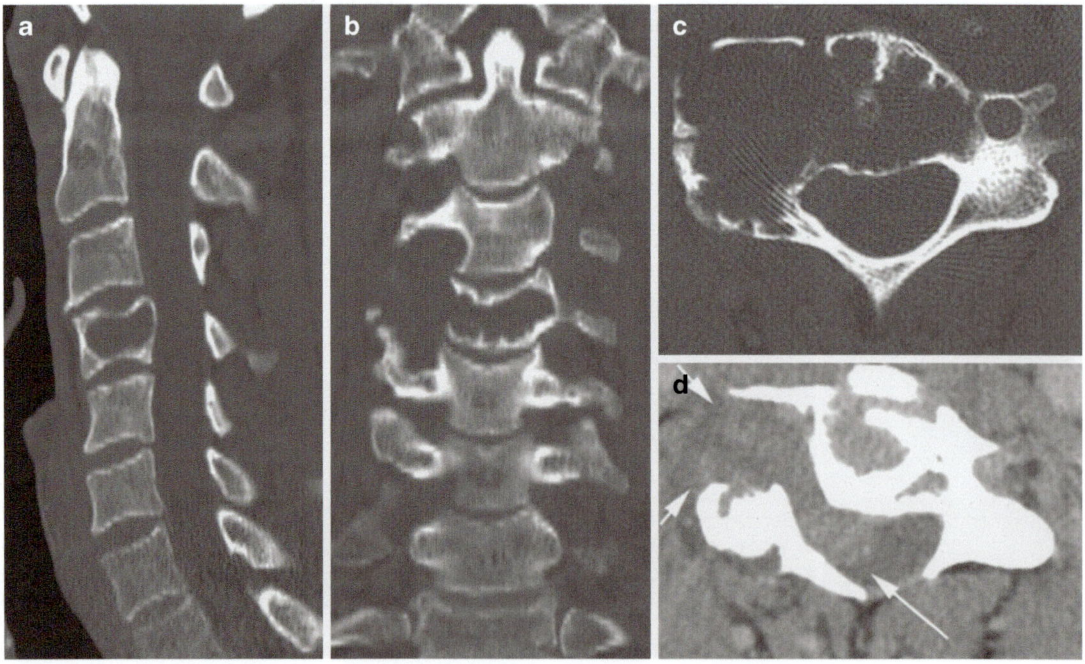

Fig. 6.11 Case 6: CT scan in 42-year-old male with large spine mass. (**a**) Sagittal CT scan reconstruction in bone technique shows lytic lesion and mild deformity at C4 vertebral body. (**b**) Coronal CT scan reconstruction in bone technique shows lytic change in C4 vertebral body and in the right-sided structures. (**c**) Axial CT scan image in bone technique shows lytic change in C4 vertebral body and in the right-sided structures back to the edge of the lamina. (**d**) Axial CT scan image in soft tissue technique shows the soft tissue mass extending from within the canal to the right paravertebral region (arrows)

However, the final histopathologic diagnosis was benign schwannoma which typically is a soft tissue mass which can affect adjacent bone due to slow growth including secondary benign pressure erosion. However, schwannoma can extend into bone or even arise within bone [31].

Case 7

In this case the imaging issues revolve around the utility of myelography and CT scan with myelographic (intrathecal) contrast. The patient is a 60-year-old male with progressive back pain and lower extremity weakness. He has had prior spine stabilization with pedicle screws and rods from T10 vertebral body to the sacrum. In such a case, MRI is often nondiagnostic or of limited diagnostic value because of metallic artifact. The routine radiographic images obtained during the myelogram show considerable epidural mass effect on the subarachnoid space at T10 level and loosening of T10 pedicle screws (Fig. 6.12). The subsequent CT scan (Figs. 6.13, 6.14, and 6.15) demonstrates fracture of the posterior T10 vertebral body and that the epidural material is soft tissue density (rather than bone or calcium). The axial CT images also show the effects of metallic artifact on CT scans: the details of the spinal canal are difficult to visualize at the level of the screws. The routine radiographic images obtained during the myelogram are not as affected by the metal and clearly show the compromise of the thecal sac (Fig. 6.12).

Therefore, in cases of spinal instrumentation, myelogram provides critical information that may not be obtained by MRI.

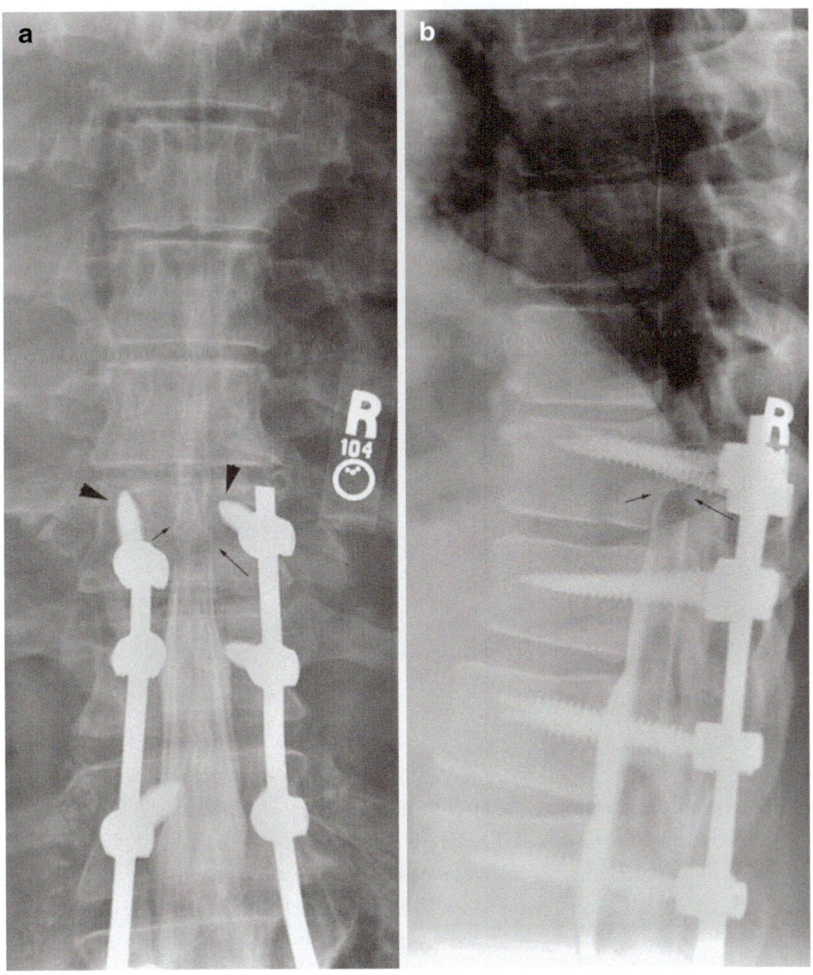

Fig. 6.12 Case 7: Myelogram in 60-year-old male with back pain and metallic spinal instrumentation. (**a**) Frontal view of lower thoracic spine after subarachnoid injection of myelographic contrast. Loosening of T10 pedicle screws (arrowheads) and epidural compromise of the subarachnoid space (small black arrows). (**b**) Lateral view of lower thoracic spine during myelogram. Circumferential epidural compromise of the subarachnoid space (small black arrows) at T10 level

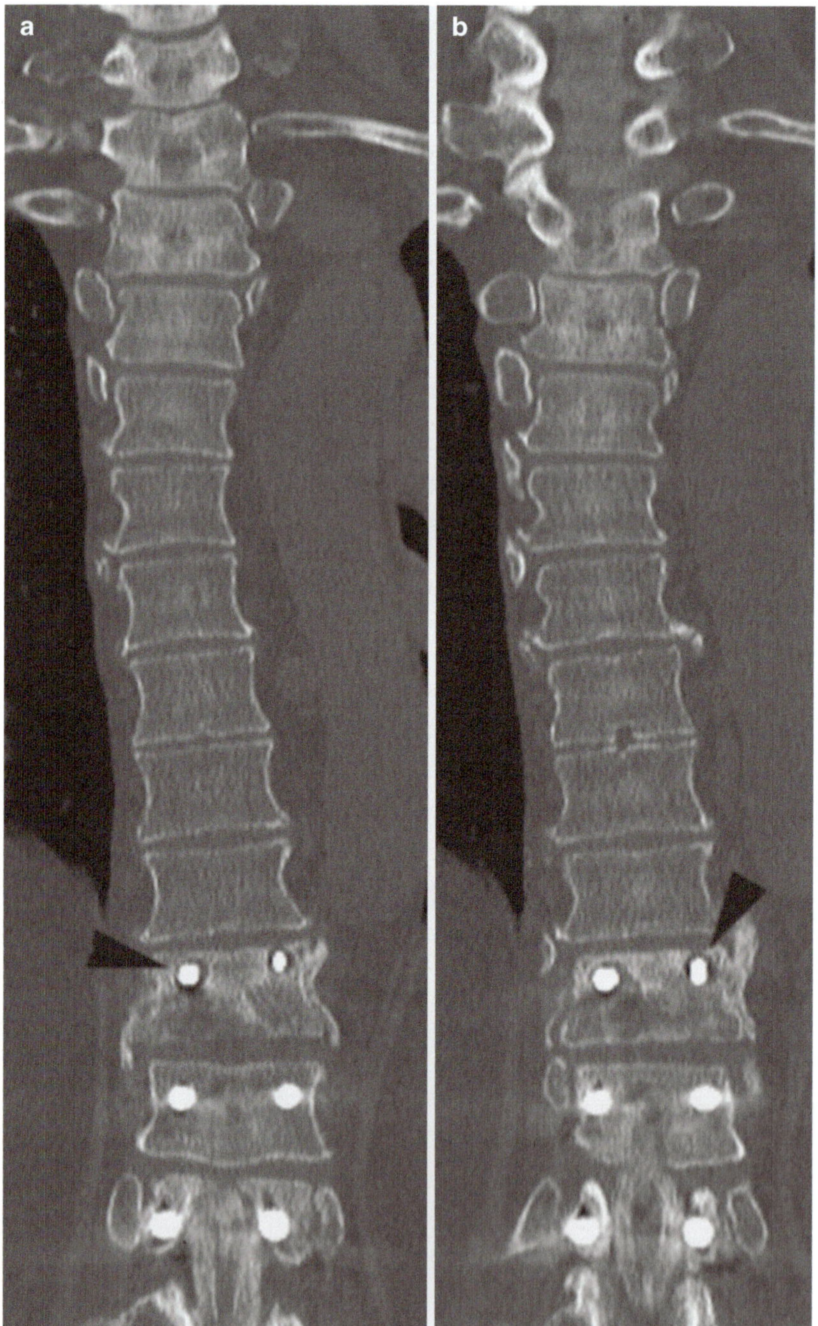

Fig. 6.13 Case 7: CT scan with myelographic contrast in 60-year-old male with back pain and metallic spinal instrumentation. (**a**, **b**) Coronal CT scan reconstructions in bone technique after myelogram. Loosening of T10 pedicle screws (arrowheads)

Case 8

This example shows how the metabolic information provided by FDG-PET can help increase specificity of imaging. A 41-year-old male with history of lymphoma underwent MRI for back pain. There is subtle abnormality in the dorsal epidural space best appreciated on the axial images (Figs. 6.16 and 6.17). However, no bone lesion is noted. Lymphoma or metastasis in the epidural space is most often the result of a spinal bone mass with secondary extension into the epidural compartment. The same issue arises when considering epidural infection: usually the result

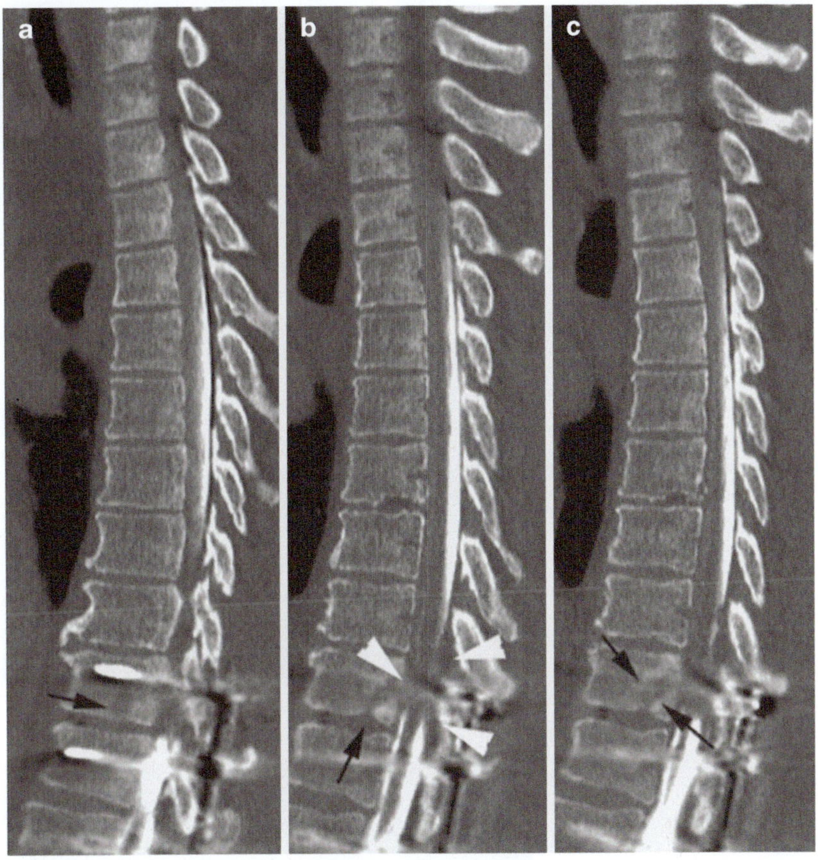

Fig. 6.14 Case 7: CT scan with myelographic contrast in 60-year-old male with back pain and metallic spinal instrumentation. (**a**–**c**) Sagittal CT scan reconstructions in bone technique after myelogram. Epidural material compromising thecal sac (white arrowheads). Fracture of posterior T10 vertebral body (black arrows)

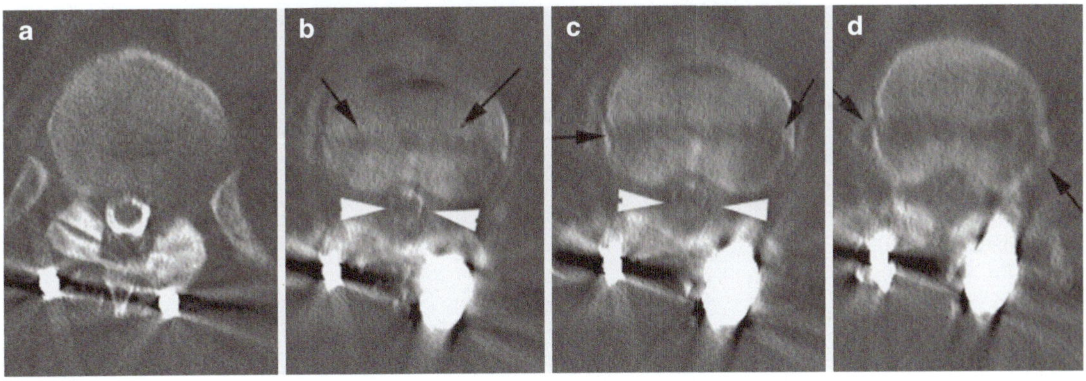

Fig. 6.15 Case 7: CT scan with myelographic contrast in 60-year-old male with back pain and metallic spinal instrumentation. (**a**–**d**) Inferior to superior axial CT scan images at T10 after myelogram. Epidural material compromising thecal sac (white arrowheads). Fracture of posterior T10 vertebral body (black arrows). Metallic artifact obscures details especially at level of pedicle screws

of secondary spread from discitis/osteomyelitis. Another consideration is that the epidural space can enlarge due to venous engorgement in the setting of intracranial (CSF) hypotension. The clinical setting can help exclude infection and intracranial hypotension. In this case, a subsequent ^{18}F-FDG PET scan (Fig. 6.18) confirmed active neoplasm as the cause of the epidural abnormality. Lymphoma can arise secondarily or even primarily in the epidural space [32].

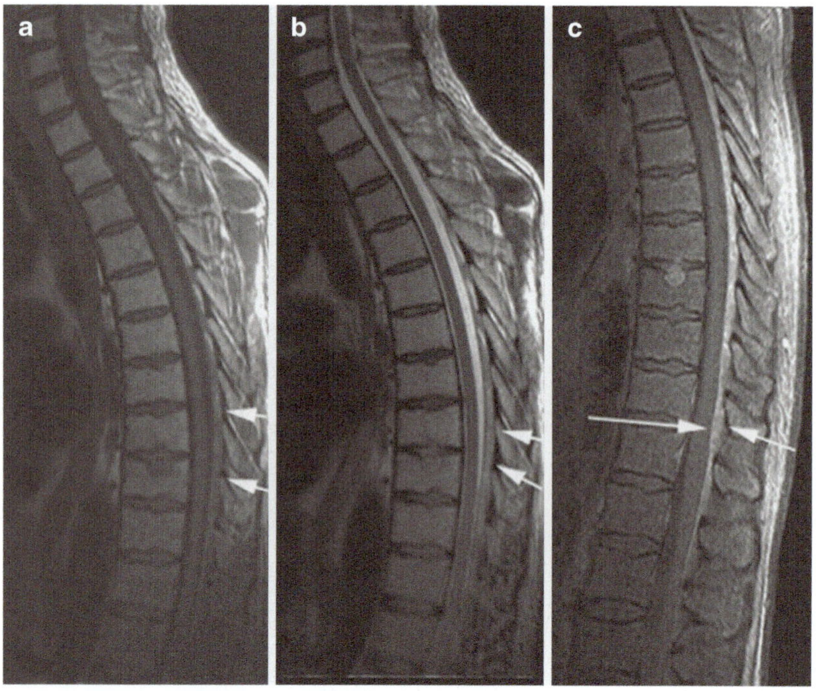

Fig. 6.16 Case 8: MRI in 41-year-old male with lymphoma. (**a**) Sagittal midline T1W image shows subtle low signal in posterior epidural space where there is usually high signal fat (arrows). (**b**) Sagittal midline T2W image without fat suppression shows subtle low signal in posterior epidural space where there is usually high signal fat (arrows). (**c**) Sagittal T1W image with fat suppression after intravenous contrast shows enhancement in posterior epidural space (arrows)

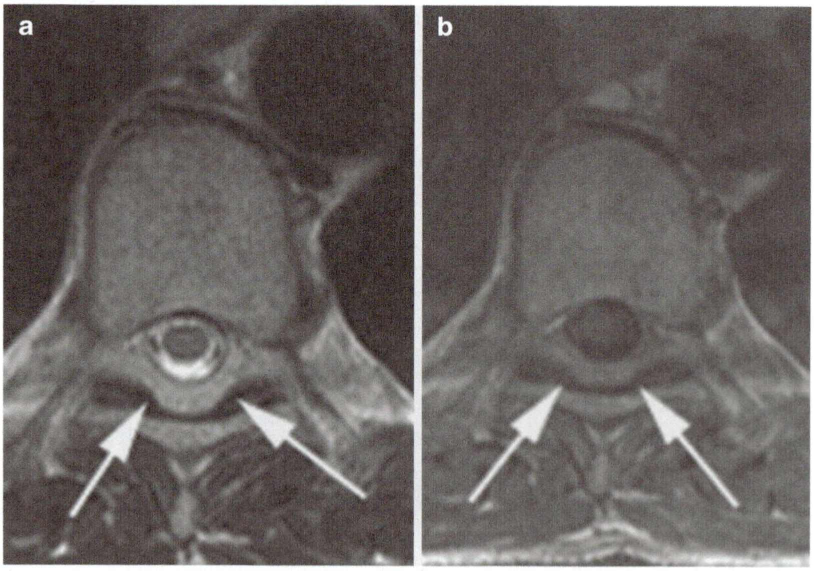

Fig. 6.17 Case 8: MRI in 41-year-old male with lymphoma. (**a**) Axial T2W image shows subtle low signal in posterior epidural space which is slightly enlarged (arrows). (**b**) Axial T1W image low signal in posterior epidural space (arrows)

Case 9

The final examples demonstrate the appearances of benign, acute fractures. The typical vertebral body acute osteoporotic fracture has band-like, almost linear edema (Fig. 6.19). A collection or cleft of fluid may be present (upper vertebral body in Fig. 6.19b). However, recent fractures usually enhance (Fig. 6.19c) which should not be confused with neoplasm. Edema or signal abnormality involving the pedicles is not exclusive to neoplasms but can occur in acute fractures (Fig. 6.20). In uncertain cases, the options include biopsy, ^{18}F-FDG PET scan, and follow-up imaging.

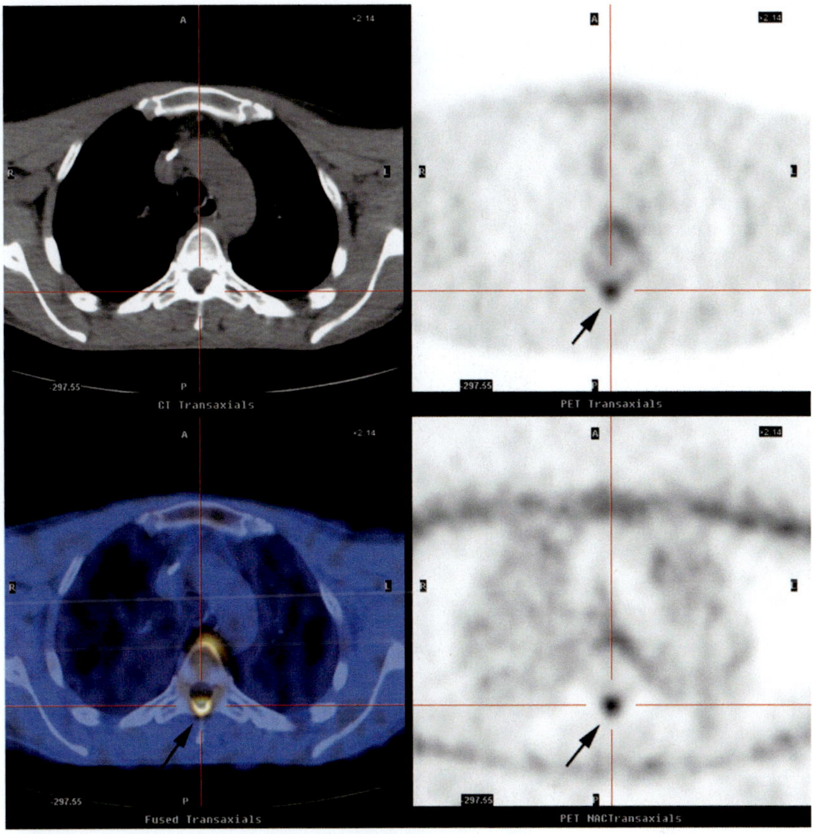

Fig. 6.18 Case 8: ^{18}F-FDG PET in 41-year-old male with lymphoma. Axial images show high metabolic activity in posterior thoracic epidural space (arrows)

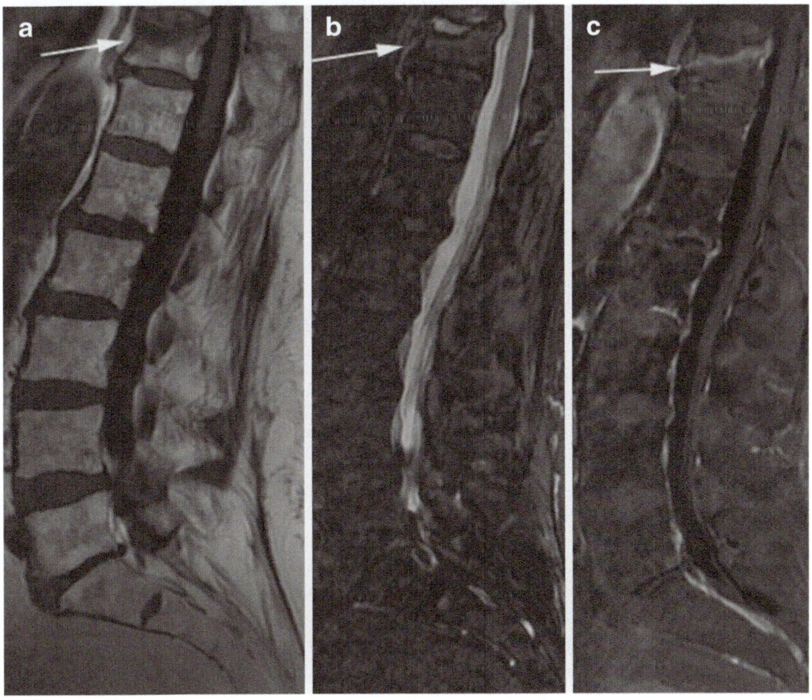

Fig. 6.19 Case 9: 70-year-female with acute back pain from benign fracture. (**a**) Sagittal midline T1W image shows low signal in deformed upper T11 vertebral body where there is usually high signal fat (arrow). (**b**) Sagittal midline STIR image shows high signal in deformed upper T11 vertebral body (arrow). (**c**) Sagittal T1W image with fat suppression after intravenous contrast shows enhancement in T11 vertebral body (arrow)

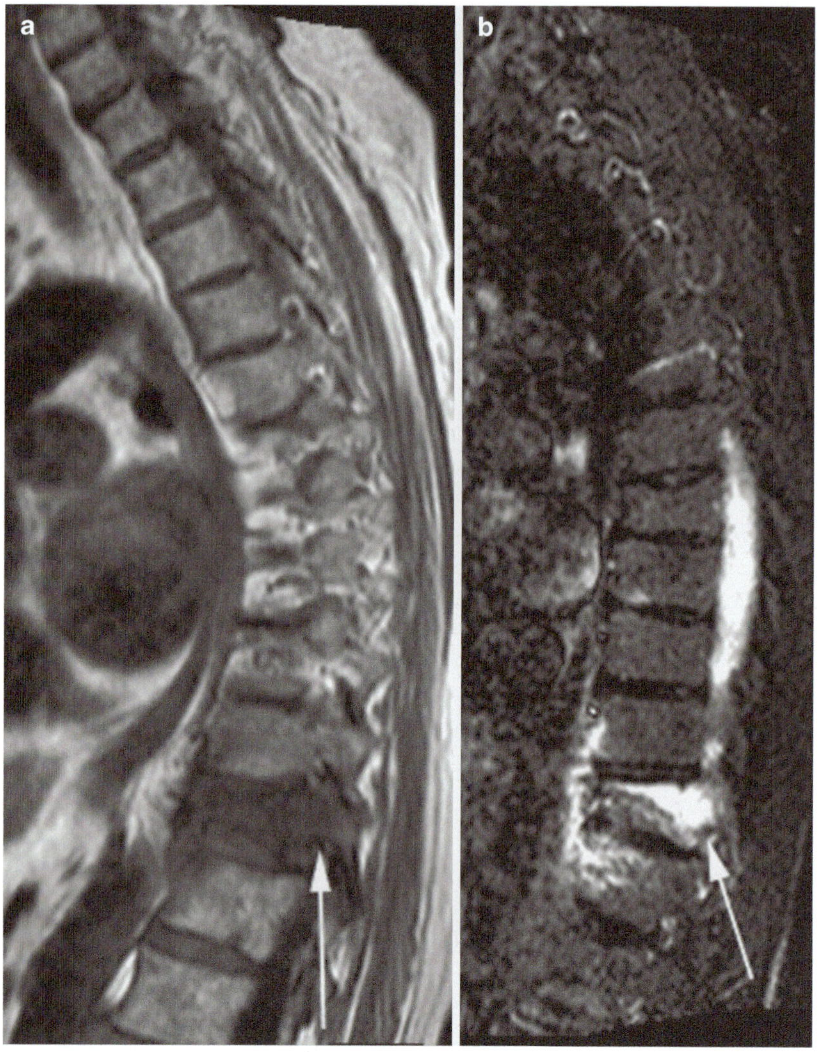

Fig. 6.20 Case 9: 82-year-old female with acute back pain from benign fracture. (**a**) Sagittal T1W image shows low signal in right T11 pedicle (arrow). The vertebral body itself shows considerable deformity and edema. (**b**) Sagittal STIR image shows high signal, edema in right T11 pedicle (arrow)

References

1. Denis F. The three column spine and its significance in the classification of acute thoracolumbar spinal injuries. Spine. 1982;8(8):817–31.
2. Rodallec MH, Feydy A, Larousserie F, et al. Diagnostic imaging of solitary tumors of the spine: what to do and say. Radiographics. 2008;28:1019–41.
3. Sutcliffe P, Connock M, Shyangdan D, et al. A systematic review of evidence on malignant spinal metastases: natural history and technologies for identifying patients at high risk of vertebral fracture and spinal cord compression. Health Technol Assess. 2013;17(42):1–274.
4. Bartels RH, van der Linden YM, van der Graaf WT. Spinal extradural metastasis: review of current treatment options. CA Cancer J Clin. 2008;58(4):245–59.
5. Batson OV. The function of the vertebral veins and their role in the spread of metastases. Ann Surg. 1940;112(1):138–49.
6. Hoey RP, Sanderson C, Iddon J, et al. The parathyroid hormone-related protein receptor is expressed in breast cancer bone metastases and promotes autocrine proliferation in breast carcinoma cells. Br J Cancer. 2003;88(4):567–73.
7. Iddon J, Bundred NJ, Hoyland J, Downey SE, Baird P, Salter D, et al. Expression of parathyroid hormone-related protein and its receptor in bone metastases from prostate cancer. J Pathol. 2000;191(2):170–4.
8. Lee YT. Breast carcinoma: pattern of metastasis at autopsy. J Surg Oncol. 1983;23(3):175–80.

9. Bubendorf L, Schopfer A, Wagner U, et al. Metastatic patterns of prostate cancer: an autopsy study of 1,589 patients. Hum Pathol. 2000;31(5):578–83.
10. Coleman RE. Clinical features of metastatic bone disease and risk of skeletal morbidity. Clin Cancer Res. 2006;12(20 Pt 2):6243s–9s.
11. Mak KS, Lee LK, Mak RH, et al. Incidence and treatment patterns in hospitalizations for malignant spinal cord compression in the United States, 1998-2006. Int J Radiat Oncol Biol Phys. 2011;80(3):824–31.
12. Roodman GD. Mechanisms of bone metastasis. N Engl J Med. 2004;350(16):1655–64.
13. Yin JJ, Pollock CB, Kelly K. Mechanisms of cancer metastasis to the bone. Cell Res. 2005;15(1):57–62.
14. Dispenzieri A. POEMS syndrome: update on diagnosis, risk-stratification, and management. Am J Hematol. 2015;90(10):951–62.
15. Sciubba DM, Petteys RJ, Dekutoski MB, Fisher CG, Fehlings MG, Ondra SL, et al. Diagnosis and management of metastatic spine disease. A review. J Neurosurg Spine. 2010;13(1):94–108.
16. Patchell RA, Tibbs PA, Regine WF, et al. Direct decompressive surgical resection in the treatment of spinal cord compression caused by metastatic cancer: a randomised trial. Lancet. 2005;366(9486): 643–8.
17. Bushberg JT, Seibert JA, Leidholdt EM Jr, Boone JM. The essential physics of medical imaging. 3rd ed. Philadelphia, PA: Lippincott Williams & Wilkins; 2012.
18. Hamaoka T, Madewell JE, Podoloff DA, Hortobagyi GN, Ueno NT. Bone imaging in metastatic breast cancer. J Clin Oncol. 2004;22(14):2942–53.
19. Gouliamos AD, Jimenez JP, Goree JA. Computed tomography and skull radiography in the diagnosis of calcified brain tumor. AJR Am J Roentgenol. 1978;130(4):761–4.
20. Lin E, Alessio A. What are the basic concepts of temporal, contrast, and spatial resolution in cardiac CT? J Cardiovasc Comput Tomogr. 2009;3(6): 403–8.
21. Yang HL, Liu T, Wang XM, Xu Y, Deng SM. Diagnosis of bone metastases: a meta-analysis comparing (18) FDG PET, CT, MRI and bone scintigraphy. Eur Radiol. 2011;21(12):2604–17.
22. Galasko CSB. The pathological basis for skeletal scintigraphy. J Bone Joint Surg Br. 1975;57:353–9.
23. Woolfenden JM, et al. Comparison of bone scintigraphy and radiography in multiple myeloma. Radiology. 1980;134(3):723–8.
24. O'Sullivan GJ, Carty FL, Cronin CG. Imaging of bone metastasis: an update. World J Radiol. 2015; 7(8):202–11.
25. Chang CY, Gill CM, Joseph Simeone F, et al. Comparison of the diagnostic accuracy of 99 m-Tc-MDP bone scintigraphy and 18 F-FDG PET/CT for the detection of skeletal metastases. Acta Radiol. 2016;57(1):58–65; Epub 2014 Dec 22.
26. Kumar R, Guinto FC, Madewell JE, David R, Shirkhoda A. Expansile bone lesions of the vertebra. Radiographics. 1988;8:749–69.
27. Raut AA, Naphade PS, Chawla A. Imaging of skull base: pictorial essay. Indian J Radiol Imaging. 2012;22(4):305–16. https://doi.org/10.4103/0971-3026.111485.
28. Fisher CG, Versteeg AL, Schouten R, Boriani S, Varga PP, Rhines LD, Heran MK, Kawahara N, Fourney D, Reynolds JJ, Fehlings MG, Gokaslan ZL. Reliability of the spinal instability neoplastic scale among radiologists: an assessment of instability secondary to spinal metastases. AJR Am J Roentgenol. 2014;203(4):869–74.
29. Han, Boo Kyung, et al. Bone SPECT imaging of vertebral hemangioma correlation with MR imaging and symptoms. Clinical Nuclear Medicine. 1995;20(10): 916–21.
30. Shanley, Dean J. Tuberculosis of the spine: imaging features. AJR. American Journal of Roentgenology. 1995;164(3):659–64.
31. Ida, Cristiane M., Scheithauer, Bernd W, Yapicier, Ozlem, et al. Primary schwannoma of the bone: a clinicopathologic and radiologic study of 17 cases. The American Journal of Surgical Pathology. 2011;35(7): 989–97.
32. Cugati G, Singh M, Pande A, et al. Primary spinal epidural lymphomas. J Craniovertebr Junction Spine. 2011;2(1):3–11.

7 Management of Metastatic Spinal Cord Compression Without Stereotactic Radiotherapy and Targeted Adjuvant Chemotherapy

Alessandro Gasbarrini, Gisberto Evangelisti, Riccardo Ghermandi, Marco Girolami, Guiseppe Tedesco, Valerio Pipola, and Stefano Boriani

Introduction

The incidence of bone metastatic deposit from carcinoma is second only to pulmonary and hepatic metastases. The most frequently affected segment of the skeleton is the vertebral column. It is estimated that more than 10% of tumor patients develop symptomatic spinal metastases and that 70% of them have evidence of metastatic disease at the time of death [1–5].

The vertebral bodies are reached largely via the bloodstream. There is evidence that blood from many anatomic sites drains directly into the axial skeleton. In a milestone postmortem study, Batson demonstrated that venous blood from the breast and the pelvis flowed not only to the vena cava but also into the venous plexus extending from the pelvis to the epidural and perivertebral veins [6].

This may explain, at least in part, the tendency of the breast, prostate, kidney, and lung to produce metastases in the axial skeleton. The molecular and cellular biology of the tumor cell and the tissue to which they metastasize also influences the pattern of metastatic spread. Tumor dissemination is a multistep process involving specific tumor and host–tissue interactions via specific molecular determinants. In recent years, many basic and translational studies focus on the effect of angiogenesis on the growth of the primary tumor and micrometastatic deposits, as well as the increased accessibility of tumor cells to the systemic circulation.

Refinement of the protocols for treating tumor patients has led to an increase in life expectancy for many patients with metastatic disease [5].

Moreover scientific progresses in the field of imaging have led to early diagnosis of secondary lesions in patients affected by a tumor. There are thus more patients with symptomatic spinal metastases who are living longer yet severely affected in terms of their quality of life [3].

The choice of the most appropriate treatment is of crucial importance for the patient who may be severely disabled by the presence of untreated spinal metastases. These spinal metastases may not only be the cause of severe deterioration in the quality of life but also the direct or indirect

A. Gasbarrini, MD · G. Evangelisti, MD
R. Ghermandi, MD · M. Girolami, MD · G. Tedesco
V. Pipola, MD
Department of Oncologic and Degenerative Spine Surgery, Rizzoli Orthopaedic Institute, Bologna, Italy

S. Boriani, MD (✉)
GSpine4 Spine Surgery Unit, IRCCS Galeazzi Orthopaedic Institute, Milan, MI, Italy
e-mail: sb@stefanoboriani.eu

R. A. W. Marco (ed.), *Metastatic Spine Disease*, https://doi.org/10.1007/978-3-319-76252-4_7

cause of death. Although there is widespread agreement in the literature regarding the need to treat symptomatic metastases, the optimal protocol to adopt is still a matter of discussion.

Bone metastases is an expression of a systemic disease, and therefore a multidisciplinary program, integrating radiotherapy (RT), chemotherapy (CHT), and surgery, is recommended [7, 8].

Our center does not currently have stereotactic radiotherapy, nor do we have access to some of the emerging adjuvant treatments for different histologic subtypes. We work with our multidisciplinary team with the treatment options available at our center. We believe that some patients who are candidates for surgery at our institution may be managed nonoperatively at other centers with access to newly developed adjuvant chemotherapy with or without stereotactic radiotherapy. It is vital, in our opinion, to underline that multidisciplinary does not mean fragmentary. It is less convenient, more time-consuming, and potentially risky for a patient with the diagnosis of SCC to be evaluated by single specialists outside of a collegial context of caregivers dedicated to the different aspects of the same disease. Our center advocates the designation of a "team leader" who works in strong collaboration with the entire multidisciplinary team. In our opinion the leader should be the medical specialist of the primary tumor, while the spine surgeon and the radiotherapist provide support for the team leader. The most common presenting symptom in patients with SCC is pain [9, 10].

The pain is often intractable and not responsive to major analgesic drugs. Although spinal tumors might be asymptomatic for relatively long periods, pain can be caused by (1) tumor expansion beyond the cortex of the vertebral body which stretches the periosteum and stimulates pain receptors (the cortex eventually breaks and the tumor invades the paravertebral tissues); (2) tumor compression of the spinal cord and/or nerve roots; (3) instability caused by progressive replacement of bone with tumor, which increases the risk of fracture of the vertebral body (impending fracture); and (4) pathological fracture in the vertebra weakened by tumor, which causes acute onset of pain. These patients do not report a history of trauma, and the fracture is thus considered a low-energy fracture. It is therefore important to consider a new onset of back or neck pain in a patient with a known history of cancer as likely due to metastatic spinal disease until proven otherwise.

Neurological deficits may be caused by both compression of the tumor on the spinal cord or nerve roots or by sudden retropulsion into the canal of tumor and bone as a result of a pathological fracture.

Metastatic epidural spinal cord compression (MESCC) is defined radiologically as an epidural metastatic lesion causing true displacement of the spinal cord from its normal position in the vertebral canal (Fig. 7.1) [11, 12]. It is estimated to occur in 5–10% of patients with cancer and in up to 40% of patients who have pre-existing bone metastases outside the spine [13].

Although the clinical progression of cord compression is not predictable, patients with motor weakness inevitably progress to complete paralysis in the absence of intervention [14].

MESCC is an oncologic emergency that, unless diagnosed early and treated promptly, can lead to permanent neurologic damage. The neurological status at the time of diagnosis, particularly motor function, has been shown to correlate with the prognosis of MESCC [15], thus supporting the concept that diagnosis and treatment before the development of a neurological deficit is of paramount importance [12].

MESCC differs from the type of compression associated with high-energy vertebral body fractures. The onset of spinal cord compression is usually slower in patients with metastatic disease, which allows the patient to

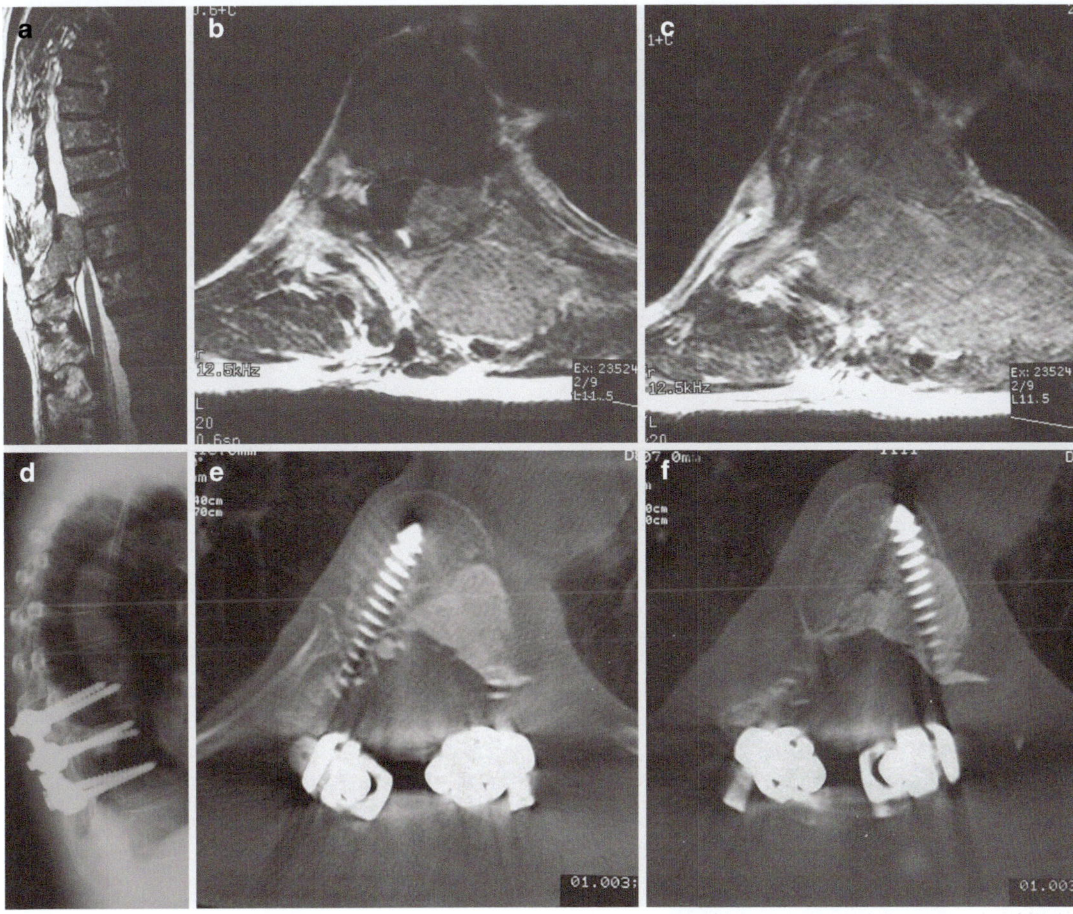

Fig. 7.1 S. A., 58 years old, solitary metastasis from hepatocarcinoma of T10 8 years after liver transplantation. Frankel class at onset: B. Surgical strategy: intralesional curettage (debulking) through a posterior approach. Frankel class at discharge: D. (**a**) Sagittal MRI shows pathologic neoplastic tissue within the spinal canal which compresses the neural structures and involves the posterior arch of the vertebra. (**b**) The axial view at T9 shows that the pathologic neoplastic tissue occupies the 50% of the vertebral canal. (**c**) MRI at T10 shows neoplastic tissue that occupies practically the entire vertebral canal and that the neural structure is confined to virtual anterolateral space. (**d**) Postoperative lateral X-ray of the T9–T11 posterior stabilization with PMMA within the vertebral body portion previously occupied by the tumor. (**e**) CT shows the T10 pedicle screw and the PMMA in the contralateral pedicle. Figure (**f**) shows the screw within the PMMA with a stabilizing function

adapt to the presence of progressive spinal cord compression. In contrast, the compression of the spinal cord is sudden, and a bony fragment is often expelled into the spinal canal in patients who sustain a high-energy vertebral body fracture. This sudden compression of the spinal cord does not allow the neurologic structures to adapt, so neurologic injury is usually instantaneous. The neural elements are also often subjected to elongation and stretching which compounds the injury sustained by these structures (Fig. 7.2).

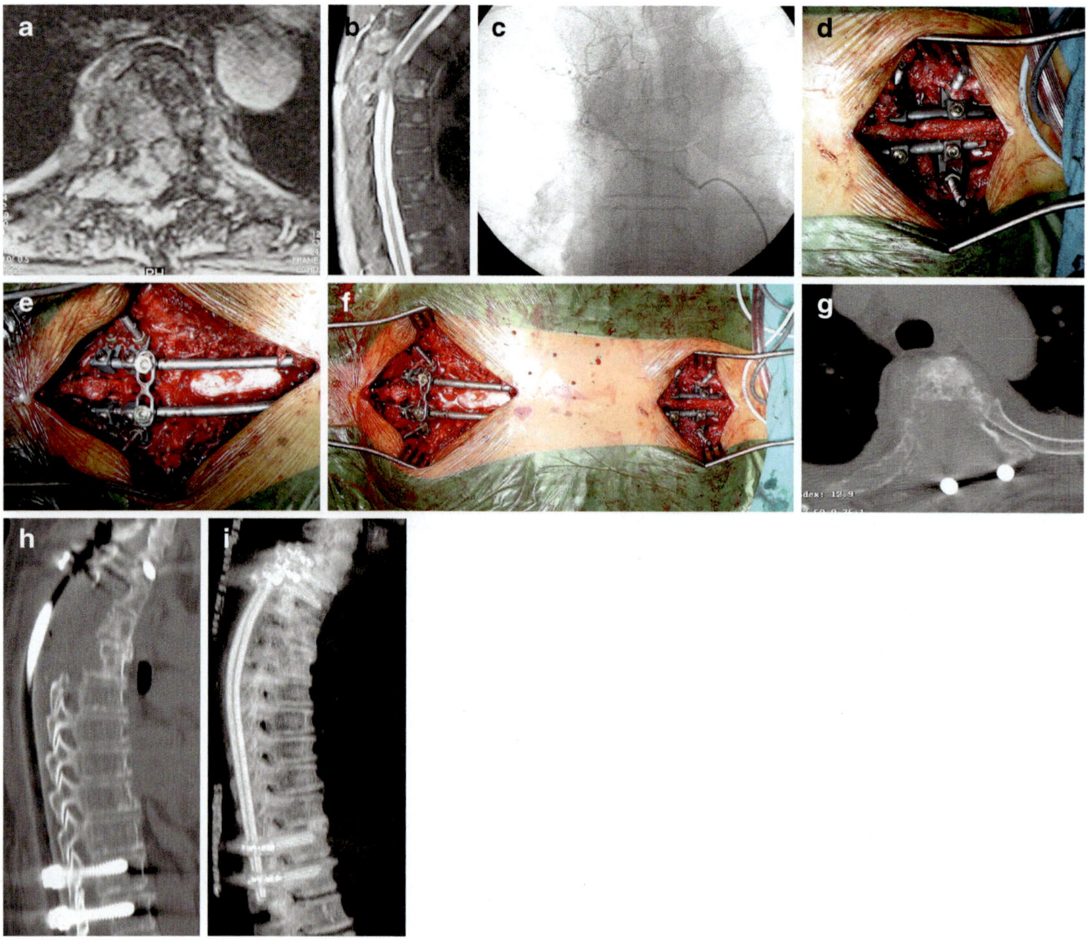

Fig. 7.2 C.G., 69 years old, multiple metastasis from breast cancer. Pathologic fractures of T4 with a medullary compression at T4–T5 level and multiple vertebral localization from T6 to T10. Onset Frankel class: B. Surgically treated with decompression and stabilization through double posterior approach. At discharge Frankel class: D. (**a**) Axial MRI at T3 showing complete anatomic disruption and medullary compression. (**b**) Sagittal MRI showing pathologic tissue compressing the neural structures at T2–T4 level and T3 fracture on segmental kyphosis; clearly visible also the metastatic localization at T5-T7-T8-T10. (**c**) Preoperative embolization of the T3 lesion in order to reduce the intraoperative bleeding. (**d**) Intraoperative 1: prone decubitus. Posterior approach to the upper thoracic spine. Pedicle screws at T1–T2, circumferential decompression at T3–T4 level with complete release of the neural structures. (**e**) Intraoperative 2: second posterior approach to the lower thoracic spine; bilateral pedicle screws at T11–T12 level. (**f**) Intraoperative 3: connection with prebent bars sliding under the paravertebral muscles. Limited blood loss and pain. Earlier start of adjuvant therapy. (**g**) Postoperative axial CT showing the circumferential decompression at T4 level. (**h**) Postoperative axial CT showing the circumferential decompression at T4 level sagittal view. (**i**) 3D reconstruction 16 months after RT and hormonotherapy

Role of Spine Surgery in Metastatic Spinal Cord Compression Treatment

The most appropriate treatment for patients with metastatic disease of the vertebral column is controversial.

As the number of patients with MESCC increases, the methods of treatment are also evolving. In the past decades, the surgical management was focused on laminectomy, in order to surgically decompress the neurological structures, followed by radiotherapy directed to achieve a more durable local control of the disease [16–21].

Initial decompression of the neural elements provided short-term pain control but did not provide spinal stability. In fact, removal of the lamina further destabilized patients with spinal cord compression associated with tumor within the vertebral body as these patients were reliant on the posterior tension band created by the ligamentous attachments to the spinous processes. Mobilization of these patients often led to progressive kyphosis, deformation of the spinal cord, progressive neurologic dysfunction, and recurrent pain. A prospective, randomized study by Young et al. [20] demonstrated equivalent outcomes for patients treated with radiation only compared to laminectomy and radiation. These results led many providers to conclude that radiotherapy was the optimal treatment for patients with MESCC. Technological advances in spinal surgery allowed surgeons to decompress and stabilize the spine, which led to a trend toward treating patients with surgery rather than conventional radiotherapy [21].

In a prospective, randomized study, Patchell et al. [22] reported that significantly more patients who underwent decompression and stabilization were able to walk after treatment (84% vs. 57%) compared to those treated with radiation and corticosteroids. These authors also reported that patients who had surgery retained their ability to walk significantly longer (153 days vs. 53 days). Critical evaluation of the Patchell study elicits several study biases that favor surgery. Knowledge of these potential biases along with patient-centered treatment algorithms and advances in chemotherapy, radiotherapy, and minimally invasive spine surgery have decreased the number of patients who currently undergo decompression and stabilization in many centers.

The first element to be considered in the decision-making process for a spine metastasis is diagnosis. In the spine, a CT-guided trocar biopsy performed through the pedicle without invading the epidural space seems to be the best way to gain the pathological diagnosis without spreading the tumor cells.

The evolution of anesthesiological techniques allowed surgical treatments that were previously considered prohibitive. The problem is to know which is the best sequential process to arrive at the most appropriate treatment considering the individual general conditions of the patient and the parameters of the metastasis.

The aim of surgery in case of cord compression might be one, or an association, of the following:

- Neurological function preservation or recovery from a neurological deficit
- Pain relief
- Spinal stability restoration
- Local control of the tumor

Even though local control of the tumor is a target of the treatment of metastases, it is not always achieved surgically. In fact, the wide variety of histotypes which may deposit in the spine differs in the sensitivity to nonsurgical treatments (such as RT, hormonal therapy, and immunotherapy). Moreover, it is intuitive that the longer the expected survival of the patient is, the greater is the possibility that the disease might relapse (with eventual compression of the spinal cord and/or pathological fracture), thus the differential importance of achieving durable local control.

It is important for the surgeon to be aware of the various options available to achieve local control of the various different histotypes, whether surgical or not.

From our prospective the surgical techniques in spine metastasis can be summarized into (1) decompression and stabilization, (2) intralesional excision (curettage or debulking), and (3) en bloc resection, these latter two followed by reconstructive procedures (with various techniques). All these operations can be performed by either the anterior, posterior, or combined approaches.

1. Decompression and stabilization: This is the quickest and least aggressive surgical procedure. It can be performed anteriorly or posteriorly through open or minimally invasive approaches or posteriorly. Combined approaches are not commonly used in this setting. A decompressive

laminectomy with or without removal of the epidural tumor is combined with posterior stabilization. The authors believe that it is mandatory to stabilize the spinal column at the same time. This procedure is indicated for patients with short-term prognosis who may have neurologic compromise and/or a pathological fracture. Surgeon familiarity and efficiency with these techniques allows this procedure to be performed in an urgent or emergent setting. Anterior decompression and stabilization is more commonly associated with visceral and vascular complications; thus fewer centers recommend this approach. Preoperative selective arterial embolization can decrease blood loss associated with vascular tumors like renal cell carcinoma and thyroid carcinoma.

2. Intralesional excision (curettage or debulking): The tumor is directly approached either anteriorly, posteriorly, or circumferentially and removed in a piecemeal fashion in order to achieve circumferential decompression of the spinal cord and decrease tumor burden. This procedure is often performed as part of a multidisciplinary approach and is preceded by selective preoperative arterial embolization for select tumors. This operation is indicated for metastases not sensitive to radiotherapy associated with a pathological fracture or spinal cord compression or when a tumor debulking is recommended to enhance oncological treatments.
3. En bloc resection: This procedure is most commonly performed for patients with primary malignant bone tumors, and it is occasionally recommended for a patient who has a middle- to long-term prognosis and a solitary metastasis from a tumor that is relatively resistant to chemotherapy and radiotherapy. The operation can be performed by a posterior approach alone or a combined anterior and posterior approach. En bloc resection is associated with a lower local recurrence rate, but the risk-to-benefit ratio is very high due to the morbidity of these long operations (8–16 h). En bloc resection is also considered in highly vascularized tumors as this type of resection may lead to less blood loss than an intralesional excision [23]. In most of the cases, a spine metastasis with such a relevant encroachment of the canal to provoke a cord symptomatic compression is not suitable to en bloc resection due to the lack of the surgical criteria to perform such kind of procedure [24]. Adjuvant treatment (i.e., RT, hormonal therapy) may decrease the incidence of local recurrence and distant progression of the tumor.

The Role of Minimally Invasive (MI) Techniques in MESCC

Various new minimally invasive techniques are emerging for treatment of spinal metastases. For a technique to be considered minimally invasive, there must be less collateral tissue damage but same exact intended surgical goal as traditional open procedure. These techniques aim to decrease morbidity and allow a quicker functional recovery but without compromising postoperative results.

Minimally invasive stabilization can be achieved using percutaneous, cannulated screws. This type of stabilization is considered for patients with an unstable spine associated with tumors that are responsive to adjuvant treatment. The instrumentation provides an internal brace, while the limited extent of the surgery potentially enhances functional recovery. Computer-assisted surgery may enhance the surgeon's ability to place percutaneous pedicle screws [25].

A minimally invasive decompression can be performed using endoscopic tubular retractors at the level of the compression. A posterior decompression is readily performed using this technique. However, a circumferential decompression may not be as thorough as an open posterolateral decompression, so it may be advisable to limit this approach to tumors with a lesser degree of spinal cord compression.

A variety of percutaneous procedures are available to improve pain and achieve stabilization, including percutaneous cement augmentation with vertebroplasty or kyphoplasty with or without radiofrequency ablation [26–29]. Video-assisted thoracoscopic surgery can be used to access the spine from T1 to T12 and perform corpectomies for resection of the tumor [12, 30].

Thoracoscopy has a steep learning curve and requires the surgeon to have a good knowledge of segmental surgical anatomy as well as the technical skills to use the long working arm of the equipment [30].

Laparoscopic approaches can also be used for retroperitoneal access to the lumbar spine for decompression and corpectomy [31].

Some authors suggest combining posterior procedures with minimally invasive anterior approaches, such as extreme lateral transpsoas (XLIF or LLIF) or anterior to psoas approaches, in order to directly decompress the anterior compression and reconstruct the anterior column.

Extreme care must be taken in patient selection when these challenging techniques for anterior column exposure are taken into consideration in this population of patients since general conditions often preclude its use (i.e., single-lung ventilation), or equal results could be achieved by multidisciplinary treatment plans (i.e., surgery + RT/CHT/hormonal/immunotherapy). In our experience, indications are so uncommon that their use can be considered anecdotal [12].

Local control of the disease can be achieved using various energy sources—i.e., high-frequency alternating current, argon gas, and plasma fields—that have been applied directly on the tumor through probes in order to produce tissue necrosis. These techniques—radiofrequency ablation, cryoablation, and cavity coblation, respectively [26–29, 32]—can be combined with stabilization techniques in order to restore segmental stability and achieve local control of the disease with the least tissue exposure possible.

Radiofrequency ablation not only produces the thermal destruction of the tumor (even if not completely histologically shown) but also thrombosis of the perivertebral venous plexus. The most severe complication of this technique is the thermal cytolysis of the neural structures, even if it seems that the integrity of the back cortical wall may be a protective barrier for the neural structures, as the presence of cortical bone can significantly reduce the temperature [32]. Indeed, the authors think that the presence of cerebrospinal fluid between the tumor mass and the spinal cord is enough to avoid some thermal damages, even if they dissuade the use of thermo-ablation in the case of wide vertebral osteolysis with invasion of the back vertebral wall.

Plasma-mediated radiofrequency, which lacks the collateral heating associated with conventional radiofrequency, has been used to ablate tissues such as intervertebral disks and cartilage and to debulk a tumor mass before vertebroplasty or kyphoplasty. The technique involves the percutaneous insertion of a cannula through which a plasma-mediated radiofrequency wand is passed. The tumor tissue can be ablated, vaporizing the mass into nitrogen and carbon dioxide. The wand has a coagulation mode for use in hypervascular tumors. When most of the tumor has been ablated, the cavity can be filled with cement [33]. Cryoablation has been used in the management of pain and rehabilitation and for posterior spinal pain syndromes arising from the facet joint or the region of the sinuvertebral nerve [34]. The successful use of cryosurgery to ablate lesions in the vertebral body has also been described [26].

Electrochemotherapy combines systemic bleomycin use with electric pulses delivered locally [28]. These electric pulses permeabilize cell membranes (electroporation) in the tissue, allowing bleomycin delivery diffusion inside the cell and its cytotoxicity. The applied electrical field is generated using stainless steel electrodes placed around the tumor tissue.

The authors include selective arterial embolization in this group even if it cannot be considered a real minimally invasive technique but rather a minimal treatment that can be used as a palliative procedure (and eventually repeated) in inoperable patients or in case of inoperable lesions. More often it is performed as adjuvant preoperative procedure in order to decrease intraoperative blood loss in case of any procedure that implies violation of the tumor pseudocapsule (decompression and stabilization with or without tumor debulking) [34–36].

Percutaneous vertebral body augmentation techniques (vertebro- or kyphoplasty) can be done in order to restore strength of the affected vertebra. Various authors report good results in terms of pain control after PMMA injection [32, 37–40].

However, its use in spinal metastases differs from that in osteoporotic vertebral compression fractures. Indeed, while osteoporosis decreases bone mass, the tumor occupying the vertebra has predominantly solid consistency, and when cement is injected inside the vertebra without having first removed it, this can go inside the spinal canal, worsening or causing compression, or anyway outside of the vertebra, causing a further dissemination of the disease.

An interesting experimental study by Reidy and collaborators [41] showed that the presence of tumor causes an increase of pressure of about eight times inside the vertebral body and this can determine the uncontrolled migration of tumor material or cement. This would be justified by the different hydraulic permeability of the neoplastic tissue so that its smaller "porosity" prevents and hinders diffusion of the PMMA within it. This also could explain the dishomogeneous distribution of cement inside the vertebral body.

Vertebroplasty does not determine a local control of the disease, even if an antineoplastic role of PMMA has been hypothesized, so if the tumor does not respond to adjuvant therapies and continues to grow, PMMA can be further displaced into the epidural space.

Some authors, trying to get local control of the disease and reduce the migration of the cement inside the perivertebral vessels, propose the combined use of techniques such as radiofrequency ablation with vertebroplasty. Some changes of the physical properties of the tumor mass and the hydraulic permeability can reduce the intravertebral pressure following vertebroplasty and therefore the risk of PMMA spillage, the most common complication.

In a recent series of 97 procedures in patients with intractable pain secondary to pathological fractures of the vertebral body marked or complete relief from pain was achieved in 84%. There were no deaths or complications related to the procedure. Precise indications are evolving for vertebroplasty and kyphoplasty in relation to metastatic spinal disease. The technique is safe and effective for treating intractable pain secondary to vertebral fractures and may be especially effective in conjunction with radiotherapy for patients with radiosensitive tumors such as multiple myeloma [42].

However, it must be emphasized that this is not a treatment for epidural compression of the cord, but provides a less invasive means of stabilization of the spine and can be useful in providing support of the anterior column when used in combination with posterior decompression and pedicle screw fixation.

Decision-Making in Case of Metastatic Spinal Cord Compression

First of all a multidisciplinary approach involving specialists in oncology, hematology, histopathology, spinal surgery, radiation oncology, and radiology is required. The treatment of MESCC is primarily palliative with the aim of restoring or preserving neurological function, relieving pain, and maintaining or restoring spinal stability.

The first element to be considered, as previously said, in the decision-making process for treatment of spine metastases is diagnosis. In the spine, a CT-guided trocar biopsy performed through the pedicle without invading the epidural space seems to be the best way to reduce the spread of the tumor cells.

While for the treatment of primary tumors a systematic approach has been accepted, there are no accepted guidelines in the treatment of spinal metastases.

Protocols of chemotherapy (CHT), hormone therapy, immunotherapy, and radiotherapy exist and are progressively increasing survival for the majority of solid and hematologic tumors. Chemotherapeutic agents can be classified into antitumor drugs and those which minimize the secondary effects of the tumor [12, 43].

Except in tumors such as Ewing's sarcoma and neuroblastoma which are chemosensitive, antitumor drugs have a limited role in the treatment of spinal metastases. However drugs which prevent or ameliorate the effects of spinal tumors, such as corticosteroids, bisphosphonates, and analgesics, are widely used.

Corticosteroids are the mainstay of the pharmacological treatment of pain associated with spinal metastases and the acute neurological deterioration that may occur. They decrease edema of the spinal cord which may have an oncolytic effect on certain tumors, such as lymphoma, myeloma, and breast cancer [44].

Observation on animal model have confirmed the clinical findings that individuals treated with dexamethasone achieve improved motor function more quickly than untreated controls [43].

The optimum dosing schedules for corticosteroids in patients with MESCC have not been determined prospectively. Indeed, it has been shown that there was no difference in outcome with regard to pain, walking, or bladder function with the administration of an initial intravenous bolus of 100 mg compared with that of 10 mg [12, 45–47].

We give 16 mg of dexamethasone per day, in four individual doses of 4 mg, preoperatively for 5–7 days to patients with MESCC, except for those with a lymphoma, and then reduce the dose over 5–7 days after operation. Bisphosphonates can be given orally or intravenously to inhibit osteoclastic activity. They do not prevent skeletal metastases, but are used to treat hypercalcemia, reduce pain, and decrease the risk of fracture by affecting bone metabolism and inhibiting osteoclastic activity, particularly in patients with myeloma and breast and prostate cancer.

However, drugs cannot effectively control pain and functional impairment from vertebral body collapse and cord compression from epidural space invasion.

Moreover, the erroneous certainty that patients with secondary skeletal localizations should be considered terminal, and therefore not of orthopedic interest, makes often surgery urgent and essential (if feasible), with increasing operative risks for the patient and difficulties to its relatives/caregivers/beloved and to the healthcare facility taking in charge of these problems.

The indications for surgery include the need to establish a diagnosis, to prevent or treat spinal instability, and to resolve epidural compression with cord dysfunction from bone or tumor and radioresistant tumors, those which recur despite radiotherapy and neurological deterioration during the latter. The timing of surgery is an important factor contributing to the likely neurological outcome. If definitive treatment of MESCC is planned, in our opinion, this should be started within 24 h. If there is rapid deterioration in the neurological state, the operation must be undertaken as soon as possible. If deterioration is gradual, surgery can be planned for the next scheduled list. Early studies comparing the efficacy of decompressive laminectomy without stabilization to that of radiotherapy found no difference in the outcome or survival [20]. This surgical approach did not address the most common site for spinal metastases, namely, in the vertebral body which causes neural compression as the tumor extends dorsally and destabilizes the spine [44]. Subsequently, surgery was usually not advocated until radiotherapy had failed. Technical advances which allow circumferential decompression of the spinal cord combined with stabilization of the spine have allowed more aggressive and more effective surgical procedures to be used for patients with MESCC. Improved results using better surgical techniques of circumferential decompression and stabilization have led to the concept that, in some circumstances, the outcome may be improved after total spondylectomy or en bloc resection [48–50].

It has been suggested that this may be a potential cure for patients with involvement at a single spinal level without metastases, in certain tumors such as renal cell carcinoma [3, 51–54].

However, a recent review recommends that for such patients stereotactic radiosurgery should be the first line of treatment rather than en bloc excision [55].

The definition of metastatic or neoplastic instability is still not clear. Fracture–dislocation, a translational deformity, and significant collapse with mechanical pain are accepted criteria for surgical stabilization. Three-column destruction, progressive deformity, and pain may also be considered for stabilization procedures. The Spine Oncology Study Group have proposed the Spinal Instability Neoplastic Score [56], which encompasses the location of the tumor, the character and type of pain related to movement, the quality of the bone, spinal alignment, vertebral collapse, and involvement of the posterior elements. This may prove to be valuable in deciphering which patients require a stabilization procedure.

Finally, it can be said that a patient with diffuse neoplastic disease, generally impaired conditions, and incipient neurological deficit should be treated with palliative decompression and stabilization followed by radiotherapy which may noticeably improve the quality of life.

On the other hand, in a patient in good general conditions suffering from a primary tumor with a relatively positive prognosis and a symptomatic isolated spinal metastasis, more aggressive treatment similar to that for a primary tumor is justified.

Sioutos et al. [5] statistically analyzed the factors influencing the incidence of complications and length of survival after surgical treatment of spinal metastases and showed that this is influenced by preoperative neurological conditions, the histotype of the primary tumor, and the number of vertebrae involved, but not by the spread of the disease or the age of the patient. On the basis of these observations, the authors recommend careful selection of both patient candidates for surgical treatment and the surgical treatment itself. Many factors must be taken into account when choosing the most appropriate surgical technique: the general conditions of the patient, the histotype of the primary tumor and its sensitivity to adjuvant treatments, the spread of the disease, and the current neurological conditions [12].

The surgical approach is dictated by the location of the tumor, the site of compression on the spinal cord, the histology of the tumor, and the type of spinal reconstruction or stabilization which will be required once the tumor has been resected. Vascular tumors, including renal cell carcinoma, thyroid carcinoma, and hepatocellular carcinoma, can be embolized preoperatively to decrease blood loss during surgery. Intraoperative neurophysiological monitoring using somatosensory and motor-evoked potentials are useful adjuncts. Anterior approaches commonly provide the best access to metastatic tumors causing compression of the cord since these frequently arise from the vertebral body and extend dorsally. The upper thoracic (T1–T4) region presents a particular challenge and may require the combination of an anterolateral cervical approach and a sternotomy, with or without thoracotomy [57].

However, a posterior transpedicular approach to decompress the ventral aspect of the spinal cord is becoming more popular because of the invasive nature of the anterior approach, particularly at these levels [58, 59].

The T5–T10 levels are best approached through a thoracotomy from the right side to avoid the great vessels and aortic arch. However, the bulk of the extravertebral tumor usually dictates the side of approach [57].

Approaches to the T11–L1 region often require a combined thoracotomy and a retroperitoneal approach, and metastases at L2–L4 can be reached through an incision in the flank. Tumor limited to L5 is most commonly managed by posterior decompression and stabilization [44].

Combined anteroposterior decompression and stabilization can be carried out either in a single setting or staged. Posterior stabilization with pedicle screw instrumentation is advocated in patients with significant kyphosis, with lesions at the thoracolumbar junction or to supplement anterior reconstruction in patients who undergo two or more adjacent vertebrectomies [44].

The editor prefers posterior decompression and stabilization with or without transpedicular excision of the tumor for the vast majority of patients indicated for decompression and stabilization of the thoracic or lumbar spine rather than subjecting these patients to a sternotomy, thoracotomy, or retroperitoneal anterior approach.

Flow Chart for Multidisciplinary Management of Metastases in the Mobile Spine

The literature proposes many preoperative scoring systems to classify patients by creating repeatable treatment protocols [18, 19, 59, 60, 61].

These scores, using a range of prognostic factors, have been devised and correlated with clinical outcomes to predict survival. They allow the recognition of patients who are unlikely to do well after surgery and the choice of suitable management. Recognized systems include that of Tomita et al. [60] and the revised scheme of Tokuhashi et al. [59]

The former uses three factors which have been shown to be significant, namely, the grade of malignancy and the presence of visceral metastases and metastases in bone. The Tokuhashi scoring system additionally differentiates the primary site of the neoplasm and the influence of the neurological status to predict survival. While these systems are tremendously useful in the planning of an elective approach to spinal metastases, they are not suitable for use in emergency cases in which the necessary informations for determining the parameters cannot be assembled quickly enough.

On the basis of our experience, we have built up an algorithm [18, 62] for treating spinal metastases in which the importance of the parameters taken in consideration varies according to when they are considered in order to tailor the best treatment available at the moment on each individual patients (Fig. 7.3). Indeed each patient follows his or her personal sequential process which does not necessarily consider all the parameters every time as some may be irrelevant for the purposes of choosing the type of treatment. For example, a patient in poor general conditions with a high American Society of Anesthesiologists (ASA) score is usually not candidate for surgery, irrespective of the histotype of the primary tumor or the number of secondary localizations. For this patient, the most important parameter will therefore be the sensitivity of the tumor histotype to adjuvant treatment. In the same way, a patient with acute and worsening spinal cord damage will undergo emergency palliative decompression and stabilization surgery without considering a more demanding operation.

Finally, we consider the patient not just in terms of the disease, reducing the choice of treatment to an overly simplistic mathematical score. Instead, we analyze the case holistically, firstly considering the individual and his or her general conditions and only subsequently the parameters of the metastases.

Without considering all the clinical and instrumental examinations which the patient undergoes on admission and forming part of preoperative staging, our treatment algorithm begins with diagnosis of spinal metastases.

The first assessment must be performed by the anesthetist who must say whether the patient is operable or not. If the patient is not operable due to a high ASA score, nonsurgical options are considered. Next, the sensitivity of the tumor histotype to adjuvant therapies (CHT, RT, hormonal therapy) is considered. If the tumor does not respond to any form of treatment, the only option for the patient is pain relief. If the patient is operable, the severity of spinal cord compression and neurological damage is evaluated by means of the Frankel score. If there is neurological deficit or paralysis, the possibility of recovery is evaluated on the basis of time from symptom onset. Finally, if in our opinion neurological recovery of the patient is not possible, sensitivity to adjuvant treatments is re-evaluated. If, on the other hand, the patient has acute and progressive spinal cord damage, emergency surgery is performed.

If there is no deficit or the damage is recoverable and stable, sensitivity to adjuvant treatments is evaluated. If the tumor histotype is not sensitive and there is a single metastasis only, resection of the lesion is chosen. On the other hand, decompression and stabilization is indicated if there are multiple metastases and they are treatable. If they are not treatable, pain relief alone is administered. When there is no deficit or the damage is recoverable and not progressive and the tumor is sensitive to some form of adjuvant treatment, pathological fracture (actual or impending) is evaluated. This parameter is, in fact, decisive in orienting the choice toward either surgical treatment with compression and stabilization or adjuvant treatment only.

Resection of the tumor may be performed en bloc with a wide margin or through debulking. Generally speaking en bloc removal is suggested for hypervascularized tumors, metastases from renal cell carcinoma and from sarcoma, and the

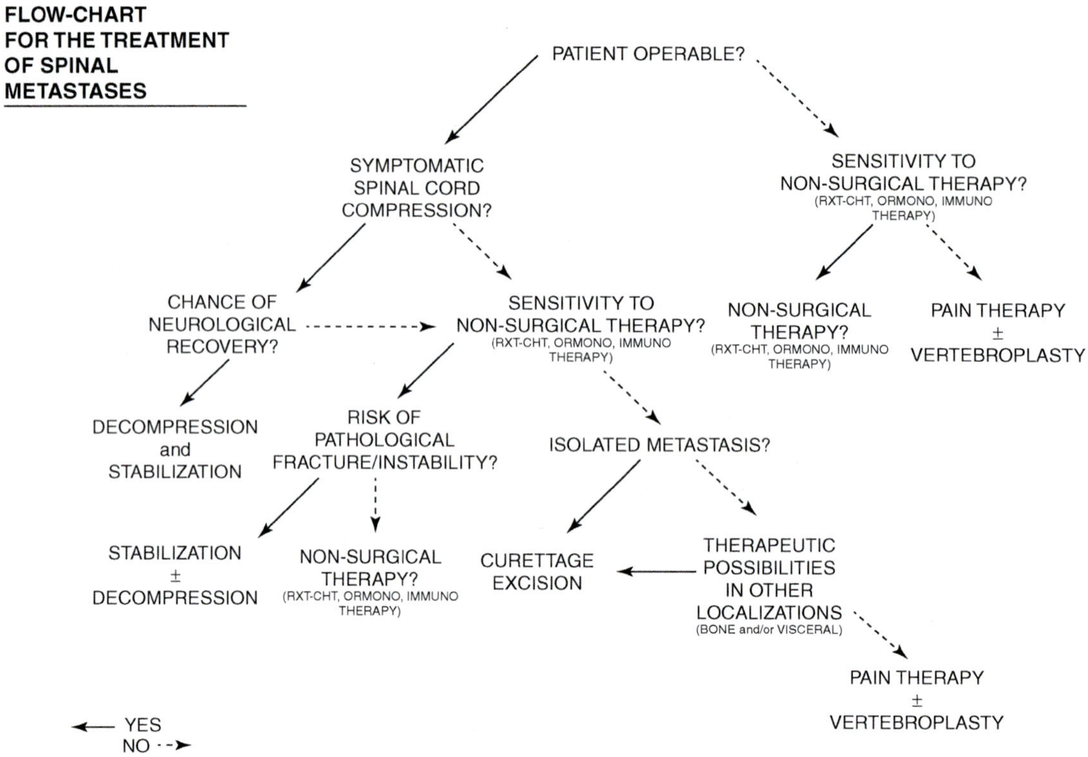

Fig. 7.3 Algorithm for the management of spinal metastasis

cases in which this type of operation is easy to perform.

Experience at Our Institution

Materials and Methods

From January 1990 to December 2016, 745 cases of spinal metastases from a solid tumor have been treated at the Rizzoli Orthopedic Institute in Bologna. One hundred twenty-two patients (16.37%) had a MESCC. Patients suffering from plasmacytoma and lymphoma were excluded from the study as the therapeutic approach and prognostic evaluation are, in our experience, different.

The patients with MESCC were 61 males and 61 females with a mean age of 58 and 22 years (range 29–81 years). We identified 25 metastases located in the cervical section, 66 in the thoracic section, and 31 in the lumbar section. The anatomical location of the primary tumor is reported in Fig. 7.2. The most frequent locations were the kidney, lung, breast, and colon. In 9.83% of the cases, the original tumor was not known at the onset of the vertebral symptoms.

The score used in the 1990s to evaluate the neurological assessment was the Frankel score. So we preferred to use this score to assess neurological impairment. No patients were classified as Frankel E. Twenty-nine patients were Frankel D3, 24 cases were D2, 38 cases were D1, 22 cases were C, 7 cases were B, and 2 cases were A.

On admission, there was a pathological fracture of the vertebra in 60 cases (49.18%). Before surgery all patients underwent an anesthesiological evaluation in order to assess comorbidities and the risks of surgery. All the patients considered in this series underwent a surgical operation.

It should be kept in mind that the patients referred to us had already been selected by the oncologists, and this explains the high number of surgical operations.

One hundred twenty-two patients have undergone one of the following surgical treatments:

1. Decompression and stabilization in 36 cases (29.5%): It was chosen for patients with short-term prognosis in cases of neurological damage as a result of pathological fracture, but also in conditions of very high sensitivity to radiotherapy or hormonal treatment.
2. Intralesional resection "debulking" in 82 cases (67.21%): This procedure was performed as part of a multidisciplinary approach to treating the metastases and was preceded by appropriate surgical planning including selective preoperative arterial embolization. We chose this operation in presence of metastases not sensitive to radiotherapy, with pathological fracture and/or signs of spinal cord compression, or when the oncologist considered it necessary to remove the tumor to enable adjuvant treatments to act more effectively on the remaining cells.
3. En bloc resection in four cases (3.27%): This was performed on patients suffering from a single spinal metastasis deriving from the primary tumor, with a long life expectancy, and already treated. The operation was performed with a double approach in two cases and a posterior approach alone in two cases. The criteria making this operation possible include tumor size, volume, and location. The Frankel classification grade of these four patients was D3 for two patients and D1 for the other two patients The primary tumor was renal cell carcinoma in three cases and a metastases from malignant schwannoma in one case. The mean follow-up has been 47 months (min 12 months, max 125 months). At the end of the follow-up, three patients had died from problems related to the tumor whereas one was still alive. One case was reoperated after 3 months for the failure of the posterior instrumentation. One case had a surgical revision of the surgery for dehiscence and a pulmonary embolism.

Results

All patients underwent periodic outpatient visits in which a clinical examination was combined with X-ray examination of the spinal column, CT and/or MRI of the operated segment and any other examinations indicated in the individual case. The main elements recorded for each patient were functional assessment of the neurological conditions according to the Frankel scale, complications associated with the operation, local recurrence or local progression of the disease, and general clinical status.

The 122 patients included in our study were followed up for a mean of 17.10 months (range 1–125 months). At the longest available follow-up, 16 (13.11%) patients had died a mean distance of 18.81 months after admission to hospital (range 1 day to 63 months).

In total, there were 10 (8.19%) intraoperative complications: one case of excessive bleeding, seven cases of dura lesion that has been sutured, one case of pleural lesion, and one case of dura resection with patch reconstruction. We had 20 (16.39%) early postoperative complications: early infection with wound dehiscence (7), screw mal-placement (1), screw mobilization (2), pleural effusion (2), hematoma (1), pulmonary embolism and cardiac arrest (1), deep vein thrombosis (1), paroxysmal supraventricular tachycardia (1), atrial fibrillation (1), bronchopneumonia (1), urinary tract infection (1), and subcutaneous emphysema (1). We had 7 (5.73%) late complications: deep infection with fistula (1), breakage of fixation devices (4), aseptic necrosis (1), and junctional syndrome (1).

Twenty-three patients (18.85%) had a local recurrence after the first surgery.

Conclusions

Appropriate surgical treatment of bone metastases and tumors in general has now become an integral part of the correct approach to the tumor patient.

The evolution of anesthetic techniques now allows more aggressive treatment of some patients with spinal metastases. These procedures can dramatically improve the patient's quality of life and may prolong the patient's life expectancy by preventing complications related to paralysis.

In the majority of cases, it is therefore possible to restore or maintain movement and control pain while maintaining sensitivity, dignity, and hope.

The surgical indication for MESCC must consider:

- The medical condition and life expectancy of the patient
- The type of cancer and its relative response to adjuvant therapy
- Timing of onset of neurological impairments and chances of recovery with a surgical decompression
- Need to improve function and stability and to limit pain
- Need for complete local control, in order to prevent recurrence
- Possibility of associating adjuvant treatments to improve the efficacy of the treatment, reducing morbidity

It is vital in our opinion to underline that the patient's health should always be the center of our main purpose. The surgeon has an important role in the team and should be consulted during the settlement of a treatment planning. Too often surgery is considered the last resort and taken into account only when other options are not available anymore. A strong and continuous collaboration between specialists can identify the exact moment in which surgery can lead to optimal results with decreased morbidity for the patient. In the context of a metastatic disease, in our opinion, the oncologist should be the team leader.

Acknowledgements The authors thank Mr. Carlo Piovani for his helpful collaboration in patients' image storage and editing.

References

1. Wise JJ, Fischgrund JS, Herkowitz HN, Montgomery D, Kurtz LT. Complication, survival rates and risk factors of surgery for metastatic disease of the spine. Spine. 1999;24(18):1943–51.
2. Ryken TC, Eichholz KM, Gerszten PC, Welch WC, Gokaslan ZL, Resnick DK. Evidence-based review of the surgical management of vertebral column metastatic disease. Neurosurg Focus. 2003;15(5):11.
3. Sundaresan N, Rothman A, Manhart K, Kelliher K. Surgery for solitary metastases of the spine: rationale and results of the treatment. Spine. 2002;27:1802–6.
4. Hosono N, Yonenobu K, Fuji T, Ebara S, Yamashita K, Ono K. Orthopaedic management of spinal metastases. Clin Orthop. 1995;312:148–59.
5. Sioutos PJ, Arbit E, Meshulam CF, Galicich JH. Spinal metastases from solid tumors. Analysis of factors affecting survival. Cancer. 1995;76(8):1453–9.
6. Batson OV. Role of vertebral veins in metastatic processes. Ann Intern Med. 1942;16:38–45.
7. Damron TA, Sim FH. Surgical treatment for metastatic disease of the pelvis and the proximal end of the femur. Instr Course Lect. 2000;49:461–70.
8. Schuster JM, Grady MS. Medical management and adjuvant therapies in spinal metastatic disease. Neurosurg Focus. 2001;11(6):e3.
9. Helweg-Larsen S, Sørenson PS. Symptoms and signs in metastatic spinal cord compression: a study from first symptom until diagnosis in 153 patients. Eur J Cancer. 1994;30:396–8.
10. Livingstone KE, Perrin RG. The neurosurgical management of spinal metastases causing cord and cauda equina compression. J Neurosurg. 1978;49:839–43.
11. Loblaw DA, Laperriere NJ, Mackillop WJ. A population-based study of malignant spinal cord compressioninOntario.ClinOncol(RCollRadiol).2003;15:211–7.
12. Quraishi NA, Gokaslan ZL, Boriani S. The surgical management of metastatic epidural compression of the spinal cord. J Bone Joint Surg. 2010;92(8):1054–60.
13. Barron KD, Hirano A, Araki S, Terry RD. Experiences with metastatic neoplasmsinvolving the spinal cord. Neurology. 1959;9:91–106.
14. Sciubba DM, Gokaslan ZL. Diagnosis and management of metastatic spine disease. Surg Oncol. 2006;15:141–51.
15. Arguello F, Baggs RB, Duerst RE, et al. Pathogenesis of vertebral metastasis and epidural spinal cord compression. Cancer. 1990;65:98–106.
16. Bradley Jacobs W, Perrin RG. Evaluation and treatment of spinal metastases: an overview. Neurosurg Focus. 2001;11(6):e10.

17. Greenberg HS, Kim JH, Posner JB. Epidural spinal cord compression from metastatic tumor: results with a new treatment protocol. Ann Neurol. 1980;8:361–6.
18. Gasbarrini A, Cappuccio M, Mirabile L, Bandiera S, Terzi S, Barbanti Bròdano G, Boriani S. Spinal metastases: treatment evaluation algorithm. Eur Rev Med Pharmacol Sci. 2004;8:265–74.
19. Harrington KD. Orthopedic surgical management of skeletal complications of malignancy. Cancer. 1997; 15(80):1614–27.
20. Young RF, Post EM, King GA. Treatment of spinal epidural metastases. Randomized prospective comparison of laminectomy and radiotherapy. J Neurosurg. 1980;53:741–8.
21. Klimo P, Schmidt MH. Surgical management of spinal metastases. Oncologist. 2004;9:188–96.
22. Patchell RA, Tibbs PA, Regine WF, et al. Direct decompressive surgical resection in the treatment of spinal cord compression caused by metastatic cancer: a randomised trial. Lancet. 2005;366:643–8.
23. Li H, Gasbarrini A, Cappuccio M, Boriani S. Outcome of excisional surgeries for the patients with spinal metastases. Eur Spine J. 2009;18:1423–30.
24. Boriani S, Bandiera S, Colangeli S, Ghermandi R, Gasbarrini A. En bloc resection of primary tumors of the thoracic spine: indications, planning, morbidity. Neurol Res. 2014;36:566–76.
25. Holly LT, Foley KT. Three-dimensional fluouroscopy-guided percutaneous thoracolumbar pedicle screw placement: technical note. J Neurosurg. 2003;99(Suppl): 324–9.
26. Callstrom MR, Dupuy DE, Solomon SB, Beres RA, Littrup PJ, Davis KW, Paz-Fumagalli R, Hoffman C, Atwell TD, Charboneau JW, Schmit GD, Goetz MP, Rubin J, Brown KJ, Novotny PJ, Sloan JA. Percutaneous image-guided cryoablation of painful metastases involving bone: multicenter trial. Cancer. 2013;119(5):1033–41.
27. Dabravolski D, Esser J, Lahm A, et al. Treatment of tumors and metastases of the spine by minimally invasive CAVITY-coblation method (plasma field therapy). J Neurosurg Sci. 2017;61(6):565–78.
28. Gasbarrini A, Campos WK, Campanacci L, et al. Electrochemotherapy to metastatic spinal melanoma: a novel treatment of spinal metastasis? Spine (Phila Pa 1976). 2015;40:E1340–6.
29. Goetz MP, Callstrom MR, Charboneau JW, Farrel MA, Maus TP, Welch TJ, Wong GY, Sloan JA, Novotny PJ, Petersen IA, Beres RA, Regge D, Capanna R, Saker MB, Groenenmeyer D, Gevargez A, Ahrar K, Choti MA, de Baere TJ, Rubin J. Percutaneous image-guided radiofrequency ablation of painful metastases involving bone: a multicenter study. J Clin Oncol. 2004;22:300–6.
30. Han PP, Kenny K, Dickman CA. Thoracoscopic approaches to the thoracic spine: experience with 241 surgical procedures. Neurosurgery. 2002;51(Suppl): 88–95.
31. Mühlbauer M, Pfisterer W, Eyb R, Knosp E. Minimally invasive retroperitoneal approach for lumbar corpectomy and anterior reconstruction: technical note. J Neurosurg. 2000;93(Suppl):161–7.
32. Groenemeyer D, Schirp S, Gevargez A. Image-guided radiofrequency ablation of spinal tumors: preliminary experience with expandable array electrode. Cancer J. 2002;8(1):33–9.
33. Gellad FE, Sadato N, Numaguchi Y, et al. Vascular metastatic lesions of the spine: preoperative embolization. Radiology. 1990;176:683–6.
34. Georgy BA, Wong W. Plasma-mediated radiofrequency ablation assisted percutaneous cement injection for treating advanced malignant vertebral compression fractures. AJNR Am J Neuroradiol. 2007;28: 700–5.
35. Sundaresan N, Choi IS, Hughes JE, et al. Treatment of spinal metastases from kidney cancer by presurgical embolization and resection. J Neurosurg. 1990; 73:548–54.
36. Prabhu VC, Bilsky MH, Jambhekar K, et al. Results of preoperative embolization for metastatic spinal neoplasms. J Neurosurg. 2003;98(Suppl 2):156–64.
37. Alvarez L, Pérez-Higueras A, Quinones D, Calvo E, Rossi RE. Vertebroplasty in the treatment of vertebral tumors: postprocedural outcome and quality of life. Eur Spine J. 2003;12:356–60.
38. Fourney DR, Schomer DF, Nader R, Chlan J, Suki D, Ahrar K, Rhines LD, Gokaslan ZL. Percutaneous vertebroplasty and kyphoplasty for painful vertebral body fractures in cancer patients. J Neurosurg Spine. 2003;98:21–30.
39. Pilitsis JG, Rengachary SS. The role of vertebroplasty in metastatic spinal disease. Neurosurg Focus. 2001;11:E9.
40. Shimony JS, Gilula LA, Zeller AJ, Brown DB. Percutaneous vertebroplasty for malignant compression fractures with epidural involvement. Radiology. 2004;232(3):846–53.
41. Reidy D, Ahn H, Mousavi P, Finkelstein J, Whine CM. A biomechanical analysis of intravertebral pressures during vertebroplasty of cadaveric spines with and without simulated metastases. Spine. 2003;28(14): 1534–9.
42. Mendel E, Bourekas E, Gerszten P, Golan JD. Percutaneous techniques in the treatment of spine tumours: what are the diagnostic and therapeutic indications and outcomes? Spine. 2009;34(Suppl):93–100.
43. Yu MK, Buys SS. Medical management of skeletal metastasis. Neurosurg Clin N Am. 2004;15:529–36.
44. Witham TF, Khavkin YA, Gallia GL, et al. Surgery insight: current management of epidural spinal cord compression from metastatic spine disease. Nat Clin Pract Neurol. 2006;2:87–94.
45. Delattre JY, Arbit E, Thaler HT, Rosenblum MK, Posner JB. A dose-response study of dexamethasone in a model of spinal cord compression caused by epidural tumor. J Neurosurg. 1989;70:920–5.
46. Turner S, Marosszeky B, Timms I, Boyages J. Malignant spinal cord compression: a prospective evaluation. Int J Radiat Oncol Biol Phys. 1993; 26:141–6.

47. Vecht CJ, Haaxma-Reiche H, van Putten WL, et al. Initial bolus of conventional versus high-dose dexamethasone in metastatic spinal cord compression. Neurology. 1989;39:1255–7.
48. Fourney DR, Gokaslan ZL. Anterior approaches for thoracolumbar metastatic spine tumours. Neurosurg Clin N Am. 2004;15:443–51.
49. Fourney DR, Abi-Said D, Rhines LD, et al. Simultaneous anterior-posterior approach to the thoracic and lumbar spine for the radical resection of tumors followed by reconstruction and stabilisation. J Neurosurg. 2001;94(Suppl):232–43.
50. Manabe S, Tateishi A, Abe M, Ohno T. Surgical treatment of metastatic tumors of the spine. Spine. 1989; 14:41–7.
51. Sakaura H, Hosono N, Mukai Y, et al. Outcome of total en bloc spondylectomy for solitary metastasis of the thoracolumbar spine. J Spinal Disord Tech. 2004;17:297–300.
52. Tomita K, Kawahara N, Baba H, et al. Total spondylectomy for solitary spinal metastases. Int Orthop. 1994;18:291–8.
53. Tomita K, Toribatake Y, Kawahara N, Ohnari H, Kose H. Total en bloc spondylectomy and circumspinal decompression for solitary spinal metastasis. Paraplegia. 1994;32:36–46.
54. Boriani S, Biagini R, De Iure F, et al. En bloc resections of bone tumors of the thoracolumbar spine: a preliminary report on 29 patients. Spine. 1996;21:1927–31.
55. Bilsky MH, Laufer I, Burch S. Shifting paradigms in the treatment of metastatic spine disease. Spine. 2009;34(Suppl):101–7.
56. Fisher CG, DiPaola CP, Ryken TC, Bilsky MH, Shaffrey CI, Berven SH, Harrop JS, Fehlings MG, Boriani S, Chou D, Schmidt MH, Polly DW, Biagini R, Burch S, Dekutoski MB, Ganju A, Gerszten PC, Gokaslan ZL, Groff MW, Liebsch NJ, Mendel E, Okuno SH, Patel S, Rhines LD, Rose PS, Sciubba DM, Sundaresan N, Tomita K, Varga PP, Vialle LR, Vrionis FD, Yamada Y, Fourney DR. A novel classification system for spinal instability in neoplastic disease: an evidence-based approach and expert consensus from the Spine Oncology Study Group. Spine (Phila Pa 1976). 2010;35(22):E1221–9.
57. Fourney DR, Gokaslan ZL. Spinal instability and deformity due to neoplastic conditions. Neurosurg Focus. 2003;14:e8.
58. Wang JC, Boland P, Mitra N, et al. Single-stage posterolateral transpedicular approach for resection of epidural metastatic spine tumors involving the vertebral body with circumferential reconstruction: results in 140 patients. J Neurosurg Spine. 2004;1:287–98.
59. Akeyson EW, McCutcheon IE. Single-stage posterior vertebrectomy and replacement combined with posterior instrumentation for spinal metastasis. J Neurosurg. 1996;85:211–20.
60. Tokuhashi Y, Matsuzaki Y, Toriyama S, Kawano H, Ohsaka S. Scoring system for the preoperative evaluation of metastatic spine tumor prognosis. Spine. 1990;15:1110–3.
61. Tomita K, Kawahara N, Kobayashi T, et al. Surgical strategy for spinal metastases. Spine. 2001;26:298–306.
62. Boriani S, Gasbarrini A. Point of view. Spine. 2005;30:2227–9.

8 Metastatic Spine Disease: Critical Evaluation of the Current Literature

Adedayo O. Ashana, Andrew B. Kay, and Justin Earl Bird

Introduction

The spine is the most common location for metastatic disease to bone [1], causing up to 20% of all cancer patients to develop symptomatic spinal metastases [2]. As novel systemic therapies change the survivorship profiles of cancer patients, the clinical burden of metastatic spinal cord compression will likely increase. Therefore it is important to periodically evaluate treatment paradigms and develop responsive, innovative management strategies that continuously improve outcomes for these patients [2, 3].

The treatment of metastatic disease to the spine has significantly evolved over time. Both operative and nonoperative treatment modalities have been emphasized at various time points, and both strategies have been used with varying degrees of success. Steroids alone had an important role in the early treatment of metastatic spine disease but now primarily serve as an adjunct along with other treatment modalities. Decompressive laminectomies were performed in the past but often found to be complicated by spinal instability. Improvements in the delivery of radiation therapy led to a paradigm shift favoring radiotherapy [4] until the development of spinal instrumentation led to a renewed interest in the role of surgery, allowing both decompression and stabilization of the spine. In a landmark randomized controlled trial, Patchell et al. demonstrated favorable outcomes in patients with metastatic spinal cord compression treated with surgery compared to those treated nonoperatively [5]. This study tilted the consensus toward surgical intervention and led to many of the treatment algorithms that are commonly used today. However, given the narrow inclusion/exclusion criteria of the study and limitations in study design, the results cannot and should not be generalized to the heterogeneous MESCC patient population. Furthermore, the development of more effective systemic therapies, especially stereotactic radiosurgery, has had a significant impact on the role of surgery and in many instances made nonoperative treatment more efficacious. In this chapter, a critical review of the literature is performed focusing on the management of patients with metastatic epidural spinal cord compression.

A. O. Ashana, MD (✉)
Department of Orthopedic Spine Surgery, OSS Health, York, PA

A. B. Kay, MD
Department of Orthopaedic Surgery, Houston Methodist Hospital, Houston, TX, USA
e-mail: abkay@houstonmethodist.org

J. E. Bird, MD
Department of Orthopaedic Oncology, The University of Texas MD Anderson Cancer Center, Houston, TX, USA
e-mail: jebird@mdanderson.org

R. A. W. Marco (ed.), *Metastatic Spine Disease*, https://doi.org/10.1007/978-3-319-76252-4_8

Steroids

Steroids are generally considered useful adjuncts in the treatment of patients with metastatic spinal cord compression. However, controversies exist due to conflicting outcomes in the literature and a long list of potential complications associated with steroid use. A randomized study comparing patients receiving high-dose dexamethasone to a control group demonstrated a significant higher percentage of ambulatory patients in the former group at 6 months (59% vs. 33% high-dose steroid vs. control group, respectively) [6]. The authors strongly recommended high-dose glucocorticoids as an adjunct in patients with metastatic spinal cord compression. A 2015 Cochrane review found a paucity of evidence for the use of corticosteroids for MESCC. Only three small trials were found, and all were inadequately powered to determine clinical benefit and optimal dosage. The trials demonstrated no difference between high and moderate dose or no corticosteroids in enhancing ambulation (60% vs. 55%, RR 1.08, 95% CI 0.81–1.45), 2-year survival rates (11% vs. 10%, RR 1.11, 95% CI 0.24–5.05), pain reduction (78% vs. 91%, RR 0.86, 95% CI 0.62–1.2), or urinary continence (63% vs. 53%, RR 1.18, 95% CI 0.66–2.13) [7]. A more recent systematic review found only six high-quality studies on the outcomes and optimal dosing of steroids for MESCC. The authors concluded that while steroids may increase the proportion of patients maintaining ambulation at 1 year, there was no clear effect on bowel or bladder function, nor survival. Additionally, there was low-level evidence for administering steroids within 12 h after MESCC was diagnosed. The authors recommended a 10 mg IV bolus of dexamethasone followed by 4 mg every 6 h, followed by definitive therapy with radiation or surgery and then weaning [8].

The negative side effects associated with use of steroids in patients with metastatic spinal cord compression are well documented. A study of 28 patients with metastatic spinal cord compression treated with high-dose dexamethasone and radiotherapy demonstrated an overall 28.6% rate of side effects and 14.3% rate of serious side effects including fatal ulcers and perforated viscera which were considered unacceptable by the authors [9]. Another retrospective review of 59 neuro-oncology patients treated with high-dose steroids revealed a 51% rate of steroid toxicity and a 19% rate of hospital admission for steroid-related complications [10]. Based on these data, the general consensus is that steroids are beneficial; however the risks of *high*-dose steroids for metastatic spinal cord compression outweigh the benefits. The authors of this chapter recommend an "intermediate dosing" strategy (10–16 mg IV bolus of dexamethasone, followed by 4–6 mg IV every 6 h) for patients with spinal cord compression with acute neurologic deficits.

Radiotherapy

It has been well documented that different tumor types demonstrate variable sensitivity to radiation therapy, leading some to investigate the efficacy of isolated treatment of MESCC with radiation therapy. Highly sensitive tumors include myeloma and lymphoma. Moderately sensitive include metastases from colon, breast, prostate, and squamous cell primary tumors. Conversely, metastatic lung, renal, melanoma, and most sarcomas demonstrate poor sensitivity to conventional radiotherapy. However, sarcomas such as Ewing's sarcoma, leiomyosarcoma, alveolar soft parts sarcoma, myxoid liposarcoma, and synovial sarcoma are all relatively radiosensitive.

Multiple studies have shown the efficacy of conventional radiation therapy alone for the treatment of metastatic spinal cord compression [4, 11–17]. In a study of 209 patients with metastatic spinal cord compression treated with different modalities, Maranzano et al. demonstrated that of those who received radiation alone, 82% experienced improved back pain relief, 76% preserved ambulation, 60% reported improvement of neurologic symptoms, and 44% recovered sphincter control. Overall, those patients with sensitive histology and early diagnosis experienced the best response to radiation therapy [11]. The 2015 Cochrane review examined trials comparing different radiotherapy doses and schedules in patients with MESCC. The authors found that single-dose (8 Gy) radiotherapy was as effective as short-course RT (16 Gy in two fractions over 1 week) in enhancing short-term ambulation, reducing analgesic and narcotic use, and maintaining urinary continence in the short term [7]. However, the authors noted that single-dose radiation may result in increased rates of local recurrence compared to short course (4% vs. 0%) but observed equivalent median survival between the different regimens. Gastrointestinal and other serious adverse effects were infrequent with each regimen chosen.

Stereotactic Radiosurgery

Recent advances in image-guided delivery of high-dose radiation therapy have led to great improvements in the treatment of patients with metastatic spine disease. Stereotactic radiosurgery (SRS) allows for delivery of high-dose radiation therapy close to the spinal cord without exceeding the radiation exposure limits of safety for the spinal cord and other adjacent vital structures. SRS often consists of 18–24 Gy single-dose radiation (higher doses are more effective) with the constraint that the spinal cord is not exposed to more than 14 Gy in a single voxel [17]. This is made possible with advances in patient immobilization, target visualization, and precise delivery methods using image-guided algorithms. Studies have reported promising clinical response greater than 85% and partial or complete pain response in 85–92% [18–22]. In a long-term study (median follow-up 6.1 years), spine radiosurgery resulted in a durable 5-year local control rate of more than 90% [23]. Other studies have reported similar findings [17].

Despite promising clinical data, histopathological data confirming local control with SRS has been limited. In the largest such series to date, the author examined histological data of patients undergoing vertebral cement augmentation for mechanical pain or instability (secondary to vertebral compression fracture) or instrumentation for radiographic evidence of tumor progression after previously undergoing SRS. Of the 582 patients treated with high-dose single-fraction SRS over a 9-year period, the authors identified 30 patients (5.1%) who underwent the aforementioned procedures. The initial diagnosis primarily included radioresistant histologies (63% radioresistant, 37% radiosensitive). There was no evidence of tumor in 78% of lesions reviewed, while a minority (22%) demonstrated residual tumor, demonstrating a tumor-ablative role for SRS in the majority of patients with metastatic lesions [24].

Nonetheless, significant variation in protocols for administration of SRS exists amongst institutions and clinical sites. Specifically, the relative efficacy and implications of single- versus multi-fraction regimens remain controversial with published data on this topic primarily limited to retrospective analyses [25].

The few available studies on this subject fail to resolve the controversy. Heron et al. performed a comparative analysis of single-fraction SBRT compared to fractionated SBRTT (mean dose of 16.3 Gy vs. 20.6–24.5 Gy in 3–5 fractions, respectively) and noted superior 2-year local control with the multifraction group. Other authors have noted improved local control with 24 Gy single-fraction treatment compared to multifraction SBRT of 25–30 Gy in 3–5 fractions for sarcoma and renal cell carcinoma [26, 27]. It remains unclear if these findings can be generalized to other histopathologies. Further studies are needed to delineate the optimal dose and fractional schedules for patients with metastatic spine disease.

Fortunately, relatively low complication rates are associated with the use of spinal stereotactic radiosurgery in the literatures. In a phase II feasibility study, Lo et al. found no cases of grade 4–5 toxicity, a 2.3% rate of grade 3 toxicity, and a 25% rate of grade 1–2 toxicity among the 44 patients undergoing spinal SRS [28]. Vertebral compression fractures (VCF) is the most commonly reported complication following spinal SRS, although significant variation exists in the reported incidence. Rose et al. reported a radiographic VCF rate of 39% and median time to VCF of 25 months for 71 lesions treated with single-fraction spinal SRS [29]. However,

Boehling et al. reported a VCF rate of 20% and a median time to VCF of 3 months for 123 lesions [30]. A pooled multi-institutional analysis involving 410 lesions demonstrated 1- and 2-year VCF rates of 12.35 and 13.5, respectively, at a median time to VCF of 2.5 months. The study demonstrated increased VCF rates with increasing dose/fraction (VCF rate of 39% for ≥24 Gy vs. 10% VCF rate for ≤19 Gy) [31]. The impact of single versus fractionated SRS on VCF remains controversial though it appears that fractionation may confer a comparatively lower VCF rate [32]. Although less common than VCF, radiation myelopathy represents permanent neurologic damage and may be the most devastating complication. Fortunately, the largest series to date (involving 1388 patients) reported a myelopathy rate of 0.4%. Further understanding of spinal cord tolerance and safe dose limits will likely further reduce this complication [33]. Other reported complications include pain flare, esophageal toxicity, and damage to great vessels. It appears that pain flare occurs more frequently with SRS compared to conventional radiotherapy. Nonetheless, prophylactic corticosteroid treatment appears to decrease this complication [25, 34]. Rates of esophageal toxicity and damage to great vessels are relatively low since recommended dose constraints for these tissues are typically higher than doses used for spinal SRS [35, 36].

Surgery

Early studies on surgery for metastatic spinal cord compression did not favor surgical treatment. Young et al. compared 16 patients treated with laminectomy and radiotherapy to 13 treated with radiotherapy alone. The study showed no significant difference in efficacy regarding pain relief, ambulatory status, or sphincter control [4]. Laminectomy alone resulted in decompression and pain control but ultimately led to spinal instability. Improvements in spinal instrumentation however led to treatment strategies combining decompressive surgeries with spinal stabilization [16]. Based on experience demonstrating the importance of spinal stability, the Spine Oncology Study Group (SOSG) proposed the Spine Instability Neoplastic Score (SINS) to help assess spinal instability preoperatively based on clinical and radiographic information [37]. The SINS uses six variables including location, type of pain, radiographic alignment, nature of the lesion (lytic vs. blastic), vertebral body collapse, and involvement of the posterior elements and gives each a numerical score. The authors considered lesions with a low score (0–6) stable and not requiring surgical intervention on their own, whereas the authors believed lesions with a high score (13–18) indicated instability and would benefit from surgical consultation. Intermediate scores (7–12) are regarded as potentially unstable. The SINS paper does not recommend any specific treatment, but rather serves as a guide to help clinicians decide which patients are at risk for further vertebral collapse and deformity. The authors found that the SINS showed excellent inter- and intra-observer reliability in determining stability, as well as high sensitivity and specificity for detecting potentially unstable or unstable at 95.7% and 79.5% [37].

However, several criticisms of this system are worth mentioning. First, the authors gave higher scores to junctional regions of the spine such as the occipito-cervical junction. In the experience of the authors of this chapter, lesions at the occipito-cervical region tend to remain stable when treated nonoperatively. For example, odontoid tumors frequently spread in a cephalocaudal direction, rarely causing spinal cord compression or instability. Second, vertebral body collapse >50% receives a higher score when, in fact, significant vertebral body collapse and even vertebral plana are often very stable and can be treated nonoperatively or with less invasive procedures such as vertebroplasty [38]. Nonetheless, the SINS criteria provided an objective means of assessing patients for spinal instability and improved our understanding regarding the indications for stabilization procedures.

One of the most challenging aspects of caring for a patient with metastatic epidural spinal cord compression is determining whether surgical intervention will indeed help the patient, given the poor prognoses and medical condition of many of these patients. Patchell and colleagues in a landmark study demonstrated that surgery can be helpful in patients with MESCC. The study was a prospective, randomized, multicentered trial comparing outcomes in patients with metastatic epidural cord compression treated with operative management to those treated nonoperatively [5]. Of 101 patients with metastatic spinal cord compression, 50 were randomized to receive steroids, circumferential decompression, stabilization, and radiation, and 51 received radiotherapy and steroids alone. Significantly more patients in the surgery group were able to walk after treatment (84% vs. 57%, $p = 0.001$), and those treated with surgery were also able to retain their ability to walk significantly longer (122 days vs. 13 days, $p = 0.003$). Of the patients who entered the study ambulatory, 32/34 (94%) treated with surgery retained their ability to walk, versus 26/35 (74%) treated with radiation alone, and those treated with surgery retained the ability to walk longer (153 days vs. 53 days). Of the 32 patients who entered the study non-ambulatory for less than 48 h, significantly more patients treated with surgery regained the ability to walk (10/16, 62% vs. 3/16, 19%), and the median length of ambulation was 59 days versus 0 days. Additionally, those treated with surgery had a significantly reduced need for corticosteroids (1.6 mg vs. 4.2 mg dexamethasone daily) and opioid pain medications (0.4 mg vs. 4.8 mg daily morphine equivalents). The 30-day mortality rates were also lower in the surgical group (6% vs. 14%), although this difference was not statistically significant ($p = 0.32$). The results led the authors to conclude that surgery followed by radiotherapy should be favored for metastatic spinal cord compression for maintaining ambulatory status and continence, increasing survival time, and decreasing steroid and opioid use [5].

However, the Patchell study has important limitations, and its conclusions should not be over generalized. When compared to historical studies of patients treated with radiotherapy [4, 39–47], the patients in the Patchell study who received nonoperative treatment had significantly worse outcomes, suggesting the possibility of study or selection bias. Even though the study was conducted at many high-volume centers, patient enrollment proceeded unusually slowly, with only a single patient being enrolled over a decade in some centers. Understanding why so few of the patients presenting to these busy centers were eligible for inclusion is important for determining the applicability of the study. Additionally, 18/51 (35%) of patients received nonoperative treatment despite presenting with an unstable spine; doing so leads to skewed results as these patients probably should have been treated with stabilization rather than randomized to the radiation-only arm. The study also excluded highly radiosensitive tumor types such as myeloma yet included generally insensitive tumor types such as sarcomas—the latter of which randomized into the radiotherapy-alone arm. The specific histologies of these sarcomas were not provided; therefore it is unclear how tumor type affected the results.

In a follow-up study, Chi et al. performed a sub-analysis of the Patchell data to examine the relevance of patient age on the outcomes. The authors found a decreasing benefit of surgery as age increased, to the point that, by age 65, there was no observable difference in outcomes between the two groups [48]. This is very relevant considering that over 60% of patients with cancer are above age 65, leading one to conclude that surgery may have a limited role in the treatment of patients with epidural spinal cord compression.

The findings of a 2015 Cochrane review by George et al. also counter the perceptions that surgery generally improves outcomes for the majority of patients with MESCC [7]. The aim of the paper was to perform a rigorous systematic review of the literature to determine the effectiveness of radiotherapy, surgery, and steroids in the treatment of patients with metastatic epidural spinal cord compression. Six randomized controlled trials of radiotherapy, surgery, and corticosteroids involving 876 adult patients were included. Relative risk ratios and the numbers needed to treat with 95% confidence intervals were calculated. When comparing laminectomy and radiotherapy to radiotherapy alone, the authors found no statistically significant difference for ambulatory capacity (37% vs. 39% at 4 months, RR 0.98). The authors concluded that patients with stable spines who are able to walk could be reasonably treated with radiotherapy alone. However, surgery was found to be beneficial for a narrow cohort, ambulatory patients with relatively radioresistant tumor histology and nonambulatory patients with a single area of involvement and paraplegia onset within 48 h, and for relatively radioresistant tumor histology and over 3 months of life expectancy. Based on these data, proper patient selection is critical to achieve acceptable outcomes after surgical intervention for MESCC.

Treatment Framework

Efforts have been made to develop comprehensive multidisciplinary frameworks to determine the role of various treatment modalities. One such framework is the neurologic, oncologic, mechanical, and systemic (NOMS) framework developed at Memorial Sloan Kettering Cancer Center [49].

The neurologic component of NOMS focuses on the degree of spinal cord compression seen on MRI, classifying it as high or low grade based on the method of Bilsky et al. [50]. After doing so, the clinician considers the oncology of the tumor, classifying it as radioresistant or radiosensitive. Stereotactic radiosurgery is recommended for patients without high-grade epidural spinal cord compression, while surgical intervention is reserved for patients with high-grade epidural spinal cord compression and radioresistant histologies [50]. These recommendations must be considered, however, in the context of other critical patient factors; and one must be careful when using this framework not to overemphasize MRI findings in the decision to perform surgery. While the algorithm helps to encourage nonoperative treatment for patients with radiosensitive tumors and low-grade spinal cord compression, there is no validation for the clinical significance of spinal cord compression seen on MRI. Additionally, the framework regards tumor types such as renal cell carcinoma, lung carcinoma, and sarcoma as radioresistant and thus surgical candidates; however, recent advances in adjuvant therapies are changing sensitivity profiles of various tumor types. For example, anti-angiogenic chemotherapeutic agents such as sunitinib, sorafenib, and pazopanib can potentially sensitize renal cell carcinoma to radiation therapy, improve local control, and improve the effectiveness of nonoperative treatment of patients who would have historically required surgical intervention [51, 52]. Moreover, several sarcomas like Ewing's sarcoma, rhabdomyosarcoma, synovial sarcoma, and myxoid liposarcoma are relatively radiosensitive. The mechanical evaluation in NOMS focuses on a determination of spinal stability. Using the Spine Instability Neoplastic Score [37], the NOMS framework allows for less invasive interventions such as vertebroplasty or kyphoplasty to address spinal instability in certain instances. The Cancer Patient Fracture Evaluation study randomized 134 patients to receive balloon kyphoplasty or usual care and then assessed outcomes with the Roland-Morris Disability Questionnaire (RMDQ). Patients treated with kyphoplasty had an 8.4 point improvement in their RMDQ scores at 1 month versus 0.1 for usual care, leading the authors to endorse its safety and efficacy for short-term outcomes [53]. Fourney et al. found marked improvement in pain in 56 patients treated with kyphoplasty or vertebroplasty as far as 1 year after the procedure [54]. Additionally, a systematic review performed by the SOSG led to a strong recommendation for percutaneous cement augmentation for the treatment of symptomatic osteolytic tumors [55]. After analyses of neurological, oncological, and mechanical considerations, the clinician draws attention to systemic considerations. This final component of NOMS addresses the patient's ability to tolerate the proposed intervention based on medical comorbidities and overall tumor burden. Prognostic scoring systems may be considered, but ultimately the treatment plan is based on individual discussions between the clinical team and the patient. While the NOMS framework addresses "systemic" factors, these factors are considered last. Therefore, if one is not thorough, the systemic factors may be inadvertently underemphasized, and the patient's ability to undergo surgery safely may be underappreciated (see MOSS Chap. 2). Consequently, the treatment decision might be skewed toward surgery based on the initial assessments of neurologic compression, radioresistance, and mechanical factors even before considering that the patient's overall medical status and life expectancy may be too poor to recommend an operation.

Conclusion

In conclusion, substantial advances in chemotherapy, radiation therapy, biological agents, and surgical technique have considerably improved outcomes in patients with metastatic spine disease. While many more patients can now be treated nonoperatively, many patients who historically were not candidates for surgical procedures due to poor prognoses may now be candidates for surgery. Given all these advances, critically reviewing the literature must be an iterative process to keep up to date with the evolving landscape of metastatic epidural spinal cord compression. Thoughtful consideration of both nonoperative and operative modalities should be given to ensure that each patient receives the best treatment possible, based on the unique set of circumstances that each patient presents with.

References

1. Aaron AD. The management of cancer metastatic to bone. JAMA. 1994;272(15):1206–9.
2. Jacobs WB, Perrin RG. Evaluation and treatment of spinal metastases: an overview. Neurosurg Focus. 2001;11(6):1–1.
3. Posner JB. Spinal metastases. In: Neurologic complications of cancer. Philadelphia, PA: FA Davis Co.; 1995. p. 111–42.
4. Young RF, Post EM, King GA. Treatment of spinal epidural metastases: randomized prospective comparison of laminectomy and radiotherapy. J Neurosurg. 1980;53(6):741–8.
5. Patchell RA, Tibbs PA, Regine WF, Payne R, Saris S, Kryscio RJ, Mohiuddin M, Young B. Direct decompressive surgical resection in the treatment of spinal cord compression caused by metastatic cancer: a randomised trial. Lancet. 2005;366(9486):643–8.
6. Sørensen PS, Helweg-Larsen S, Mouridsen H, Hansen HH. Effect of high-dose dexamethasone in carcinomatous metastatic spinal cord compression treated with radiotherapy: a randomised trial. Eur J Cancer. 1994;30(1):22–7.
7. George R, Jeba J, Ramkumar G, Chacko AG, Leng M, Tharyan P. Interventions for the treatment of metastatic extradural spinal cord compression in adults. Cochrane Database Syst Rev. 2015;9:CD006716.
8. Kumar A, Weber MH, Gokaslan Z, Wolinsky JP, Schmidt M, Rhines L, Fehlings MG, Laufer I, Sciubba DM, Clarke MJ, Sundaresan N. Metastatic spinal cord compression and steroid treatment: a systematic review. Clin Spine Surg. 2017;30(4):156–63.
9. Heimdal K, Hirschberg H, Slettebø H, Watne K, Nome O. High incidence of serious side effects of high-dose dexamethasone treatment in patients with epidural spinal cord compression. J Neuro-Oncol. 1992;12(2):141–4.
10. Weissman DE, Dufer D, Vogel V, Abeloff MD. Corticosteroid toxicity in neuro-oncology patients. J Neuro-Oncol. 1987;5(2):125–8.
11. Maranzano E, Latini P. Effectiveness of radiation therapy without surgery in metastatic spinal cord compression: final results from a prospective trial. Int J Radiat Oncol Biol Phys. 1995;32(4):959–67.
12. Aabo K, Walbon-Jørgensen S. Central nervous system complications by malignant lymphomas: radiation schedule and treatment results. Int J Radiat Oncol Biol Phys. 1986;12(2):197–202.
13. Gilbert RW, Kim JH, Posner JB. Epidural spinal cord compression from metastatic tumor: diagnosis and treatment. Ann Neurol. 1978;3(1):40–51.
14. Greenberg HS, Kim JH, Posner JB. Epidural spinal cord compression from metastatic tumor: results with a new treatment protocol. Ann Neurol. 1980;8(4):361–6.
15. Posner JB. Back pain and epidural spinal cord compression. Med Clin North Am. 1987;71(2):185.
16. Siegal T, Siegal T. Current considerations in the management of neoplastic spinal cord compression. Spine. 1989;14(2):223–8.
17. Yamada Y, Bilsky MH, Lovelock DM, Venkatraman ES, Toner S, Johnson J, Zatcky J, Zelefsky MJ, Fuks Z. High-dose, single-fraction image-guided intensity-modulated radiotherapy for metastatic spinal lesions. Int J Radiat Oncol Biol Phys. 2008;71(2):484–90.
18. Gerszten PC, Mendel E, Yamada Y. Radiotherapy and radiosurgery for metastatic spine disease: what are the options, indications, and outcomes? Spine. 2009;34(22S):S78–92.
19. Gerszten PC, Burton SA, Ozhasoglu C, Welch WC. Radiosurgery for spinal metastases: clinical experience in 500 cases from a single institution. Spine. 2007;32(2):193–9.
20. Ryu S, Fang Yin F, Rock J, Zhu J, Chu A, Kagan E, Rogers L, Ajlouni M, Rosenblum M, Kim JH. Image-guided and intensity-modulated radiosurgery for patients with spinal metastasis. Cancer. 2003;97(8):2013–8.

21. Ryu S, Rock J, Rosenblum M, Kim JH. Patterns of failure after single-dose radiosurgery for spinal metastasis. J Neurosurg. 2004;101:402–5.
22. Gerszten PC, Burton SA, Ozhasoglu C, Vogel WJ, Welch WC, Baar J, Friedland DF. Stereotactic radiosurgery for spinal metastases from renal cell carcinoma. J Neurosurg Spine. 2005;3(4):288–95.
23. Moussazadeh N, Lis E, Katsoulakis E, Kahn S, Svoboda M, DiStefano NM, McLaughlin L, Bilsky MH, Yamada Y, Laufer I. Five-year outcomes of high-dose single-fraction spinal stereotactic radiosurgery. Int J Radiat Oncol Biol Phys. 2015;93(2):361–7.
24. Katsoulakis E, Laufer I, Bilsky M, Agaram NP, Lovelock M, Yamada Y. Pathological characteristics of spine metastases treated with high-dose single-fraction stereotactic radiosurgery. Neurosurg Focus. 2017;42(1):E7.
25. Huo M, Sahgal A, Pryor D, Redmond K, Lo S, Foote M. Stereotactic spine radiosurgery: review of safety and efficacy with respect to dose and fractionation. Surg Neurol Int. 2017;8:30.
26. Folkert MR, Bilsky MH, Tom AK, Oh JH, Alektiar KM, Laufer I, Tap WD, Yamada Y. Outcomes and toxicity for hypofractionated and single-fraction image-guided stereotactic radiosurgery for sarcomas metastasizing to the spine. Int J Radiat Oncol Biol Phys. 2014;88(5):1085–91.
27. Ghia AJ, Chang EL, Bishop AJ, Pan HY, Boehling NS, Amini B, Allen PK, Li J, Rhines LD, Tannir NM, Tatsui CE. Single-fraction versus multifraction spinal stereotactic radiosurgery for spinal metastases from renal cell carcinoma: secondary analysis of phase I/II trials. J Neurosurg Spine. 2016;24(5):829–36.
28. Lo SS, Sahgal A, Chang EL, Mayr NA, Teh BS, Huang Z, Schefter TE, Yao M, Machtay M, Slotman BJ, Timmerman RD. Serious complications associated with stereotactic ablative radiotherapy and strategies to mitigate the risk. Clin Oncol. 2013;25(6):378–87.
29. Rose PS, Laufer I, Boland PJ, Hanover A, Bilsky MH, Yamada J, Lis E. Risk of fracture after single fraction image-guided intensity-modulated radiation therapy to spinal metastases. J Clin Oncol. 2009;27(30):5075–9.
30. Boehling NS, Grosshans DR, Allen PK, McAleer MF, Burton AW, Azeem S, Rhines LD, Chang EL. Vertebral compression fracture risk after stereotactic body radiotherapy for spinal metastases. J Neurosurg Spine. 2012;16(4):379–86.
31. Sahgal A, Atenafu EG, Chao S, Al-Omair A, Boehling N, Balagamwala EH, Cunha M, Thibault I, Angelov L, Brown P, Suh J. Vertebral compression fracture after spine stereotactic body radiotherapy: a multi-institutional analysis with a focus on radiation dose and the spinal instability neoplastic score. J Clin Oncol. 2013;31(27):3426–31.
32. Guckenberger M, Mantel F, Gerszten PC, Flickinger JC, Sahgal A, Létourneau D, Grills IS, Jawad M, Fahim DK, Shin JH, Winey B. Safety and efficacy of stereotactic body radiotherapy as primary treatment for vertebral metastases: a multi-institutional analysis. Radiat Oncol. 2014;9(1):226.
33. Hall WA, Stapleford LJ, Hadjipanayis CG, Curran WJ, Crocker I, Shu HK. Stereotactic body radiosurgery for spinal metastatic disease: an evidence-based review. Int J Surg Oncol. 2011;2011:979214.
34. Khan L, Chiang A, Zhang L, Thibault I, Bedard G, Wong E, Loblaw A, Soliman H, Fehlings MG, Chow E, Sahgal A. Prophylactic dexamethasone effectively reduces the incidence of pain flare following spine stereotactic body radiotherapy (SBRT): a prospective observational study. Support Care Cancer. 2015;23(10):2937–43.
35. Gomez DR, Hunt MA, Jackson A, O'Meara WP, Bukanova EN, Zelefsky MJ, Yamada Y, Rosenzweig KE. Low rate of thoracic toxicity in palliative paraspinal single-fraction stereotactic body radiation therapy. Radiother Oncol. 2009;93(3):414–8.
36. Xue J, Kubicek G, Patel A, Goldsmith B, Asbell SO, LaCouture TA. Validity of current stereotactic body radiation therapy dose constraints for aorta and major vessels. Semin Radiat Oncol. 2016;26(2):135–9.
37. Fourney DR, Frangou EM, Ryken TC, DiPaola CP, Shaffrey CI, Berven SH, Bilsky MH, Harrop JS, Fehlings MG, Boriani S, Chou D. Spinal instability neoplastic score: an analysis of reliability and validity from the spine oncology study group. J Clin Oncol. 2011;29(22):3072–7.
38. Hentschel SJ, Rhines LD, Shah HN, Burton AW, Mendel E. Percutaneous vertebroplasty in vertebra plana secondary to metastasis. Clin Spine Surg. 2004;17(6):554–7.
39. Cassady JR, Sagerman RH, Chang CH. Radiation therapy for lymphoma of the spinal canal 1. Radiology. 1967;89(2):313–5.
40. Friedman M, Kim TH, Panahon AM. Spinal cord compression in malignant lymphoma—treatment and results. Cancer. 1976;37(3):1485–91.
41. Khan FR, Glicksman AS, Chu FC, Nickson JJ. Treatment by radiotherapy of spinal cord compression due to extradural metastases 1. Radiology. 1967;89(3):495–500.
42. Martin WE, Heller P. Radiation therapy for paraplegia due to multiple myeloma. JAMA. 1965;191(3):247–9.
43. Mones RJ, Dozier D, Berrett A. Analysis of medical treatment of malignant extradural spinal cord tumors. Cancer. 1966;19(12):1842–53.
44. Murphy WT, Bilge N. Compression of the spinal cord in patients with malignant lymphoma 1. Radiology. 1964;82(3):495–501.
45. Raichle ME, Posner JB. The treatment of extradural spinal cord compression. Neurology. 1970;20(4):391.
46. Rubin P, Miller G. Extradural spinal cord compression by tumor: part I: experimental production and treatment trials 1. Radiology. 1969;93(6):1243–8.
47. Rubin P, Mayer E, Poulter C. Part II: High daily dose experience without laminectomy 1. Radiology. 1969;93(6):1248–60.
48. Chi JH, Gokaslan Z, McCormick P, Tibbs PA, Kryscio RJ, Patchell RA. Selecting treatment for patients with malignant epidural spinal cord compression—does age matter?: results from a randomized clinical trial. Spine. 2009;34(5):431–5.

49. Laufer I, Rubin DG, Lis E, Cox BW, Stubblefield MD, Yamada Y, Bilsky MH. The NOMS framework: approach to the treatment of spinal metastatic tumors. Oncologist. 2013;18(6):744–51.
50. Bilsky MH, Laufer I, Fourney DR, Groff M, Schmidt MH, Varga PP, Vrionis FD, Yamada Y, Gerszten PC, Kuklo TR. Reliability analysis of the epidural spinal cord compression scale: clinical article. J Neurosurg Spine. 2010;13(3):324–8.
51. Lim ZD, Mahajan A, Weinberg J, Tannir NM. Outcome of patients with renal cell carcinoma metastatic to the brain treated with sunitinib without local therapy. Am J Clin Oncol. 2013;36(3):258–60.
52. Rousseau B, Kempf E, Desamericq G, Boissier E, Chaubet-Houdu M, Joly C, Saldana C, Boussion H, Neuzillet C, Macquin-Mavier I, Oudard S. First-line antiangiogenics for metastatic renal cell carcinoma: a systematic review and network meta-analysis. Crit Rev Oncol Hematol. 2016;107:44–53.
53. Berenson J, Pflugmacher R, Jarzem P, Zonder J, Schechtman K, Tillman JB, Bastian L, Ashraf T, Vrionis F, Cancer Patient Fracture Evaluation (CAFE) Investigators. Balloon kyphoplasty versus non-surgical fracture management for treatment of painful vertebral body compression fractures in patients with cancer: a multicentre, randomised controlled trial. Lancet Oncol. 2011;12(3):225–35.
54. Fourney DR, Schomer DF, Nader R, Chlan-Fourney J, Suki D, Ahrar K, Rhines LD, Gokaslan ZL. Percutaneous vertebroplasty and kyphoplasty for painful vertebral body fractures in cancer patients. J Neurosurg Spine. 2003;98(1):21–30.
55. Mendel E, Bourekas E, Gerszten P, Golan JD. Percutaneous techniques in the treatment of spine tumors: what are the diagnostic and therapeutic indications and outcomes? Spine. 2009;34(22S):S93–100.
56. Rompe JD, Hopf CG, Eysel P. Outcome after palliative posterior surgery for metastatic disease of the spine–evaluation of 106 consecutive patients after decompression and stabilisation with the Cotrel-Dubousset instrumentation. Arch Orthop Trauma Surg. 1999;119(7–8):394–400.

Indications for En Bloc Spondylectomy for Metastatic Spine Disease

9

Raphaële Charest-Morin and Charles G. Fisher

Background

The field of spinal oncology has undergone dramatic changes over the last two decades. Our understanding of spine stability evolved and was coupled with improved surgical techniques that enabled circumferential decompression and reconstruction of the spinal column. High levels of evidence confirmed that using these techniques resulted in better pain control, improved neurological function, and even better survival when compared to radiation therapy alone [1]. At the same time, our ability to perform oncological resection for primary spine tumors grew, and leaders in the field transposed these resection strategies to metastatic spine disease. In a restricted and carefully selected subset of patients with spinal metastasis, it was suggested that these oncological or "en bloc" resections could improve local control and potentially lead to cure even in the face of a bony metastasis to the spine; selecting the correct patient, however, remained the challenge. Furthermore, advances in the field of stereotactic spinal radiation therapy provided another option to treatment algorithms, reporting good local control rates without the morbidity associated with en bloc resections. This chapter discusses when en bloc resection of spinal metastasis should be considered, along with other treatment alternatives and strategies.

En bloc resection refers to a procedure in which the tumor is excised in a single piece without entering the tumor capsule, as opposed to a curettage, which is a piecemeal removal of the tumor. The oncologic goals of the former are to decrease the risk of local recurrence and improve disease-free survival. An en bloc procedure is meaningless if not reported with specimen margins. Different types of margins can be achieved. A wide margin is when a healthy cuff of tissue surrounds the excised specimen. Dissection through the reactive layer also known as the pseudocapsule occurs with marginal margins. In the spine, this is frequently observed at the dura, as taking dura with the specimen carries significant risk. Finally, an intralesional margin is when the resection occurs through the lesion as seen in a piecemeal resection. Achieving wide or marginal margins should be sought when undergoing an en bloc resection. This terminology and the principles of oncologic resection are largely derived from the Enneking classification in musculoskeletal oncology published in 1980 [2]. Its application in the spine is far more recent, and respect of

R. Charest-Morin, MD, FRCSC (✉)
Department of Orthopaedic, Centre Hospitalier Universitaire de Québec, Quebec City, QC, Canada
e-mail: Raphaele.charest-morin.1@ulaval.ca

C. G. Fisher, MD, MHSc, FRCSC
Division of Spine, Department of Orthopaedics, The Combined Neurosurgical and Orthopaedic Spine Program at Vancouver Coastal Health, Vancouver, BC, Canada
e-mail: Charles.fisher@vch.ca

R. A. W. Marco (ed.), *Metastatic Spine Disease*, https://doi.org/10.1007/978-3-319-76252-4_9

these principles has been shown to be safe and feasible for primary bone tumor [3]. Improved local control rate and survival have furthermore been demonstrated when following these principles in this population [4–9].

Initially, given the complexity and morbidity associated with these oncologic resections, their use was limited to primary bone tumors and even with this pathology, not universally adopted. More recently, with better training, advanced technology, and acceptable outcomes from a safety and efficacy perspective, indications have expanded to patients with metastatic spine disease (MSD). The metastatic spine population differs significantly from the primary tumor one. First and foremost, the surgical objective in primary tumor patients is curative, whereas in metastatic patients, the goals are to relieve pain, improve neurology, and enhance quality of life for the patient's remaining time. Primary tumor patients are usually younger, are healthier, and have localized disease. In contrast, patients with MSD are older, they frequently experience multiple metastases with a high systemic burden, and their functional status may be declining. In addition they are often undergoing or have undergone chemotherapy and/or radiation therapy. It would be futile and even harmful for these patients to undergo an aggressive procedure such as en bloc resection.

Overall accepted surgical indications in the metastatic spine population encompass mechanical instability, neurologic compromise, and pain relief, providing histologic diagnosis. Controversial but expanding indications are en bloc resections for patients with solitary or limited metastasis for cure or prolonged local control. With advances in radiation oncology, specifically the widespread use of stereotactic body radiotherapy (SBRT), improved and more prolonged local control is commonly observed [10, 11]. This along with evolving targeted systemic therapy has made the indications for an en bloc resection in the metastatic spine population even more difficult to standardize.

Indications

En bloc spondylectomy has generally been reserved for patients with a solitary metastasis and specific histology. Selecting the right patient for this type of surgery is challenging, as prognosis is hard to predict. Several classification systems have been developed to help the surgeon in the decision-making process. The most commonly used are the Tomita and the Revised Tokuaski Prognostic Scores. Tomita et al. [12] developed a system based on three factors: the rate of growth of the primary tumor, the presence of bony metastasis, and the presence of visceral metastasis (Table 9.1). Adding the scores of the three components produces a final score (2–10, from good to poor prognosis). Tomita et al. [12] suggested treatment according to the calculated score. For prognostic score of 2–3, wide or marginal excision for long-term local control is suggested, a score between 4 and 5 mandates a marginal or intralesional resection for midterm local control, a 6–7 score indicates a palliative surgery, and a score greater than 8 orients the surgeon toward non-operative measures. This scoring system is derived from a study of 67 patients between 1987 and 1991. Histology was an important predictor, and tumors were broadly classified as being slow growth (breast, thyroid, prostate), moderate growth (kidney, uterus), and rapid growth (lung, stomach, liver, colon).

The other score that has been widely used is the Revised Tokuashi Prognostic Score [13] (Table 9.2). This scoring system used six variables that are given a score between 0 and 5. Variables included the primary site of cancer, the

Table 9.1 Tomita score (adapted from Tomita et al. [12])

Score	1 point	2 points	4 points
Primary tumor	Slow growth	Moderate growth	Rapid growth
Visceral metastases	–	Treatable	Untreatable
Bone metastases	Solitary	Multiple	–

Table 9.2 Revised Tokuashi score (adapted from Tokuashi et al. [13])

Score	0	1	2	3	4	5
KPS	10–40%	50–70%	80–100%	–	–	–
Extraspinal bone metastases	≥3	1–2	0	–	–	–
Spinal metastasis	≥3	2	1	–	–	–
Metastasis to major organs	Unremovable	Removable	No metastasis	–	–	–
Frankel grade	A–B	C–D	E	–	–	–
Primary site of cancer	Lung Stomach Bladder Esophagus Pancreas Osteosarcoma	Liver Gallbladder Unidentified	Others	Kidney Uterus	Rectum	Thyroid Prostate Breast Carcinoid tumor

Karnofsky performance status (KPS), the number of extraspinal bone metastasis, spinal and visceral metastasis, and the Frankel Score. A score is calculated from the sum of each category, with a higher score being a good prognosis. Again, histology was a strong predictor of survival. A score of 5 is given for the less aggressive histology such as thyroid, breast, and carcinoid tumor. A score of 4 is given for a rectal tumor and a 3 for a renal cell carcinoma. At the far end, a score of 0 is given for the lung, pancreas, osteosarcoma, bladder, esophagus, and stomach. Based on this study, a wide en bloc excision is recommended for the higher score (12–15), a palliative surgery for the intermediate score (9–11), and a conservative approach for the lower scores (0–8). Although these classification systems have been widely used, criticisms have been raised, questioning their validity and reliability [13–17]. Furthermore, inability to differentiate good and moderate prognosis using these scores has been reported [15]. These scoring systems do not consider recent advances in the oncological field such as molecular targeted therapies and SBRT. Furthermore, life expectancy has changed over the last decade for some tumors, especially patients with renal cell carcinoma (RCC) whose survival improved from 2005 to 2010, due to newer treatments [18]. Ultimately, tumor histology, patient performance status, and the systemic burden of the disease will guide the surgeon in the decision-making process. So, for an en bloc procedure to be considered, an oligometastasis from a histology with favorable long-term prognosis must be present. Therefore, the classical indications are an isolated metastasis from a renal cell carcinoma, a thyroid cancer, and more recently from breast cancer because of the potential for long-term survival and poor local control from adjuvant treatments.

Poor response to conventional therapy has led surgeons to perform en bloc resection for isolated RCC spinal metastasis to achieve satisfactory local control. For RCC spinal metastasis, several factors have been identified to predict prolonged survival. Grade of the original nephrectomy specimen (the higher Furham grade (3, 4) is associated with worse prognosis) activity of the systemic disease and neurological status has been shown to predict survival. Patients with an isolated metastasis had a significantly better survival (overall survival (OS) 19 months, 95% CI 9.8–28.2 months) compared to those who had more than one metastasis (OS 9.7 months, 95% CI 8.1–11.3 months, $p < 0.001$). Also, recently, a higher Tokuhashi Score correlated with improved survival. Of 30 patients, a high score (12–15) survived a median of 32.9 months compared to the lower score (0–8) who survived 5.4 months ($p = 0.006$). The Memorial Sloan Kettering Cancer Center (MSKCC/Motezer) Score using time of diagnosis to systemic treatment, hemoglobin, calcium, LDH, and KPS score also has been shown to predict life expectancy for metastatic renal cell carcinoma

[19]. Patients with a "favorable risk" (time from diagnosis to systemic treatment <1 month, KPS >80, LDH <1.5× upper limit of normal, hemoglobin > lower limit of normal, calcium <10 mg/dL) have a median survival of 25 months compared to 2 months for those with a "poor risk." Careful patient selection is of paramount importance when attempting an en bloc resection due to the increased morbidity and resource utilization associated with the procedure.

The introduction and dissemination of SBRT produced a significant change in clinical practice with respect to spinal metastases; tumors that were previously radioresistant were now radiosensitive due to the higher doses of conformal radiation that could be safely delivered. In a systematic review published in 2009, Bilsky et al. [11] reported that local control rates after an en bloc resection compared with SBRT were similar. Following en bloc resection, a 7.5% local recurrence rate was observed at a median follow up of 16 months. For SBRT, a radiologic control failure or symptomatic progression ranged between 6% and 13% at comparable median follow-up. Recently, however, the actuarial local control following SBRT for renal carcinoma has been reported to be 82% at 1 year and 68% at 2 years. The actuarial overall survival at 1 year was 79% and decreased to 49% at 2 years [20]. In the systematic review published by Bilsk et al. [11], they reported results of an unpublished series by Boriani et al. where 25 patients were treated with en bloc procedure for a solitary metastasis. Fifty-two percent of these patients progressed or died at 8–20 months (32% mortality at 8 months), underlining our inability to select long-term survivors in whom the potentially improved local control rate conferred by an oncological resection would be beneficial. Based on this data, the Spine Oncology Study Group (SOSG) recommended that an isolated renal cell carcinoma metastasis without epidural compression should undergo SBRT as a first line of treatment rather than an en bloc resection (strong recommendation). The rationale was to avoid the morbidity of the surgery in patients who would have progressed over a relatively short period regardless of their treatment and would be better served by a less invasive strategy. If local recurrence occurs after SBRT and the patient is well with no other metastases, en bloc resection can be considered because of the potential for long-term survival.

SBRT does however have limitations. To be eligible for SBRT, epidural disease should be minimal to be able to maximize dose and avoid cord toxicity. Local recurrence usually happens in the epidural space because of underdosing [21]. The degree of epidural cord compression (ESCC) is classified with the Bilsky classification [22]. In the ESCC scale, grade 0 denotes bone-only disease, 1a denotes epidural impingement without deformation of the thecal sac, 1b denotes deformation of the thecal sac but without spinal cord abutment, 1c denotes deformation of the thecal sac with spinal cord abutment but without cord compression, 2 denotes spinal cord compression but with cerebrospinal fluid (CSF) visible around the cord, and 3 denotes spinal cord compression without CSF visible around the cord. Following SBRT, higher failure rates have been observed with ESCC grade 2 and 3 due to progression at the epidural space [21]. Another prerequisite is that the metastatic lesion must be stable as SBRT does not address mechanical instability. Mechanical instability is determined with the Spinal Instability Neoplastic Score (SINS) using six variables: location, type of lesion, pain, radiographic spinal alignment, vertebral body collapse, and posterolateral involvement of the spinal element [23]. A score of 13 or greater indicates mechanical instability. More details about the SINS are provided in previous chapters.

En bloc resection for patients with isolated spinal metastasis from a thyroid cancer has also been reported with successful outcomes [24]. In a series of eight patients, at final follow-up (average 6.4 years), all patients were alive, and five had no evidence of disease [25]. However, as with RCC, good local control has been achieved with SBRT. Local control of 88% at 2 years and 79% at 3 years have been reported [26]. With these results, SBRT should be considered as the first line of treatment for isolated thyroid spinal metastasis. Poor prognostic factors for surgically treated spinal metastasis from thyroid carcinoma included progressive systemic disease but also occurrence of postoperative complications such as wound infection, pseudomeningocele, and also urinary tract infection [27]. In the same study, Sellin et al. [27] did not show a correlation between tumor histology and overall survival. However, a trend toward improved survival was observed with favorable histology such as follicular, follicular-papillar, and follicular-columnar.

Although focus on en bloc resection for RCC and thyroid isolated spine metastasis has been emphasized, other histologies may be candidates if certain factors are present. Patients with oligometastasis from breast cancer or a functional secreting metastasis (e.g., pheochromocytoma) may be indicated depending on the risk/benefit ratio. Nonetheless, the decision to proceed to an en bloc resection should be multidisciplinary, with all possible treatments and patient preferences considered.

Surgical Considerations

Once the patient has been staged both locally and systemically, and eligibility for an en bloc resection has been determined, the feasibility of the surgery should be assessed. Magnetic resonance imaging and CT scan are essential to detail local anatomy and planned margins. Even with a known primary, a biopsy should be performed when uncertainty remains about the diagnosis. Trocar biopsy should be favored over open or incisional biopsy as it has been shown to negatively impact outcomes in the rare event of a primary malignant bone tumor [28].

The Weinstein-Boriani-Biagini (WBB) surgical staging system was developed for primary spine tumors to help with planning of the en bloc surgical resection [29], but its principles can be applied in the treatment of spinal metastasis. On axial presentation, the WBB divides the vertebra into 12 zones (Fig. 9.1). Zone 1 represents the left half of the spinous process followed by the others in a counterclockwise sense. Lastly, according to the WBB, the vertebra is further divided into five layers: from layer A representing the tissue surrounding the vertebra to layer E corresponding to an intradural involvement. Different types of resection can be performed depending on tumor location. A sagittal resection, which is a wedge resection of the vertebral body, is indicated when the tumor is eccentrically located (Fig. 9.2). A posterior resection is performed when only the posterior elements are

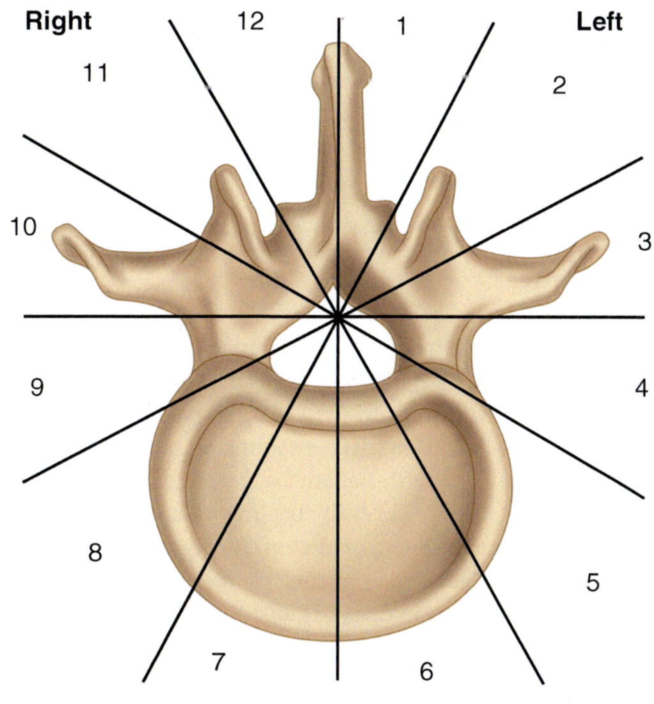

Fig. 9.1 12 zones of Weinstein-Boriani-Biagini surgical staging system

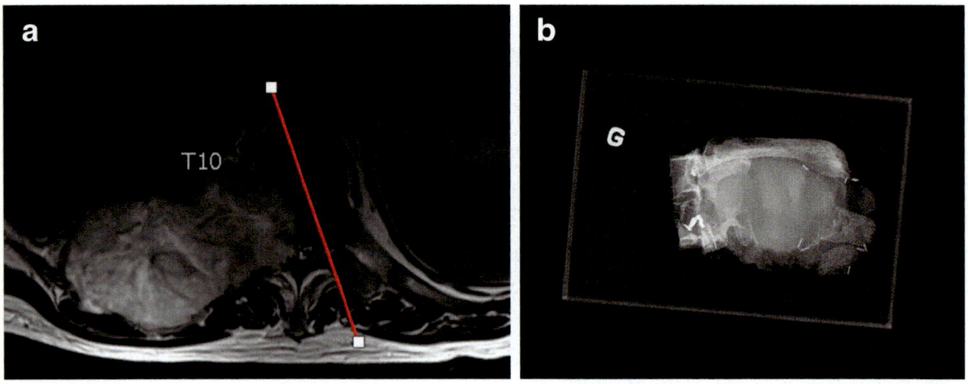

Fig. 9.2 Sagittal resection for isolated thyroid cell metastasis at T9–T10. (**a**) Planned sagittal resection at T10. (**b**) Intraoperative radiograph of the specimen

involved which is rare with metastatic disease. A corpectomy is a resection of the vertebral body. And finally, a spondylectomy or vertebrectomy is the removal of the vertebra. However, to be technically feasible, enough bone in the posterior ring (formed by the lamina and pedicles) needs to be free of disease to allow clearance of the thecal sac during resection, and an access to the nerve roots is required (Fig. 9.3). In the thoracic spine, resection can be performed through a posterior-only approach if there is no significant soft tissue extension, as nerve roots can be sacrificed without altering function. In the cervical and lumbar spine, two stages (anterior and posterior) are usually required. Detailed surgical techniques are beyond the scope of this chapter, and a specific expertise is required to perform this type of surgery.

Outcomes

Complications are common after surgery in the metastatic spine population. In a prospective study of the MSD, up to 76% of the patients experienced at least one adverse event after emergent spine surgery [30]. Patients selected for an en bloc procedure are generally healthier than the general metastatic spine population. By itself, en bloc resection carries significant morbidity. As described by Yamazaki et al. [3], distortion of the anatomy, epidural veins/tumor bleeding, nervous and vascular manipulation/sacrifice, adherence from previous surgery, and radiation therapy are risk factors highly prevalent in this population. Most studies on en bloc resection included both primary and metastatic spine tumors as this procedure is a rare. Overall complication rate for a mobile location ranged from 13 to 73.4% and complication-related death ranged from 0 to 7.7%. Significant blood loss can be anticipated. Due to the complexity of the surgery, prolonged operative times are common. Iatrogenic dural tears are not infrequent. Neurologic deterioration due to ischemic cord injury following segmental artery ligation has also been reported [6, 31].

Omeis et al. [32] reported a 9.5% infection rate after en bloc resection for MSD. The most common organism was staphylococcus aureus. Complex plastic closure, previous spinal surgery, multiple comorbidities, the presence of an infection at the time of previous surgery, and increased length of hospital stay were associated with postoperative infection. Hardware failure is a common cause of revision following en bloc resection. Amendola et al. [33] reported that hardware failure requiring revision was 9.7%. The largest series on en bloc resection has been recently published and reports on 220 patients (primary bone tumor and MSD) [34]. Combined approach, neoadjuvant chemotherapy, and neoadjuvant radiotherapy were associated with adverse events. Surprisingly, metastatic spine disease was not associated with adverse events more than primary

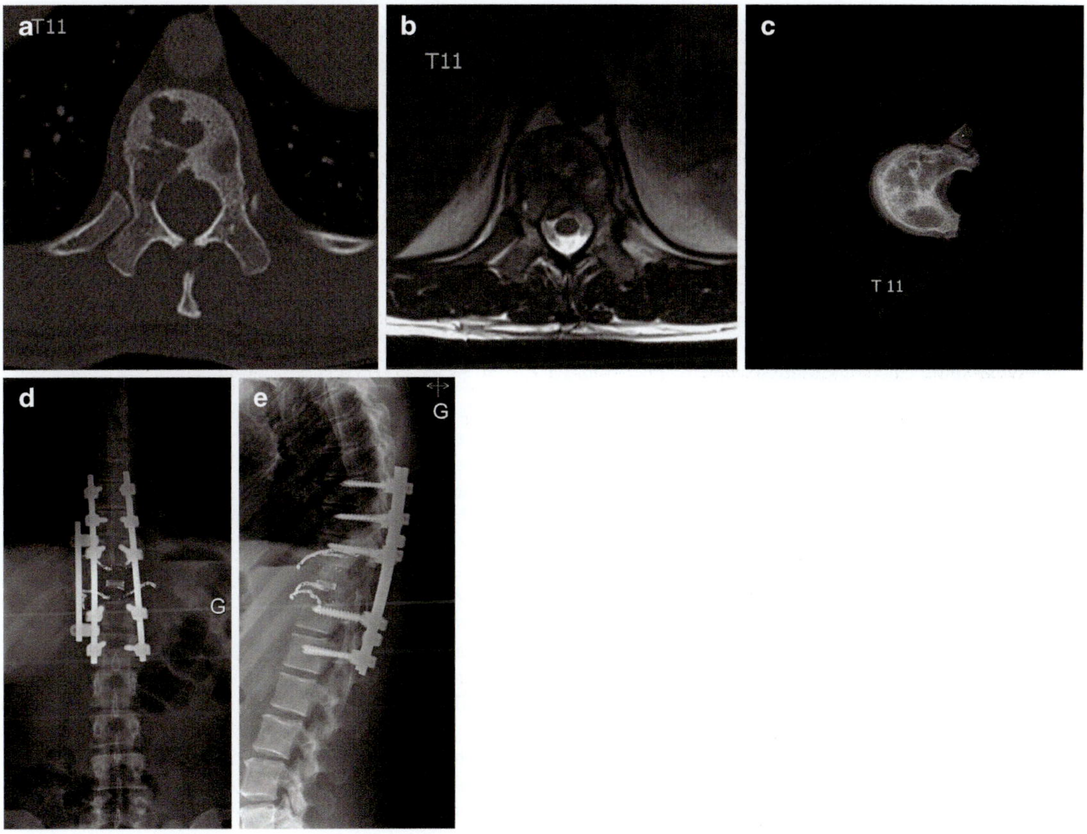

Fig. 9.3 En bloc resection for an isolated rectum metastasis. (**a**, **b**) Preoperative MRI and CT scan showing feasibility of an en bloc resection with a pedicle free of disease. (**c**) Intraoperative radiograph of the specimen. (**d**, **e**) Postoperative AP and lateral radiographs showing posterior instrumentation from T8–L1 with anterior reconstruction with a peek cage

tumor. However, it was an independent risk factor for patient's death (OR 2.67, $p = 0.042$).

Lastly, the impact of an oncologic resection on health-related quality of life (HRQOL) should be acceptable for the patient, especially in the metastatic spine population where life expectancy is generally reduced. Literature specifically on en bloc resection in the patient with MSD is limited; however, when cure is achieved, results can be extrapolated from the primary tumor literature. In a recent systematic review, HRQOL after surgical treatment of a primary bone tumor has been reported to be close the general population when long follow-up is available. As expected, HRQOL tends to improve over time as the patient recovers from surgery [35]. Only one study included patients with MSD (three patients) [36]. Both their SF-36 and Oswestry disability index were close to the normative values at a minimum of 3 years postoperatively. Not surprisingly, in this series, patients operated for a primary bone tumor performed better than patients with metastatic spine disease.

Acceptable oncologic results can be obtained after an en bloc resection for solitary spinal metastases. However, knowledge is lacking regarding patient-reported outcomes following this type of procedure. Selecting the right patient, for the right operation, is pivotal. Adequate HRQOL can probably be achieved with careful patient selection through a multidisciplinary team and experienced specialized center.

References

1. Patchell RA, Tibbs PA, Regine WF, Payne R, Saris S, Kryscio RJ, et al. Direct decompressive surgical resection in the treatment of spinal cord compression caused by metastatic cancer: a randomised trial. Lancet. 2005;366(9486):643–8.
2. Enneking WF, Spanier SS, Goodman MA. A system for the surgical staging of musculoskeletal sarcoma. Clin Orthop Relat Res. 1980;153:106–20.
3. Yamazaki T, McLoughlin GS, Patel S, Rhines LD, Fourney DR. Feasibility and safety of en bloc resection for primary spine tumors: a systematic review by the Spine Oncology Study Group. Spine (Phila Pa 1976). 2009;34(22):S31–8.
4. Charest-Morin R, Fisher CG, Varga PP, Gokaslan ZL, Rhines LD, Reynolds JJ, et al. En bloc resection versus intralesional surgery in the treatment of giant cell tumor of the spine. Spine (Phila Pa 1976). 2017;42(18):1383–90.
5. Dekutoski MB, Clarke MJ, Rose P, Luzzati A, Rhines LD, Varga PP, et al. Osteosarcoma of the spine: prognostic variables for local recurrence and overall survival, a multicenter ambispective study. J Neurosurg Spine. 2016;25(1):59–68.
6. Fisher CG, Keynan O, Boyd MC, Dvorak MF. The surgical management of primary tumorsof the spine: initial results of an ongoing prospective cohort study. Spine (Phila Pa 1976). 2005;30(16):1899–908.
7. Fisher CG, Saravanja DD, Dvorak MF, Rampersaud YR, Clarkson PW, Hurlbert J, et al. Surgical management of primary bone tumors of the spine: validation of an approach to enhance cure and reduce local recurrence. Spine (Phila Pa 1976). 2011;36(10):830–6.
8. Fisher CG, Versteeg AL, Dea N, Boriani S, Varga PP, Dekutoski MB, et al. Surgical management of spinal chondrosarcomas. Spine (Phila Pa 1976). 2016;41(8):678–85.
9. Gokaslan ZL, Zadnik PL, Sciubba DM, Germscheid N, Goodwin CR, Wolinsky J-P, et al. Mobile spine chordoma: results of 166 patients from the AOSpine Knowledge Forum Tumor database. J Neurosurg Spine. 2016;24(4):644–51.
10. Gerszten PC, Yamada Y. Radiotherapy and radiosurgery for metastatic spine disease what are the options, indications, and outcomes? Spine (Phila Pa 1976). 2009;34(22):78–92.
11. Bilsky MH, Laufer I, Burch S. Shifting paradigms in the treatment of metastatic spine disease. Spine (Phila Pa 1976). 2009;34(22 Suppl):S101–7.
12. Tomita K, Kawahara N, Kobayashi T, Yoshida A, Murakami H, Akamaru T. Surgical strategy for spinal metastases. Spine (Phila Pa 1976). 2001;26(3):298–306.
13. Tokuhashi Y, Matsuzaki H, Oda H, Oshima M, Ryu J. A revised scoring system for preoperative evaluation of metastatic spine tumor prognosis. Spine (Phila Pa 1976). 2005;30(19):2186–91.
14. Lee C-H, Chung CK, Jahng T-A, Kim K, Kim CH, Hyun S-J, et al. Which one is a valuable surrogate for predicting survival between Tomita and Tokuhashi scores in patients with spinal metastases? A meta-analysis for diagnostic test accuracy and individual participant data analysis. J Neuro-Oncol. 2015;123(2):267–75.
15. Wibmer C, Leithner A, Hofmann G, Clar H, Kapitan M, Berghold A, et al. Survival analysis of 254 patients after manifestation of spinal metastases: evaluation of seven preoperative scoring systems. Spine (Phila Pa 1976). 2011;36(23):1977–86.
16. Bollen L, Wibmer C, Van der Linden YM, Pondaag W, Fiocco M, Peul WC, et al. Predictive value of six prognostic scoring systems for spinal bone metastases: an analysis based on 1379 patients. Spine (Phila Pa 1976). 2016;41(3):E155–62.
17. Gregory TM, Coriat R, Mir O. Prognostic scoring systems for spinal metastases in the era of anti-VEGF therapies. Spine (Phila Pa 1976). 2013;38(11):965–6.
18. Morgen SS, Lund-Andersen C, Larsen CF, Engelholm SA, Dahl B. Prognosis in patients with symptomatic metastatic spinal cord compression: survival in different cancer diagnosis in a cohort of 2321 patients. Spine (Phila Pa 1976). 2013;38(16):1362–7.
19. Bakker NA, Coppes MH, Vergeer RA, Kuijlen JMA, Groen RJM. Surgery on spinal epidural metastases (SEM) in renal cell carcinoma: a plea for a new paradigm. Spine J. 2014;14(9):2038–41.
20. Ghia AJ, Chang EL, Bishop AJ, Pan HY, Boehling NS, Amini B, et al. Single-fraction versus multifraction spinal stereotactic radiosurgery for spinal metastases from renal cell carcinoma: secondary analysis of Phase I/II trials. J Neurosurg Spine. 2016;24(5):829–36.
21. Al-Omair A, Masucci L, Masson-Cote L, Campbell M, Atenafu EG, Parent A, et al. Surgical resection of epidural disease improves local control following postoperative spine stereotactic body radiotherapy. Neuro-Oncology. 2013;15(10):1413–9.
22. Bilsky MH, Laufer I, Fourney DR, Groff M, Schmidt MH, Varga PP, et al. Reliability analysis of the epidural spinal cord compression scale. J Neurosurg Spine. 2010;13(3):324–8.
23. Fisher CG, DiPaola CP, Ryken TC, Bilsky MH, Shaffrey CI, Berven SH, et al. A novel classification system for spinal instability in neoplastic disease: an evidence-based approach and expert consensus from the Spine Oncology Study Group. Spine (Phila Pa 1976). 2010;35(22):E1221–9.
24. Kato S, Murakami H, Demura S, Fujimaki Y, Yoshioka K, Yokogawa N, et al. The impact of complete surgical resection of spinal metastases on the survival of patients with thyroid cancer. Cancer Med. 2016;5(9):2343–9.
25. Matsumoto M, Tsuji T, Iwanami A, Watanabe K, Hosogane N, Ishii K, et al. Total en bloc spondylectomy for spinal metastasis of differentiated thyroid cancers: a long-term follow-up. J Spinal Disord Tech. 2013;26(4):E137–42.

26. Bernstein MB, Chang EL, Amini B, Pan H, Cabanillas M, Wang XA, et al. Spine stereotactic radiosurgery for patients with metastatic thyroid cancer: secondary analysis of phase I/II trials. Thyroid. 2016;26(9):1269–75.
27. Sellin JN, Suki D, Harsh V, Elder BD, Fahim DK, Mccutcheon IE, et al. Surgery for spinal metastases from thyroid carcinoma. J Neurosurg Spine. 2015;23:419–28.
28. Boriani S, Saravanja D, Yamada Y, Varga PP, Biagini R, Fisher CG. Challenges of local recurrence and cure in low grade malignant tumors of the spine. Spine (Phila Pa 1976). 2009;34(22):S48–57.
29. Boriani S, Weinstein JN, Biagini R. Primary bone tumors of the spine. Terminology and surgical staging. Spine (Phila Pa 1976). 1997;22(9):1036–44.
30. Dea N, Versteeg A, Fisher C, Kelly A, Hartig D, Boyd M, et al. Adverse events in emergency oncological spine surgery: a prospective analysis. J Neurosurg Spine. 2014;21(5):698–703.
31. Liljenqvist U, Lerner T, Halm H, Buerger H, Gosheger G, Winkelmann W. En bloc spondylectomy in malignant tumors of the spine. Eur Spine J. 2008;17(4):600–9.
32. Omeis IA, Dhir M, Sciubba DM, Gottfried ON, McGirt MJ, Attenello FJ, et al. Postoperative surgical site infections in patients undergoing spinal tumor surgery: incidence and risk factors. Spine (Phila Pa 1976). 2011;36(17):1410–9.
33. Amendola L, Cappuccio M, De Iure F, Bandiera S, Gasbarrini A, Boriani S. En bloc resections for primary spinal tumors in 20 years of experience: effectiveness and safety. Spine J. 2014;14(11):2608–17. https://doi.org/10.1016/j.spinee.2014.02.030; Epub 2014 Feb 20.
34. Boriani S, Gasbarrini A, Bandiera S, Ghermandi R, Lador R. En bloc resections in the spine: the experience of 220 patients during 25 years. World Neurosurg. 2017;98:217–29.
35. Dea N, Charest-Morin R, Sciubba DM, Bird JE, Disch AC, Mesfin A, et al. Optimizing the adverse event and HRQOL profiles in the management of primary spine tumors. Spine (Phila Pa 1976). 2016;41(20S):S212–7.
36. Mazel C, Owona P, Cogan A, Balabaud L, Grunenwald D. Long-term quality of life after en-bloc vertebrectomy: 25 patients followed up for 9 years. Orthop Traumatol Surg Res. 2014;100(1):119–26.

10 Occipitocervical and Upper Cervical Metastatic Spinal Disease

Jared Fridley, Adetokunbo Oyelese, and Ziya L. Gokaslan

Introduction

Cancer was diagnosed in an estimated 1.7 million people in the United States during 2016 [1]. When cancer metastasizes, it tends to spread to the lung, liver, and bone. The spine is the most common skeletal structure affected. Nearly 40% of cancer patients at autopsy have pathologic evidence of spinal metastases [2]. An estimated 5–10% of patients with metastatic spine disease will become symptomatic and require treatment during their lifetime [3]. The most common spinal segment to be affected is the thoracic spine due to its substantial number of vertebrate and adjacent vascular plexus. This is followed by the lumbar spine and then the cervical spine. Involvement of the CVJ accounts for only 0.5% of spinal metastases [4] and are usually asymptomatic. Patients with symptomatic CVJ tumors can present a management challenge to the treating physician owing to its unique bony anatomy, adjacent neurovascular structures, and unique biomechanics. Any comprehensive treatment plan for CVJ tumors must consider not only the tumor itself, but also how the tumor affects these three factors.

J. Fridley, MD
Department of Neurosurgery, The Warren Alpert Medical School of Brown University, Providence, RI, USA
e-mail: Jared.Fridley@Lifespan.org

A. Oyelese, MD, PhD, FAANS
Department of Neurosurgery, The Warren Alpert Medical School of Brown University, Providence, RI, USA

Department of Neurosurgery, Rhode Island Hospital, Providence, RI, USA
e-mail: aoyelese@lifespan.org

Z. L. Gokaslan, MD, FAANS, FACS (✉)
Department of Neurosurgery, The Warren Alpert Medical School of Brown University, Providence, RI, USA

Department of Neurosurgery, Rhode Island Hospital and The Miriam Hospital, Providence, RI, USA
e-mail: ziya_gokaslan@brown.edu; ziya.gokaslan@lifespan.org

Epidemiology

The most common primary sources of metastatic spinal disease are breast carcinoma (35%), non-small-cell lung carcinoma (15%), and prostate carcinoma (10%) [4]. Other sources include renal, gastrointestinal, thyroid, sarcoma, lymphoma, and multiple myeloma. The CVJ seems to be affected by a similar proportion of primary tumors, albeit less frequently than other spinal segments [4]. Rarely is an isolated CVJ tumor the primary presentation of metastatic disease. When symptomatic, CVJ metastases tend to occur within the C2 vertebral body/dens, the C1–2 articular processes, or the occipital condyle [5, 6].

R. A. W. Marco (ed.), *Metastatic Spine Disease*, https://doi.org/10.1007/978-3-319-76252-4_10

Presentation

Pain is the most common presenting symptom in patients with tumors of the CVJ and upper cervical spine. When describing the pain, it is helpful to categorize it as either focal pain or mechanical pain. Focal neck pain is often described as achiness or stiffness at a specific segment in the spine and is often worse at night. Mechanical neck pain refers to aggravation of pain with neck movement. Direct compression by tumor of the C2 nerve roots, or tumor destruction of the atlantoaxial facet causing local inflammation or bony compression of C2 nerve roots, can lead to occipital neuralgia. Occipital neuralgia is described as a sharp shooting pain that travels from the upper neck toward the suboccipital and posterior auricular area of the scalp. Flexion or extension of the neck can sometimes exacerbate symptoms.

Weight loss, night sweats, and chills are often associated with widespread metastatic disease. Tumor spread into other organ systems can lead to bleeding diathesis, pulmonary dysfunction, abdominal pain, gastrointestinal bleeding, constipation, focal neurologic deficits, and/or extremity pain among others. Determination of the degree of metastatic spread and the subsequent physiologic effects of multi-organ involvement is important not only in terms of patient prognosis but also when assessing the risk of various treatment options including surgical intervention.

Very rarely does a tumor of the CVJ cause direct spinal cord compression leading to symptoms/signs of myelopathy. This is due in part to the relatively large spinal canal at C1 and C2. Moreover, the authors believe that myelopathy is less likely to occur because the stout cruciate ligament prevents spinal cord compression by tumor involving the CVJ. When myelopathy is present, this is usually due to a tumor of significant size or tumor extension through the foramen magnum. Bony erosion of the atlantoaxial junction may also lead to segmental instability and subluxation which can cause cord injury. Lower cranial nerve dysfunction may result from tumor compression of the medulla, spinal accessory nerve, and very rarely the hypoglossal nerve. The spinal accessory nerve is the most common cranial nerve affected by CVJ tumors because of its length and recurrent looping anatomy. Deficits of the spinal accessory nerve include weakness when turning the head or shrugging the shoulders due to its innervation of the trapezius/sternocleidomastoid muscles. Alternatively, patients might present with torticollis which is a dystonia of the muscles that can be very painful. Swallowing dysfunction from vagus nerve or glossopharyngeal nerve is not common but can be seen with cranial tumor extension.

In some patients, a CVJ metastasis may have no associated symptoms, but rather the tumor is found incidentally on a metastatic imaging workup. A thorough patient history and physical examination after the tumor is visualized may elicit symptoms that the patient felt at the time to be innocuous or secondary to degenerative spinal disease.

Diagnostic Workup

Patients with symptoms/signs of an upper cervical/CVJ tumor should first obtain imaging to confirm clinical suspicion, and if confirmed, determine tumor characteristics. Magnetic resonance imaging (MRI) with and without contrast is typically the first-line imaging modality for workup. Multiplane reconstructions in axial, sagittal, and coronal planes are helpful for defining the relationship of tumor to neural elements and adjacent soft tissue structures. Computed tomography (CT) is used to evaluate the extent of osseous disease and whether the tumor is osteolytic or osteoblastic. Attention is paid to the articular surfaces of the CVJ and whether there is any evidence of atlantoaxial subluxation or tumor-associated destruction of the bony anatomy. Imaging of the chest, abdomen, and pelvis using CT with and without contrast is mandatory to evaluate the extent of disease and help determine patient prognosis.

Vascular imaging, with either CT angiography or conventional angiography, is recommended to evaluate the course of the vertebral arteries and their involvement with tumor if surgical treatment is being contemplated. Determining the patency and dominance of the vertebral arteries is necessary if one of the vertebral arteries is planned for sacrifice or if preoperative embolization is planned. Angiographic assessment of collateral blood flow and filling of the posterior inferior cerebellar arteries is helpful to determine the risk of infarction prior to vertebral artery embolization. A balloon occlusion test of the involved vertebral artery is recommended in the case of dominant vertebral artery involvement. Tumor blush on angiography indicates hypervascularity, in which case preoperative particle or glue embolization can be useful to minimize both blood loss and operative time. Renal cell carcinoma, thyroid carcinoma, melanoma, and hepatocellular carcinoma can be particularly vascular and should be considered for embolization if surgery is planned.

Laboratory Studies

Laboratory studies can provide useful information to assist in the diagnoses of a CVJ metastasis, particularly if solitary. For example, elevations in serum prostate-specific antigen (PSA) or carcinoembryonic antigen (CEA) can point toward a prostate or gastrointestinal primary tumor, respectively. Hematopoietic malignancies, such as multiple myeloma, may be suspected with abnormalities in hematocrit or platelet count. If suspected, a serum protein electrophoresis (SPEP) or urine protein electrophoresis (UPEP) is performed to look for a monoclonal gammopathy. Definitive diagnosis may ultimately require bone marrow biopsy.

If multiple lesions are found on imaging, but the primary is not certain, needle biopsy of an accessible lesion can be performed. This is done either with CT guidance, as is the case with abdominal or retroperitoneal masses, or with endoscopic guidance for masses in the gastrointestinal track or bronchial tree. Needle biopsy of a CVJ mass is not recommended due to the surrounding neurovascular anatomy and risk of injury to these structures. If systemic workup is negative for signs of a source of metastatic disease, and there is a solitary lesion of the CVJ, consideration must be given for a primary malignancy and a CT guided biopsy is indicated.

Treatment Strategy

The treatment of a CVJ neoplasm is personalized based on information gathered from history and physical examination, primary pathology, tumor location and involvement of adjacent neurovascular structures, and presence of spinal instability. If metastatic disease of the CVJ is suspected, the first treatment decision to make is whether to perform surgery or radiation as first-line therapy. It should always be kept in mind that the treatment of spinal metastases is palliative and should be focused on patient quality of life and functional outcome.

A useful method for spinal metastases treatment decision making is based on the NOMS framework described by Laufer et al. [7]. This framework is based on patient neurologic, oncologic, mechanical, and systemic considerations. If a patient with a spinal metastasis has significant neurologic dysfunction and/or significant spinal cord compression, surgical decompression is generally recommended. Very rarely is this the case for a CVJ metastasis. Oncologic considerations are based on primary pathology and whether it is sensitive to external beam radiotherapy. Lymphoma and multiple myeloma are considered especially radiosensitive, whereas renal cell carcinoma and non-small-cell lung carcinoma are not. Mechanical stability is based on the location of the lesion, presence and type of spinal pain, whether the tumor is osteolytic or osteoblastic, presence of deformity or subluxation, degree of vertebral body collapse, and whether there is posterolateral element involvement. These variables can be combined to calculate the spinal instability neoplastic score (SINS) [8] used to ascertain whether there might be mechanical instability. The CVJ is a mobile segment of the spine with a significant amount of flexion-extension between occiput and C1 and rotation between C1 and C2. Disruption of the occipital-C1 or atlantoaxial facets can lead to significant radiographic and clinical instability.

The editor and authors believe that spinal instability is uncommon in this region of the spine. The editor thus believes that the SINS classification overestimates the likelihood of instability associated with tumor involving the CVJ. The last portion, but perhaps most important part, of the NOMS framework is systemic considerations. These include the extent of disease spread, patient performance status, and overall medical condition. The editor is in agreement that systemic considerations are probably the most important factors to consider in the treatment of these patients. The editor thus believes that MOSS is a more practical framework to provide treatment recommendations for these patients.

Radiation

In the absence of significant neural compression or spinal instability, radiation can be a viable first-line treatment option. Conventional fractionated external beam radiotherapy (EBRT) of the spine has historically been given as a palliative option in patients that either were not surgical candidates or who had radiosensitive neoplasms. EBRT is typically given at a dose of 300 cGy over 10 fractions. It can be an effective means of pain relief in patients with CVJ metastases as shown in a small series of 33 patients with CVJ metastases by Bilsky et al. In this study series, there were 23 patients without evidence of radiographic instability (defined as less than 5 mm of atlantoaxial subluxation and less than 11° of odontoid angulation) who underwent initial treatment with EBRT [9]. Over 90% of these patients had either significant relief or resolution of their neck pain. There were two patients that underwent eventual surgical intervention for spinal stabilization.

Within the last several decades, technological innovation in radiation delivery has culminated in the development of stereotactic spinal radiosurgery (SRS). This radiation method is characterized by single or hypofractionated high-dose radiation, delivered in a precise, conformal, 3-dimensional manner to the spinal tumor or tumor resection cavity of interest. SRS has recently been demonstrated to be efficacious in the treatment of CVJ metastases, both in terms of pain relief and local tumor control [10, 11]. Azad et al. reported a series of 25 patients with CVJ metastases who underwent SRS [10]. The metastases originated from various primaries, and no patient had a SINS score >12. At a median of 18 months of post-radiation follow-up, there was resolution or improvement in neck pain in approximately 50% of patients with preoperative pain. Sixteen out of nineteen patients at last follow-up either had no change or a decrease in the size of the radiated tumor. Only 2 out of 25 patients ultimately underwent surgical stabilization. In large SRS series for spinal metastases, not specific to the CVJ, local control rates of nearly 90% are common, making it a viable first-line treatment option with minimal morbidity [12, 13]. As discussed below, surgical intervention for CVJ metastases is usually reserved for a specific set of circumstances given the recent success of SRS therapy.

Surgery

The primary goals of surgical intervention for spinal metastases are palliative in nature and include relief of pain, maintenance or improvement in ambulation, and improvement in patient quality of life. Patients with metastatic disease, in general, succumb to the systemic effects of cancer and not from the morbidity associated from spinal disease. Present day indications for surgical intervention are primarily limited to surgical decompression for neural element impingement causing neurologic dysfunction or spinal stabilization for signs/symptoms of mechanical instability. CVJ metastases do not often cause metastatic epidural spinal cord compression partly due to the capacious size of the spinal canal at the CVJ. This means that in many patients, radiation can be offered as first-line therapy, often with minimal risk of radiation-induced myelopathy. When tumor does cause high-grade epidural compression, with possible clinical evidence of myelopathy, surgical decompression may be warranted.

Decompression of the CVJ from metastases is dictated primarily by whether the tumor is causing compression ventrally or dorsally. Tumor arising from the posterior elements can be easily accessed through a simple posterior cervical approach to the CVJ, with exposure of the relevant CVJ bony anatomy. A laminectomy of C1 and/or C2, followed by direct tumor resection, may suffice to decompress the spinal cord without causing iatrogenic instability. Unfortunately, ventral cord compression is more common, and requires more thoughtful deliberation prior to any intervention. The morbidity of any anterior approach to the CVJ, such as the transoral or high retropharyngeal approach, must be weighed against not only other surgical approaches, but also radiation alone, especially if the risk to the patient from surgery is felt to be too great [14]. A middle ground option that is sometimes considered in light of the success of SRS is surgical resection of a subtotal amount of tumor to create separation between it and the spinal cord. The goal in doing so is to allow postoperative SRS to be safely delivered to the tumor while minimizing radiation toxicity to the spinal cord. This strategy is referred to as "separation surgery" [15]. An example strategy for separation surgery for a CVJ metastasis would be to incorporate a posterior or posterolateral approach to a ventral CVJ metastasis causing cord compression. A posterior or posterolateral approach may be chosen over an anterior approach to minimize surgical approach-related morbidity. Once the relevant bony anatomy is exposed, C1 and C2 laminectomies are performed, followed by identification of the C1–2 facet joints and C2 nerve roots. Sacrifice of one or both C2 nerve roots can be very helpful for exposure of ventral tumor. This is generally well tolerated as the C2 root is a purely sensory root, resulting in unilateral suboccipital scalp numbness postoperatively. Only rarely do patients develop postoperative occipital neuralgia because of C2 root sacrifice. Ventral epidural tumor can create a surgical corridor by displacing thecal sac, allowing a wider approach window.

One of the primary concerns with a posterior approach for resection of a CVJ tumor, especially if there is lateral tumor extension, is injury to the adjacent vertebral artery. Study of the vertebral artery on preoperative imaging is essential to minimize surgical risk. Determination of the dominant vertebral artery, the course of the vessel, its relationship to the surrounding bony anatomy, and ascertainment of its involvement with tumor are important not only for tumor resection, but also to help determine instrumentation plans if needed. If the vertebral artery is encased by tumor, residual disease can be reasonably left behind with the intention to radiate this area postoperatively. Hypervascular metastases in which resection is planned, such as renal cell carcinoma, may benefit from preoperative embolization to reduce intraoperative blood loss. If fed from branches of the dominant vertebral artery, then care should be taken to ascertain collateral vasculature and location of the posterior inferior cerebellar arteries. Errant embolization of the posterior circulation vasculature can result in brain stem or cerebellar infarct leading to significant neurologic deficit.

In patients with clinical or radiographic evidence of atlantoaxial instability related to either metastatic disease or from surgical insult, posterior surgical stabilization is recommended. Clinical instability may be defined as an inability of the CVJ to function under physiologic loads without pain, neurologic deficit, or spinal deformity [16]. Radiographic evidence of atlantoaxial subluxation, angulation of the dens, rotatory subluxation, and destruction of the occipitoatlantal/atlantoaxial facet complex are indications for stabilization (Fig. 10.1). Occipitocervical instrumented fusion is preferred over atlantoaxial stabilization, even in the case of isolated C1 or C2 metastases, primarily because of the unpredictable course of metastatic disease and the concern that involvement of adjacent areas may lead to possible construct failure and need for additional surgery (Fig. 10.2). Even in the absence of gross radiographic instability, we generally recommend posterior instrumented stabilization in patients with mechanical neck pain. In a published series by Fourney et al. [5], occipitocervical stabilization in 19 patients with CVJ

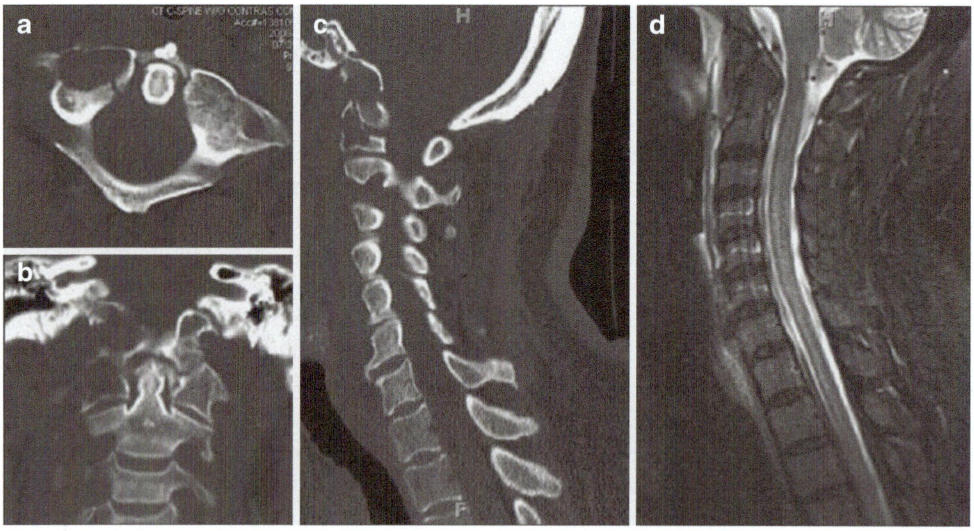

Fig. 10.1 Imaging from a 66-year-old with non-small-cell lung carcinoma and severe axial neck pain. Computed tomography (CT) and magnetic resonance imaging (MRI) of the atlanto-occipital junction. (**a**) An axial CT image shows significant hypodense areas in the right occipitocervical junction, demonstrating extensive tumor infiltration. (**b**) The coronal CT image again illustrates the scope of metastatic disease in both the right atlas and occipital condyle, with both being almost entirely consumed by the tumor. (**c**) A sagittal view shows hypodense destructive lytic masses in both the occipital condyle and atlas. (**d**) A T2-weighted MR image shows normal cerebral spinal fluid distribution with no evidence of spinal cord compression. From Xu R, Sciubba D, Gokaslan Z, Bydon A. Metastasis to the occipitocervical junction: A case report and review of the literature. Surgical neurology international. 2010 Jan 1;1(1):16

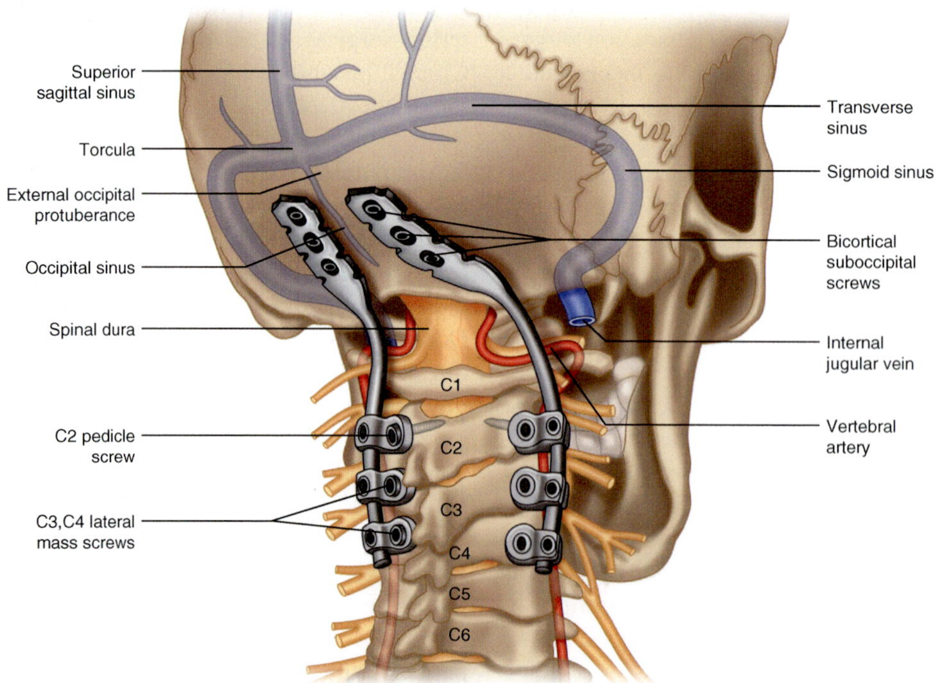

Fig. 10.2 Artist rendering of an occipitocervical fusion construct. From Fourney DR, York JE, Cohen ZR, Suki D, Rhines LD, Gokaslan ZL. Management of atlantoaxial metastases with posterior occipitocervical stabilization. Journal of Neurosurgery: Spine. 2003 Mar;98(2):165–70

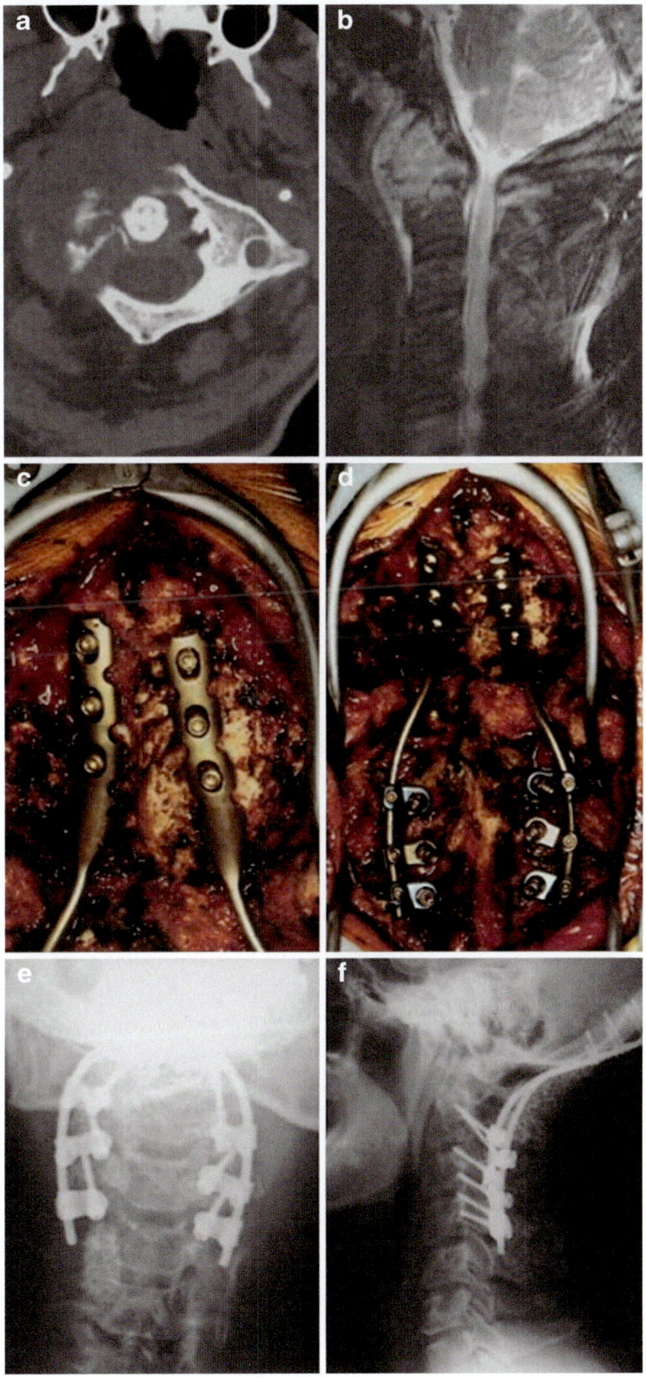

Fig. 10.3 Imaging studies obtained in a 43-year-old man who presented with neck pain, torticollis, and lower cranial nerve deficits; a renal cell carcinoma, metastatic to the right occipital condyle and lateral mass of C1, caused rotatory atlantoaxial subluxation. (**a**) Axial computerized tomography scan and (**b**) sagittal T2-weighted MR image demonstrating lytic tumor. (**c, d**) Intraoperative photographs demonstrating the instrumented occipitocervical fusion. (**e**) Postoperative anteroposterior and (**f**) lateral plain X-ray films revealing the bicortical occipital and lateral mass (C3 and C4) screws, as well as C2 pedicle screws. From Fourney DR, York JE, Cohen ZR, Suki D, Rhines LD, Gokaslan ZL. Management of atlantoaxial metastases with posterior occipitocervical stabilization. Journal of Neurosurgery: Spine. 2003 Mar;98(2):165–70

metastases resulted in a significant improvement in neck pain with minimal surgical morbidity (Fig. 10.3). Reduction of motion at tumor-affected spinal segments in the cervical spine can significantly improve patient quality of life by mechanical neck pain reduction. Despite the relatively short survival of many patients with metastatic cancer, we will often perform a posterolateral arthrodesis to help mitigate potential future hardware failures, with minimal operative time and cost added to the overall surgery.

References

1. Society AC. Cancer Facts and Figures 2016. 2016. https://old.cancer.org/acs/groups/content/@research/documents/document/acspc-047079.pdf.
2. Wong DA, Fornasier VL, MacNab I. Spinal metastases: the obvious, the occult, and the impostors. Spine (Phila Pa 1976). 1990;15(1):1–4.
3. Sundaresan N, Boriani S, Rothman A, Holtzman R. Tumors of the osseous spine. J Neuro-Oncol. 2004; 69(1–3):273–90.
4. Moulding HD, Bilsky MH. Metastases to the craniovertebral junction. Neurosurgery. 2010;66(suppl_3): A113–A8.
5. Fourney DR, York JE, Cohen ZR, Suki D, Rhines LD, Gokaslan ZL. Management of atlantoaxial metastases with posterior occipitocervical stabilization. J Neurosurg. 2003;98(2 Suppl):165–70.
6. Xu R, Sciubba DM, Gokaslan ZL, Bydon A. Metastasis to the occipitocervical junction: a case report and review of the literature. Surg Neurol Int. 2010;1:16.
7. Laufer I, Rubin DG, Lis E, Cox BW, Stubblefield MD, Yamada Y, et al. The NOMS framework: approach to the treatment of spinal metastatic tumors. Oncologist. 2013;18(6):744–51.
8. Fisher CG, DiPaola CP, Ryken TC, Bilsky MH, Shaffrey CI, Berven SH, et al. A novel classification system for spinal instability in neoplastic disease: an evidence-based approach and expert consensus from the Spine Oncology Study Group. Spine (Phila Pa 1976). 2010;35(22):E1221–9.
9. Bilsky MH, Shannon FJ, Sheppard S, Prabhu V, Boland PJ. Diagnosis and management of a metastatic tumor in the atlantoaxial spine. Spine (Phila Pa 1976). 2002;27(10):1062–9.
10. Azad TD, Esparza R, Chaudhary N, Chang SD. Stereotactic radiosurgery for metastasis to the craniovertebral junction preserves spine stability and offers symptomatic relief. J Neurosurg Spine. 2015:1–7.
11. Tuchman A, Yu C, Chang EL, Kim PE, Rusch MC, Apuzzo ML. Radiosurgery for metastatic disease at the craniocervical junction. World Neurosurg. 2014;82(6):1331–6.
12. Gerszten PC, Burton SA, Ozhasoglu C, Welch WC. Radiosurgery for spinal metastases: clinical experience in 500 cases from a single institution. Spine (Phila Pa 1976). 2007;32(2):193–9.
13. Ryu S, Rock J, Rosenblum M, Kim JH. Patterns of failure after single-dose radiosurgery for spinal metastasis. J Neurosurg. 2004;101(Suppl 3):402–5.
14. Jones DC, Hayter JP, Vaughan ED, Findlay GF. Oropharyngeal morbidity following transoral approaches to the upper cervical spine. Int J Oral Maxillofac Surg. 1998;27(4):295–8.
15. Laufer I, Iorgulescu JB, Chapman T, Lis E, Shi W, Zhang Z, et al. Local disease control for spinal metastases following "separation surgery" and adjuvant hypofractionated or high-dose single-fraction stereotactic radiosurgery: outcome analysis in 186 patients. J Neurosurg Spine. 2013;18(3):207–14.
16. White AA 3rd, Panjabi MM. The clinical biomechanics of the occipitoatlantoaxial complex. Orthop Clin North Am. 1978;9(4):867–78.

Mid-cervical Metastatic Spinal Disease

11

Syed Uzair Ahmed, Zane Tymchak, and Daryl R. Fourney

Epidemiology

The spine is the most common site of bony metastasis in cancer patients. The cervical spine accounts for 8–20% of cases of spinal metastasis [1–3]. As such, it is the least common location for the presence of spinal metastasis. A large variation in the rate of cervical metastasis likely relates to whether asymptomatic lesions are reported [1]. Men are more likely to be affected than women, with the highest incidence occurring between the fourth and sixth decades. The most common pathologies are breast, prostate, and non-small-cell lung carcinoma.

Pathology

The cervical spine is the site of metastatic deposits in up to 8–15% of cases of spinal metastatic disease [1, 4, 5]. This proportion is generally thought to reflect the lesser amount of vascular cancellous bone present in the cervical spine [6, 7]. Anatomically, the vertebral body, specifically the junction of the pedicle and vertebral body, is the most common site of metastatic spread [7]. The posterior elements are not as frequently involved, and involvement is usually due to direct extension of vertebral body lesions [8]. The most common primary malignancies responsible for bony metastases in this region are breast, prostate, and non-small-cell lung carcinoma (NSCLC) [9, 10]. Spread to the cervical spine is attributable to direct invasion, hematogenous, or dissemination though cerebrospinal fluid (CSF) pathways. Hematogenous spread is responsible for the majority of cervical spine metastases [7, 9]. CSF dissemination is by far the least common method of spread but may rarely be seen after surgical treatment of a primary or metastatic brain lesion (so-called intradural "drop metastases") [9]. Of the common primary cancers with predilection for the spine, only breast cancer has been shown to preferentially affect the cervical spine [11]. Although uncommon, intramedullary metastasis to the cervical spinal cord occur in roughly 2% of autopsied cancer patients [12]. Isolated metastasis to the cervical spine is uncommon, occurring in only 11% of cases [13].

In contrast to the atlantoaxial spinal cord, the subaxial cervical spinal cord is more susceptible to compression by epidural disease due to a number of clinical and anatomic factors described by

S. U. Ahmed, MD
Division of Neurosurgery, University of Saskatchewan, Saskatoon, SK, Canada
e-mail: Uzair.ahmed@usask.ca

Z. Tymchak, MD
Royal University Hospital, Saskatoon, SK, Canada
e-mail: zat318@mail.usask.ca

D. R. Fourney, MD, FRCSC, FACS (✉)
Department of Neurosurgery, University of Saskatchewan, Royal University Hospital, Saskatoon, SK, Canada
e-mail: daryl.fourney@usask.ca

R. A. W. Marco (ed.), *Metastatic Spine Disease*, https://doi.org/10.1007/978-3-319-76252-4_11

Molina and colleagues [3]. These factors include the higher incidence of metastatic disease in the subaxial spine [2], the less capacious area of the subaxial spinal canal, and the robust ligamentous complex at C1–2. Spinal epidural disease is more common in the subaxial cervical spine than the atlantoaxial spine [3].

Clinical Presentation

Pain is the most common presenting feature of metastatic spinal lesions [2]. Almost all patients presenting with spinal metastases have pain symptoms [14, 15]. Patients may encounter two types of pain: mechanical (axial) pain or biological (localized) pain. Mechanical pain is due to instability, worsens with axial loading and ambulation, and is relieved with laying down. Biological pain is typically attributed to stretching of the vertebral body periosteum and is the classic nighttime pain in cancer patients.

Neurological symptoms of compression may comprise of radiculopathy or myelopathy. Radicular pain from compression of C2–C4 nerve roots presents as pain in the suboccipital, retroauricular, or retro-orbital regions. Radiculopathy from the C5 to C8 nerve roots may manifest as radicular pain, paresthesia, sensory deficits, or weakness in the distribution of the affected nerve root. Radicular symptoms are usually ipsilateral to the compression [2]. Myelopathy as a presentation is more common in the mid-cervical spine than the occipitocervical region, due to the smaller diameter of the spinal canal in the mid-cervical region. Symptoms of myelopathy may depend on the location of the compression. Symptoms may consist of a loss of fine motor skills, such as handwriting or buttoning. Symptoms in the lower extremities may include a loss of balance and gait instability. Abnormal reflexes, such as the Hoffman reflex, and up-going toes on the Babinski test, may be present, along with a progressive increase in tone and hyperreflexia. Progressive upper and lower extremity weakness will develop with worsening compression. Bowel and bladder changes may occur and manifest as urinary retention or incontinence.

Diagnosis

If a diagnosis of cervical spine metastasis is suspected, patients should go on to have a thorough clinical history and detailed neurological examination. Patients with prior history of cancer and new onset neck pain should be investigated for spinal metastasis. Diagnostic work-up includes basic blood work, imaging of the entire spine, and systemic evaluation for burden of disease [16]. When subaxial metastasis occurs in the presence of an unknown primary, which occurs in 10–20% of metastatic spine cases [17], the patient should first undergo a metastatic work-up to determine the site and extent of primary malignancy. When possible, pathologic confirmation should be obtained prior to surgical management of the spinal lesion (Fig. 11.1). In the subaxial cervical spine, computed tomographic (CT)-guided biopsy via an anterolateral approach can be safely utilized to obtain a diagnosis with good diagnostic yield [1, 16, 18, 19]. Plain radiographs have limited diagnostic utility as >50% of a vertebral body needs to be involved in the case of lytic tumors before they can be detected [20]. Imaging of the cervical spine generally includes magnetic resonance imaging (MRI) with gadolinium enhancement as well as CT [16]. Dynamic radiographs can be used to assess for instability. Bone scintigraphy can be useful for evaluating systemic burden of disease. Digital subtraction angiography (DSA) can be used to evaluate the potency of the vertebral arteries if involved, and balloon test occlusion can be performed to determine collateral flow if vertebral artery sacrifice or bypass techniques are being considered [3, 21].

Indications for Surgery

The primary indications for surgery are neurological dysfunction, spinal instability, and pain. While palliation is the usual goal in surgical management of subaxial metastatic disease, curative resections can rarely be considered. Validated scoring systems and decision-making tools can be utilized in subaxial metastases and are useful in educating patients. These include the Tomita system [22], the Tokuhashi scoring system [23], the Spinal Instability Neoplastic Disease Score (SINS) [24, 25], and the LMNOP decision-making framework [26, 27]. The LMNOP framework takes into account disease location (L), mechanical instability (M) as graded by SINS, the patient's neurological status (N), and the oncologic diagnosis (O). The "P" in LMNOP includes patient factors such as medical fitness, wishes, prognosis (life expectancy), and prior therapies (e.g., previous radiation therapy, response to chemotherapy) [26].

Accurate pathological diagnosis is perhaps the most important consideration as tumor pathology

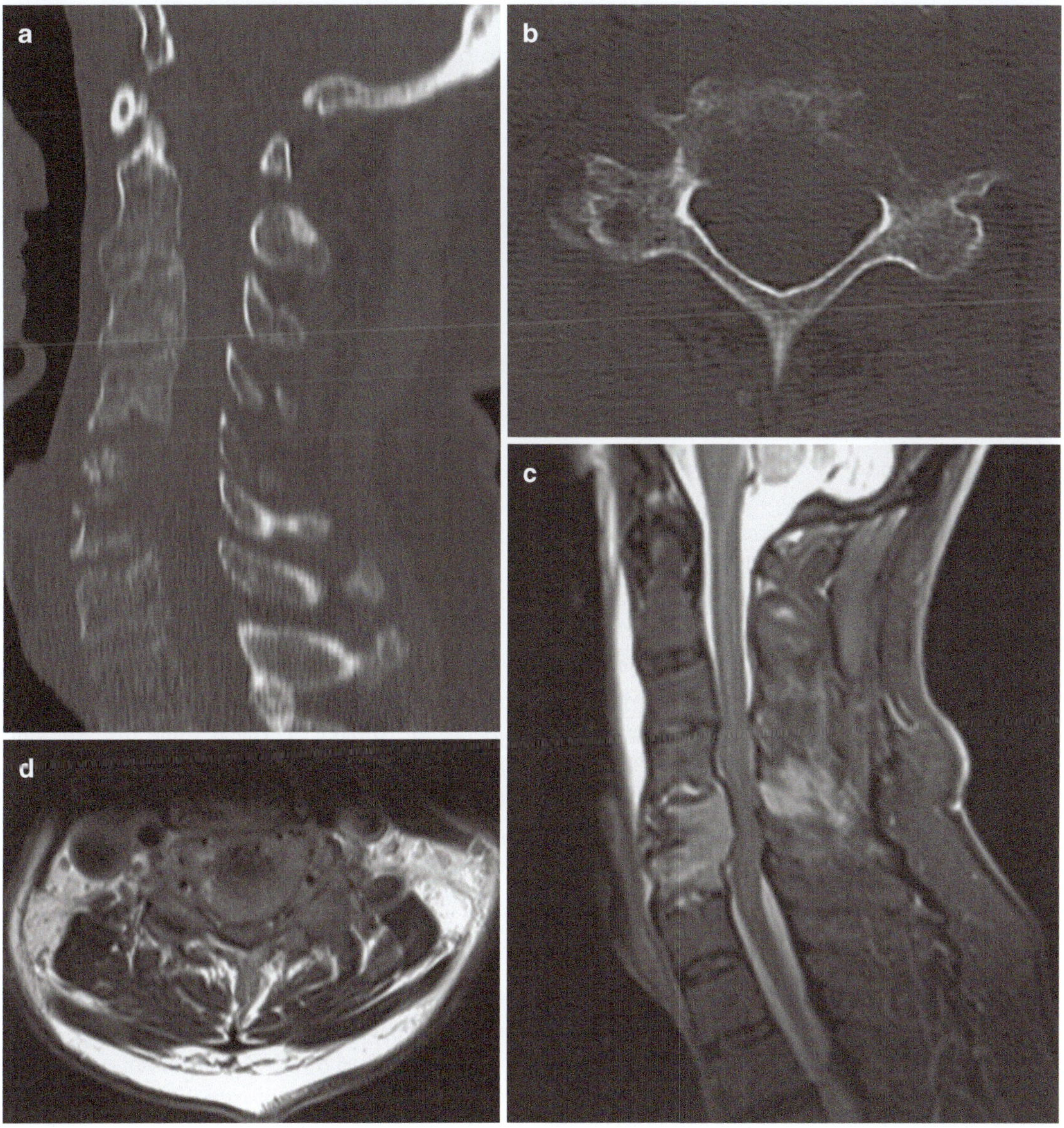

Fig. 11.1 Importance of biopsy. This 75-year-old man presented with numbness and loss of dexterity in his hands as well as mild gait difficulty marked by increased tone. (**a**) Sagittal CT shows lysis at C5/6. (**b**) Axial CT through C6 shows relative preservation of the posterior elements. (**c**) Sagittal post-contrast MRI shows posterior column invasion by tumor. (**d**) Axial MRI at C6 shows severe spinal cord compression. (**e**) CT-guided biopsy determined the diagnosis was B-cell lymphoma. (**f**) Sagittal CT scan 4 months after radiation therapy shows bony healing. The patient completely recovered from myelopathic symptoms without surgery

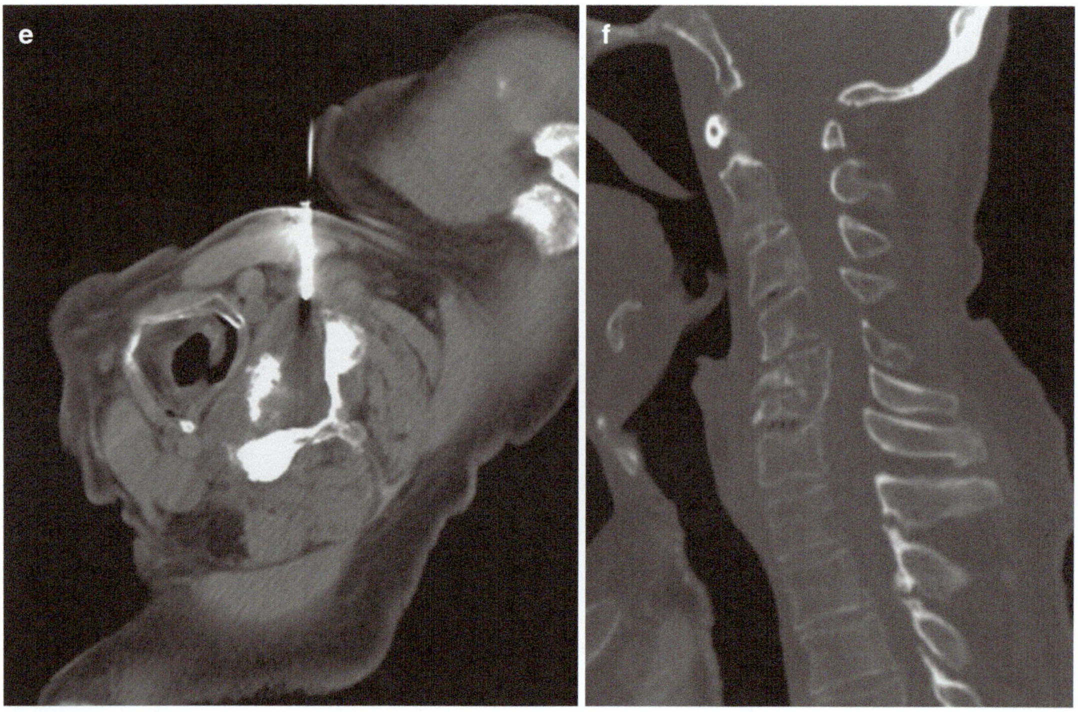

Fig. 11.1 (continued)

remains the most significant prognostic factor [1, 16]. In general, surgical intervention is not recommended when the patient's anticipated survival is less than 3 months; however, this is difficult to determine in practice and so should only be used as a guide [2, 3, 16, 26, 28].

The goals of surgery are to decompress the neural elements, reduce tumor burden, restore alignment, achieve rigid stabilization, and obtain the histopathological diagnosis if not already known.

Due to multiple patient, disease, and treatment-related factors, obtaining fusion in this patient population is unlikely. The goal of surgery instead is to achieve durable stabilization for the remaining life expectancy of the patient. The survival time in patients with metastatic spine disease is limited, therefore providing less time to achieve fusion across the affected levels. Progressive disease also affects the rate of fusion directly through continued bony destruction as well as indirectly through generalized deconditioning of the patient. Adjuvant treatment with chemotherapy and radiation therapy also affects bone healing.

Surgical Approaches

Anterior

The anterior approach to the cervical spine is the most commonly employed surgical option for metastatic subaxial cervical spine disease, since most metastatic disease occurs in the vertebral bodies, making it amenable to direct anterior decompression of neural elements as well as reduction of tumor volume. The anterior approach also allows for stabilization and fusion of diseased segments, reducing the pain from instability. The subaxial cervical spine is readily accessible from the anterior approach, in contrast to the craniocervical and cervicothoracic junctions.

The standard Smith-Robinson approach to the cervical spine is employed [29]. A transverse incision is created over the affected vertebral body, centered on the anterior edge of the sternocleidomastoid muscle. We prefer to incise the platysma muscle vertically rather than transversely, so that exposure can easily be extended proximally or distally, if required. The sternocleidomastoid muscle is retracted laterally to expose the mid-cervical fascia. The omohyoid muscle is encountered in the subaxial spine and may be retracted or transected. There is no reason to open the carotid sheath. The carotid sheath is identified and the mid-cervical fascia is incised medial to it. The carotid sheath is retracted laterally and the trachea and esophagus medially, to expose the anterior cervical spine. The prevertebral fascia is incised in the midline, and the longus colli muscles are dissected from their attachments along the lateral aspects of the vertebral bodies bilaterally, which allows for better anchoring of self-retaining retractors. Care should be taken to incise the fascia in the midline, as lateral dissection can place the vertebral artery and sympathetic chain at risk.

Decompression in the form of corpectomy of the tumor-infiltrated vertebral bodies is then carried out. The posterior longitudinal ligament is also resected as part of the decompression, and the midline dura is identified. The nerve roots may then be decompressed laterally, and the tumor may be dissected from the vertebral arteries (VA). Perioperative imaging of the vertebral arteries to confirm patency of the contralateral VA is necessary for these purposes. Infiltration of the VAs may limit aggressive dissection.

The recurrent laryngeal nerve (RLN) should also be evaluated perioperatively using fiberoptic laryngoscopy, as palsy may occur secondary to tumor infiltration. Unilateral RLN palsy should lead to the surgical approach from the ipsilateral side [30].

Anterior stabilization options include titanium mesh or expandable cages, fibular strut auto- or allograft, polymethyl methacrylate, and an anterior plate [2] (Fig. 11.2).

Posterior

The posterior approach is less often used in isolation for subaxial metastatic disease given that most metastases spread to the vertebral body [7]. However, it remains a useful approach for achieving decompression of the posterior aspect of the spinal cord and nerve roots as well as for addressing multilevel instability.

The patient is positioned prone on a Jackson table with the neck in neutral position and head fixed with a Mayfield head clamp. Consideration should be given to the number of levels requiring arthrodesis as the suboccipital region and/or the cervicothoracic junction may need to be exposed. A standard midline approach is utilized. Adequate bony exposure includes diseased levels as well as sufficient levels above and below to accommodate instrumentation. Typically, instrumentation is performed first followed by decompression and intralesional resection of tumor to decompress the neural elements and aid in cytoreduction. Lateral mass screw-rod constructs are most popular and achieve adequate arthrodesis. During highly destabilizing maneuvers, unilateral screw-rod instrumentation should be placed to avoid intraoperative translation of the subaxial spine and injury to the neural elements. Once decompression and arthrodesis are adequate, decortication of the lateral masses and onlay of morcelized allograft bone is recommended to aid in fusion. Lateral mass screws are usually satisfactory at levels C3–C6; however, pedicle screws are often recommended at C7 because the lateral mass at C7 is often very small.

Closure should be carefully performed in a multilayered fashion to avoid wound dehiscence, particularly as many patients will go on to have radiation.

As with anterior approaches, an important consideration is the vertebral arteries (VA). Lateral extension of tumor and posterior instrumentation of the subaxial spine have been identified as risk factors for VA injury during surgery [31–33]. Although the VA enters the foramen transversarium at C6 in up to 94.9% of patients, it can course extra-foraminally as high as C4 before entering the foramen [34]. Careful preoperative evaluation of the anatomic course of the VAs and their location to the pathology of interest is recommended to avoid VA injury. In addition, preoperative angiography ± embolization of tumor feeders can be utilized (Fig. 11.3).

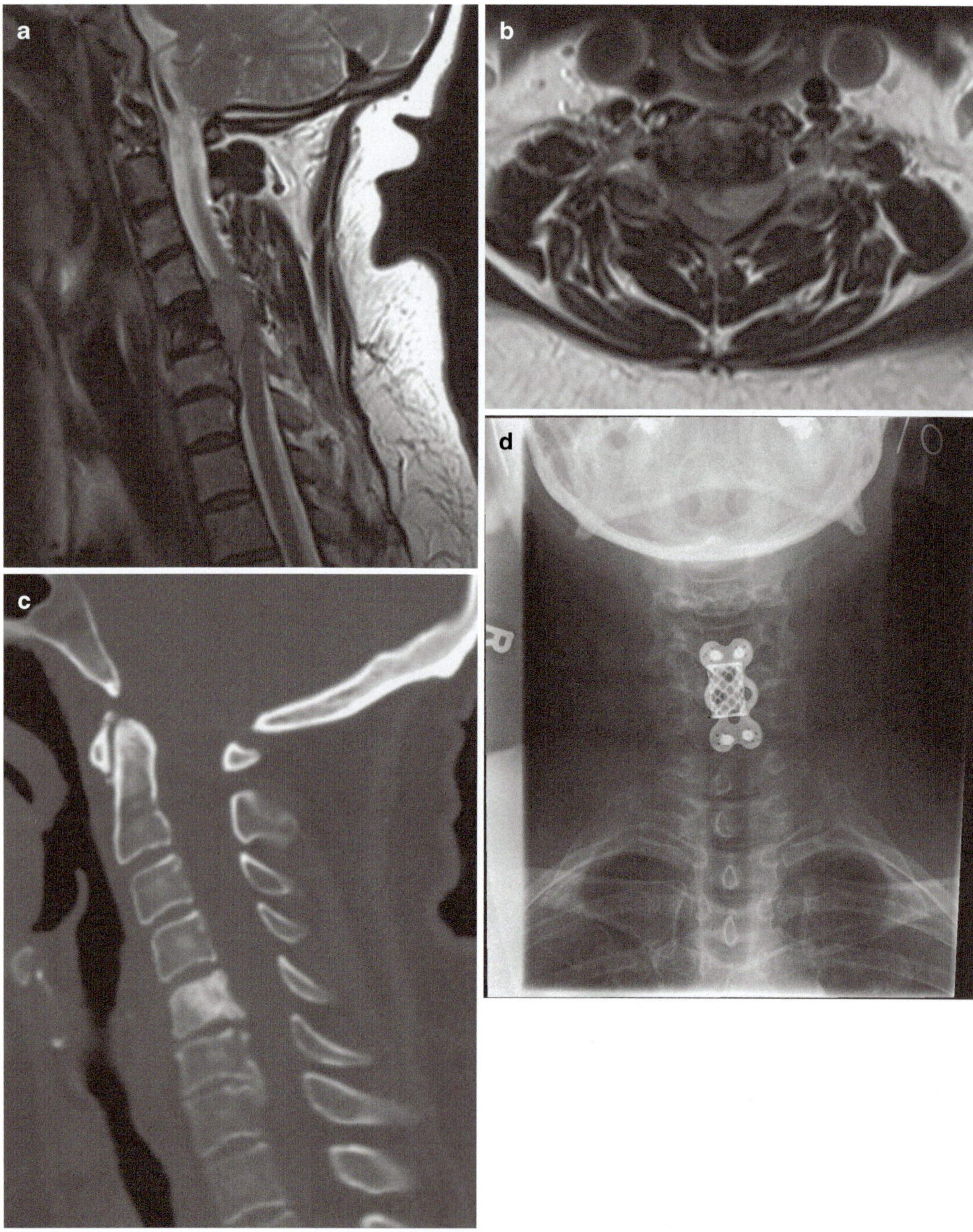

Fig. 11.2 Anterior approach. This 57-year-old woman presented with cervical myeloradiculopathy due to metastatic leiomyosarcoma. (**a**) Sagittal MRI shows severe cord compression. (**b**) Axial MRI shows epidural tumor compressing the spinal cord on the left side. (**c**) Sagittal CT scan shows osteoblastic response at C5. Postoperative AP (**d**) and lateral (**e**) X-ray films show cage and plate after C5 corpectomy. One-year postoperative sagittal (**f**) and axial (**g**) MRI scans show spinal cord decompression

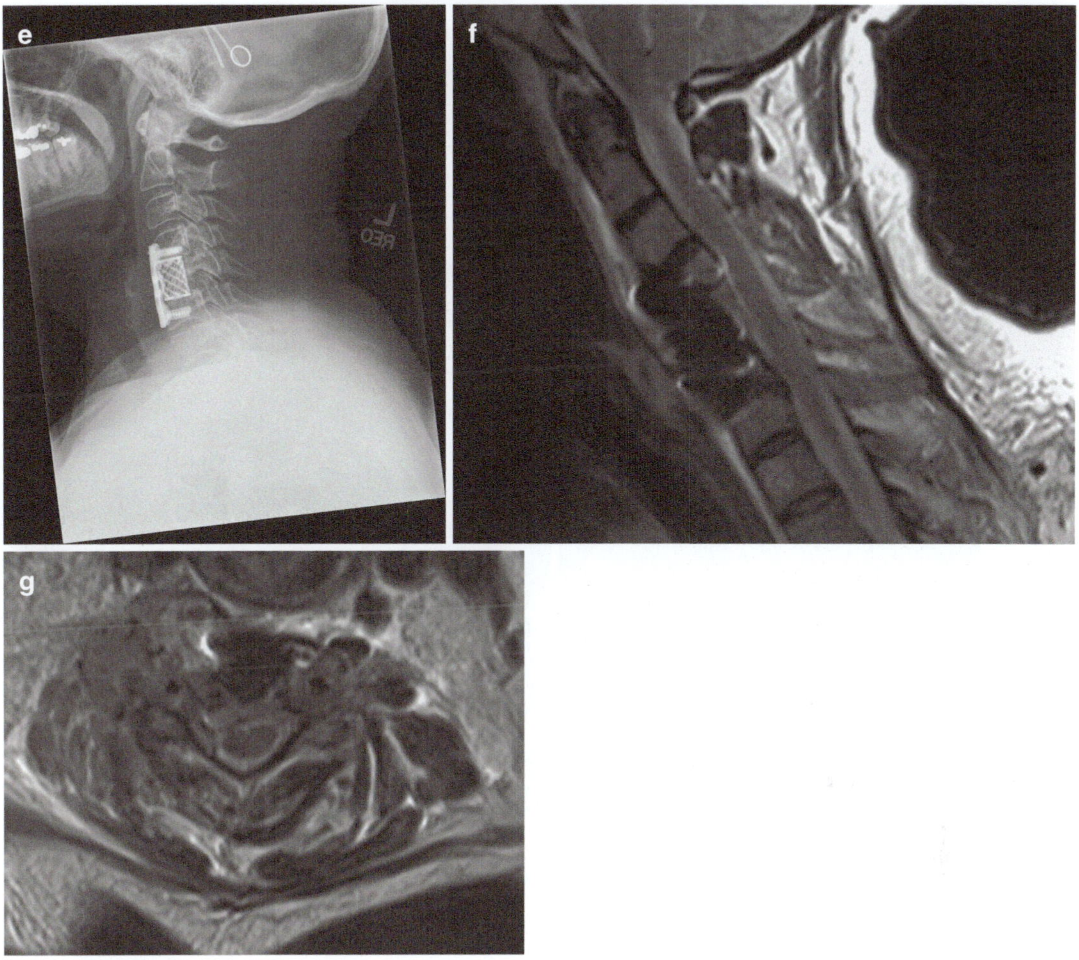

Fig. 11.2 (continued)

Preoperative CT scans should be evaluated for bony quality and lateral mass anatomy when planning instrumentation of the subaxial spine from a posterior approach. It can also be useful for planning the number of levels to include in your construct. Generally, the decision to include more levels is based on the extent of tumor involvement and proximity to junctional anatomy as well as intraoperative findings. As with all spinal instrumentation in the setting of metastatic neoplasia, careful attention to achieving a solid construct is of the utmost importance, as we prefer to not use collars or other external immobilization devices in this palliative patient population.

Combined Anterior and Posterior Approaches

Augmentation of anterior decompression with a posterior approach should be given consideration in all cases. Indications for adding a posterior procedure to anterior decompression and fusion include multilevel disease, circumferential metastases causing dorsal compression or destruction, and translational kyphotic deformity (Fig. 11.4). Vertebral body disease requiring excision of more than one vertebral body usually requires additional posterior stabilization [2, 35].

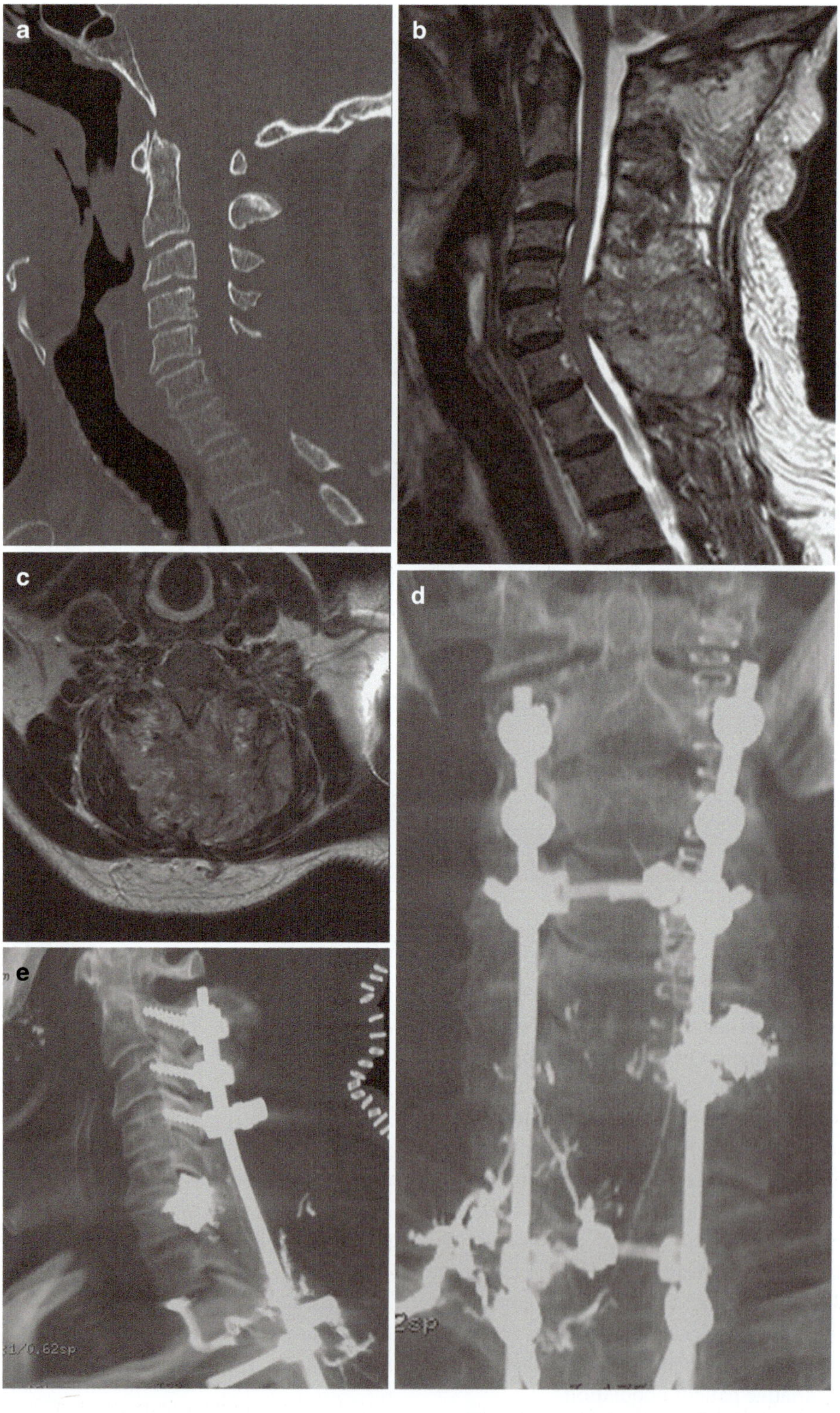

Fig. 11.3 Posterior approach. This 70-year-old man with metastatic renal cell carcinoma presented with severe mechanical type neck pain due to a very large renal cell metastasis that had destroyed most of the posterior elements of the subaxial cervical spine. (**a**) Sagittal CT shows loss of posterior elements from C5 to C7. Sagittal (**b**) and axial (**c**) MRI shows massive metastasis involving the posterior elements of the cervical spine. Postoperative AP (**d**) and lateral (**e**) CT reconstructed images show materials used for endovascular embolization as well as posterior instrumentation

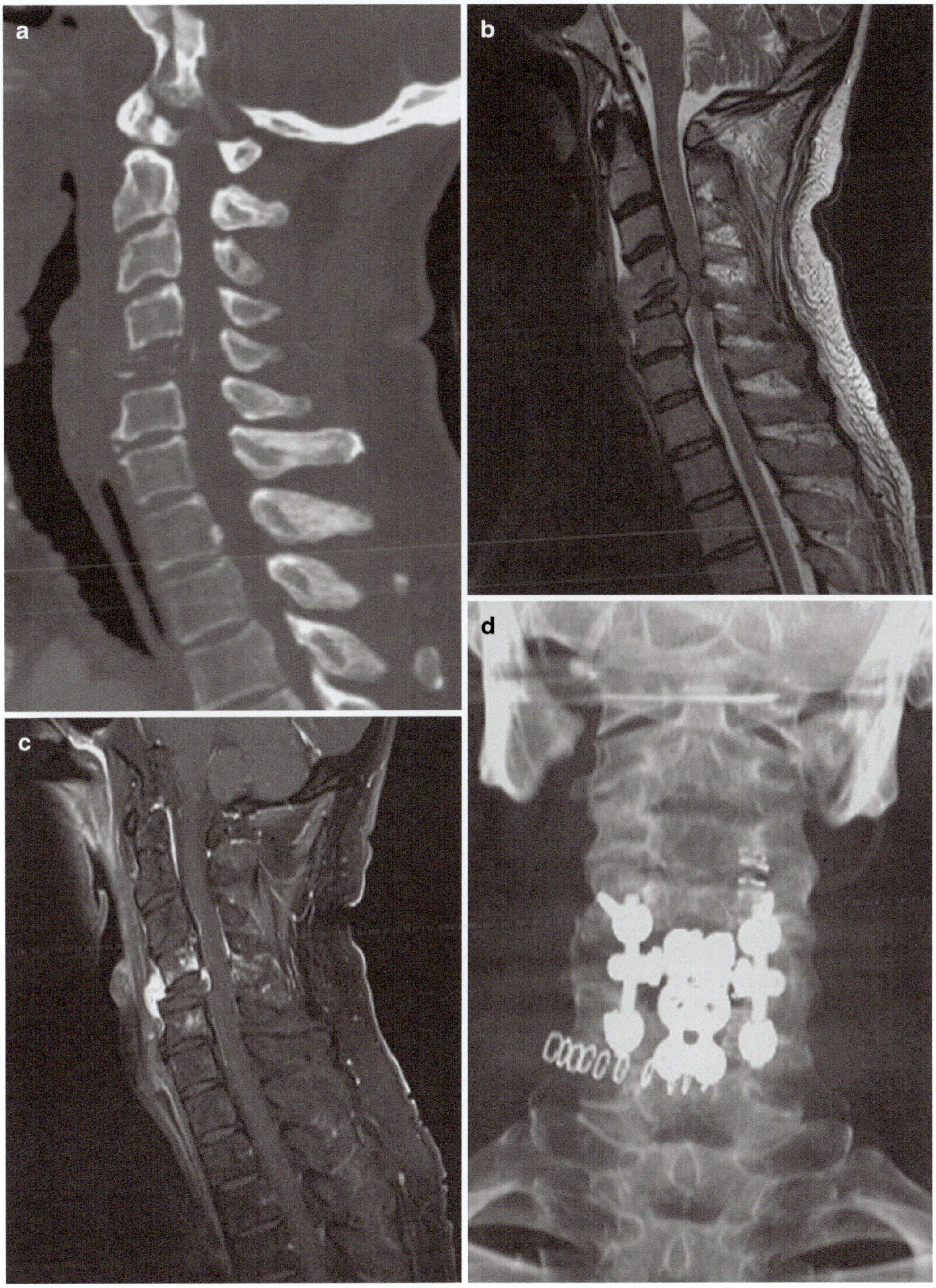

Fig. 11.4 Combined approach. This 69-year-old man presented with severe mechanical type neck pain and myeloradiculopathy due to lytic non-small-cell lung cancer metastasis at C5. (**a**) Sagittal CT shows pathologic fracture at C5. Sagittal T2-weighted (**b**) and post-contrast (**c**) MRI show ventral spinal cord compression, involvement of the posterior elements, and kyphosis. Postoperative AP (**d**) and lateral (**e**) reconstructed CT images show two-staged anterior/posterior decompression, reconstruction, and stabilization with C5 cage/plate and C4–6 lateral mass screws

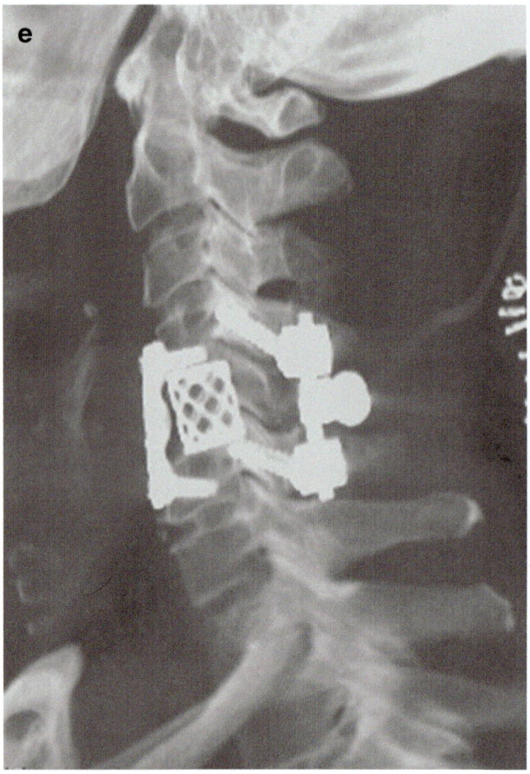

Fig. 11.4 (continued)

Complication Avoidance

Since palliation is the overall goal of surgery in metastatic spine disease, avoidance of surgical complications is of the utmost importance, as these may significantly impact the patient's quality of life. Significant complications include surgical site infection (SSI), vascular or neurological injury, and failure of instrumentation with continued or recurrent instability.

Surgical site infection (SSI) is the most common perioperative complication of spinal tumor surgery, with an overall rate of 9.5% [2, 36]. Risk factors for SSI include adjuvant radiation therapy, diabetes mellitus, prior surgery in the same area, complex wound closure, involvement of multiple surgical teams, and blood transfusions [2, 36]. Techniques to reduce infection risk have been studied, including the placement of vancomycin powder into the wound, but a large-scale study has not been completed [2, 37].

As discussed, the vertebral arteries are at risk during both anterior and posterior approaches to the mid-cervical spine. These arteries should be evaluated preoperatively using MRI or CT angiography.

Neurological injury during decompression or instrumentation is a significant risk of surgery. This risk is increased in the presence of significant epidural disease. Intraoperative neuromonitoring in the form of somatosensory evoked potentials (SSEP), electromyography (EMG), and motor evoked potentials (MEP) may be carried out to monitor and avoid neurological injury. A study of 152 consecutive cases of epidural spine disease with multimodality monitoring showed high specificity of signal changes intraoperatively. Of two patients with postoperative deficits, one had transient MEP changes and the other had no signal changes intraoperatively. Other patients showed transient signal changes that reversed with correction of hypotension [38].

The failure of instrumentation is a significant complication, with ongoing instability having a significant impact on patient quality of life. As discussed, the goal of surgery should be to provide stability for the patient's life expectancy, and constructs should be planned with this goal in mind. We plan our constructs to avoid the use of external orthotics in the cancer population.

Tumor recurrence may occur in a significant number of patients and may contribute to poor patient outcomes. A study of 46 patients undergoing surgery for subaxial cervical spinal metastasis showed a 39% rate of tumor recurrence. Postoperative adjuvant therapy was found to be the only factor to reduce recurrence rates [14].

References

1. Jenis LG, Dunn EJ, An HS. Metastatic disease of the cervical spine. A review. Clin Orthop Relat Res. 1999;359:89–103.
2. Mesfin A, Buchowski JM, Gokaslan ZL, Bird JE. Management of metastatic cervical spine tumors. J Am Acad Orthop Surg. 2015;23(1):38–46.
3. Molina CA, Gokaslan ZL, Sciubba DM. Diagnosis and management of metastatic cervical spine tumors. Orthop Clin North Am. 2012;43(1):75–87, viii–ix.
4. Brihaye J, Ectors P, Lemort M, Van Houtte P. The management of spinal epidural metastases. Adv Tech Stand Neurosurg. 1988;16:121–76.
5. Constans JP, de Divitiis E, Donzelli R, Spaziante R, Meder JF, Haye C. Spinal metastases with neurological manifestations. Review of 600 cases. J Neurosurg. 1983;59(1):111–8.
6. Jonsson B, Jonsson H Jr, Karlstrom G, Sjostrom L. Surgery of cervical spine metastases: a retrospective study. Eur Spine J. 1994;3(2):76–83.
7. Yuh WT, Quets JP, Lee HJ, Simonson TM, Michalson LS, Nguyen PT, et al. Anatomic distribution of metastases in the vertebral body and modes of hematogenous spread. Spine (Phila Pa 1976). 1996;21(19):2243–50.
8. Jacobs WB, Perrin RG. Evaluation and treatment of spinal metastases: an overview. Neurosurg Focus. 2001;11(6):e10.
9. Arguello F, Baggs RB, Duerst RE, Johnstone L, McQueen K, Frantz CN. Pathogenesis of vertebral metastasis and epidural spinal cord compression. Cancer. 1990;65(1):98–106.
10. Moulding HD, Bilsky MH. Metastases to the craniovertebral junction. Neurosurgery. 2010;66(suppl_3): A113–A8.
11. Chaichana KL, Pendleton C, Sciubba DM, Wolinsky JP, Gokaslan ZL. Outcome following decompressive surgery for different histological types of metastatic tumors causing epidural spinal cord compression. Clinical article. J Neurosurg Spine. 2009;11(1):56–63.
12. Costigan DA, Winkelman MD. Intramedullary spinal cord metastasis. A clinicopathological study of 13 cases. J Neurosurg. 1985;62(2):227–33.
13. Rao S, Badani K, Schildhauer T, Borges M. Metastatic malignancy of the cervical spine. A nonoperative history. Spine (Phila Pa 1976). 1992;17(10 Suppl): S407–12.
14. Cho W, Chang UK. Neurological and survival outcomes after surgical management of subaxial cervical spine metastases. Spine (Phila Pa 1976). 2012;37(16):E969–77.
15. Quan GM, Vital JM, Pointillart V. Outcomes of palliative surgery in metastatic disease of the cervical and cervicothoracic spine. J Neurosurg Spine. 2011;14(5):612–8.
16. Sciubba DM, Petteys RJ, Dekutoski MB, Fisher CG, Fehlings MG, Ondra SL, et al. Diagnosis and management of metastatic spine disease. A review. J Neurosurg Spine. 2010;13(1):94–108.
17. Cahill DW. Surgical management of malignant tumors of the adult bony spine. South Med J. 1996;89(7):653–65.
18. Lis E, Bilsky MH, Pisinski L, Boland P, Healey JH, O'Malley B, et al. Percutaneous CT-guided biopsy of osseous lesion of the spine in patients with known or suspected malignancy. AJNR Am J Neuroradiol. 2004;25(9):1583–8.
19. Rimondi E, Rossi G, Bartalena T, Ciminari R, Alberghini M, Ruggieri P, et al. Percutaneous CT-guided biopsy of the musculoskeletal system: results of 2027 cases. Eur J Radiol. 2011;77(1):34–42.
20. Edelstyn GA, Gillespie PJ, Grebbell FS. The radiological demonstration of osseous metastases. Experimental observations. Clin Radiol. 1967;18(2): 158–62.
21. Mazel C, Balabaud L, Bennis S, Hansen S. Cervical and thoracic spine tumor management: surgical indications, techniques, and outcomes. Orthop Clin North Am. 2009;40(1):75–92, vi–vii.
22. Tomita K, Kawahara N, Baba H, Tsuchiya H, Fujita T, Toribatake Y. Total en bloc spondylectomy. A new surgical technique for primary malignant vertebral tumors. Spine (Phila Pa 1976). 1997;22(3):324–33.
23. Tokuhashi Y, Matsuzaki H, Oda H, Oshima M, Ryu J. A revised scoring system for preoperative evaluation of metastatic spine tumor prognosis. Spine (Phila Pa 1976). 2005;30(19):2186–91.
24. Fisher CG, DiPaola CP, Ryken TC, Bilsky MH, Shaffrey CI, Berven SH, et al. A novel classification system for spinal instability in neoplastic disease: an evidence-based approach and expert consensus from the Spine Oncology Study Group. Spine (Phila Pa 1976). 2010;35(22):E1221–9.
25. Fourney DR, Frangou EM, Ryken TC, Dipaola CP, Shaffrey CI, Berven SH, et al. Spinal instability neoplastic score: an analysis of reliability and validity from the spine oncology study group. J Clin Oncol. 2011;29(22):3072–7.

26. Ivanishvili Z, Fourney DR. Incorporating the spine instability neoplastic score into a treatment strategy for spinal metastasis: LMNOP. Global Spine J. 2014;4(2):129–36.
27. Paton GR, Frangou E, Fourney DR. Contemporary treatment strategy for spinal metastasis: the "LMNOP" system. Can J Neurol Sci. 2011;38(3):396–403.
28. Heidecke V, Rainov NG, Burkert W. Results and outcome of neurosurgical treatment for extradural metastases in the cervical spine. Acta Neurochir. 2003;145(10):873–80; discussion 80–1.
29. Robinson RA, Riley LH Jr. Techniques of exposure and fusion of the cervical spine. Clin Orthop Relat Res. 1975;109:78–84.
30. McLain RF. Cancer in the spine: comprehensive care. Totowa, NJ: Humana Press; 2006. p. 379.
31. Smith MD, Emery SE, Dudley A, Murray KJ, Leventhal M. Vertebral artery injury during anterior decompression of the cervical spine. A retrospective review of ten patients. J Bone Joint Surg Br. 1993;75(3):410–5.
32. Sen C, Eisenberg M, Casden AM, Sundaresan N, Catalano PJ. Management of the vertebral artery in excision of extradural tumors of the cervical spine. Neurosurgery. 1995;36(1):106–15; discussion 15-6.
33. Zhao L, Xu R, Hu T, Ma W, Xia H, Wang G. Quantitative evaluation of the location of the vertebral artery in relation to the transverse foramen in the lower cervical spine. Spine (Phila Pa 1976). 2008;33(4):373–8.
34. Hong JT, Park DK, Lee MJ, Kim SW, An HS. Anatomical variations of the vertebral artery segment in the lower cervical spine: analysis by three-dimensional computed tomography angiography. Spine (Phila Pa 1976). 2008;33(22):2422–6.
35. Acosta FL Jr, Aryan HE, Chou D, Ames CP. Long-term biomechanical stability and clinical improvement after extended multilevel corpectomy and circumferential reconstruction of the cervical spine using titanium mesh cages. J Spinal Disord Tech. 2008;21(3):165–74.
36. Omeis IA, Dhir M, Sciubba DM, Gottfried ON, McGirt MJ, Attenello FJ, et al. Postoperative surgical site infections in patients undergoing spinal tumor surgery: incidence and risk factors. Spine (Phila Pa 1976). 2011;36(17):1410–9.
37. Pahys JM, Pahys JR, Cho SK, Kang MM, Zebala LP, Hawasli AH, et al. Methods to decrease postoperative infections following posterior cervical spine surgery. J Bone Joint Surg Am. 2013;95(6):549–54.
38. Avila EK, Elder JB, Singh P, Chen X, Bilsky MH. Intraoperative neurophysiologic monitoring and neurologic outcomes in patients with epidural spine tumors. Clin Neurol Neurosurg. 2013;115(10):2147–52.

Cervicothoracic Metastatic Spine Disease

12

Darryl Lau, Joseph A. Osorio, and Christopher Pearson Ames

General Spinal Metastasis

Therapeutic approaches to cancer treatment and management have continued to advance greatly over the recent years, notably in the realms of radiotherapy [1], chemotherapy [2, 3], and surgical intervention [4]. However, even with such improvements, about half of the patients with spinal metastasis will succumb to their primary malignancy, a rate which is relatively unchanged from the past [5]. Patients who succumb to their cancers ultimately expire from cancer invasion and widespread metastasis, and many times it is these secondary lesions that cause significant debilitation and decreased quality of life [6, 7]. One of the most common bony areas that metastasis is identified within is the spinal column, specifically the anterior spinal elements such as the vertebral body [8]. Metastatic lesions can be found at all levels of the spinal column, but the thoracic spine is the most commonly affected region given its high vascularity and its greatest number of vertebrae [9–11]. It has been estimated that 80–90% of symptomatic spinal metastasis are located in the thoracic and lumbar levels [12]. Some of the most common primaries of spinal metastatic lesions (from most frequent to least frequent) are the breast, lung, renal cell, prostate, sarcoma, colon, hepatocellular carcinoma, multiple myeloma, thyroid, melanoma, and lymphoma [13].

D. Lau, MD · J. A. Osorio, MD, PhD
Department of Neurosurgery, University of California, San Francisco, San Francisco, CA, USA
e-mail: darryl.lau@ucsf.edu; joseph.osorio@ucsf.edu

C. P. Ames, MD (✉)
Department of Neurological Surgery, University of California, San Francisco, San Francisco, CA, USA
e-mail: Christopher.ames@ucsf.edu; AmesC@neurosurg.ucsf.edu

Patient Presentation

Clinical presentation of spinal metastasis involving the cervical and thoracic region is highly dependent on the extent of disease, presence of spinal instability, and/or ongoing neural compression (nerve root and spinal cord). Patients may present asymptomatically with spinal metastasis seen as an incidental finding on imaging (Fig. 12.1). On the other hand, patients can present with a variety of symptoms that manifest as intractable axial pain, radiculopathy, myelopathy, or focal neurological deficit [14–17]. These symptomologies are the result of specific pathological processes. Aggressive proliferation, invasion, and erosion of metastatic spinal lesions can lead to spinal column destruction, instability, deformity (Fig. 12.2), and neural compression

R. A. W. Marco (ed.), *Metastatic Spine Disease*, https://doi.org/10.1007/978-3-319-76252-4_12

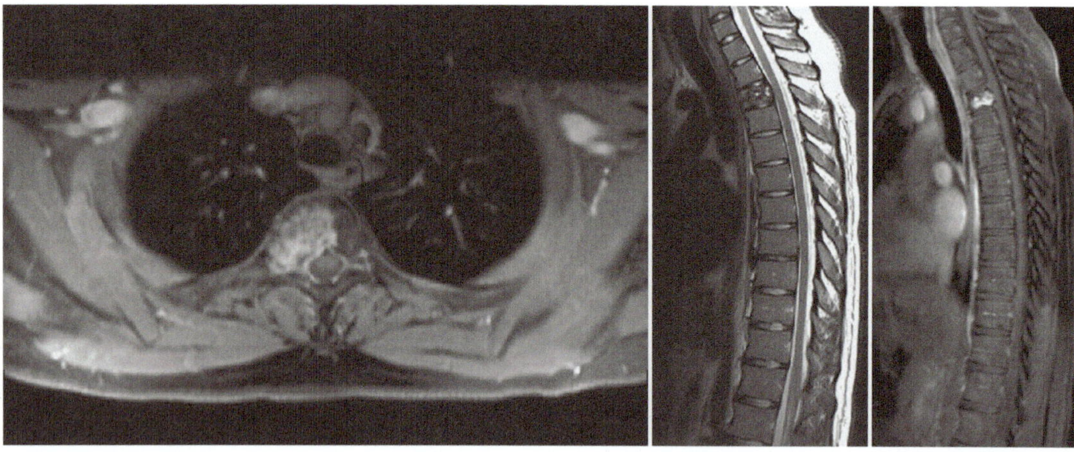

Fig. 12.1 Incidental T3 vertebral body metastasis from testicular cancer without nerve root and spinal cord compression. The patient underwent staging MRI and was found to have a contrast enhancing tumor within the vertebral body. There is no spinal cord compression or nerve root compression

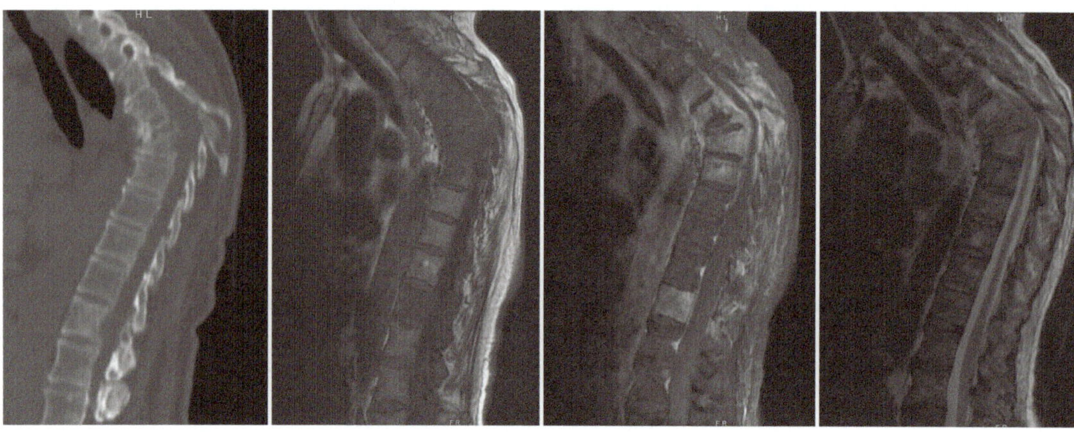

Fig. 12.2 Destructive T4 to T6 metastatic breast cancer causing significant spinal deformity and instability. CT and MRI show a destructive spinal metastasis spanning T4 to T6 causing significant thoracic kyphosis and spinal instability. There is spinal cord compression secondary to violation of the central canal by the tumor and severity of spinal deformity

[18]. Axial neck and back pain is the result of spinal instability, direct compression of neural elements, and/or inflammatory tumor response. Specifically in the cervical and thoracic spine, myelopathy and radiculopathy occur in the setting of active spinal cord and spinal nerve compression, respectively (Fig. 12.3). Other general signs of systemic metastasis such as weight loss, cachexia, and organ-based symptoms are more commonly a result of the primary lesion (i.e., hemoptysis with lung cancer).

Evaluation, Imaging, and Work-Up

Patients should undergo a full physical examination, including a detailed neurological examination. The neurological examination should emphasize testing strength, sensation, and reflexes, in particular, examining for hyperreflexia and pathological reflexes such as Hoffman's sign and clonus. In regard to imaging of the spine, patients should undergo at least a magnetic resonance imaging (MRI) with and without gadolinium and

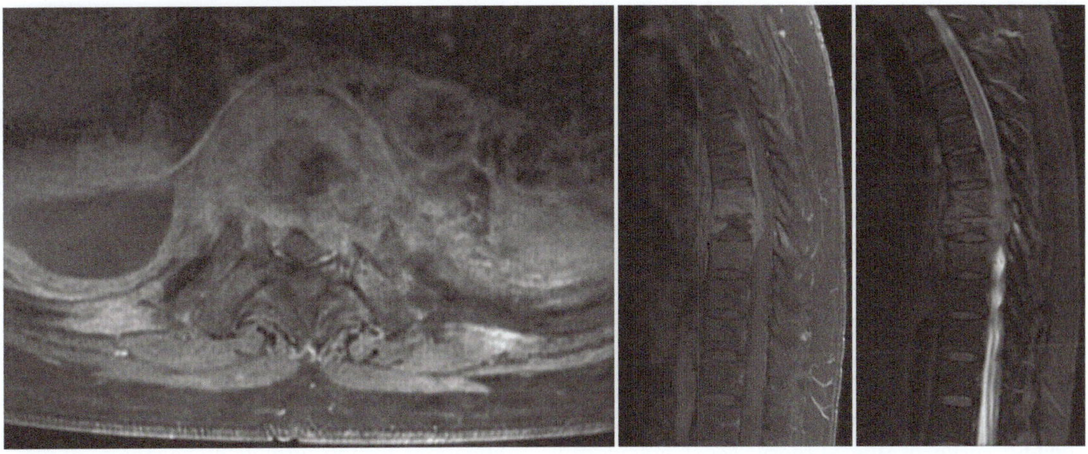

Fig. 12.3 T7 to T8 lung metastasis causing severe central stenosis and spinal cord compression. MRI demonstrates a T7-based metastasis that extends inferiorly to T8 resulting in severe narrowing of the central canal and active spinal cord compression. There is no significant spinal deformity

computed tomography (CT) of the spine to further characterize the lesion. Sagittal reconstruction CT images and midsagittal MRIs can help determine the feasibility of an anterior approach to C7, T1, and T2. If destruction of the spinal column is present and deformity is a concern, the patient should undergo a standing scoliosis X-ray series. Other additional exams should include a general metastatic work-up if there is no known cancer diagnosis, as this will guide medical and surgical management of the spinal metastasis.

General Indications for Surgery

The most common indications for surgical intervention for cervicothoracic metastasis are the presence of lesions resistant to radiation or chemotherapy, intractable pain, neurological deficit, spinal instability, and/or presence of spinal cord compression. Unlike the lumbar spine, the presence of radiological evidence for ongoing spinal cord compression may be an indicator for surgical decompression, especially in the setting of T2 signal abnormality within the spinal cord and/or an abnormal neurological examination. Surgery can also be considered in patients with spinal metastasis resulting only in nerve root compression and radiculopathy.

Considerations and Decision-Making in Selection of Surgical Candidates

The timing and type of management of spinal metastasis involving the cervical and thoracic spine are dependent on a variety of factors. In the absence of nerve root compression, spinal cord compression (i.e., tumor involves only bony elements), and significant spinal deformity resulting in instability, surgical management could be deferred and non-operative management can be considered such as radiation and chemotherapies if the tumor pathology is appropriate. However, in the setting of an abnormal examination with evidence of neural compression and/or spinal instability, surgery should be considered. The timing of when to intervene surgically is highly dependent on whether there is spinal cord compression and the duration of the patient's neurological deficit. The decision to operate is case based, but in general more acute neurological deficits secondary to spinal cord compression and/or injury warrant a more urgent decompression to optimize outcomes.

In patients who have indications for surgery and do not require immediate surgical attention, the initial step in deciding whether to offer surgery is to determine the type of metastasis that is being treated (i.e., tumor primary). This is one of the most important factors when making treatment decisions. It is important to consider the histology and radiosensitivity of the metastasis. Many studies have a common consensus that tumor origin has the most important role in influencing survival after surgery. Most noteworthy were metastatic lesions of lung origin because of its grave prognosis even after surgery. The World Health Organization (WHO) now recognizes four main subtypes of lung cancer which are categorized into two general categories: small-cell carcinoma and non-small-cell carcinoma (squamous cell carcinoma, adenocarcinoma, and large-cell carcinoma) [19]. Overall, lung cancer has a 5-year survival rate of about 10%, and it is worse with small-cell carcinoma [20]. The inherent capability for lung cancer to cause massive dissemination and early death may be one of the explanations why these patients tend to fare significantly less well in terms of survival after surgery. Radio-resistant metastatic lesions of the spine are more likely to recur after surgical resection and are associated with worse prognosis [21–24]. Therefore, radiation and chemotherapy sensitivity should be considered when evaluating a patient for surgery in the management of spinal metastasis.

Next, it is important to decide which patients will benefit most from surgery, based on a benefit (improved functionality) to risk (morbidity and mortality) profile; this is especially true in surgical treatment of cervicothoracic spine metastasis. In the setting of such symptoms, select patients may undergo surgical intervention, and the Patchell Criteria is a commonly used guideline in determining which patients are appropriate for surgery. In 2005, Patchell et al. performed a randomized prospective trial in the treatment of spinal metastasis [25]. In their study of 101 patients, surgical decompression with adjuvant radiation was shown to be superior to radiation alone in the treatment of spinal metastasis. The patient selection criteria for this study included radiological evidence of epidural compression, at least one neurologic sign or symptom, and an expected survival of at least 3 months. Other studies also emphasized that patients with at least a 3-month life expectancy should undergo surgical intervention [26–36]. Since the publication of the study, these criteria have been utilized as a guide in the selection process of evaluating candidates for surgical management of spinal metastasis. Therefore, among many of the identified studies, indications for the surgical management of metastatic tumors in the cervicothoracic spine were based on clinical presentation, predicted life expectancy, and oncological history.

Some studies have examined the outcomes of patients who underwent surgery for neurological deficit as the main indication for surgery. A study by Jansson et al. used neurological deficit as the main indication (rather than pain) for surgical intervention for thoracic and lumbar spinal metastasis [37]. The authors' view regarding this treatment scheme was that pain associated with spinal metastasis can be addressed with advanced pain management and radiation therapy and that surgical intervention has not been shown to improve survival. One article by Kim et al. examined the surgical outcomes of patients who were non-ambulatory prior to surgery (Nurick Grades 4 and 5) [38]. In their study they showed that 68% of patients who could not walk resumed the ability to ambulate postoperatively. They concluded that if patients maintain motor strength of at least four out of five on strength testing, and surgery is done in a timely manner, most non-ambulatory patients can walk after surgery.

Other general factors that should be considered when offering surgery to patients with cervicothoracic spinal metastasis—older age (greater than 40 years); poor nutritional status; the presence of cardiac, pulmonary, hepatic, or renal function impairments; and the presence of metastasis involving three or more contiguous vertebral levels—have been shown to increase the risk for surgical morbidity [31, 39].

Surgical Goals and Approaches

Although surgical treatment of metastatic and primary tumors of the spine may be associated with significant morbidity, surgery for metastatic tumors has been proven to offer significant improvement in Karnofsky performance scores (KPS) and overall survival [13]. Spinal metastases most commonly affect the vertebral bodies of the spinal column and can lead to vertebral body destruction causing spinal cord compression or spinal instability [5]. In such cases, surgical intervention is warranted, and the goals of surgery are to relieve compression upon the spinal cord, facilitate local control (if possible), and stabilize the spine [25, 40]. As previously mentioned, most metastatic lesions are located anterior in the vertebral body and can extend posteriorly. Therefore removal of the vertebral body via corpectomy or vertebral body resection is commonly the treatment of choice when possible. Following the removal of the vertebral body, the anterior column in general is reconstructed with a cage and supplemented with posterior instrumentation and fusion. If a corpectomy cannot be performed, or ventral decompression is not deemed warranted, a posterior-only approach to decompression can be utilized both in the cervical and thoracic spine.

Cervical Spine

In general approaches to corpectomy in the cervical region are done through an anterior approach (Fig. 12.4). This technique is established and well tolerated by patients. A single-level corpectomy with anterior column reconstruction may not need additional posterior supplementation, but in cases with poor bone quality and/or correction of deformity, posterior fixation should be considered. Posterior spinal instrumentation should be considered for patients who have multilevel corpectomies to ensure adequate spinal fixation. There are cases where a posterior-only approach is indicated due to multilevel disease, previous radiation, and swallowing difficulty with difficulty in retraction of the trachea and esophagus and where circumferential fusion cannot be done due to the patients' poor medical condition [15]. *Ames* et al. reported three cases in which a posterior transpedicular technique, adapted for the cervical spine, was

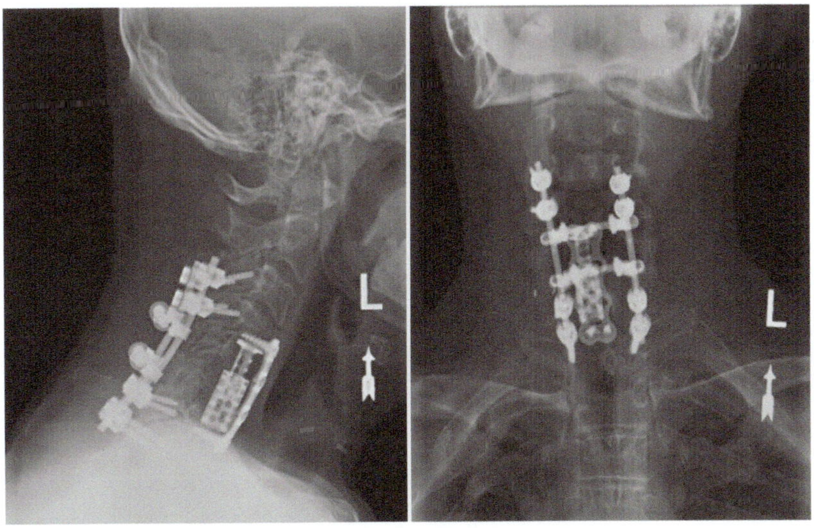

Fig. 12.4 Combined anterior cervical corpectomy with spinal column reconstruction and posterior spinal fusion for melanoma spinal metastasis. As seen in the cervical X-ray, this patient underwent an anterior approach to C5 to C6 corpectomy and placement of an expandable metal cage for reconstruction. He then underwent a supplemental posterior spinal fusion from C3 to T1 with lateral mass and pedicle screw fixation

used for intralesional resection of metastatic tumors involving C2 vertebral body [41]. Their technique involved skeletonizing the C2 pedicle, sacrifice of the C2 nerve root, mobilization of the vertebral artery, and reconstruction of the vertebral body with pins and methyl methacrylate. These authors did not report any perioperative complications or instrumentation failures. Similarly, *Eleraky* et al. reported their experience of posterior transpedicular corpectomy for malignant cervical spine tumors [15]. A total of eight patients underwent surgery and six underwent anterior column reconstruction. They did not experience perioperative complications and achieved gross total resection in all cases.

Thoracic Spine

A corpectomy of the upper thoracic spine can be performed through either an anterior-only approach, posterior-only approach, or combined anterior-posterior approach (Fig. 12.5) [42, 43]. Some surgeons prefer to use posterior-only approaches (such as transpedicular corpectomies, costotransversectomies, or lateral extracavitary approaches) to perform thoracic corpectomies [42, 44–47]. This is because posterior-only approaches avoid the morbidity of the anterior approach and obviate the need for an access surgeon [42, 46, 48, 49]. In addition, posterior-only approaches treat multiple spinal levels and anterior-posterior pathology all in a single-stage surgery [46]. There is also a transition to utilizing less invasive approaches such as mini-open corpectomies [50]. Mini-open corpectomy is performed with a midline facial incision over only the corpectomy level of interest and percutaneous instrumentation above and below that level. This less invasive approach offers less blood loss, shorter hospital stays, and possibly lower infection rates as well.

The specific approach used also has a large influence on perioperative and surgically related postoperative outcomes such as blood loss, operative time, complications, and length of stay [42]. More recently, a series of recommendations have emerged for approaches to the thoracolumbar spine for metastatic lesions [12]. For levels T2–T5, there is a strong recommendation for a posterolateral approach because anterior access to the spine can be limited by the heart, great vessels, esophagus, trachea, vagus nerve, recurrent laryngeal nerve, phrenic nerve, and thoracic duct [28, 51]. Posterolateral approaches also obviate the need to detach periscapular muscles compared to traditional high thoracotomy approaches to the cervicothoracic spine. Bernstein et al. have recently described a muscle-sparing high thoracotomy approach which can be used for lesions with large soft tissue components extending into the thoracic cavity or for patients with Pancoast tumors [52]. The posterior approach can be used

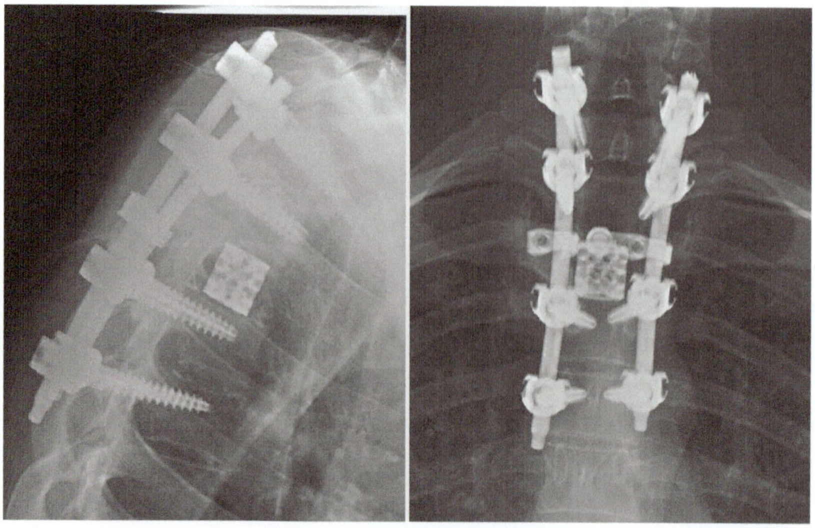

Fig. 12.5 Posterior-only approach to upper thoracic corpectomy with spinal reconstruction and posterior spinal fusion. As seen in the thoracic X-rays, this patient underwent a T3 transpedicular corpectomy with mesh cage placement for spinal metastasis from renal cell carcinoma. At the same time, he underwent pedicle screw fixation and fusion

to treat multiple levels, and long segmental fixation can be performed to correct deformity when present [27, 46].

Tumor Resection Strategies and Extent of Resection

In terms of the extent of tumor removal and resection strategies in removing metastatic lesions, there are multiple studies reporting the risk and benefits of complete tumor removal [27–30, 33, 34, 43, 53–60], partial resection [39, 61–73], and simple posterior decompression (no tumor resection) [21, 26, 36, 38, 74–84]. There are three studies that directly compared varying extents of tumor removal and resection strategies [55, 56, 85]. *Ibrahim* et al. performed a large multicenter prospective study of 223 adult patients with metastatic spinal tumors to answer the question of whether surgical intervention has the ability to impact and improve the quality of life [85]. In their analysis, they categorized three types of resection strategies: en bloc (defined as vertebrectomy, corpectomy, or spondylectomy), debulking (intralesional piecemeal or partial resection), and palliative (minimal resection and mainly simple posterior decompression). Of the 223 patients, 74% underwent excisional surgery (debulking or en bloc resection). Compared to palliative surgery, excisional surgery was associated with better pain control (72% vs. 61%), higher rates of regaining mobility (72% vs. 45%), higher rates of sphincter function (55% vs. 21%), and higher rates of improved neurological status (74% vs. 41%). There was no significant difference in complication rate: 16% in excision group and 12% in palliative group. The median overall survival was significantly higher among patients who underwent en bloc resection (18.8 months), compared to patients that underwent debulking surgery (13.4 months) and palliative decompression (3.7 months). Selection bias toward performing excisional surgery for patients with a longer life expectancy may explain the improved outcomes in these patients compared to patients who underwent palliative surgery. *Li* et al. compared outcomes of en bloc resection and debulking surgery among 131 adult patients with spinal metastasis [55]. In their study, they found that en bloc resection was significantly associated with longer operative time (8 h vs. 4 h) and larger blood loss (1537 mL vs. 954 mL) compared to the partial resection surgery. However, there was no significant difference in complication rate (9% vs. 11%), and patients who underwent en bloc resection had a higher median survival compared to partial resection (41 months vs. 25 months). Conversely, Park et al. performed a comparative retrospective study of 103 patients with spinal metastasis who underwent either posterior decompression (defined as partial resection) with fixation or circumferential decompression (defined as gross total resection) with fusion [56]. Their outcome of interest was postoperative ambulation and overall survival; they found no significant difference between operative strategies for both outcomes.

A new concept and less aggressive surgical approach to spinal metastasis treatment has emerged over the past 5 years. The treatment concept is called "separation surgery" in which circumferential spinal cord decompression and separation of the thecal sac from the epidural tumor is achieved in order to optimize radiation therapy [86, 87]. In the study by *Bilsky* et al., dorsal separation and decompression is done via laminectomy, facetectomy, and/or partial tumor resection [87]. Ventral separation and decompression is done via tumor resection and limited vertebral body resection. The reported outcomes to this technique are promising especially in patients at higher risk for invasive surgery, but complete corpectomy is not performed nor is anterior column reconstruction. Moreover, separation surgery relies heavily on stereotactic radiosurgery, and this treatment modality may not be available at all hospitals [87].

Surgical Complications

Because the overall goal of surgery for spinal metastases is to maintain and/or improve quality of life, it is important to minimize the morbidity related to surgery and hasten recovery time [13, 25]. The morbidity and complication rates can be relatively high in patients who undergo surgery for spinal metastasis [31, 32, 74, 88–90]. Surgical complication rates for metastasis involving the cervical spine range from 13% to 26%, and in the thoracic spine, rates range from 18% to 61% [31, 91, 92]. Specific intraoperative complications include neurological deficits and high blood loss requiring transfusions (especially when treating hemorrhagic tumors such as renal cell carcinoma, melanoma, and thyroid adenocarcinoma). The most common reported postoperative surgical complications are wound-related issues (infections and dehiscence) [93].

When assessing patients with symptomatic spinal metastasis, knowledge of potential risk factors for increased risk for complication is highly valuable in terms of counseling patients on expectations and weighing the benefits of surgery. Preoperative factors associated with higher risk for complications include older age (especially greater than 65 years), metastatic disease involving three or more contiguous vertebral levels, poor baseline neurological function, and history of radiation to the operative area [31, 90].

Conclusion

The most common spinal column tumor type is metastasis from a secondary site. Spinal metastases involving the cervical and thoracic region have the ability to cause not only nerve root compression but also spinal cord compression. In the C6, C7, and T1 levels, anterior-only or combined anterior-posterior approaches can be performed for decompression and stabilization. From T2 to T5, there has been a push toward utilizing posterior-only approaches for corpectomy and spinal instrumentation. However, in certain cases an anterior or lateral approach can be used to access the vertebral body for tumor resection.

It is clear that patients with a reasonable life expectancy may gain significant functional and symptomatic benefit from surgery of spinal metastasis. There is some evidence that patients who undergo surgery may have improved survival, but further investigation is required to further delineate which subgroup of patients will have improved survival [13].

References

1. Ahmad SS, Duke S, Jena R, Williams MV, Burnet NG. Advances in radiotherapy. Br Med J. 2012;345:e7765.
2. Chan BA, Coward JI. Chemotherapy advances in small-cell lung cancer. J Thorac Dis. 2013;5(Suppl 5):S565–S78.
3. Ali I, Rahis U, Salim K, Rather MA, Wani WA, Haque A. Advances in nano drugs for cancer chemotherapy. Curr Cancer Drug Targets. 2011;11(2):135–46.
4. Dohrmann GJ, Byrne RW. What's new in neurosurgery: advances in neurovascular and spine surgery, epilepsy surgery, surgery for movement disorders and intraoperative imaging. Med Princ Pract. 2010;19(5):328–9.
5. Sciubba DM, Petteys RJ, Dekutoski MB, Fisher CG, Fehlings MG, Ondra SL, et al. Diagnosis and management of metastatic spine disease. A review. J Neurosurg Spine. 2010;13(1):94–108.
6. Yachida S, Jones S, Bozic I, Antal T, Leary R, Fu B, et al. Distant metastasis occurs late during the genetic evolution of pancreatic cancer. Nature. 2010;467(7319):1114–7.
7. Costa L, Major PP. Effect of bisphosphonates on pain and quality of life in patients with bone metastases. Nat Clin Pract Oncol. 2009;6(3):163–74.
8. Arguello F, Baggs RB, Duerst RE, Johnstone L, McQueen K, Frantz CN. Pathogenesis of vertebral metastasis and epidural spinal cord compression. Cancer. 1990;65(1):98–106.
9. Fornasier VL, Horne JG. Metastases to the vertebral column. Cancer. 1975;36(2):590–4.
10. Ono K, Galasko CS. Skeletal metastases. Clin Orthop Relat Res. 1995;312:2–3.
11. Harrington KD. Metastatic disease of the spine. J Bone Joint Surg Am. 1986;68(7):1110–5.
12. Polly DW Jr, Chou D, Sembrano JN, Ledonio CG, Tomita K. An analysis of decision making and treatment in thoracolumbar metastases. Spine. 2009;34(22 Suppl):S118–27.
13. Lau D, Leach MR, La Marca F, Park P. Independent predictors of survival and the impact of repeat surgery in patients undergoing surgical treatment of spinal metastasis. J Neurosurg Spine. 2012;17(6):565–76.
14. Togao O, Mihara F, Yoshiura T, Noguchi T, Kuwabara Y, Yoshimitsu K, et al. Percutaneous vertebroplasty in the treatment of pain caused by metastatic tumor. Fukuoka Igaku Zasshi. 2005;96(4):93–9.
15. Eleraky M, Setzer M, Vrionis FD. Posterior transpedicular corpectomy for malignant cervical spine tumors. Eur Spine J. 2010;19(2):257–62.
16. Alvarez L, Perez-Higueras A, Quinones D, Calvo E, Rossi RE. Vertebroplasty in the treatment of vertebral tumors: postprocedural outcome and quality of life. Eur Spine J. 2003;12(4):356–60.
17. Ryken TC, Eichholz KM, Gerszten PC, Welch WC, Gokaslan ZL, Resnick DK. Evidence-based review of

the surgical management of vertebral column metastatic disease. Neurosurg Focus. 2003;15(5):E11.
18. Mazel C, Hoffmann E, Antonietti P, Grunenwald D, Henry M, Williams J. Posterior cervicothoracic instrumentation in spine tumors. Spine. 2004;29(11):1246–53.
19. Edwards SL, Roberts C, McKean ME, Cockburn JS, Jeffrey RR, Kerr KM. Preoperative histological classification of primary lung cancer: accuracy of diagnosis and use of the non-small cell category. J Clin Pathol. 2000;53(7):537–40.
20. Grivaux M, Zureik M, Marsal L, Asselain B, Peureux M, Chavaillon JM, et al. Five-year survival for lung cancer patients managed in general hospitals. Rev Mal Respir. 2011;28(7):e31–8.
21. King GJ, Kostuik JP, McBroom RJ, Richardson W. Surgical management of metastatic renal carcinoma of the spine. Spine. 1991;16(3):265–71.
22. Missenard G, Lapresle P, Cote D. Local control after surgical treatment of spinal metastatic disease. Eur Spine J. 1996;5(1):45–50.
23. Sundaresan N, Galicich JH, Lane JM, Bains MS, McCormack P. Treatment of neoplastic epidural cord compression by vertebral body resection and stabilization. J Neurosurg. 1985;63(5):676–84.
24. Lau D, Than KD, La Marca F, Park P. Independent predictors for local recurrence following surgery for spinal metastasis. Acta Neurochir. 2014;156(2):277–82.
25. Patchell RA, Tibbs PA, Regine WF, Payne R, Saris S, Kryscio RJ, et al. Direct decompressive surgical resection in the treatment of spinal cord compression caused by metastatic cancer: a randomised trial. Lancet. 2005;366(9486):643–8.
26. Chen LH, Niu CC, Fu TS, Lai PL, Wong CB, Chen WJ. Posterior decompression and stabilization for metastatic spine diseases. Chang Gung Med J. 2004;27(12):903–10.
27. Fourney DR, Abi-Said D, Rhines LD, Walsh GL, Lang FF, McCutcheon IE, et al. Simultaneous anterior-posterior approach to the thoracic and lumbar spine for the radical resection of tumors followed by reconstruction and stabilization. J Neurosurg. 2001;94(2 Suppl):232–44.
28. Gokaslan ZL, York JE, Walsh GL, McCutcheon IE, Lang FF, Putnam JB Jr, et al. Transthoracic vertebrectomy for metastatic spinal tumors. J Neurosurg. 1998;89(4):599–609.
29. Holman PJ, Suki D, McCutcheon I, Wolinsky JP, Rhines LD, Gokaslan ZL. Surgical management of metastatic disease of the lumbar spine: experience with 139 patients. J Neurosurg Spine. 2005;2(5):550–63.
30. Jackson RJ, Loh SC, Gokaslan ZL. Metastatic renal cell carcinoma of the spine: surgical treatment and results. J Neurosurg. 2001;94(1 Suppl):18–24.
31. Lau D, Leach MR, Than KD, Ziewacz J, La Marca F, Park P. Independent predictors of complication following surgery for spinal metastasis. Eur Spine J. 2013;22(6):1402–7.
32. Quan GM, Vital JM, Aurouer N, Obeid I, Palussiere J, Diallo A, et al. Surgery improves pain, function and quality of life in patients with spinal metastases: a prospective study on 118 patients. Eur Spine J. 2011;20(11):1970–8.
33. Shehadi JA, Sciubba DM, Suk I, Suki D, Maldaun MV, McCutcheon IE, et al. Surgical treatment strategies and outcome in patients with breast cancer metastatic to the spine: a review of 87 patients. Eur Spine J. 2007;16(8):1179–92.
34. Sundaresan N, Digiacinto GV, Hughes JE, Cafferty M, Vallejo A. Treatment of neoplastic spinal cord compression: results of a prospective study. Neurosurgery. 1991;29(5):645–50.
35. Vrionis FD, Small J. Surgical management of metastatic spinal neoplasms. Neurosurg Focus. 2003;15(5):E12.
36. Wang JC, Boland P, Mitra N, Yamada Y, Lis E, Stubblefield M, et al. Single-stage posterolateral transpedicular approach for resection of epidural metastatic spine tumors involving the vertebral body with circumferential reconstruction: results in 140 patients. Invited submission from the Joint Section Meeting on Disorders of the Spine and Peripheral Nerves, March 2004. J Neurosurg Spine. 2004;1(3):287–98.
37. Jansson KA, Bauer HC. Survival, complications and outcome in 282 patients operated for neurological deficit due to thoracic or lumbar spinal metastases. Eur Spine J. 2006;15(2):196–202.
38. Kim CH, Chung CK, Jahng TA, Kim HJ. Resumption of ambulatory status after surgery for nonambulatory patients with epidural spinal metastasis. Spine J. 2011;11(11):1015–23.
39. Chen LH, Chen WJ, Niu CC, Shih CH. Anterior reconstructive spinal surgery with Zielke instrumentation for metastatic malignancies of the spine. Arch Orthop Trauma Surg. 2000;120(1–2):27–31.
40. Bhatt AD, Schuler JC, Boakye M, Woo SY. Current and emerging concepts in non-invasive and minimally invasive management of spine metastasis. Cancer Treatment Rev. 2013;39(2):142–52.
41. Ames CP, Wang VY, Deviren V, Vrionis FD. Posterior transpedicular corpectomy and reconstruction of the axial vertebra for metastatic tumor. J Neurosurg Spine. 2009;10(2):111–6.
42. Lu DC, Lau D, Lee JG, Chou D. The transpedicular approach compared with the anterior approach: an analysis of 80 thoracolumbar corpectomies. J Neurosurg Spine. 2010;12(6):583–91.
43. Sundaresan N, Steinberger AA, Moore F, Sachdev VP, Krol G, Hough L, et al. Indications and results of combined anterior-posterior approaches for spine tumor surgery. J Neurosurg. 1996;85(3):438–46.
44. Chou D, Wang VY, Gupta N. Transpedicular corpectomy with posterior expandable cage placement for L1 burst fracture. J Clin Neurosci. 2009;16(8):1069–72.
45. Chou D, Wang VY. Trap-door rib-head osteotomies for posterior placement of expandable cages after transpedicular corpectomy: an alternative to lateral extracavitary and costotransversectomy approaches. J Neurosurg Spine. 2009;10(1):40–5.

46. Lau D, Song Y, Guan Z, Sullivan S, La Marca F, Park P. Perioperative characteristics, complications, and outcomes of single-level versus multilevel thoracic corpectomies via modified costotransversectomy approach. Spine. 2013;38(6):523–30.
47. Shen FH, Marks I, Shaffrey C, Ouellet J, Arlet V. The use of an expandable cage for corpectomy reconstruction of vertebral body tumors through a posterior extracavitary approach: a multicenter consecutive case series of prospectively followed patients. Spine J. 2008;8(2):329–39.
48. Jarrett CD, Heller JG, Tsai L. Anterior exposure of the lumbar spine with and without an "access surgeon": morbidity analysis of 265 consecutive cases. J Spinal Disord Tech. 2009;22(8):559–64.
49. Han SJ, Lau D, Lu DC, Theodore P, Chou D. Anterior thoracolumbar corpectomies: approach morbidity with and without an access surgeon. Neurosurgery. 2011;68(5):1220–5; discussion 5–6.
50. Lau D, Chou D. Posterior thoracic corpectomy with cage reconstruction for metastatic spinal tumors: comparing the mini-open approach to the open approach. J Neurosurg Spine. 2015;23(2):217–27.
51. Anderson TM, Mansour KA, Miller JI Jr. Thoracic approaches to anterior spinal operations: anterior thoracic approaches. Ann Thorac Surg. 1993;55(6):1447–51; discussion 51–2.
52. Bernstein DT, Zhuge W, Blackmon SH, Marco RAW. A novel muscle-sparing high thoracotomy for upper thoracic spine resection and reconstruction. Eur Spine J. 2017 (Epub ahead of print).
53. Akeyson EW, McCutcheon IE. Single-stage posterior vertebrectomy and replacement combined with posterior instrumentation for spinal metastasis. J Neurosurg. 1996;85(2):211–20.
54. Boriani S, Bandiera S, Donthineni R, Amendola L, Cappuccio M, De Iure F, et al. Morbidity of en bloc resections in the spine. Eur Spine J. 2010;19(2):231–41.
55. Li H, Gasbarrini A, Cappuccio M, Terzi S, Paderni S, Mirabile L, et al. Outcome of excisional surgeries for the patients with spinal metastases. Eur Spine J. 2009;18(10):1423–30.
56. Park JH, Rhim SC, Jeon SR. Efficacy of decompression and fixation for metastatic spinal cord compression: analysis of factors prognostic for survival and postoperative ambulation. J Korean Neurosurg Soc. 2011;50(5):434–40.
57. Street J, Fisher C, Sparkes J, Boyd M, Kwon B, Paquette S, et al. Single-stage posterolateral vertebrectomy for the management of metastatic disease of the thoracic and lumbar spine: a prospective study of an evolving surgical technique. J Spinal Disord Tech. 2007;20(7):509–20.
58. Sundaresan N, Rothman A, Manhart K, Kelliher K. Surgery for solitary metastases of the spine: rationale and results of treatment. Spine. 2002;27(16):1802–6.
59. Villavicencio AT, Oskouian RJ, Roberson C, Stokes J, Park J, Shaffrey CI, et al. Thoracolumbar vertebral reconstruction after surgery for metastatic spinal tumors: long-term outcomes. Neurosurg Focus. 2005;19(3):E8.
60. Zhang D, Yin H, Wu Z, Yang X, Liu T, Xiao J. Surgery and survival outcomes of 22 patients with epidural spinal cord compression caused by thyroid tumor spinal metastases. Eur Spine J. 2013;22(3):569–76.
61. Bilsky MH, Boland P, Lis E, Raizer JJ, Healey JH. Single-stage posterolateral transpedicle approach for spondylectomy, epidural decompression, and circumferential fusion of spinal metastases. Spine. 2000;25(17):2240–9, discussion 250.
62. Chataigner H, Onimus M. Surgery in spinal metastasis without spinal cord compression: indications and strategy related to the risk of recurrence. Eur Spine J. 2000;9(6):523–7.
63. Chen YJ, Hsu HC, Chen KH, Li TC, Lee TS. Transpedicular partial corpectomy without anterior vertebral reconstruction in thoracic spinal metastases. Spine. 2007;32(22):E623–6.
64. Di Martino A, Vincenzi B, Denaro L, Barnaba SA, Papalia R, Santini D, et al. 'Internal bracing' surgery in the management of solid tumor metastases of the thoracic and lumbar spine. Oncol Rep. 2009;21(2):431–5.
65. Hammerberg KW. Surgical treatment of metastatic spine disease. Spine. 1992;17(10):1148–53.
66. Hosono N, Yonenobu K, Fuji T, Ebara S, Yamashita K, Ono K. Vertebral body replacement with a ceramic prosthesis for metastatic spinal tumors. Spine. 1995;20(22):2454–62.
67. Huang TJ, Hsu RW, Li YY, Cheng CC. Minimal access spinal surgery (MASS) in treating thoracic spine metastasis. Spine. 2006;31(16):1860–3.
68. Metcalfe S, Gbejuade H, Patel NR. The posterior transpedicular approach for circumferential decompression and instrumented stabilization with titanium cage vertebrectomy reconstruction for spinal tumors: consecutive case series of 50 patients. Spine. 2012;37(16):1375–83.
69. Onimus M, Papin P, Gangloff S. Results of surgical treatment of spinal thoracic and lumbar metastases. Eur Spine J. 1996;5(6):407–11.
70. Viswanathan A, Abd-El-Barr MM, Doppenberg E, Suki D, Gokaslan Z, Mendel E, et al. Initial experience with the use of an expandable titanium cage as a vertebral body replacement in patients with tumors of the spinal column: a report of 95 patients. Eur Spine J. 2012;21(1):84–92.
71. Walter J, Reichart R, Waschke A, Kalff R, Ewald C. Palliative considerations in the surgical treatment of spinal metastases: evaluation of posterolateral decompression combined with posterior instrumentation. J Cancer Res Clin Oncol. 2012;138(2):301–10.
72. Weigel B, Maghsudi M, Neumann C, Kretschmer R, Muller FJ, Nerlich M. Surgical management of symptomatic spinal metastases. Postoperative outcome and quality of life. Spine. 1999;24(21):2240–6.
73. Yen D, Kuriachan V, Yach J, Howard A. Long-term outcome of anterior decompression and spinal fixation after placement of the Wellesley Wedge for

thoracic and lumbar spinal metastasis. J Neurosurg. 2002;96(1 Suppl):6–9.
74. Arrigo RT, Kalanithi P, Cheng I, Alamin T, Carragee EJ, Mindea SA, et al. Predictors of survival after surgical treatment of spinal metastasis. Neurosurgery. 2011;68(3):674–81; discussion 81.
75. Bauer HC. Posterior decompression and stabilization for spinal metastases. Analysis of sixty-seven consecutive patients. J Bone Joint Surg Am. 1997;79(4):514–22.
76. Cho DC, Sung JK. Palliative surgery for metastatic thoracic and lumbar tumors using posterolateral transpedicular approach with posterior instrumentation. Surg Neurol. 2009;71(4):424–33.
77. Crnalic S, Hildingsson C, Wikstrom P, Bergh A, Lofvenberg R, Widmark A. Outcome after surgery for metastatic spinal cord compression in 54 patients with prostate cancer. Acta Orthop. 2012;83(1):80–6.
78. Crnalic S, Lofvenberg R, Bergh A, Widmark A, Hildingsson C. Predicting survival for surgery of metastatic spinal cord compression in prostate cancer: a new score. Spine. 2012;37(26):2168–76.
79. Jonsson B, Sjostrom L, Olerud C, Andreasson I, Bring J, Rauschning W. Outcome after limited posterior surgery for thoracic and lumbar spine metastases. Eur Spine J. 1996;5(1):36–44.
80. Kato S, Hozumi T, Takeshita K, Kondo T, Goto T, Yamakawa K. Neurological recovery after posterior decompression surgery for anterior dural compression in paralytic spinal metastasis. Arch Orthop Trauma Surg. 2012;132(6):765–71.
81. Kato S, Murakami H, Minami T, Demura S, Yoshioka K, Matsui O, et al. Preoperative embolization significantly decreases intraoperative blood loss during palliative surgery for spinal metastasis. Orthopedics. 2012;35(9):e1389–95.
82. Kim CH, Chung CK, Jahng TA, Kim HJ. Surgical outcome of spinal hepatocellular carcinoma metastases. Neurosurgery. 2011;68(4):888–96.
83. Park JH, Jeon SR. Pre- and postoperative lower extremity motor power and ambulatory status of patients with spinal cord compression due to a metastatic spinal tumor. Spine. 2013;38(13):E798–802.
84. Quraishi NA, Rajagopal TS, Manoharan SR, Elsayed S, Edwards KL, Boszczyk BM. Effect of timing of surgery on neurological outcome and survival in metastatic spinal cord compression. Eur Spine J. 2013;22(6):1383–8.
85. Ibrahim A, Crockard A, Antonietti P, Boriani S, Bunger C, Gasbarrini A, et al. Does spinal surgery improve the quality of life for those with extradural (spinal) osseous metastases? An international multicenter prospective observational study of 223 patients. Invited submission from the Joint Section Meeting on Disorders of the Spine and Peripheral Nerves, March 2007. J Neurosurg Spine. 2008;8(3):271–8.
86. Amankulor NM, Xu R, Iorgulescu JB, Chapman T, Reiner AS, Riedel E, et al. The incidence and patterns of hardware failure after separation surgery in patients with spinal metastatic tumors. Spine J. 2014;14(9):1850–9.
87. Laufer I, Iorgulescu JB, Chapman T, Lis E, Shi W, Zhang Z, et al. Local disease control for spinal metastases following "separation surgery" and adjuvant hypofractionated or high-dose single-fraction stereotactic radiosurgery: outcome analysis in 186 patients. J Neurosurg Spine. 2013;18(3):207–14.
88. Finkelstein JA, Zaveri G, Wai E, Vidmar M, Kreder H, Chow E. A population-based study of surgery for spinal metastases. Survival rates and complications. J Bone Joint Surg Br. 2003;85(7):1045–50.
89. Williams BJ, Fox BD, Sciubba DM, Suki D, Tu SM, Kuban D, et al. Surgical management of prostate cancer metastatic to the spine. J Neurosurg Spine. 2009;10(5):414–22.
90. Wise JJ, Fischgrund JS, Herkowitz HN, Montgomery D, Kurz LT. Complication, survival rates, and risk factors of surgery for metastatic disease of the spine. Spine (Phila Pa 1976). 1999;24(18):1943–51.
91. Yang J, Jia Q, Peng D, Wan W, Zhong N, Lou Y, et al. Surgical treatment of upper cervical spine metastases: a retrospective study of 39 cases. World J Surg Oncol. 2017;15(1):21.
92. Lei M, Liu Y, Yan L, Tang C, Liu S, Zhou S. Posterior decompression and spine stabilization for metastatic spinal cord compression in the cervical spine. A matched pair analysis. Eur J Surg Oncol. 2015;41(12):1691–8.
93. Bakar D, Tanenbaum JE, Phan K, Alentado VJ, Steinmetz MP, Benzel EC, et al. Decompression surgery for spinal metastases: a systematic review. Neurosurg Focus. 2016;41(2):E2.

Surgical Treatment for Patients with Thoracic Spinal Metastasis

13

Robert F. McLain

Introduction

Time has long passed when spinal metastasis was considered the principal sign of impending death, with nothing more to offer than comfort and pain medications. With better radiotherapeutic modalities, more effective chemotherapy, and overall advances in management and health maintenance, patients—even when they cannot expect cure—have an excellent chance for continued life and activity so long as (1) we prevent paralysis and (2) control pain.

Although most metastatic lesions respond well to radiotherapy, radioresistant tumors and those causing fracture can result in bony compression of the spinal cord and require direct surgical decompression to preserve function and eliminate neuropathic pain. Metastatic lesions, and most primary tumors for that matter, usually arise in the vertebral body, predisposing to both anterior vertebral collapse and instability and anterior cord compression. Because the cord is compressed from the anterior surface, simple laminectomy is usually not beneficial, and anterior decompression, carried out through thoracotomy, is often needed to correct both the mechanical and the neurological problems [1–14]. In the upper thoracic spine, the direct surgical approach can be challenging in the best of circumstances. Patients with advanced pulmonary disease and limited pulmonary reserve may not tolerate either the thoracotomy approach or the temporary loss of lung capacity associated with MIS procedures. In patients with extensive disease or marginal bone quality, a second-stage posterior operation is usually needed to provide stability necessary to allow early mobilization.

Posterolateral decompression of the thoracic spine offers potential advantages over traditional anterior/posterior procedures, including decreased operative time, decreased morbidity, and reduced hospital stay. While early studies could not demonstrate the same neurological benefit for posterolateral decompression as for direct anterior decompression, technical advances make contemporary dorsal approaches far more appealing [15, 16].

Drawbacks to the traditional posterolateral decompression included poor access to any tumor immediately anterior to the spinal cord. This was the tumor most responsible for neural compression and most likely to cause problems after local recurrence, and the need to manipulate the spinal cord to completely remove both adjacent tumor and tumor adherent to the dura was hampered by poor visualization and increased surgical risks.

Using standard endoscopic instruments, subtotal and total vertebrectomy, cord decompression,

R. F. McLain, MD
Spine and Orthopaedic Institute, St Vincent Charity Medical Group, Cleveland, OH, USA

Biomedical Engineering, Cleveland State University, Cleveland, OH, USA
e-mail: robertfmclain@gmail.com

R. A. W. Marco (ed.), *Metastatic Spine Disease*, https://doi.org/10.1007/978-3-319-76252-4_13

and anterior reconstruction can be accomplished through the same incision used for the posterior instrumentation, with a dramatic reduction in morbidity, and reduced intensive care unit and inpatient hospitalization. This approach has proven useful for a variety of metastatic tumors and essentially extends the utility of traditional costotransversectomy approaches familiar to most neurosurgeons and orthopedic surgeons. Variations on this approach provide current surgeons a spectrum of options that can be selected to provide the best exposure and margins for tumors involving any quadrant of the vertebral column and the surrounding soft tissues.

Preoperative Planning

Identify the Problem

Patients presenting with thoracic spinal metastases undergo a routine battery of tests to determine their medical status, the extent of their disease, and to elucidate the individual risk and benefit of surgical care [17]. Patients indicated for surgical treatment include those who have radioresistant tumors such as renal cell carcinoma, those who have failed previous radiotherapy, patients with bony compression of the neural elements, and those with segmental instability due to bone destruction. The decompression techniques typically applied to metastatic lesions involve intralesional resections, always leaving some tumor behind, and are not ideal for patients with primary malignancies [18].

Establish Reasonable Goals

Skeletal metastases can be produced by almost any kind of malignant disease but are most commonly associated with breast, lung, prostate, and, less frequently, renal, thyroid, and gastrointestinal carcinomas. Multiple myeloma and lymphoma are common sources of disseminated skeletal lesions, though hematopoietic neoplasms are often considered primary lesions rather than metastases. Breast, lung, prostate, and plasma cell disease account for almost 60% of all spinal column tumors. The patient's sex and age, the location of metastases, and the interval between initial diagnosis and appearance of metastases are correlated with outcome, but the primary prognostic determinant is tumor type. Patients with breast, renal, and prostate carcinoma frequently survive long enough to require treatment of their spinal disease, while patients with pulmonary malignancies frequently succumb before surgical treatment is needed. More effective medical treatment now allows more patients to live long enough to require treatment of spinal metastases. In the past, gastrointestinal carcinoma patients often died of the liver and lung metastases long before their spinal lesion became clinically apparent. Multiple myeloma was often rapidly fatal, and patients with spinal involvement had a poor chance for 2-year survival. Great advances in medical treatment have changed the prognosis for these patients, and the goals of treatment have changed as well.

While radiotherapy remains the mainstay for treating spinal metastases, mechanical instability still requires surgical treatment in patients who are healthy enough to undergo surgery. Similarly, radioresistant tumors or those with extensive bony destruction may benefit from tumor removal and reconstruction of the anterior weight-bearing column [19]. Occasionally, a patient with a solitary metastasis presents a special circumstance in which en bloc vertebrectomy offers potential for long-term survival or local "cure" [20].

Neurologic compromise consistently indicates the need for prompt treatment, irrespective of tumor type. If the tumor is radiosensitive and neural progression is gradual, radiotherapy is the initial treatment of choice. If progression is rapid, however, or the neural compression is caused by bony rather than soft tissue encroachment or the tumor is known to be radioresistant, surgical decompression of the cord or roots is called for in any but the sickest patients.

Select an Approach

The surgical approach must provide sufficient access for both tumor excision and spinalstabilization, depending on the patient's needs. If both goals cannot be achieved through the same incision, the surgeon may need to plan a combined approach.

Metastatic lesions rarely require a true margin for best local control; postoperative radiotherapy and chemotherapy determine the long-term survival of the patient. Even if gross tumor is left behind in the field, a satisfactory decompression of the spinal cord is important to neurologic outcome, and the correct surgical approach is important to achieving this goal. Dorsal lesions are uncommon in metastatic disease but are easily approached posteriorly. The same is true for metastases primarily involving the pedicle or nerve root. Because extensive or multilevel laminectomies in the thoracic spine can lead to postoperative kyphosis, posterior instrumentation is commonly applied to restore the posterior column tension band, using the same midline exposure.

Lesions isolated to the vertebral body should be approached anteriorly if they are radioresistant or if there is a chance for long-term local control. Larger lesions should be carefully analyzed preoperatively to identify invasion or adherence to the great vessels. Reconstruction may be performed with or without anterior internal fixation depending on the extent of the resection and the inherent stability of the residual elements, but most often benefits from posterior reinforcement with segmental instrumentation.

Lesions of the upper thoracic segments can be managed through a combined anterior and posterior surgical approach. These lesions involve the most inaccessible region of the vertebral column, however, and are the most difficult lesions to reconstruct. Complete excision can be obtained, though tumor margins must be crossed. Failure to accomplish solid reconstruction and an adequate anterior column support may result in loss of fixation, with catastrophic neurologic complications if hardware migrates into the canal or if excessive kyphosis develops [21, 22]. Minimally invasive and video-assisted techniques that permit wide and adequate anterior decompression and reconstruction through the posterolateral window have significantly improved the ability to accomplish treatment goals with less morbidity and fewer hospital days.

Establish the Surgical Plan and a Backup Plan

Select the approach that gives the best opportunity to accomplish all goals at one setting. However, be prepared with a backup plan. Poor bone quality or progression of disease in the adjacent vertebra may make anterior column reconstruction more difficult or may require extension of the corpectomy further than initially planned. Uncontrolled bleeding, despite preoperative embolization, may curtail the resection or necessitate a staged procedure when a combined operation was planned. Occasionally, frozen section will reveal that the lesion is not what was expected, requiring a change in thinking with respect to the surgical goals and approach [23].

Optimize the Patient

In addition to the usual cardiopulmonary optimization required for any extensive spine procedure, give attention to nutritional status. Wound healing is compromised in irradiated tissues already; patients need adequate nutrition for healing the soft tissue injury associated with surgery, to maintain metabolic balance and to allow postoperative mobilization and skin care. Patients with severe albumin and total protein deficits are likely to have wound healing, skin care, and medical complications after any invasive procedure.

Surgical Techniques

The anterior cervicothoracic junction and upper thoracic spine are difficult to access surgically. Traditional options have included sternal splitting approaches, sternoclavicular excisions, posterolateral extracavitary approach, and costotransversectomy. Splitting the sternum causes much morbidity, and sternoclavicular approaches provide limited exposure. Endoscopic techniques useful in the mid-thoracic segments provide a poor angle for vertebrectomy and anterior decompression in cases where the working space is confined to the apex of the thoracic cavity.

In selecting an approach for the metastatic lesion, we have one advantage: en bloc excision is typically not necessary [24]. Midline posterior approaches can be applied in the cervicothoracic and upper thoracic spine so long as the surgeon is careful to complete the tumor removal from directly anterior to the cord, and they provide simultaneous access for instrumentation often required to stabilize the operated segments. Over the past two decades, a variety of endoscopic and imaging systems have been developed that provide improved viewing of the anterior cord during video-assisted decompression, whether from the posterolateral approach or a transthoracic portal. [25].

Biopsy Technique

The choice of biopsy technique depends on the location of the lesion, the integrity of the overlying bone, proximity to the spinal cord and nerve roots, and the internal consistency of the tumor [26]. The best site for biopsy is usually the advancing edge or the extraosseous portion of the tumor. The center of the lesion may be necrotic and provide minimal or no diagnostic tissue. To obtain a diagnostic result, multiple sites within the tumor should be sampled. Prior to finishing the procedure, the surgeon or radiologist should communicate with the pathologist to insure that the representative tissue has been obtained and enough is available to allow the histopathologic as well as complementary immunohistochemical analyses or karyotyping.

Fine Needle Aspiration Biopsy

Fine needle aspiration biopsy is best suited to lesions that are composed of soft tissue and/or fluid. Once the tumor tissue has been triangulated by fluoroscopy or CT, the needle is inserted into the desired location and placement confirmed prior to obtaining tissue. Although cytology techniques provide reliable diagnosis of soft tissue neoplasms, there are limitations inherent to the technique. FNAB provides only a small amount of cellular material from each biopsy site, and a significant percentage of aspirates are inconclusive. FNAB is usually adequate for metastatic lesions, even though its utility in diagnosing primary malignant tumors is limited.

Core Needle or Trephine Biopsy

The image-guided core biopsy is most reliable for obtaining tissue samples from soft tissue and bone tumors. Biopsy trephines are designed to obtain a core of tissue from calcified tissue and bone, without distorting its architecture. Advantages of core biopsy over open biopsy include the potential to avoid surgery, earlier institution of radiotherapy, ability to obtain tissue from deeper areas in the lesion, decreased risk of pathologic fracture, use of local rather than general anesthesia, cost savings, and rapid differentiation of primary from metastatic lesions. Compared to open biopsy, core needle or trephine biopsy contaminates very little tissue, making subsequent resection of the track at definitive surgery a simple matter when local control is an issue. The trephine technique is particularly well suited for lesions that are sclerotic, calcified, or contained within intact bone. To optimize the diagnostic yield, surgeons should obtain a minimum of three specimens in bone lesions and four in soft tissue lesions. While frozen-section analysis is not possible with bone biopsy specimens, it is usually possible to obtain diagnostic information from a "touch prep" to insure you have obtained diagnostic tissue at the time of the biopsy.

A posterolateral approach is most commonly used in the thoracic spine, particularly for lesions with extraosseous extension into the paraspinal tissues. For lesions confined within the vertebral body, the transpedicular approach popularized for kyphoplasty provides a safe alternative with decreased risks of pulmonary or nerve root injury. The needle is advanced through a stab wound placed 4–8 cm off the midline at the level of the involved vertebra. To access a vertebral body lesion, the needle is directed to the junction of the transverse process and the lateral facet and then driven through the cortex into the lateral aspect of the pedicle. The needle can then be passed under fluoroscopic control into the tumor mass, or a guidewire can be placed and a working cannula positioned to allow a Craig needle biopsy trocar, capable of harvesting larger pieces of ossified tissue, to be passed.

Posterolateral Decompression and Fusion in the Upper Thoracic Spine

When treated for lesions causing ventral spinal cord compression, only 40% of traditional laminectomy patients have retained or regained the ability to walk, compared to 80% of the patients undergoing vertebrectomy [8]. With this in mind, a formal anterior approach is the gold standard for spinal cord decompression in metastatic disease. While posterior stabilization is often required to supplement the anterior reconstruction and improving pain control and neurologic function, it typically requires a second major operation after the anterior tumor surgery.

Traditionally, posterolateral decompression and costotransversectomy results have not been as good as with the open anterior approach, even when combined with posterior, segmental instrumentation [27]. The likely reason was, in many cases, the inability to successfully control residual tumor postoperatively. The likelihood that small amounts of tumor left anterior to the cord would rapidly extend and cause recurrent cord compression led surgeons to excessively manipulate the cord in places where visualization was difficult, leading to cord trauma and dural tears [28]. In the past, surgeons concluded that it was impossible to adequately decompress the cord through the posterior or posterolateral approach, removing retropulsed vertebral fragments and tumor, without traumatizing the cord [29].

With advances in contemporary radiotherapy, this is less of a concern. In fact, the improvement in radiosurgical techniques has led to shift in goals in some patients: for radiosensitive tumors, the surgery can be carried out simply to gain an interval between the main tumor mass and the spinal cord, so that focal beam radiotherapy can be more safely applied [30].

Surgical Techniques

The surgical incision is longitudinal and midline, centered over the involved segment. Dissection is carried laterally to the costotransverse articulation at the site of the tumor, on the side of greatest compromise. The proximal origin of the rib and any rib invaded by tumor is excised, exaggerating the traditional costotransversectomy approach. A wide laminectomy should be performed, removing the dorsal elements across to the far facet, and cranially and caudally to provide a sufficient decompression of the involved cord. On the side of most extensive tumor involvement, the pedicle is resected down to the back of the vertebral body, completing standard transpedicular approach (Fig. 13.1a–d). Bipolar cautery is needed to control normal and some enlarged epidural vessels. The tumor anterior to the pedicle is then debulked under direct visualization until a cavity is formed in the vertebral body. The spinal nerves may be retracted gently during tumor excision or be ligated and excised if they are invested with neoplastic tissue.

If endoscopic visualization is desired, maintain suction in the base of the initial corpectomy cavity, irrigating frequently, and introduce a standard 4 mm arthroscope or spinal endoscope into the cavity. A 30-degree scope can be used initially, providing light, magnification, and visualization of the posterior vertebral cortex along with the tumor and bone immediately anterior to the spinal cord. Curettes and pituitary rongeurs can be used together to remove soft tissue and bone fragments from the central vertebral body, across to the far pedicle, creating a large void anterior to the cord. A 70-degree scope is then introduced, providing a view across the surface of the spinal cord and posterior longitudinal ligament. With a direct view of the interval between the dura and the tumor tissue directly in front of the cord, fine curettes and dissectors can be used to develop the interval between the dura and posterior vertebral body, moving all compressive tissues away from the spinal cord. Under endoscopic control, the surgeon can collapse the posterior cortex and tumor tissue into the vertebral cavity without actually touching the spinal cord. Any

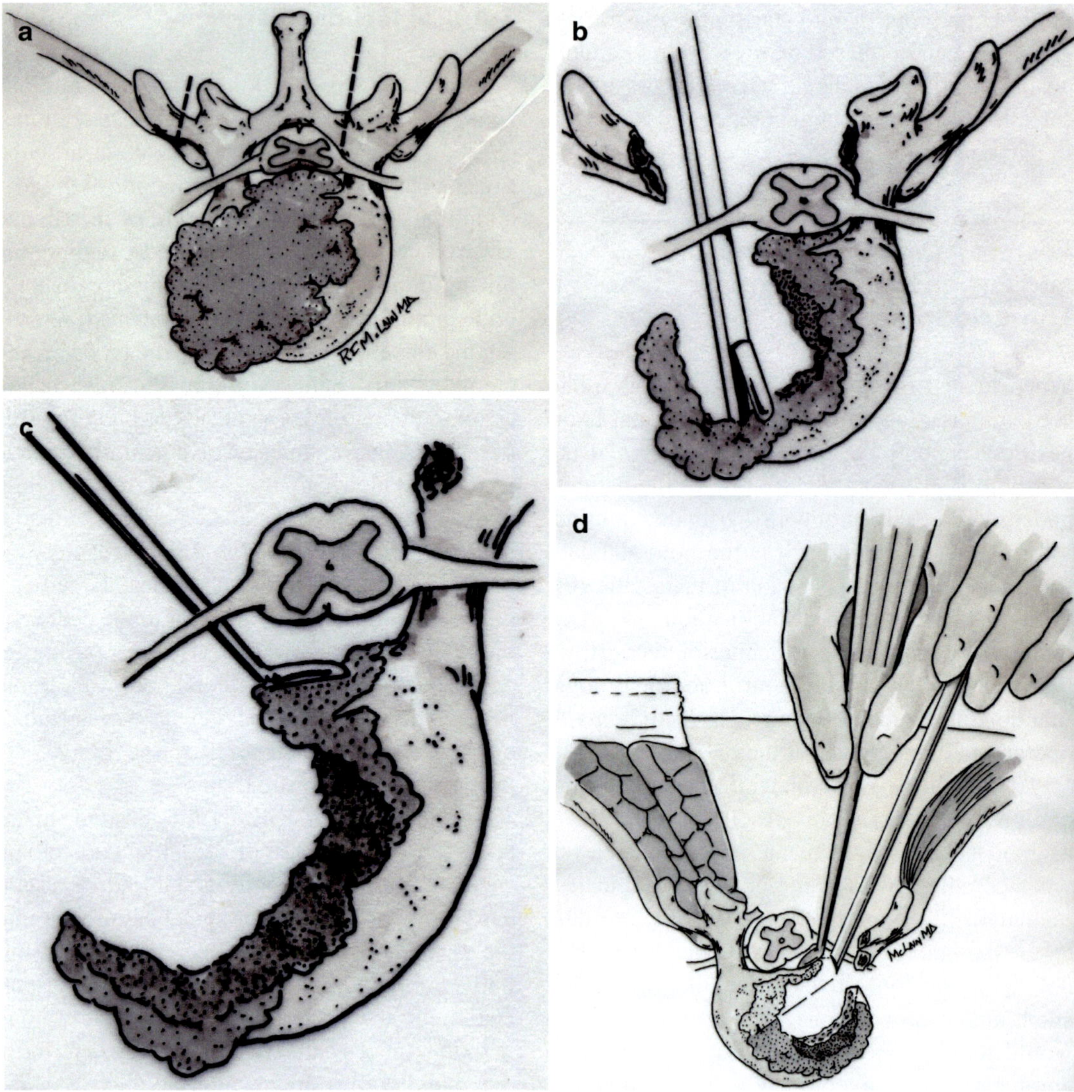

Fig. 13.1 (**a**) Transpedicular corpectomy: resect the lamina and pedicle down to the back of the vertebral body, mobilizing the nerve root. Use bipolar cautery to control epidural vessels and neovasculature. (**b**) Debulk the tumor anterior to the pedicle under direct visualization, using curettes and pituitaries, until a cavity is formed in the vertebral body. The spinal nerves may be retracted gently or be ligated and excised if they are invested with tumor. (**c**) If endoscopic visualization is desired, maintain suction in the base of the initial corpectomy cavity, irrigating frequently, and introduce a standard 4 mm endoscope into the cavity. Curettes and pituitary rongeurs can be used together to remove soft tissue and bone fragments from the central vertebral body, across to the far pedicle, creating a large void anterior to the cord. (**d**) A 70-degree scope can be introduced to provide a view across the volar surface of the spinal cord and posterior longitudinal ligament

remaining tumor tissue can be meticulously debrided from the surface of the exposed dura under direct vision (Fig. 13.2a, b).

Epidural veins can be visualized and controlled with an angled bipolar cautery. If the tumor involves the far pedicle, a bilateral approach can be used; otherwise, the contralateral pedicle and lamina remain intact for posterior grafting and fusion. After completing the decompression, the adjacent end plates are debrided of disc material and prepared for reconstruction (Fig. 13.3).

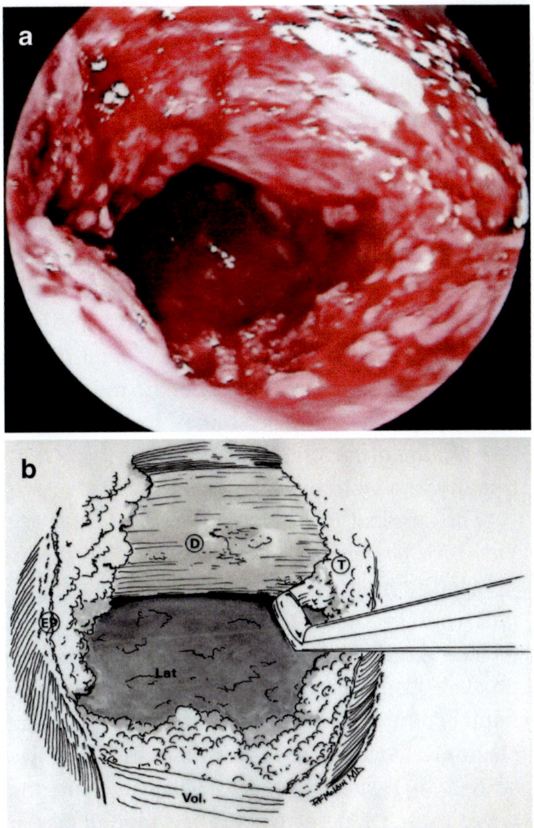

Fig. 13.2 (**a**) Endoscopic view of the volar surface of the dura after removal of impinging tumor and posterior vertebral cortex. (**b**) Schematic view through transpedicular portal using 70-degree scope. With care, surgeon can carry out meticulous removal of tumor tissue and careful preparation of end plates without manipulating the spinal cord or resecting the exiting nerve root. *EP* end plate, *D* dura, *T* tumor, *Vol* volar soft tissues, *Lat* far lateral wall of vertebral body

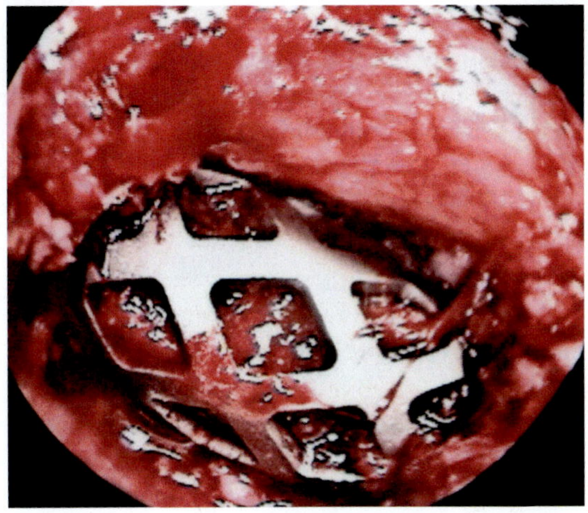

Fig. 13.3 Endoscopic view with 70-degree scope offers an unparalleled view of the vertebral defect after instrumentation, with cage firmly anchored in end plates, insuring the best possible fixation for the anterior column

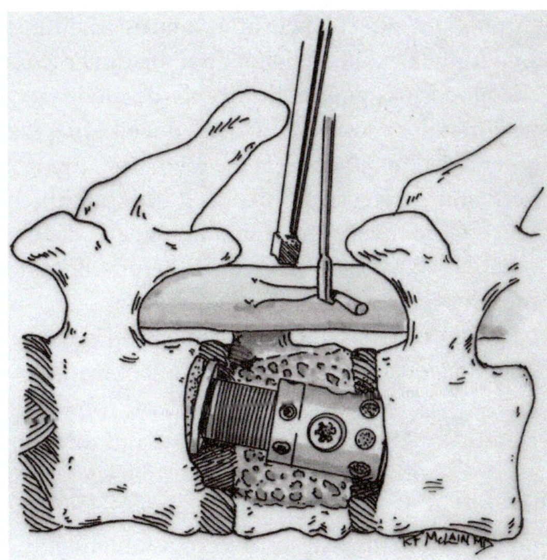

Fig. 13.4 Expandable titanium reconstruction cage is placed following vertebrectomy. End plate preparation is carried out with curved curettes, and collapsed cage is inserted end-on and turned into the long axis of the spine. Once aligned, the cage is expanded to fill the gap and then correct the kyphotic collapse as needed

A titanium cage filled with autograft bone provides immediate axial stability with maximum potential for fusion, important for patients with potential for survival greater than 3 months. The cage is maneuvered into place, while the cord is viewed with the 70-degree scope and then expanded to fill the interval and restore vertebral body height (Fig. 13.4). Segmental fixation is then applied through the dorsal exposure, using a construct that will stabilize the level of the lesion and any adjacent spinal lesions, and gently compressing the anterior strut. When the wound is closed, a chest X-ray obtained in the operating room confirms that a pneumothorax has not occurred.

In patients with metastatic disease, the ability to avoid a thoracotomy significantly reduces the need for postoperative ventilation and ICU care. In patients with existing pulmonary disease, avoiding the need to deflate either lung reduces pulmonary complications and postoperative respiratory distress. Considering that many patients may not live long enough to establish a full and durable fusion, there is some logic in considering more minimally invasive techniques for stabilization that do not require exposing the spinal elements above or below the level of the decompression.

MIS Fixation Techniques

The ability to reliably place thoracic pedicle screws using image guidance techniques has allowed surgeons performing fusion surgery, scoliosis fusions, and tumor surgery to significantly reduce operative blood loss and hospital stays while still instrumenting the needed segments of the thoracic and lumbar spine [31, 32]. Pedicle screws can be placed percutaneously or through the intact fascia after a more traditional longitudinal skin incision, but in either case, the blood loss and morbidity associated with a traditional exposure can be reduced. In cases where decompression is needed, the thoracic vertebral body can be exposed along with the level immediately above and below and decompressed as discussed above. If there is no compressive lesion, the tumor is radiosensitive, and stability is the overriding concern, posterior percutaneous vertebroplasty can be carried out along with percutaneous fixation, providing stability without great morbidity and allowing early transition to radiotherapy. Balloon kyphoplasty has been widely used in thoracolumbar and thoracic metastases and myelomatous disease and has been used cautiously in upper thoracic (T1–T5) lesions with good results as long as there is residual integrity to the posterior vertebral cortex [33, 34]. Clinically apparent myelopathy is considered a contraindication to balloon kyphoplasty, however, and decompression is recommended.

Separation Surgery

The concept of separation surgery has grown with our confidence that stereotactic radiosurgery (SRS) can kill most any tumor tissue it can safely reach. "Safely" being the operative word, radiation oncologists have a very difficult time windowing tumors that are directly compressing nerve root or spinal cord tissue and must either accept a suboptimal tumor exposure or risk direct and permanent injury to the cord. Moulding et al. initially reported a pilot study of 21 patients undergoing "separation surgery" in anticipation of postoperative, single-fraction SRS [35] and demonstrated a significant improvement in local control compared to traditional radiotherapy techniques. Subsequent studies have confirmed this treatment benefit, even in tumor types traditionally known to be radioresistant [30].

The surgical technique is similar to that provided for posterolateral corpectomy, but there is no need to aggressively resect tumor that is distant from the spinal cord.

The surgical decompression is, again, accomplished from the posterolateral approach, via laminectomy including unilateral or bilateral facetectomy. Bony elements are carefully removed with a high-speed bur, exposing the dura and nerve root at a point where the tissue planes are still normal. Working toward the point of maximal compression, the surgeon then sequentially resects the tumor tissue from the epidural space to create a free space circumferentially around the spinal cord. Typically, only a small portion of the vertebral body, just ventral to the cord, is resected, but the PLL and all epidural tumor must be removed to provide a physical separation between the remaining involved tissue and the dura and spinal cord [36]. If more than 50% of the vertebral body must be resected or if the bone involved is mechanically insubstantial, a gross resection of the involved vertebral body and adjacent discs should be completed, and the adjacent level discs removed back to the adjacent healthy end plates. The interval can then be reconstructed with an expandable titanium or PEEK cage inserted through the posterolateral access. In this approach, there is no need to attempt a complete or gross-total resection of anterior vertebral or paraspinal tumor tissue.

Postoperative irradiation therapy (SRS) is the key to obtaining local control and surgical success. As the radiation dose involved in SRS is delivered deep to the healing surgical wounds, high-dose hypofractionated or single-fraction "ablative" RT can be initiated within 2–3 weeks after the open surgical procedure. Local control with this technique has been observed in between 75 and 90% of treated patients [37], including those with tumors traditionally considered radioresistant [38].

Mid-thoracic Metastases: Combined Anterior and Posterior Reconstruction

Rapid and complete cord decompression can provide dramatic improvement even in advanced states of neurologic compromise, depending on the rate of progression and the interval from paralysis to treatment. While radiotherapy has been the traditional standard for treatment of most patients with metastatic disease, patients with radioresistant tumors, cord compression secondary to bony impingement, and those who have reached the maximum dose of radiation are frequently indicated for surgical decompression.

Because the results of laminectomy are often no better than those of radiotherapy alone, surgical decompression through a direct anterior approach has become widely regarded as the standard of care in spinal cord decompression and spinal stabilization for mid-thoracic and thoracolumbar lesions.

While the posterior approach is the recommended choice in the upper cervical spine [39] and for tumors of the posterior elements in the lower cervical, thoracic, and lumbar spine, the anterior approach addresses the majority of lower cervical, thoracic, and lumbar lesions, as most tumors in these regions arise in the vertebral body [4, 6, 40].

As noted above, alternative posterolateral approaches provide important options in many patients, particularly those with medical factors that preclude thoracotomy, but the principles of decompression and stabilization are rooted in the formal anterior/posterior strategy [24, 41]. The formal anterior and posterior combined approach is particularly important for cases warranting en bloc spondylectomy or when the tumor involves multiple adjacent levels [42–46].

Solitary or locally aggressive tumors that require or may benefit from a complete or en bloc excision must be managed through a combined anterior and posterior surgical approach. These lesions involve the most inaccessible region of the vertebral body and provide major technical challenges to the surgeon considering tumor resection. Thoracic lesions with soft tissue extension should be carefully analyzed preoperatively to anticipate possible invasion or adherence to the great vessels of the thoracic cavity, retroperitoneal structures of the abdomen, or critical neurovascular elements of the cervicothoracic junction. In patients undergoing corpectomy, both anterior and posterior stabilization is usually necessary. Failure to provide a balanced and secure reconstruction can result in loss of fixation, with serious neurologic complications if hardware migrates into the canal or if excessive kyphosis develops [21, 22].

The anterior cervicothoracic junction and upper thoracic spine present an anatomic challenge in any case where a formal anterior corpectomy is needed. For the cervicothoracic junction and T1 vertebra, the low anterior approach (a caudal extension of the Southwick-Robinson approach) can be used in most cases and stabilized with an anterior cervical plate supplemented with posterior cervicothoracic fixation. Bridging the junction is usually wise, and a posterior construct transitioning from lateral mass cervical fixation to upper thoracic pedicle screws is reliable.

Other options for upper thoracic corpectomy include the sternal splitting approach and the sternoclavicular excision, but these are rarely needed in patients with metastatic disease, as they can cause considerable morbidity.

The anterior approach to the thoracic spine is by way of thoracotomy and rib resection [40]. Typically, the rib above the level involved is selected and excised from its base to the costochondral cartilage. Save the rib for autograft material. The approach through the eleventh rib bed, with extrapleural-retroperitoneal dissection, provides access to the thoracolumbar junction [47].

The left-sided thoracotomy approach is generally preferred, as the aorta is a tougher tissue than the vena cava, but scarring, chest wall invasion, or previous pneumonectomy can dictate which side is available for the approach. While the anterior approach in scoliotic and young trauma patients is familiar to most spine surgeons and can be accomplished with a little experience, the approach in tumor patients can be quite challenging and fraught with danger. Whether from tumor involvement or the effects of radiation, vascular structures can be friable or buried in abnormal tissue, and neovasculature is often extensive. Erosions into the mediastinum or into the chest cavity can directly invest the pleura or the lung itself, and block the approach in cases. The assistance of an experienced cardiothoracic surgeon during the exposure and closure would never be criticized.

Once the lung and pleura are reflected out of the way, the segmental vessels can be isolated, mobilized, and ligated and clipped before cutting and dissecting them out of the way. The normal paired vessels are easy to see and manage in healthy adolescents, but there may be numerous additional small vessels running through the tumor margin in these cases, and additional ties and clips should be applied as often as needed. Before digging in to the tumor itself, find the lateral aspect of the disc above and below and dissect anteriorly over the front of the column to establish working planes and then work bluntly to the midportion of the involved tumor to insure that there are no dense adhesions to the vascular trunks (Fig. 13.5). The discs can then be incised and resected to expose the vertebral end plates, exposing the body and tumor more fully, so that excision can be carried out more quickly and surely with less blood loss. Do as much work on the adjacent end plates as you can before violating the tumor, as bleeding may be brisk thereafter.

Bleeding from the tumor is most aggressive when the surgeon is in the midst of the pathological bone. Rapid removal of involved bone back to the cortical shell and pedicles will usually control blood loss, but areas of persistent bony bleeding can be dressed with bone wax and, before closure, with PMMA to seal vascular voids in the diseased bone. Bleeding from the associated soft tissue mass also slows as the mass is removed, but control at the margins of the invasive tumor is more difficult and dangerous. Proper preoperative treatment can make a huge difference to the safety and control during excision of the anterior thoracic metastasis.

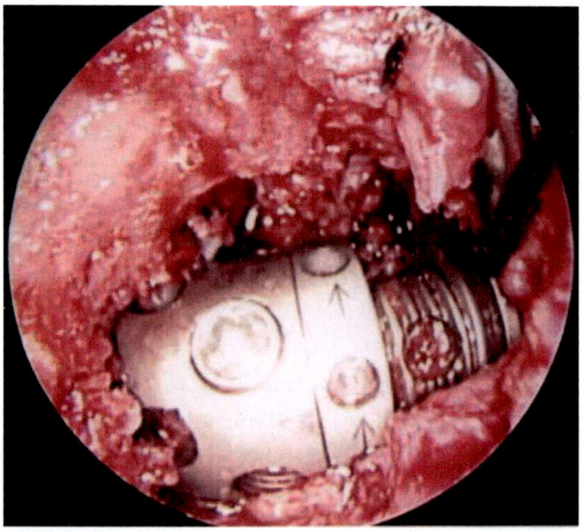

Fig. 13.5 Patient with T4 breast metastasis immediately after corpectomy and anterior column reconstruction using endoscopic assistance. Adequate space between the cage and cord can be insured by direct inspection using the endoscope

Complete radiographic evaluation prior to surgery, including CT and MRI, allows accurate determination of the tumor location and extension and can show adhesions and invasion of adjacent tissues that may need to be addressed during resection. Angiography, along with preoperative embolization, should be considered to assess whether any tumor will be highly vascular and certainly when tumors of metastatic renal cell, melanoma, or thyroid carcinoma are encountered.

Reconstruction of the Thoracic Spine

After tumor resection, spinal column reconstruction must restore mechanical stability and compensate for the loss of bony elements. Any construct chosen must restore the anterior weight-bearing column. Without a stable reconstruction, thoracic collapse and kyphosis will result in pain and neurologic compromise. Posterior instrumentation may restore the posterior tension band after extensive laminectomy and will help to prevent kyphosis. Anterior reconstruction restores the weight-bearing column and supplements posterior instrumentation in resisting torsional and translational deforming forces. When bone quality is marginal to poor or when residual disease is inevitable, problems can be avoided by including more levels in the fixation construct above and below the tumor, combining anterior and posterior instrumentation, and by maximizing fixation points. Whenever the patient has more than 3 months of expected survival, promote biologic fusion by using autograft or allograft bone to span the construct.

Posterior Instrumentation

The superior strength and resiliency of contemporary fixation systems allow them to be used in cases where posterior elements have been resected or eroded by tumor. The surgeon can contour rods to restore sagittal alignment and can either compress or distract separately at each intercalary level. Pedicle screws offer more secure anchorage than old hook systems, can provide fixation at each operated level, and can be used in the thoracic spine with reliably good results. [48].

When the anterior column is intact, pedicle screw and lateral mass screw fixation can bridge the cervicothoracic or thoracolumbar junctions and provide satisfactory stabilization without the need of an anterior approach (Fig. 13.6). In situations where the anterior and middle load-bearing columns are compromised, posterior implants can fatigue and fail, and anterior reconstruction is required (Fig. 13.7) [49]. Pedicle screw fixation can be augmented in poor-quality bone with polymethyl methacrylate applied down the pedicle into the prepared vertebral body [50].

Anterior Reconstruction

Anterior spinal reconstruction using polymethyl methacrylate (PMMA) remains an option, as it is quick, easy, and inexpensive, but this role has

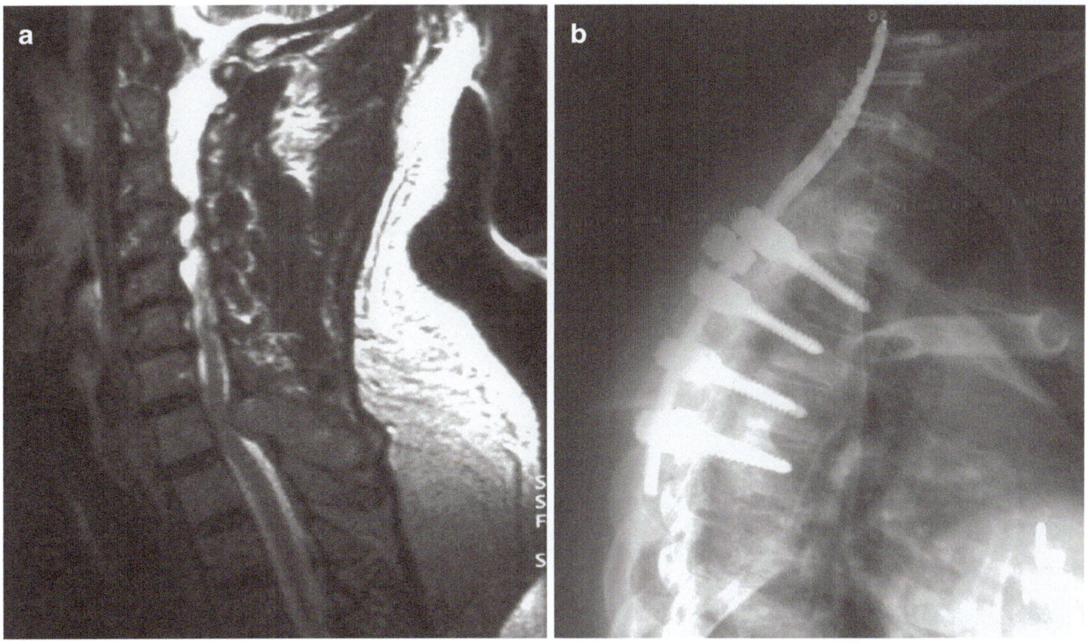

Fig. 13.6 (**a**) T1–T2 thoracic metastasis from colon carcinoma, with focal cord compression and paraparesis. Vertebral body involvement is minimal, but dorsal elements and pedicles are involved. Radiotherapy provided no neurological improvement. (**b**) Wide laminectomy provided excellent neurological recovery and removed all local tumor. Transitional construct allowed segmental fixation above and below the lesion with lateral mass screws above and pedicle screws below. Patient survived 4 years after surgery without local recurrence or neurologic compromise

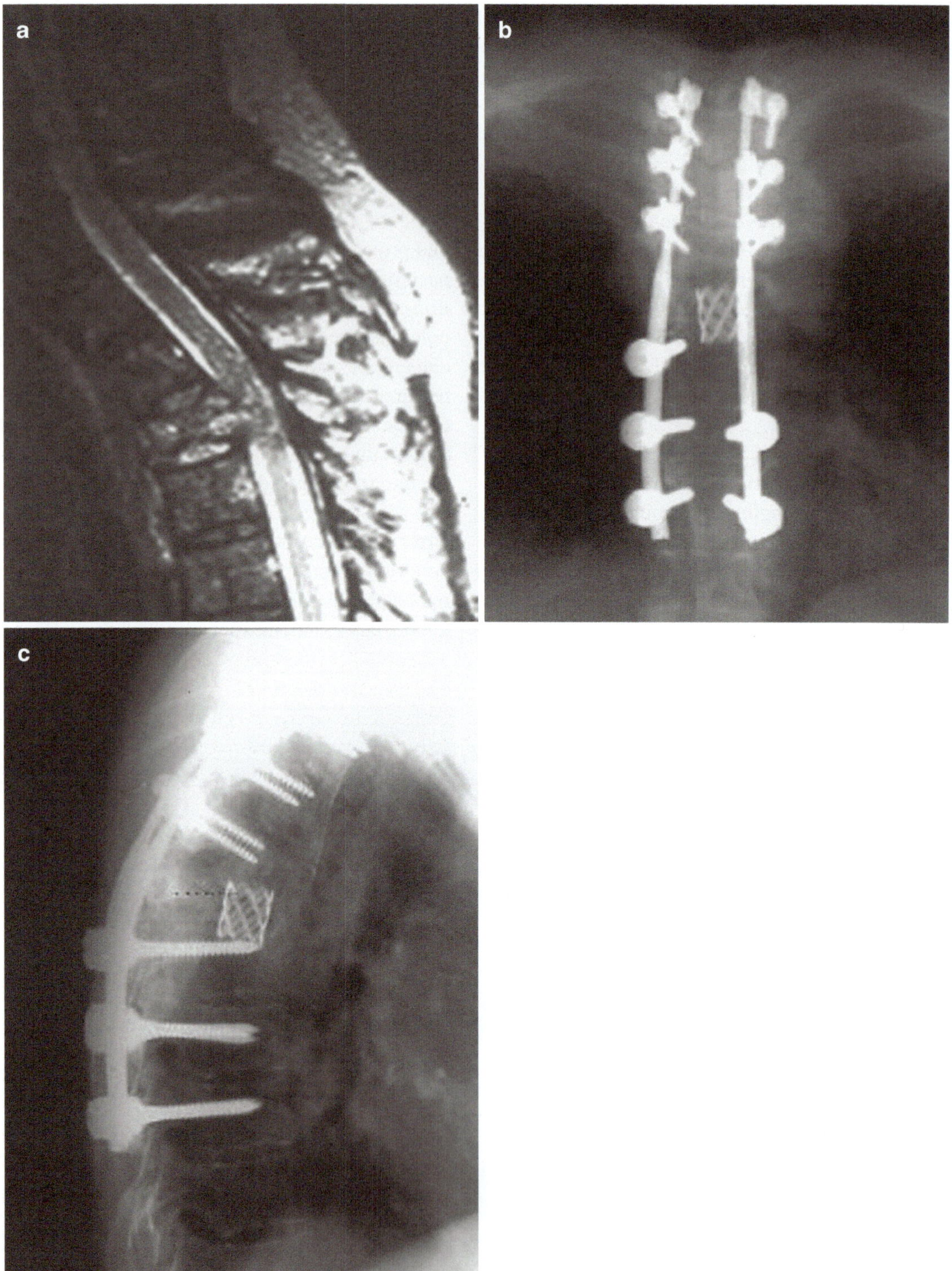

Fig. 13.7 (**a**) T4 thoracic metastasis from breast carcinoma. Patient with severe pain and paraparesis due to pathologic fracture and focal cord compression. Traditional anterior approach through either sternotomy or T3–T4 thoracotomy is challenging, with considerable risk and morbidity. (**b**, **c**) AP and lateral radiographs following endoscopically assisted corpectomy and posterior pedicle screw reconstruction. Patient was discharged to home on the sixth postoperative day, ambulating independently. Postoperative radiotherapy and medical management provided successful 5-year survival

become more limited as better alternatives have become available. PMMA is resilient in compression but has no potential for biologic fixation. It serves as a spacer, providing a temporary internal splint in anticipation of eventual bony arthrodesis or inevitable demise; only patients with a very limited life expectancy should be indicated for methacrylate fixation without bone grafting. Longitudinal Steinmann pins may be incorporated into the adjacent vertebra prior to applying the PMMA to enhance both the stability of the construct and its fixation to the adjacent vertebral bodies [51].

Once the involved vertebra is resected, with its adjacent discs, the full width of the adjacent levels is available for interbody stabilization. Prosthetic cages can be used with morcellized autograft, tricortical strut grafts, and allograft bone in patients with a greater anticipated survival. Autograft may be keyed into the vertebral end plates, when fusion is a sufficient concern to warrant graft harvest, but the end plates should not be violated when using titanium or PEEK cages [52, 53].

Anterior fixation can restore sagittal, coronal, and torsional rigidity following vertebrectomy, eliminating the need for posterior instrumentation in some patients [54]. Fixation reduces the chance that the strut graft or cage will loosen or shift. Since the fixation prevents the graft from shifting, the graft does not need to be keyed into the end plates, and since the graft rests on intact end plates, there is less chance of subsidence over time.

Carbon fiber, titanium, and PEEK vertebral replacement prostheses have become available which can expand to fill the vertebrectomy space, providing both the mechanical support necessary for axial stability and restoring axial height of the collapsed vertebra to correct kyphosis [55].

MIS Techniques for the Lower Thoracic and Thoracolumbar Spine

Improvements in intraoperative imaging and guidance, and in retractor design, have facilitated significant advances in minimally invasive approaches to tumors of the lower thoracic and thoracolumbar spine. This will be discussed in more detail in the chapter on Thoracolumbar Metastases but should be mentioned here.

The direct lateral approach to the involved vertebral body builds off experience with the direct lateral interbody fusion (DLIF) technique and has proven useful in selected cases. The approach is carried out in the decubitus position, taking care to orient the image intensifier so that true lateral and PA projections can be obtained of the involved segment. A short oblique incision, based over the rib of the involve vertebra, allows access to the pleural cavity between the ribs. For vertebral resection, a larger exposure is often needed and a segment of rib may be resected and retained for graft. If the rib is dissected subperiosteally, the retropleural space can be developed without violating the pleura, and the plane between the vertebral body and the pleura bluntly developed. The lateral side of the vertebral body, the pedicle, and the adjacent discs can be directly visualized along with the segmental vessels, which are clipped. A table-mounted expandable retractor system can then be inserted, oriented, and locked in position to provide reliable exposure of the diseased vertebra and its adjacent interspaces. Corpectomy and reconstruction can be carried out from this approach, along with lateral plate fixation, and—if indicated—the dura can be opened for removal of intradural tumor and repaired directly with suture and fibrin glue [56].

Vertebroplasty and Kyphoplasty

Cement augmentation may be carried out with or without laminectomy and for patients with either poor prognosis and advanced disease or reasonably good prognosis with radio- or chemosensitive but destructive lesions.

Certain patients require vertebral augmentation simply to maintain architectural stability while medical management successfully eradicates the tumor. No other surgical treatment is necessary to get a satisfactory result. Patients with solitary plasmacytoma or multiple myeloma often present with multiple impending fractures, and percutaneous kyphoplasty can provide the needed structural support, while medical management holds the disease in check [57]. Patients who have already experienced more severe vertebral destruction, particularly those too ill to tolerate extensive reconstruction and instrumentation, may gain good benefit from simple laminectomy of costotransversectomy, followed by vertebral body augmentation with PMMA. In these cases, laminectomy allows the surgeon to directly observe that no cement extravasates from diseased bone into the spinal canal, and allows a margin of safety if there is no cement encroachment of swelling of neoplastic tissues. The cement then stabilizes the fractured and collapsing vertebral body, or bodies, and prevents progressive kyphosis and vertebral plana.

Conclusion

The goal of spinal tumor surgery, in metastatic disease, is to restore/maintain neurologic function and reduce pain, thereby extending independent, high-quality survival. By reducing morbidity, decreasing hospitalization and ICU stays, while providing comparable neurologic outcomes and stability, video-assisted and image-guided posterolateral approaches provide an attractive alternative to open combined procedures. Newer techniques do not change the prognosis for systemic disease; advances in medical management and radiotherapy are managing that. But newer minimally invasive techniques, in combination with radiotherapeutic advances such as stereotactic radiosurgery, can provide excellent local control even in patients with advanced disease who might not tolerate traditional surgery. Properly planned and executed surgical care continues to be integral to protecting neurological elements, restoring neurologic function, and controlling and eliminating pain in cases where metastatic disease invades the thoracic spinal column.

Disclosure The author has received nothing of value from any entity, industrial agency, or sponsor in relation to any aspect of the study presented here.

References

1. Fidler MW. Anterior decompression and stabilization of metastatic spinal fractures. J Bone Joint Surg. 1986;68B(1):83–90.
2. Gilbert RW, Kim JH, Posner JB. Epidural spinal cord compression from metastatic tumor: diagnosis and treatment. Ann Neurol. 1978;3(1):40–51.
3. Hall AJ, MacKay NNS. The results of laminectomy for compression of the cord or cauda equina by extradural malignant tumor. J Bone Joint Surg. 1973;55B(3):497–505.
4. Harrington KD. Anterior decompression and stabilization of the spine as a treatment for vertebral collapse and spinal cord compression from metastatic malignancy. Clin Orthop Relat Res. 1988;233:177–97.
5. Kostuik JP, Errico TJ, Gleason TF, Errico CC. Spinal stabilization of vertebral column tumors. Spine. 1988;13(3):250–6.
6. Kostuik JP. Anterior spinal cord decompression for lesions of the thoracic and lumbar spine, techniques, new methods of internal fixation, results. Spine. 1983;8(5):512–31.
7. Manabe S, Tateishi A, Abe M, Ohno T. Surgical treatment of metastatic tumors of the spine. Spine. 1989;14(1):41–7.
8. McLain RF, Weinstein JN. Tumors of the spine. Semin Spine Surg. 1990;2:157–80.
9. Nather A, Bose K. The results of decompression of cord or cauda equina compression from metastatic extradural tumors. Clin Orthop. 1982;169:103–8.
10. Sherman RMP, Waddell JP. Laminectomy for metastatic epidural spinal cord tumors. Clin Orthop. 1986;207:55–63.
11. Siegal T, Tiqva P, Siegal T. Vertebral body resection for epidural compression by malignant tumors. J Bone Joint Surg. 1985;67A(3):375–82.
12. Sundaresan N, Galicich JH, Lane JM, Bains MS, McCormick P. Treatment of neoplastic epidural cord compression by vertebral body resection and stabilization. J Neurosurg. 1985;63:676–84.
13. White WA, Patterson RH, Bergland RM. Role of surgery in the treatment of spinal cord compression by metastatic neoplasm. Cancer. 1971;27(3):558–61.
14. Wright RL. Malignant tumors in the spinal extradural space: results of surgical treatment. Ann Surg. 1963;157(2):227–31.
15. Bridwell KH, Jenny AB, Saul T, Rich KM, Grubb RL. Posterior segmental spinal instrumentation (PSSI) with posterolateral decompression and debulking for metastatic thoracic and lumbar spinal disease. Spine. 1988;13:1383–94.
16. Lemons VR, Wagner FC Jr, Montesano PX. Management of thoracolumbar fractures with accompanying neurological injury. Neurosurgery. 1992;30:667–71.
17. Weinstein JN, McLain RF. Tumors of the spine. In: Rothman RH, Simeone FA, editors. The spine. 3rd ed. Philadelphia: WB Saunders Company; 1992. p. 1279–318.
18. Weinstein JN, McLain RF. Primary tumors of the spine. Spine. 1987;12(9):843–51.
19. Jackson RJ, Gokaslan ZL, Loh SC. Metastatic renal cell carcinoma of the spine: surgical treatment and results. J Neurosurg. 2001;94(1 Suppl):18–24.

20. Sundaresan N, Rothman A, Manhart K, et al. Surgery for solitary metastases of the spine: rationale and results of treatment. Spine. 2002;27(16):1802–6.
21. Shives TC, McLeod RA, Unni KK, et al. Chondrosarcoma of the spine. J Bone Joint Surg. 1989;71(A):1158–65.
22. McAfee PC, Bohlman HH, Ducker T, et al. Failure of stabilization of the spine with methylmethacrylate. J Bone Joint Surg. 1986;68(8):1145–57.
23. Lewandrowski K, Togawa D, Bauer TW, McLain RF. The role of vertebral biopsy in selected patients with known malignancy. J Bone Joint Surg. 2005;87A:1348–53.
24. McLain RF. Endoscopically assisted decompression for metastatic thoracic neoplasms. Spine. 1998;23(10):1130–5.
25. McLain RF, Lieberman IH. Endoscopic approaches to metastatic thoracic disease. Spine. 2000;25(14):1855–8.
26. Talac R, McLain RF. Biopsy principles and techniques for spinal tumors. Semin Spine Surg. 2009;21:70–5.
27. DeWald RL, Bridwell KH, Prodromas C, Rodts MF. Reconstructive spinal surgery as palliation for metastatic malignancies of the spine. Spine. 1985;10(1):21–6.
28. Martin NS, Williamson J. The role of surgery in the treatment of malignant tumours of the spine. J Bone Joint Surg. 1970;52B(2):227–37.
29. Findlay GFG. The role of vertebral body collapse in the management of malignant spinal cord compression. J Neurol Neurosurg Psychiatry. 1987;50:151–4.
30. Laufer I, Iorgulescu JB, Chapman T, et al. Local disease control for spinal metastases following "separation surgery" and adjuvant hypofractionated or high-dose single-fraction stereotactic radiosurgery: outcome analysis in 186 patients. J Neurosurg Spine. 2013;18:207–14.
31. Gu Y, Dong J, Jiang X, Wang Y. Minimally invasive pedicle screws fixation and percutaneous vertebroplasty for the surgical treatment of thoracic metastatic tumors with neurologic compression. Spine. 2016;41(19B):B14–22.
32. Lau D, Chou D. Posterior thoracic corpectomy with cage reconstruction for metastatic spinal tumors: comparing the mini-open approach to the open approach. J Neurosurg Spine. 2015;23:217–27.
33. Dudeney S, Lieberman IH, Reinhardt MK, Hussein M. Kyphoplasty in the treatment of osteolytic vertebral compression fractures as a result of multiple myeloma. J Clin Oncol. 2002;20:2382–7.
34. Eleraky M, Papanastassiou I, Setzer M, et al. Balloon kyphoplasty in the treatment of metastatic tumors of the upper thoracic spine. J Neurosurg Spine. 2011;14:372–6.
35. Moulding HD, Elder JB, Lis E, et al. Local disease control after decompressive surgery and adjuvant high-dose single-fraction radiosurgery for spinal metastases. J Neurosurg Spine. 2010;13:87–93.
36. Wang JC, Boland P, Mitra N, et al. Single-stage posterolateral transpedicular approach for resection of epidural metastatic spine tumors involving the vertebral body with circumferential reconstruction: results in 140 patients. J Neurosurg Spine. 2004;1:287–98.
37. Harel R, Angelov L. Spinal metastases: current treatments and future directions. Eur J Cancer. 2010;46:2696–707.
38. Angelov L. Stereotactic spine radiosurgery (SRS) for pain and tumor control in patients with spinal metastasis from renal cell carcinoma: a prospective study. Int J Radiat Oncol Biol Phys. 2009;75(3):S112–3.
39. Bilsky MH, Shannon FJ, Sheppard S, et al. Diagnosis and management of a metastatic tumor in the Atlantoaxial spine. Spine. 2002;27(10):1062–9.
40. Gokaslan ZL, York JE, Walsh GL, et al. Transthoracic vertebrectomy for metastatic spinal tumors. J Neurosurg. 1998;89(4):599–609.
41. Bilsky MH, Boland P, Lis E, et al. Single-stage posterolateral trans-pedicle approach for spondylectomy, epidural decompression, and circumferential fusion of spinal metastases. Spine. 2000;25(17):2240–50.
42. Stener B. Total spondylectomy in chondrosarcoma arising from the seventh thoracic vertebra. J Bone Joint Surg. 1971;53B(2):288–95.
43. Fourney DR, Abi-Said D, Rhines LD, et al. Simultaneous anterior-posterior approach to the thoracic and lumbar spine for the radical resection of tumors followed by reconstruction and stabilization. J Neurosurg. 2001;94(2 Suppl):232–44.
44. Heary RF, Vaccaro AR, Benevenia J, et al. *En bloc* vertebrectomy in the mobile lumbar spine. Surg Neurol. 1998;50(6):548–56.
45. Krepler P, Windhager R, Bretschneider W, et al. Total vertebrectomy for primary malignant tumours of the spine. J Bone Joint Surg. 2002;84(B):712–5.
46. Tomita K, Kawahara N, Baba H, et al. Total *en bloc* spondylectomy: a new surgical technique for primary malignant vertebral tumors. Spine. 1997;22(3):324–33.
47. Kim M, Nolan P, Finkelstein JA. Evaluation of the 11th rib extrapleural-retroperitoneal approach to the thoracolumbar junction. Technical note. J Neurosurg. 2000;93(1 Suppl):168–74.
48. Fourney DR, Abi-Said D, Lang FF, et al. Use of pedicle screw fixation in the management of malignant spinal disease: experience in 100 consecutive procedures. J Neurosurg. 2001;94(1 Suppl):25–37.
49. McLain RF, Sparling E, Benson DR. Failure of short segment pedicle instrumentation in thoracolumbar fractures: complications of Cotrel-Dubousset instrumentation. J Bone Joint Surg. 1993;75(2):162–7.
50. Jang JS, Lee SH, Rhee CH, et al. Polymethylmethacrylate-augmented screw fixation for stabilization in metastatic spinal tumors. Technical note. J Neurosurg. 2002;96(1 Suppl):131–4.
51. Miller DJ, Lang FF, Walsh GL, et al. Coaxial double-lumen methylmethacrylate reconstruction in the anterior cervical and upper thoracic spine after tumor resection. J Neurosurg. 2000;93(2 Suppl):181–90.

52. Akamaru T, Kawahara N, Tsuchiya H, et al. Healing of autologous bone in a titanium mesh cage used in anterior column reconstruction after total spondylectomy. Spine. 2002;27(13):E329–33.
53. Munting E, Faundez A, Manche E. Vertebral reconstruction with cortical allograft: long-term evaluation. Eur Spine J. 2001;10(Suppl 2):S153–7.
54. Hall DJ, Webb JK. Anterior plate fixation in spine tumor surgery. Indications, technique, and results. Spine. 1991;16:580–3.
55. Boriani S, Biagini R, Bandiera S, et al. Reconstruction of the anterior column of the thoracic and lumbar spine with a carbon fiber stackable cage system. Orthopedics. 2002;25(1):37–42.
56. Uribe JS, Dakwar E, Le TVL, et al. Minimally invasive surgery treatment for thoracic spine tumor removal. Spine. 2010;35:S347–54.
57. McLain RF, Weinstein JN. Solitary plasmacytomas of the spine: a review of 84 cases. J Spinal Disord. 1989;2(2):69–74.

Thoracolumbar Metastatic Spinal Disease

14

Charles A. Hogan and Robert F. McLain

Introduction

The thoracolumbar spine presents unique anatomical and biomechanical challenges for the treatment of spinal metastases. Physiologically, certain tumor types have predisposition for this region of the spine given Batson venous plexus drainage patterns. Anatomically, considerations include the transition into the stiffer thoracic cage from the more mobile lumbar spine, a relatively flat segment from T10 to L2 between regions of kyphosis and lordosis, transition from cord level to cauda level with the presence of the conus medullaris, costovertebral joints with rib heads blocking direct access to anterior structures, location of the great vessels and solid organs including the liver and kidneys, vascular perfusion as it pertains to the artery of Adamkiewicz [1], and, perhaps of most technical consideration, the presence of the diaphragm. Mechanically, the transition from coronally oriented thoracic facets (coupled with the stiffness of the rib cage) to sagittally oriented lumbar facets (with flexion/extension arcs transitioning to lateral bending and twisting arcs) increases mechanical load and potentially predisposes to increased mechanical construct failure.

When addressing the thoracolumbar junction, the anterolateral or lateral corridors provide access to anteriorly based tumor and epidural compression, allowing resection and spinal stabilization through anterior column support. Advances in surgical technology have allowed us to develop more minimally invasive strategies based on the established, well-validated principles of traditional open procedures.

Anterolateral Corridor Techniques

Various approaches through the anterolateral corridor include:

1. The traditional open transthoracic or retropleural thoracotomy (if working above the diaphragm) or open retroperitoneal approach (if working strictly below the diaphragm) approached via a lateral decubitus positioning.
2. The combined, open thoracoabdominal approach allowing access to the lateral thoracolumbar junction above and below the diaphragm (retroperitoneal below and intrathoracic above the diaphragm).

C. A. Hogan, MD (✉)
Department of Orthopaedic Surgery, Houston Methodist Hospital, Houston, TX, USA
e-mail: spinedoctorhogan@gmail.com

R. F. McLain, MD
Spine and Orthopedic Institute, St Vincent Charity Medical Group, Cleveland, OH, USA

Biomedical Engineering, Cleveland State University, Solon, OH, USA

R. A. W. Marco (ed.), *Metastatic Spine Disease*, https://doi.org/10.1007/978-3-319-76252-4_14

3. The extracoelomic approach connecting the retroperitoneal and retropleural cavities by taking down the diaphragm by mobilizing the parietal pleura off the chest wall along with the diaphragmatic origin, as opposed to splitting the diaphragm at its base, staying truly retropleural.
4. A minimal access open combination of the above using a short segment of the traditional incision and exposure.
5. A true minimally invasive access strategy using specialized retractors and innovative light sources or endoscopy to access and treat only the segments requiring anterior resection or stabilization.

Anterolateral Corridor Obstacles

The lateral approach to the thoracolumbar junction is situated well above the level of the lumbar roots at risk of injury during direct lateral (DLIF) or extreme lateral (XLIF) approaches to the lower lumbar segments [2]. Sacrifice of a T11 or T12 root, if tumor involvement makes it necessary, is a minor consideration compared to loss of roots at L2 and lower, but entry into the canal at this level threatens the spinal cord and conus medullaris as opposed to spinal nerve roots [3].

When working from T10 to L2, the diaphragm is the most complicated structure [4, 5]. Its attachments consist of three major muscle groups (sternal, costal, and lumbar) and a central tendon consisting of three leaflets (right, left, middle). Major structures pass through three major openings: the vena caval opening (on the right, at T8), the esophageal hiatus (centrally, T10), and the aortic hiatus (paracentral to the left, T12). The thoracic duct and the azygous vein also pass through the aortic hiatus. The most relevant diaphragmatic attachments to the spine are the medial and lateral arcuate ligaments and left and right crura. Laterally the diaphragm is anchored to the parietal pleura over the ribs: anteriorly at ribs 7 and 8, laterally at ribs 9 and 10, and posteriorly at ribs 11 and 12. The more lateral of the posterior diaphragmatic structures are confluent with the fascia that trails distally to envelop the origin of the quadratus lumborum (lateral arcuate ligament) and the psoas (medial arcuate ligament). These arcuate ligaments are important landmarks for the surgeon approaching L1, as they both invest the transverse process of L1 [3, 6]. Sharp release of the arcuate ligaments off the tip of the L1 transverse process releases a key tether of the diaphragm and provides access to the lateral L1 vertebral body during the anterolateral approach. This permits the diaphragm release via the extracavitary or extracoelomic approach (i.e., staying entirely in the retroperitoneal and retropleural corridor, yet anterior to the quadratus lumborum and psoas).

The most medial structures are the crura, which anchor the central diaphragm to the spine itself. The right crus is wider and attaches to the transverse processes between L1 and L3. It runs cranial alongside the aortic hiatus (T12), loops up over the esophageal hiatus (T10), and then runs caudal to blend back into itself between the esophageal hiatus and the aortic hiatus (between T10 and T12). The left crus attaches in the vicinity of L1–L2, runs cranial alongside the aorta as it comes through its hiatus (T12), and then loops over the esophageal hiatus (T10) where it blends into the central tendon. In reality these structures are seen surgically as thickenings of connective tissue, becoming confluent with annulus and ALL.

Kawahara and Tomita et al., in their work with en bloc spondylectomy, found that the great vessels mobilize fairly easily from T1 to T12 but proved particularly challenging to mobilize at the L1 and L2 levels, primarily because of the crural attachments adherent and confluent with the vertebral periosteum and the anterior longitudinal ligament. They also demonstrated that the first two lumbar arteries and veins consistently run in the mesh of tissues between the medial crus and the vertebral column here [4].

Finally, vascular control—difficult in any case—can be dramatically more challenging when neovasculature and epidural hypertrophy are associated with a thoracolumbar tumor. Not only can the native vessels be hard to localize and control, duplicate vasculature and intramuscular neovasculature can be quite extensive in tumors such as renal cell, melanoma, or thyroid carcinoma. Angiography and preoperative embolization, sometimes twice, can determine whether tumor excision can be accomplished at all.

Patient Selection

While open approaches allow en bloc excision, when indicated, they also allow more certain vascular control. Intralesional approaches are more amenable to MIS techniques, which are most useful when local control can be reliably augmented by radiation or medical management, and vascular control is assured. The best candidates for consideration of lateral corpectomy approach would be those with predominantly anterior column disease and possibly unilateral pedicular involvement and a life expectancy/medical fitness to warrant surgery. Patients with true spinal instability and epidural cord compression, presenting with progressive neurologic deficit, would be clear candidates for surgical decompression to maintain or restore neurological function. Structural restoration may be possible through the primary anterior approach itself or may be carried out through a separate posterior approach with posterior segmental fixation [7].

Separation surgery, carried out through an MIS approach to debride tumor tissue immediately adjacent to radiosensitive neurological structures (roots and cord), allows more aggressive and effective use of stereotactic spinal radiosurgery and is an increasingly popular treatment algorithm. However, when dealing with traditionally radioresistant tumors and true spinal instability, surgical intervention in the form of corpectomy, anterior column support, and instrumented stabilization is still the soundest consideration.

Surgical Approaches: Localization

For tumors at the thoracolumbar junction, compare a preoperative X-ray to MRI or CT to establish the operative level in relation to a structure you will be able to identify on fluoroscopy—the most distal rib or a compressed, fractured vertebra. Alternatively, use live fluoro on a lateral, counting vertebra cranially from the sacrum. Regardless of the strategy, localization of the proper operative level is important to initiating the exposure at the best level and critical to MIS approaches. Some advocate a preoperative marker in the level of the operative pedicle placed by interventional radiology; if the patient is going for angiography or preoperative embolization, this may be reasonable.

Much MIS lateral work relies on satisfactory fluoroscopic imaging. It is exceedingly important to have the lateral fluoro view you see on the monitor correlate to a truly perpendicular trajectory to the floor. Passing instruments perfectly perpendicular to the horizontal helps avoid misadventures anteriorly into the vessels and posteriorly into the canal or exiting nerve roots. With the patient carefully positioned on the operating table, mark the outline of the superior and inferior endplates, anterior and posterior vertebral borders of the target vertebra using a metallic wand under fluoroscopy, and sketch the positions on the skin surface. Palpate the overlying rib and mark this as well. The intended incision is now drawn out in accordance with technique and goals of the case at hand. For an open approach, extend a line in line with your planned incision projecting anteriorly across the abdomen and posteriorly down the back (Fig. 14.1).

When planning the incision, considerations include number of levels for the corpectomy, need to place a laterally based plate and screws vs. corpectomy and anterior column support alone, and plan to stay extrapleural proximally vs. commit to being intrathoracic. For a mini-open one-level corpectomy, an oblique to transverse incision, crossing the midportion of the body (cranio-caudal), should suffice. For multi-level work, a longer oblique incision following the angle of the rib resection (running from cranial posteriorly to caudal anteriorly) is preferred.

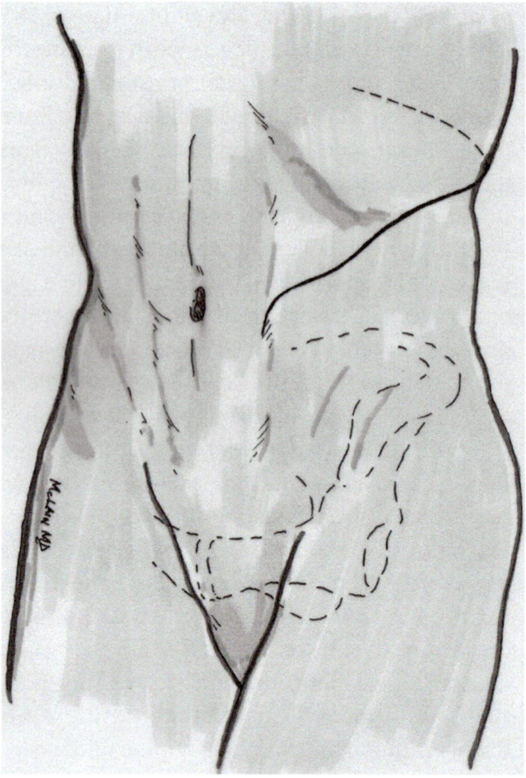

Fig. 14.1 Surgical incision for thoracolumbar exposure. Incision begins posteriorly over the costovertebral angle and is carried forward to the rectus sheath, turning distally there. For mini-open exposure, the midportion of this same incision is usually sufficient

Planning the Surgical Incision

Traditional mantra of taking the rib two levels above the surgical lesion provides wide exposure through the traditional open approach and thoracolumbar combined approaches but is less relevant for a minimal access open approach; take whichever rib is in the path to the spine with the patient in a perfectly lateral position [8, 9]. For MIS and minimally open procedures, specialized retractors provide focal retraction down a directly lateral corridor and in line with the targeted disc(s) and vertebra. If simply performing a vertebrectomy and placing a cage, exposure from disc to disc may be adequate. When applying a lateral plate and screws after a corpectomy, it is always easier to access the vertebral body below the defect than it is to place screws transversely across the endplate of the vertebral body above, which lies at or above the diaphragm.

Classic thoracoabdominal anterolateral approach to the thoracolumbar junction (transthoracic, retroperitoneal) involves taking the ninth or tenth rib [9]. This gives consistently good exposure but requires entrance into the chest cavity and chest tube placement. Extracoelomic approaches stay retropleural and may reduce morbidity by obviating need for chest tube placement, limiting duropleural fistula in setting of CSF leak, and decreasing potential for pleural adhesions, effusions, atelectasis, pneumonia, and pneumothorax [10, 11]. However, pleural adhesions or parietal pleura deficiency may make chest tube placement necessary in any case. Generally, taking a single well-planned rib allows access for the corpectomy and laterally based instrumentation. Techniques to extend access to an adjacent level would include an osteotomy of the rib above, hinging on the intact cortex to allow more exposure, segmental resection of another rib, or an extension of the primary incision and taking more rib posteriorly. If additional disc spaces must be accessed, either the subjacent rib may be osteotomized and retracted distally or a second rib may be incised distally or proximally to give access to additional disc spaces. A second rib incision will also facilitate the application of anterior spinal instrumentation such as rod and screw constructs. This second rib incision is performed through the same skin incision by simply retracting the skin distally over the bed of the selected rib two or three levels above or below the initial resection. The second periosteal incision is made through the bed of the rib but the rib is not resected.

Open Thoracoabdominal Approach (Retroperitoneal, Intrathoracic)

Traditionally, most spine surgeons accessing the thoracolumbar junction have used the open thoracoabdominal approach. Plan the incision directly overlying the rib that will allow access to the involved vertebra. Thoracoabdominal exposure is generally performed by taking the 9th, 10th, or 11th rib and consistently gives access from T11 to L2. The curvilinear incision starts posteriorly, in line with the rib; runs anterior along the rib itself, crossing the costochondral junction; and heads obliquely either toward the rectus sheath or more vertically and distally toward the ASIS. If instrumenting anteriorly down to L3, the incision should curve more distally. If performing a one-level corpectomy at L1 without plating, you won't need to complete the full distal extent of the incision. Come through the latissimus and posterior serratus in the center or top half of the rib so as to stay clear of the neurovascular bundle that runs inferiorly along the rib. Dissect the rib subperiosteally back toward the costovertebral joints and anteriorly all the way to the costochondral junction (AO or Cobb elevator). We prefer large straight and curved curettes to gain access around the rib and then a Doyen periosteal elevator to develop the plane along the deep surface of the rib. Disarticulate the rib tip from the costochondral junction; this small cartilaginous landmark will be the reapproximation start point for the multiple layers to be closed later. Generally take the rib as far back as the incision will allow the rib cutter to pass, to the posterior rib angle.

Intrathoracic Portion

Proximally, the endothoracic fascia lies just deep to the rib periosteum, and this is closely adherent to the parietal pleura. Vertical incision in line with the spine through both these layers takes you onto the lateral spine. The lung is clearly seen cranially and can be retracted with a deep broad retractor and moist lap sponge. The dome of the diaphragm is clearly seen caudally.

Retroperitoneal Portion

Initiate abdominal exposure via the bleb of retroperitoneal fat that directly underlies the cartilaginous anterior 10th rib tip. Abdominal muscular layers are taken sequentially with Kelly clamp and Bovie, in line with the wound. The junction of the transversalis abdominis and the cartilaginous rib tip is the key: this signifies the convergence of the abdominal musculature, the retroperitoneal space, and the diaphragm. Once the extraperitoneal fat is seen, bluntly develop the plane between peritoneum and posterior abdominal wall with a sponge stick or finger and sponge. The diaphragm is incised with a 1–2 cm cuff laterally around the rib attachment (to repair upon closure). Paired tag sutures should be placed in the anterior abdominal musculature and the free edge of the diaphragm, alternating black and green suture color, to facilitate anatomic closure. Reflect around the back of the peritoneal cavity, hugging peritoneum, onto the origin of the psoas and quadratus lumborum. Roll the dissecting finger anteriorly over the psoas onto the ventrolateral surface of the spine. The ureter is usually engulfed in retroperitoneal fat and falls away with the peritoneum, but in revision retroperitoneal surgery where scarring may be present, take care to identify this structure. Some consider urological consult to place ureteral stents to help ease identification. Avoid falling into the interval behind the psoas—"no man's land"—which leads to the transverse processes and neuroforamina and not the vertebral body. Protect the genitofemoral nerve running along the top of the psoas (Fig. 14.2).

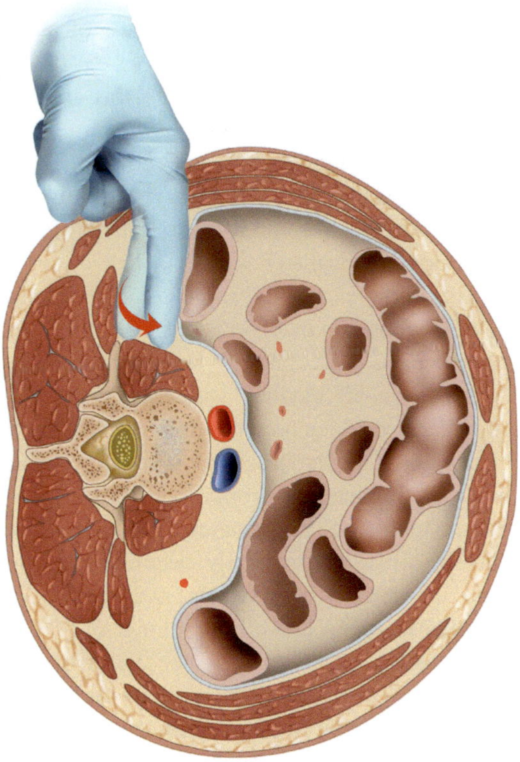

Fig. 14.2 Anterior surgical approach. The digital dissection is carried down to the surface of the psoas and then bluntly develops the plane over the surface of the psoas onto the lateral surface of the vertebral body. The plane between the anterior longitudinal ligament and the great vessels can be developed bluntly, but the vessels cannot be mobilized until the segmental vessels are isolated, ligated, and divided

Table-based retractors such as a Bookwalter or Omni are helpful, but a "C"-shaped malleable retractor inserted against the psoas to hold the viscera away and frame the surgical site helps keep hands free in the depth of the wound. Powerful retractors placed high in the flank can easily injure the spleen against the ribs. Moist lap sponges behind the broad blades protect skin edges and neurovascular bundles from hours of pressure and retraction.

Extracoelomic Approach Technique

The extracoelomic, or extracavitary, approach is extensile, provides a true anterior exposure, and simplifies the management of the diaphragm in thoracolumbar approaches. It may reduce the incidence of some complications commonly seen in transthoracic procedures, including intrapleural migration of bone graft and formation of pleural adhesions.

The principles for success with this approach remain the same as for any other: careful assessment of the patient, fundamental knowledge of the three-dimensional spinal anatomy, recognition of complicating factors and hazards, and skillful and meticulous surgical technique [10, 12].

This modification of the classic thoracoabdominal approach involves working purely in the extrathoracic (retropleural) and extraabdominal (retroperitoneal) cavities and connecting these two spaces by detaching the diaphragm from the chest wall. The diaphragm attaches in a straight line radiating laterally from the lower sternum to the arcuate ligaments that anchor off the L1 transverse process. It essentially becomes confluent with the intercostal muscles and the internal oblique muscles laterally, fanning out at the perimeter at each point. Since the ribs slant anteroinferior as they come around the chest, it makes sense that the posterior diaphragmatic attachment points correlate with the lowest vertebrae, and the lateral (costal) attachment points correspond to progressively higher ribs as you move anteriorly. The diaphragm doesn't lie under any one rib. For different patients the same direct lateral approach at T12 may put you into the chest in one patient and the retroperitoneum in another [3]. The goal of the extracoelomic approach is to find the plane between the retropleural space above and the retroperitoneal space below and never enter the chest. This is easier done by finding the retropleural space posteriorly and then working caudally and anteriorly, taking the diaphragm down off the lateral chest wall as it blends into the superior portion of the ribs as you work anteriorly [13]. The fibrous inflammatory rind and possible pleural invasion may limit technical feasibility in some tumors; carefully scrutinize the MRI for extraspinal tumor involvement before planning this approach.

The thoracic cavity is opened through the bed of the 10th rib, carrying the incision across the costochondral junction before turning obliquely across the abdominal wall toward the lateral border of the rectus sheath. The parietal pleura is dissected away from the inner thoracic wall as described above. The rib is disarticulated from the costochondral junction, and the costal cartilage is split longitudinally to enter the abdominal cavity. Split the external oblique muscle along the line of its fibers, and then divide the internal oblique muscle with electrocautery. The transversus abdominis fascia is entered near the rectus sheath where it is thinnest. After developing the interval between the fascia and the peritoneum, dissect bluntly along the abdominal wall while splitting the fascia with electrocautery. If there is scarring in the retroperitoneum, the surgeon must identify the ureter before introducing electrocautery. Identify and stay anterior to the psoas muscle.

By dissecting proximally and distally through the retroperitoneal and the extrapleural space, the attachment of the diaphragm is identified along the insertion into the chest wall. The diaphragm can now be bluntly detached from the chest wall and dissection carried posteriorly to the crus. Wet sponges are applied over the exposed pleural and peritoneal surfaces, which can then be retracted with a fan retractor to hold the lung, diaphragm, and peritoneal contents anteriorly away from the spine. This allows exposure from the mid-lumbar to the mid-thoracic spine through a single incision (Fig. 14.3).

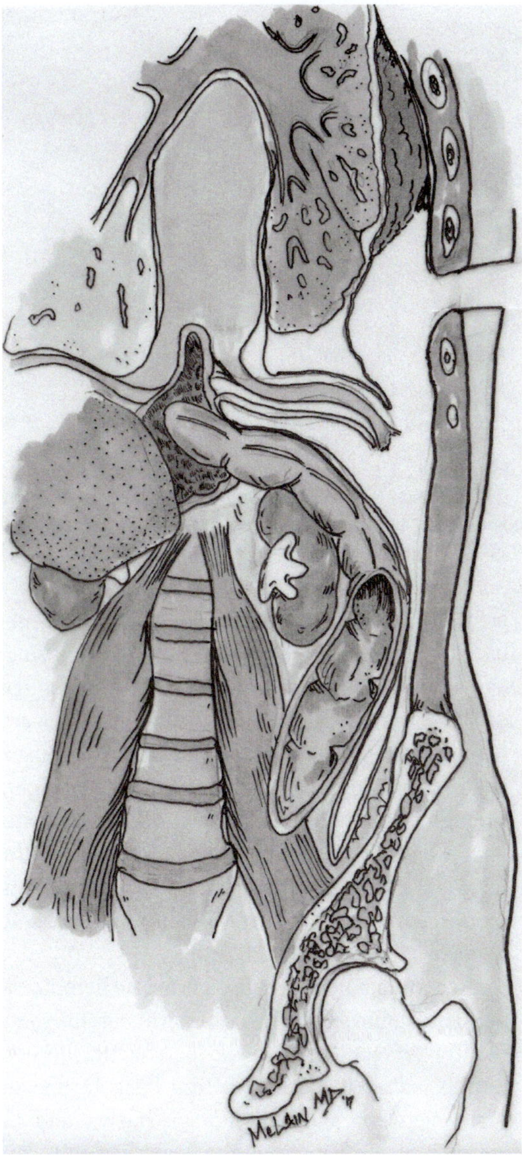

Fig. 14.3 The extracavitary or extracoelomic exposure elevates the parietal pleura from the chest wall, along with the diaphragmatic insertion, and then develops the plane from the diaphragm into the retroperitoneal cavity in the abdomen

On completion of the spinal procedure, the pleural and peritoneal tissues are allowed to fall back into their normal position. The diaphragm is not directly reattached to the chest wall but is allowed to re-approximate to the wall through the adhesion of peritoneal and pleural tissues.

Chest Tube Placement

When required, place a chest tube between the anterior and midaxillary line, via a stab incision one or two interspaces above the incision. Palpate the acromion or the ASIS under the drapes as a proxy to estimate your anterior to posterior position on the chest wall. Make the stab wound through the skin and fascia, off the superior aspect of the inferior rib (spare the neurovascular bundle). Spread muscle and puncture through the pleura with a Kelly clamp. Kelly clamp is used on sharp-angled end of the chest tube to guide this deeper into the chest to the desired location. We aim this cranially and posterior to the lung. Commonly use a 24F to 32F chest tube. Drain stitch anchoring the chest tube to the skin is helpful, as is petroleum gauze to act as a sealant about the borders of the stab wound. If known pleural violation, place to 20 cm wall suction. If placing prophylactically as a drain, place to water seal. Obtain CXR in PACU and the following morning. If concerned for a pleural violation, fill the thoracic cavity with saline and Valsalva: bubbles indicate pleural violation and should warrant consideration of chest tube placement especially if the pleural rent cannot be identified and repaired.

Red Rubber Catheter Technique for Evacuation of Retropleural Air

We recommend placement of a chest tube when knowingly performing a transthoracic approach (lateral transthoracic thoracotomy, thoracoabdominal approach) or when parietal pleural violation has inadvertently occurred (lateral retropleural thoracotomy, extracoelomic approach). If pleural violation is repairable and confirming no bubbles upon filling the chest with saline and intraoperative Valsalva, consider leaving only a drain. Intraoperative decision balances morbidity of chest tube placement with potential need for chest tube placement in the ensuing hours to days on the floor. In cases with low suspicion of having entered the parietal pleura, consider placement of a retropleural suction drain. Alternatively, retropleural air can be evacuated prior to final closure without a drain. A red rubber catheter is placed deep in the wound, between the layers of the endothoracic fascia and parietal pleura. These layers are closed with running stitch starting on either end and working toward the middle where the catheter lies. The external tip is placed under a water bath, anesthesia provides a Valsalva, and the air in this layer is evacuated while simultaneously removing the catheter and tying the last stitch.

Minimal Access Lateral Corpectomy Approach

A minimal access open approach (or mini-open) to the thoracolumbar junction affords access precisely to the target area, minimizing dissection through adjacent tissues and abdominal wall. The minimal access open approach uses a segment of the classic open incision, placing a 4- to 6-in. oblique incision over the 10th or 11th rib, extending from the proximal angle of the rib to the distal tip of the rib. As with the open approach, the rib is dissected subperiosteally and divided at the proximal angle and dislocated from the chondral cartilage. For a traditional intracavitary approach, the pleural cavity is entered just above the diaphragm and the retroperitoneal space, just below [14]. After separating the diaphragm from its lateral rim, self-retaining rib retractors can be placed to allow exposure of T11–T12 disc, down to the L1 vertebral body (Fig. 14.4).

Mini-open, left side up lateral, T12 corpectomy with anterior epidural decompression and placement of expandable interbody prosthesis from T11 to L1.

Approach

For mini-open lateral T12 corpectomy, position perfectly lateral in the right decubitus, mark the T11, T12, and L1 vertebral bodies (T11–T12 and T12–L1 discs) using preoperative fluoroscopy, and plan a surgical incision running obliquely following the trajectory of the rib that directly overlies the level to be approached, usually the 10th rib for T12. Dissect onto the rib and expose subperiosteally, undermining soft tissues anterior and

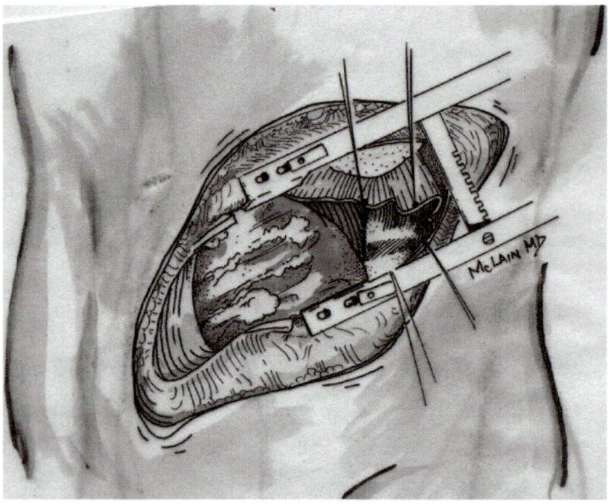

Fig. 14.4 The minimally open approach uses the mid-portion of the T10 rib resection to access the cavity above and below the diaphragm, taking down just enough diaphragm to allow corpectomy and plate fixation

posterior to the incision. Protect the neurovascular bundle, and resect the rib cleanly to prevent sharp and jagged edges that would make blunt finger dissection challenging. Ensure the rib is taken sufficiently posterior to allow a working exposure and remove bony spikes. Wax bleeding rib bone. Though ultimately the retractor will be expanded only a few inches and wanded at depth depending on working location, adequate rib resection and mobilization of the planes will allow easier retractor placement with less tension.

An extracavitary approach is useful here. Incise the periosteum in the bed of the rib carefully, and bluntly dissect between the periosteum and the loosely adherent parietal pleura [12]. Define the plane between the endothoracic fascia and the parietal pleura, and mobilize this carefully and bluntly, cranially and caudally, using a digit and then a sponge stick. Use care to develop this plane widely as this will keep you retropleural and decrease the chances of making this a transthoracic transperitoneal approach. A wide fan retractor and moist lap sponge are placed to retract the parietal pleura, the visceral pleura, and the lung anteriorly in one envelope. Dissection continues along the posterior rib cage onto the lateral spine (cranial to the level of the psoas and crura) at the T12 level. With the parietal pleura reflected, the segmental vessels are more easily identified and isolated. Particularly in the mini-open approach, segmentals must be carefully ligated before they

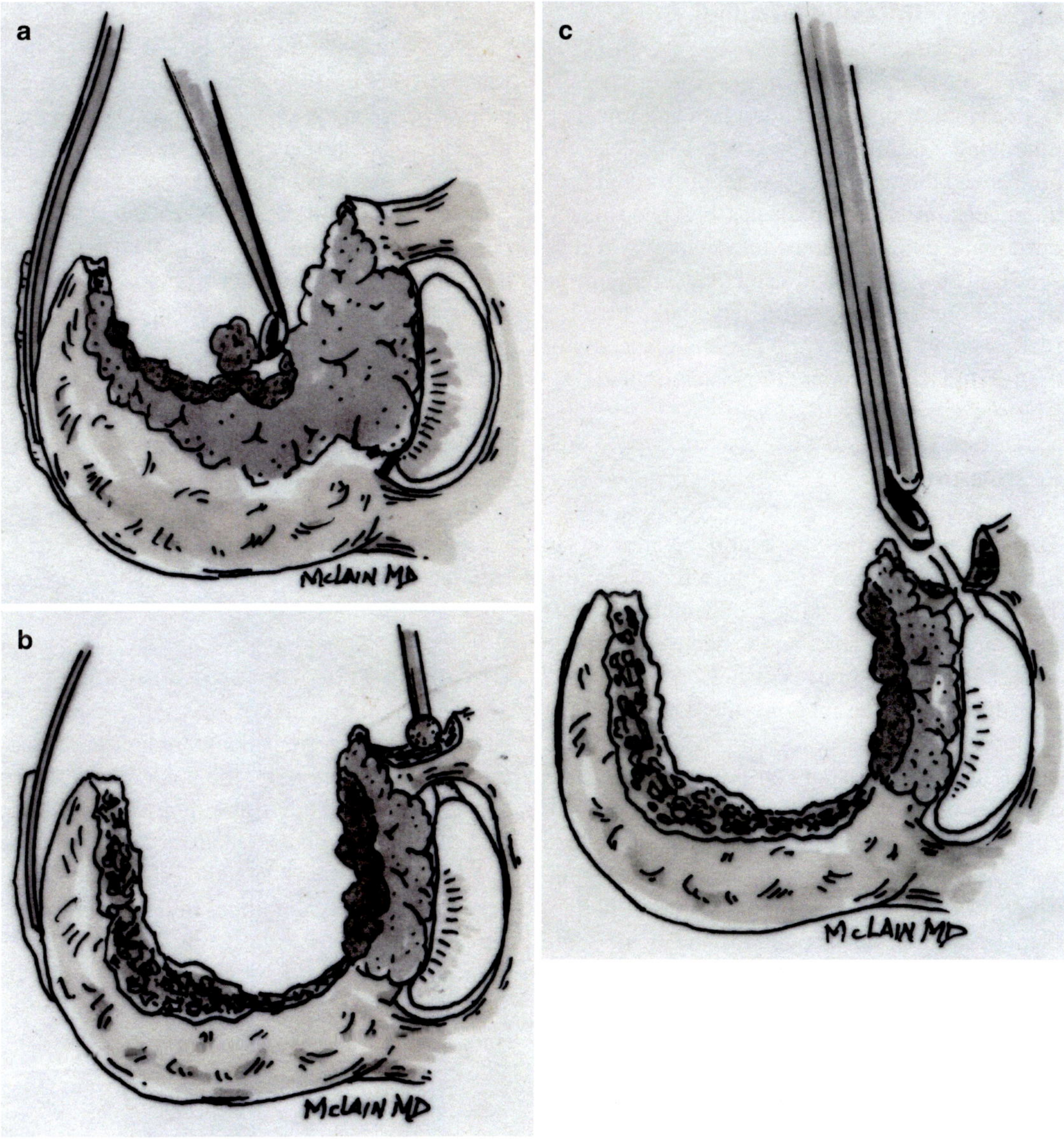

Fig. 14.5 (**a**) Corpectomy through the minimally open or fully open exposure begins by elevating the ALL and placing a malleable retractor to shield the great vessels and expose the lateral surface of the vertebra invested with tumor. Rongeurs and curettes can then quickly debulk the tumor and central vertebral cancellous bone to create a cavity ventral to the spinal canal. (**b**) If tumor is difficult to free from the spinal canal, and cord compression is significant to start with, a diamond burr can be used to take down the left-sided pedicle to allow entry into the canal from the side, avoiding blind curettage over the surface of the compressed cord and dura. (**c**) After thinning the pedicle to its medial cortex, a fine Kerrison can be inserted between the cortex and dura to complete the exposure, revealing the nerve root and the uninvolved dura and providing lateral access to the compressing tumor

are divided. Usually a silk tie ligature is placed on either side of the division and is supplemented with a hemoclip. The anterior longitudinal ligament can be raised off the surface of the vertebral bodies and discs using a sharp elevator and cautery. Once this interval is developed, a deep retractor, such as a malleable with a small reverse curve, can be inserted between the body and the ALL and toed back away from the involved vertebra, providing a shield for the great vessels during corpectomy (Fig. 14.5a–c). Corpectomy and stabilization can proceed as planned from here.

Minimally Invasive Surgical Approaches

With advent of improved retractors and imaging, improving visability, the ability to access the lumbar and thoracolumbar segments through true minimally invasive approaches has been developed to the point that some tumor surgery can be accomplished safely and effectively through an incision only a few centimeters long. In these cases, patient positioning can dictate success or failure, and particular attention is warranted.

Positioning

Turn the patient directly lateral on a reversed radiolucent slider bed with ability for lateral tilt, Trendelenburg and reverse Trendelenburg. Slide the patient as far cranial on the bed as is possible so the fluoroscopy unit will not be blocked by the table base when imaging the thoracolumbar junction. An axillary roll limits the brachial plexus and prevents shoulder issues. Place up the arm on a biplane arm holder or on pillows, with elbows and shoulders neutral and well padded but cranial to the path of fluoroscopic imaging. The neck is neutrally aligned and carefully handled by anesthesia throughout the positioning process (Fig. 14.6).

Flex the down leg only slightly at the hip and knee to balance the patient. Flex the up leg more acutely, as in Fig. 14.6, at the hip and the knee with pillows between the legs for support and to prevent pressure between bony prominences. While DLIF technique for mid-lumbar degenerative disease calls for breaking the bed in the so-called jackknife position to allow better access to the lateral spine, this is not recommended for pathological fractures and structurally unsound vertebrae affected by metastatic disease. Additionally, lateral bending has little effect on the thoracolumbar junction and lower thoracic segments targeted here. Maintaining the patient in side-bending for prolonged periods (particularly as required for corpectomy as opposed to discectomy and fusion) may also contribute to postoperative hip flexion weakness and anterior/anterolateral thigh neuropraxia [15].

Optimizing Fluoroscopic Imaging

After positioning the patient, but before securing the patient and prepping the flank, check fluoroscopic imaging to confirm orthogonal orientation of the spinal segments. On cross-Table AP at the operative level, observe pedicles in upper 1/3 of vertebral body, symmetrical in appearance, with the spinous processes bisecting pedicles directly in midline. On lateral fluoro, observe overlapping

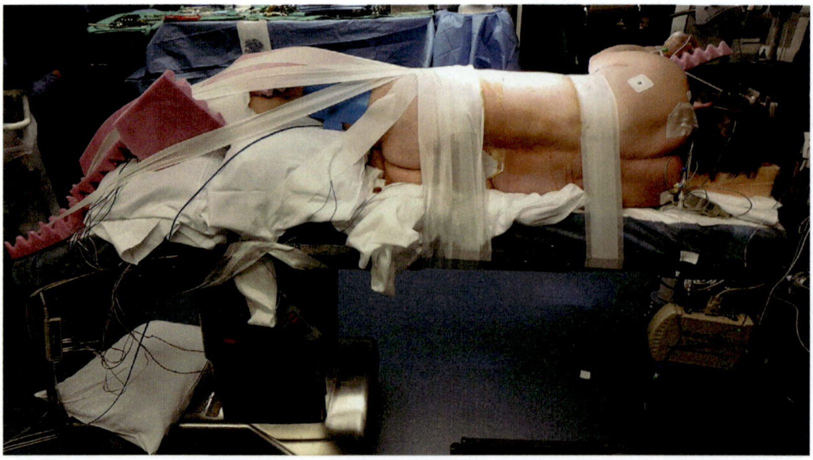

Fig. 14.6 Positioning the patient on the operating table for any of the exposures discussed; allowing access to the flank, room for an emergent extensile exposure if complications arise; and facilitating precise and reliable fluoroscopic imaging

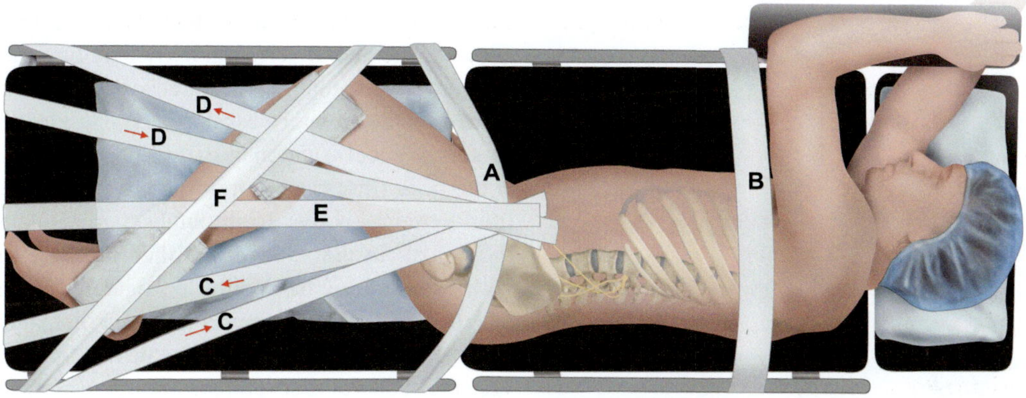

Fig. 14.7 Once the patient is in optimal position, 3″ silk tape is used, as shown, to immobilize the lower extremities and pelvis and the upper extremities and trunk to prevent shifting and malalignment during surgery

pedicles, crisp superior and inferior endplates, and crisp posterior vertebral lines. Once satisfied, secure the patient in final position and recheck orientation (Fig. 14.7). The surgeon can now tilt or elevate the table slightly to obtain the perfect cross-Table AP and lateral image with the C-arm in fixed positions.

The importance of having the patient anchored securely to the operating table without rotation of the torso relative to the pelvis cannot be overstated.

Use wide silk tape to circumferentially secure the chest to the OR table. Stay as cranial from planned surgical incision as is possible. Ensure chest excursion and lung tidal volumes are unchanged. Pad the knee and lateral malleolus on the upper leg, and secure the lower one half of the patient with wide silk tape running across the OR table in line with the lower leg and the femur, respectively. After taping across the iliac crest, the patient should not shift even if the table is tilted slightly side to side.

Retractor Placement

Place the table-mounted base for the expandable retractor of choice. Different options exist, but the effective retractor has 3–4 blades that expand, toe out, and translate slightly based off the initial chosen position, anchored off the table through a flexible arm (Fig. 14.8). They also often have an intradiscal shim or vertebral body pin that can be placed to anchor the system deep to the spine while working. This may permit the surgeon to translate the retractor anterior or posterior, cranial and caudal from the initial starting position. Placement of an expandable cage through an expandable retractor with fiber-optic lighting becomes less of a struggle as the surgeon gains

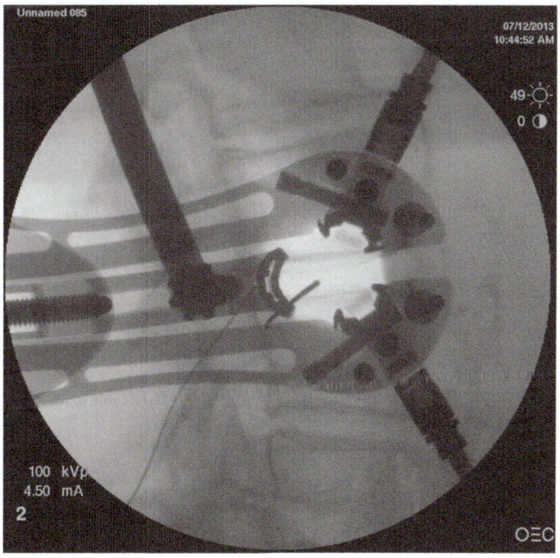

Fig. 14.8 Top-down lateral view through the upper lumbar spinal column showing image quality through a radiolucent retractor

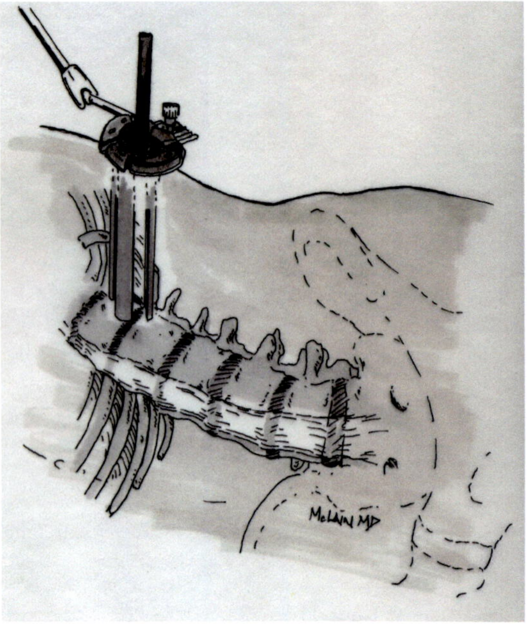

Fig. 14.9 Positioning the typical MIS retractor system over the thoracolumbar junction requires rib resection and elevation or takedown of the diaphragm. Breaking the table is not helpful in this exposure and could interfere with alignment when cage placement is performed

familiarity [16]. Placement of even the smallest MIS retractor at the thoracolumbar junction requires osteotomy or removal of the T12 and T11 ribs overlying the target vertebra below (Fig. 14.9).

Surgeons with extensive experience with DLIF and XLIF approaches for degenerative disease will have an advantage when taking on this kind of approach, and surgeons who have not used these systems may be better served through a traditional open approach. Managing bleeding, from bone, tumor, or a vessel, can be daunting through a small portal, and any surgeon should be prepared to immediately convert their minimally invasive approach to an open procedure if complications arise.

Corpectomy and Tumor Resection

Exposure of T12

Once the operative level is confirmed and retractor is placed, ensure adequate exposure cranial to caudal, anterior to posterior. Ideally one can see both discs and the intervening T12 body with retractor deployed and toed out. Our preference is to expose from T11–T12 disc to T12–L1 disc first. Loosen and reposition the retractor arm as needed. The lateral vertebral body may be soft if infiltrated with tumor, but care is first taken to isolate the segmental vessels via Bovie electrocautery vertical incision at the mid-body starting at the peak (disc) and working toward the valley (mid-vertebral body). Right-angle clamp isolates the vessels in the valley, and then tie these off with silk suture; hemoclips or ligature/bipolar may be less reliable or may come loose. Palpation with a Penfield can help to delineate the posterior vertebral body border: palpate along lateral body until you fall into the neuroforamen underneath the pedicle. Thrombin-gelatin matrix, thrombin-soaked Gelfoam, and cottonoids can tamp off radiculomedullary artery bleeding stirred up with the Penfield.

Exposure of L1

Recall the diaphragmatic attachments in this region: the left-sided lateral crus becomes confluent with ALL from L1 to L3, the medial arcuate ligament (investing fascia over the psoas) attaches to the lateral L1 vertebral body and the L1 transverse process, and the lateral arcuate ligament (investing fascia over the quadratus lumborum) attaches to the L1 TP and then along the posterior-most aspect of the 12th rib. Once the arcuate ligament attachments onto L1 TP are released, the confluence of ALL, crus, and arcuate ligament is released off the lateral L1 body with electrocautery. Particular care is taken to identify the segmental artery and vein as they run under the crus [7]. A Steinman pin can be placed transversely through the adjacent vertebra, just caudal to the L1 pedicle, to retract the psoas. Angle the pin anteriorly away from the canal as it advances, check the length on fluoroscopy, and dress the exposed, sharp end with a red rubber catheter tip to avoid surgeon or visceral injury. As one moves caudally, be aware of the confluence of lumbar nerve roots within the psoas and ensure that the psoas is swept posteriorly in its entirety before placing the retracting Steinman pin.

Discectomies

Discectomies are performed as per typical lateral interbody fusion discectomy at the T11–T12 and T12–L1 levels. Ensure thorough preparation of the endplates that will accommodate the anterior column support (fibular strut, expandable or structural cage, etc.) [17]. Complete the discectomies before starting corpectomy to minimize intraoperative bleeding; as long as the vertebra is intact, little blood is lost during discectomy, and once the discs are out, the corpectomy can be accomplished with much greater speed and safety, further minimizing bleeding.

T12 Corpectomy

Some surgeons prefer to start the corpectomy with an osteotome to mark the area of the corpectomy anteriorly, leaving a thin, protective shell of bone anteriorly and along the contralateral side. The cranial, caudal, and anterior borders of the corpectomy are now defined. The body remains attached by the contralateral pedicle. Rongeur away the remaining soft, tumor-ridden vertebral bone [18, 19]. The bone will often bleed briskly until the bulk of the tumor and pathological bone is removed. Pack the field intermittently as needed with hemostatic thrombin foam and dress bleeding bone with wax. Communicate with anesthesia prior to beginning the corpectomy. They should be caught up (if not ahead) before beginning the highest blood loss portion of the procedure. The final, posterior rim or rind of bone and tumor volar to the cord is carefully mobilized away from the canal, using fine curettes and pituitary rongeurs, working from the left to the right across the canal until the dura is free and clear.

Direct decompression of the canal may be very necessary in radioresistant tumors and compressive lesions already causing neurological symptoms. Soft or viscous tumors may be debrided away with a Penfield and suction, but fibrous and bony tumor needs to be carefully separated from the dura and pulled out of the canal and into the corpectomy defect without damaging the threatened neural tissues. Dense bony tissue can be thinned with a burr before mobilizing, and a long thin curette can be inserted behind the residual flap of tumor to reflect it piecemeal into the corpectomy defect. Curettes and pituitaries work across the surface of the dura to complete the dissection from pedicle to pedicle, endplate to endplate.

If the margin between the tumor and the vertebral cortex and PLL is difficult to reach, a diamond burr can be used to take down the lateral cortex of the pedicle at its junction with the vertebral body. As the cancellous bone of the pedicle is removed, the thin inner cortex can be separated from the underlying dura with a small curved curette, then resected with a Kerrison, exposing the exiting nerve root and the lateral surface of the dura from the lamina dorsally to the floor of the vertebral canal. From here decompression of the volar dura can proceed gently but under direct vision.

Place Anterior Column Support With or Without Side Plate and Screw Instrumentation

Once the corpectomy is complete, irrigate thoroughly with antibiotic-laden irrigation. Ensure adequate decompression of the anterior epidural space. Measure between neighboring T11 and L1 endplates, and select the cage or fabricate the strut graft that will be used for anterior column support. Select, pack, and place the cage with care to ensure the selected implant will fit through the retractor. As life expectancy warrants, pay attention to fusion techniques (pack contralateral allograft bone, pack the prosthesis with bone, etc.). Although radiation and disease may impair successful fusion, any of these TL approaches used for corpectomy will provide access to autograft rib. While not sufficient to bear loads on its own, rib struts stacked with a structural cage can dramatically improve the likelihood of anterior fusion and long-term construct survival.

If placing a locking side plate and screws, start the transverse screws in the posterior lateral corner of the vertebral body above or below and angle 10–20° away from the canal and parallel to the endplate itself. If the table has been broken at any time during the resection, return to neutral before placing the plate or locking the fixation in place. Place a small suction drain deep in the wound.

Posterior Pedicle Screw Fixation

If placing an interbody cage without a locking side plate, it is usually wise to augment spinal stability through bilateral posterior pedicle screw fixation. In highly unstable situations, these can be placed with the patient in the lateral decubitus position, but more commonly the patient can be rolled directly onto a radiolucent prone frame to complete the procedure. For a T12 corpectomy, percutaneously placed pedicle screws from T11 to L1 (with unilateral screw fixation in T12 on the contralateral side) are mechanically sufficient, but the surgeon may extend this cranially or caudally if there is any question about integrity of the anterior column support or bone quality. Anterior column support combined with bilateral posterior pedicle screw fixation has been shown sufficient in three-column reconstructions [17].

Disclosure The authors have received nothing of value from any entity, industrial agency, or sponsor in relation to any aspect of the work presented here.

References

1. Lazorthes G, Gouaze A, Zadeh J, Jacques Santini J, Lazorthes Y, Burdin P. Arterial vascularization of the spinal cord. J Neurosurg. 1971;35(3):253–62.
2. Uribe J, Arredondo N, Dakwar E, Vale F. Defining the safe working zones using the minimally invasive lateral retroperitoneal transpsoas approach: an anatomical study. J Neurosurg Spine. 2010;13(2):260–6.
3. Dakwar E, Ahmadian A, Uribe J. The anatomical relationship of the diaphragm to the thoracolumbar junction during the minimally invasive lateral extracoelomic (retropleural/retroperitoneal) approach. J Neurosurg Spine. 2012;16(4):359–64.
4. Kawahara N, Tomita K, Baba H, Toribatake Y, Fujita T, Mizuno K, et al. Cadaveric vascular anatomy for total en bloc spondylectomy in malignant vertebral tumors. Spine. 1996;21(12):1401–7.
5. Maish M. The diaphragm. Surg Clin N Am. 2010;90(5):955–68.
6. Baaj A, Papadimitriou K, Amin A, Kretzer R, Wolinsky J, Gokaslan Z. Surgical anatomy of the diaphragm in the anterolateral approach to the spine. A cadaveric study. J Spin Disord Tech. 2014;27:220–3.
7. McLain RF. Video assisted spinal cord decompression reduces surgical morbidity and speeds recovery in patients with metastasis. J Surg Oncol. 2005;91:212–6.
8. Walsh G, Gokaslan Z, McCutcheon I, Mineo M, Yasko A, Swisher S, et al. Anterior approaches to the thoracic spine in patients with cancer: indications and results. Ann Thorac Surg. 1997;64(6):1611–8.
9. Watkins RG. Tenth rib: thoracoabdominal approach. In: Watkins RG, editor. Surgical approaches to the spine. New York: Springer; 1983. p. 83–8.
10. Moskovich R, Benson D, Zhang Z, Kabins M. Extracoelomic approach to the spine. J Bone Joint Surg. 1993;75(6):886–93.
11. Kinnear W, Kinnear G, Watson L, Webb J, Johnston I. Pulmonary function after spinal surgery for idiopathic scoliosis. Spine. 1992;17(6):708–13.
12. McLain RF. Extracavitary approaches to the thoracolumbar spine. In: Weinstein SL, editor. Pediatric spine surgery. 2nd ed. Philadelphia: Lippincott, Williams and Wilkins; 2000. p. 179–84.
13. Kim M, Nolan P, Finkelstein J. Evaluation of the 11th rib extrapleural-retroperitoneal approach to the thoracolumbar junction. J Neurosurg Spine. 2000;93:168–74.
14. Zdeblick TA. Anterior thoracolumbar corpectomy and stabilization. In: Bradford DS, Zdeblick TA, editors. The spine: master techniques in orthopaedic surgery. Philadelphia: Lippincott, Williams and Wilkins; 2004. p. 195–207.
15. Molinares D, Davis T, Fung D, Liu J, Clark S, Daily D, et al. Is the lateral jack-knife position responsible for cases of transient neurapraxia? J Neurosurg Spine. 2016;24(1):189–96.
16. Scheufler K. Technique and clinical results of minimally invasive reconstruction and stabilization of the thoracic and thoracolumbar spine with expandable cages and ventrolateral plate fixation. Neurosurgery. 2007;61(4):798–809.
17. Altaf F, Weber M, Dea N, Boriani S, Ames C, Williams R, et al. Evidence-based review and survey of expert opinion of reconstruction of metastatic spine tumors. Spine. 2016;41:S254–61.
18. Park M, Deukmedjian A, Uribe J. Minimally invasive anterolateral corpectomy for spinal tumors. Neurosurg Clin N Am. 2014;25(2):317–25.
19. Uribe J, Dakwar E, Le T, Christian G, Serrano S, Smith W. Minimally invasive surgery for thoracic spine tumor removal. Spine. 2010;35(26S):S347–54.

Indications and Techniques for Anterior Thoracolumbar Resections and Reconstructions

15

Benjamin D. Elder, Wataru Ishida, and Jean-Paul Wolinsky

Introduction

Metastatic spinal tumors are by far the most prevalent spinal neoplasms [1] and are oftentimes associated with significant morbidity, including progressive paralysis, sensory loss, sphincter dysfunction, and severe axial pain [2, 3]. Treatment strategies require multidisciplinary, comprehensive approaches involving spinal surgeons, oncologists, radiation oncologists, pain management teams, and social workers, both for the patient's quality of life and for oncological outcomes [4]. In the last three decades, several technical advancements in the field of spinal oncology have allowed for a variety of surgical and nonsurgical options in the treatment of metastatic spinal tumors. The widespread use of novel devices such as expandable cages, titanium mesh cages, polyetheretherketone (PEEK) cages, and polymethylmethacrylate (PMMA), has significantly altered the options for spinal column reconstruction [5–8]. Also, with the advent of stereotactic body radiation therapy (SBRT), the rates of local control as well as pain relief have improved significantly [9–13]. Lastly, given the efficacy of SBRT, the role of less invasive "separation surgery" plus posterior screw fixation prior to SBRT has been extensively discussed [14–16].

Despite the aforementioned progress in the field of spinal oncology, en bloc resections of spinal tumors such as vertebrectomy or spondylectomy with spinal reconstruction still remain an important surgical option, though these are typically reserved for patients with primary tumors. En bloc resections oftentimes require anesthesiologic expertise such as double-lumen intubation tubes and unilateral lung ventilation as well as complex neurosurgical techniques with potential operative complications and thus should be indicated cautiously [14, 16–18]. Given the rarity that this technique is required, a full discussion of the approach is beyond the scope of this chapter. Here, we will review the indications and techniques for anterior thoracolumbar resections and reconstructions.

Indications

First, although there are no well-established guidelines for surgical decision-making, the type and location of the pathology and any neural

B. D. Elder, MD, PhD (✉)
Department of Neurosurgery, The Mayo Clinic, Rochester, MN, USA
e-mail: elder.benjamin@mayo.edu

W. Ishida, MD
Department of Neurosurgery, Johns Hopkins Hospital, Baltimore, MD, USA
e-mail: wishida1@jhmi.edu; wi2113@cumc.columbia.edu

J.-P. Wolinsky, MD
Department of Neurosurgery, Northwestern University, Chicago, IL, USA
e-mail: Jean-paul.wolinsky@northwestern.edu

R. A. W. Marco (ed.), *Metastatic Spine Disease*, https://doi.org/10.1007/978-3-319-76252-4_15

compression should be considered first when deciding on a surgical approach. Indications for resection of thoracolumbar tumors generally include intractable pain, impending spinal instability, progressive compression of the spinal cord or cauda equina by bony elements (irrespective of radiosensitivity of the tumor), and symptomatic compression of neural structures by radioresistant tumors [4]. Furthermore, the predicted oncological survival based on clinical characteristics (i.e., Tokuhashi score [19–21]) and the probability of neurological recovery after resection and decompression should be taken into account individually. For instance, a recent systematic review reported that, although supported by low-quality evidence, the duration of ambulation loss and severity of neurologic deficit (i.e., muscle strength and bladder function) were the greatest predictors of postoperative neurological recovery in patients with metastatic epidural spinal cord compression [22].

After considering all of the relevant factors above, it should be carefully determined for each individual as to which surgical approach (anterior versus posterior versus combined) is optimal. For instance, although conventionally in the thoracolumbar spine posterior approaches have been frequently chosen due to spinal surgeon's familiarity with the anatomy and potential operative morbidity tied to anterior approaches such as vascular injury, atelectasis, pulmonary embolus, pneumothorax, and intercostal neuralgia [18, 23, 24], anterior approaches allow for wider surgical corridors for decompression of the spinal cord ventrally. Additionally, anterior approaches can spare the posterior elements of the spine, which could obviate the need to additionally reconstruct the spinal column via posterior approaches.

Additionally, when using posterior approaches to the lumbar spine, particularly at or below L2, the nerve roots cannot be sacrificed without a motor deficit, which makes it difficult for us to insert vertebral body replacement (VBR) devices of sufficient height. Although expandable cages have been increasingly used for this reason, it can still be a substantial challenge to access this space, obtain an adequate correction of any kyphotic deformity, and restore the full height of the collapsed vertebrae. Hence, we often select anterior approaches for these cases. This is contrary to thoracic spine pathology, where the nerve roots can be sacrificed and an optimal surgical view and wide working channel can be obtained via posterior approaches. However, in the lower lumbar spine, the thecal sac can be manipulated and retracted to allow for increased access and visualization from a posterior approach, whereas in the thoracic spine and conus, the surgeon must carefully work around the spinal cord with minimal manipulation.

To summarize, the location of the tumor pathology, the need for wide surgical corridors to secure negative margins, the targeted correction of the deformity, and general conditions of the patients (tolerability to potential cardiorespiratory complications from anterior approaches) are the determinant factors.

Biomechanics

In terms of the biomechanics related to anterior thoracolumbar resections and reconstructions, special attention should be paid to transitional zones, namely, the cervicothoracic junction and thoracolumbar junction. They transition zones between the mobile lordosis of the cervical spine, the rigid kyphosis of the thoracic spine, and the mobile lordosis of the lumbar spine are at higher risk for instability both preoperatively and postoperatively. On the contrary, the thoracic spine has additional protection from destabilization due to the stability of the rib cage and thus may be less vulnerable to pre- or postoperative regional instability [25, 26].

Recently, the Spinal Instability Neoplastic Score (SINS) scoring system was proposed by the Spinal Oncology Study Group (SOSG), which allows for quantification of the potential spinal instability of patients with spinal tumors [27] and stratification of patients who may benefit from stabilization [28, 29]. Briefly, the SINS system takes a wide variety of relevant factors into consideration, such as tumor location (junctional, mobile spine, semirigid, and rigid), mechanical pain, bone lesion (lytic, mixed, and blastic), radiographical spinal alignment, vertebral body collapse, and posterolateral involvement of spinal elements, and scores spinal instability on a scale of 0–18. It serves as a useful screening tool for medical oncologists and radiation oncologists, as a recent systematic review proposed that consultation of spine surgeons is recommended for patients with a SINS score above 7 [29]. It was also stated that the role of the SINS score still remained somewhat controversial as several clinical studies have not identified the SINS score as a prognostic factor for spinal instability [30–32]. Furthermore, it should be noted that the original SINS score did not factor in the use of SBRT [33–35]. The biomechanics related to spinal reconstructions will be detailed in the next section.

Instrumentation Options and Reconstruction Techniques

With the advent of various novel spinal instrumentation systems, there have been more varied reconstruction strategies following tumor resection. Conventionally, structural bone graft with or without a vascularized pedicle (either autologous or allogenic) [36, 37] had been almost exclusively utilized in the setting of a thoracolumbar corpectomy, although the merits of vascularized bone grafts remain controversial [38]. Nowadays, in addition to structural bone grafts, a multitude of VBR devices exist, including titanium mesh cages, PEEK, carbon fiber PEEK, expandable cages, and PMMA ("chest tube technique") [39]. They are often utilized in conjunction with morselized autologous/allogenic bone graft [38], demineralized bone matrices, beta-tricalcium phosphate, or cellular bone matrices such as Osteocel or Trinity [40–42]. Furthermore, supplementary posterior/lateral instrumentations, including lateral plates and lateral pedicle screw/rod constructs, are also available [7, 8, 38]. There is not necessarily a universally optimal system, and the choice of instrumentation is clearly defined by the surgical approach utilized, dependent on anatomy, pathology, adjunctive treatment (radiation and chemotherapy), and predicted oncological and functional outcomes.

In terms of VBR selection, Zhou et al. biomechanically compared PEEK cage-rod constructs with titanium cage-rod constructs in the setting of an L1 corpectomy and demonstrated that the PEEK cage-rod construct allowed more motion compared to the titanium cage-rod construct but resulted in higher stability in flexion and lateral bending without preloading and flexion and extension under the preloading condition [43]. Conversely, a systematic review by Li et al. maintained that there was no clinically significant difference between these two constructs [44]. To study the effects of different VBRs on subsidence, Pekmezci et al. evaluated ten human thoracolumbar spines (T10–L2, L3–L5) biomechanically in vitro after a single-level corpectomy and reconstruction with an expandable or fixed cage plus anterior dual-rod instrumentation and demonstrated that, in spite of larger surface contact area, expandable cages had a tendency for more frequent subsidence than fixed cages and also that, in the presence of edge loading, as is clinically observed in the setting of hyperlordotic cages, there was an even higher risk of subsidence and intraoperative fracture at the moment of deployment [45]. This finding is compatible with other in vitro/in silico studies and several prospective/retrospective clinical series reported in the literature [46–48]. Additionally, Eleraky et al. described their retrospective clinical series of 16 patients with PMMA and 16 patients with expandable cages after corpectomy for tumors in thoracolumbar regions and concluded that both approaches allow for adequate correction of the kyphotic deformity and spinal stabilization with comparable functional and performance status outcomes [49]. In short, currently there is no scientific or clinical evidence which definitively supports one specific type of VBR device.

In terms of supplemental fixation, Viljoen et al. investigated the in vitro biomechanical strength of (1) expandable cages + lateral instrumentation, (2) expandable cages + short-segment pedicle screw fixation (one level above and below), and (3) expandable cages + long-segment pedicle screw fixation (two levels above and below) following an L1 corpectomy; in flexion, extension, and left/right lateral bending, supplemental posterior long-segment fixation had significantly less motion compared with the other constructs and even the intact state [50], which was in agreement with a cadaveric study by Disch et al. [48] Similarly, Liu et al. advocated for the use of supplemental bilateral pedicle screw fixation over unilateral pedicle screws or lateral plates in the setting of lumbar interbody fusion [51].

With regard to indications for attempting bony fusion and bone graft options, there is no clear agreement in the literature [7, 8, 38], but generally speaking, fusion should be attempted for patients with estimated life expectancies more than 6–12 months, when fusion may be achieved [8, 38].

In summary, although there is no clear consensus on this issue and thus treatment strategies should be tailored for each individual, anterior reconstruction with vertebral body replacement devices with or without attempted anterior bony fusion plus posterior fixation (more than two levels above and below) is recommended if a corpectomy is required or if the loading of the anterior column is significantly compromised by the tumor.

Operative Techniques and Approaches

Cervicothoracic Junction Approaches

Patient Positioning and Approaches

The surgical approach is selected based on the level of the lesion: (1) low anterior approaches allow for access down to T2 in some patients (with limited applicability in patients with short necks), (2) modified anterior approaches allow for anterior access as low as T4, and (3) sternal-splitting approaches allow for access from C3 to T4. Usually, due to the unpredictability of the course of the right recurrent laryngeal nerve, a left-sided approach is preferable. Thus, the patient is positioned supine with their neck extended and tilted slightly to the right in a low anterior approach and hyperextended and turned 60° to the right in modified anterior approaches and sternal-splitting approaches.

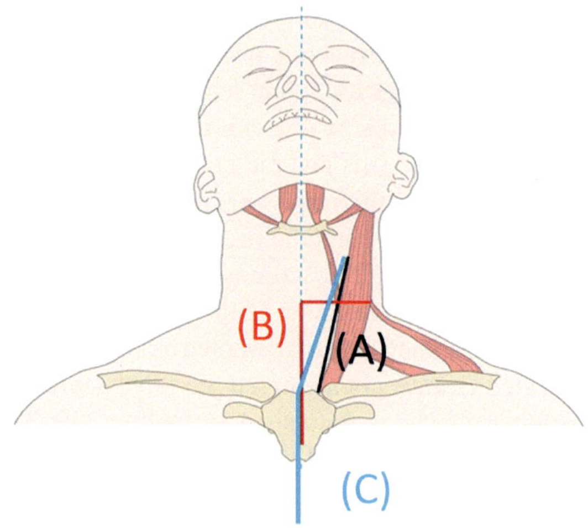

Fig. 15.1 Skin incisions for the three anterior approaches to the cervicothoracic junction (**a**) low anterior approach, (**b**) modified anterior approach, and (**c**) sternal-splitting approach

Low Anterior Approach

This approach is essentially the inferior extension of an ordinary anterior cervical approach. A paramedian transverse skin incision or a longitudinal skin incision just medial to the sternocleidomastoid (SCM) muscle down to the level of the manubrium is performed (Fig. 15.1a). The platysma and superficial fascia are dissected sharply. Cautious blunt dissection provides a plane between the carotid sheath laterally and the trachea and esophagus medially. Then, the longus colli muscles and anterior longitudinal ligament are identified, followed by the level confirmation with the use of X-ray and needles. Cauterization of the longus colli muscles allows for access as low as the T1–T2 disc space in some patients.

Modified Anterior Approach

A wider exposure at the cervicothoracic junction can be obtained via the modified anterior approach. First, a transverse skin incision is made from the lateral border of the left SCM muscle to the midline at the level of approximately 2 cm above the left clavicle. Second, the medial end of the initial skin incision is extended caudally to the junction of the sternum and the manubrium (Fig. 15.1b). Then, the platysma, both heads of the SCM muscle, and the inferior strap muscles are elevated and retracted. Next, the medial third of the left clavicle is resected with special attention to the subclavian vein. Again, by establishing a plane between the carotid sheath and the trachea and esophagus, the brachiocephalic vessels can be identified, which are then retracted caudally. These maneuvers allow for exposure from C4 to T4.

Sternal-Splitting Approaches

If further exposure is necessary, a sternal-splitting approach may facilitate exposure of the cervicothoracic junction. Sundaresan et al. [52] described a procedure that removed a rectangular portion of the manubrium to enhance exposure of this region of the spine. Sar et al. [53] described the use of this rectangular piece of manubrium to reconstruct the anterior column. Darling et al. [54] described an approach that involved a midline split of the manubrium with lateral division of the synostosis between the manubrium and the body of the sternum. The manubrium was then wired together so that neither the clavicle nor the manubrium was resected. These authors believed that this exposure may have less morbidity associated with it compared to procedures involving resection of the medial clavicle or manubrium. Lehman et al. [55] described an extensile sternal-splitting approach that allowed exposure from C4 to T3, while Kraus et al. [56] further extended this procedure by extending the incision laterally through the rib cage resulting in a trap door, or clamshell, of the chest wall.

Cohen et al. [57] described an anterior approach to T3 via an "interaortocaval subinnominate window." The first part of the skin incision commences from the medial border of the left SCM muscle at the level of C3 and ends at the sternal notch and then proceeds to the caudal end of the sternum in the midline (Fig. 15.1c). After obtaining the same plane between the carotid sheath and the trachea, blunt dissection is performed to create space between the sternum and the pleura. The sternum is split down to the xiphoid process with the use of an oscillating saw. The left innominate artery is identified following division of the thymus and mobilized down to the superior vena cava. The upper pericardial reflection is incised, allowing for identification and mobilization of the ascending aorta and proximal innominate artery. Following mobilization of the great vessels, a window is created with the aorta rotated to the left and the SVC mobilized to the right. This allows for a window for access to the T1–T3 vertebral bodies. York et al. [58] have also described high thoracotomy approaches to the upper thoracic spine.

Reconstruction Techniques

Depending on the working space available, the insertion of VBR devices with or without anterior plates and screws is usually feasible. This is often supplemented with posterior instrumentation depending on biomechanical factors as discussed previously.

Complications

Complications of anterior approaches to the cervicothoracic junction include risk of injury to the recurrent laryngeal nerve, the esophagus, the thoracic duct, and the phrenic nerve. When a clavicle osteotomy is added, the possibility of vascular injury (subclavian vessels and brachiocephalic vessels) as well as non-union of the clavicle are of importance.

Thoracic/Thoracolumbar Approaches

Patient Positioning and Approaches

Various factors such as cardiopulmonary function and the level, location, and extension of pathology should be considered thoroughly in order to determine (1) a thoracotomy approach (T3–T11) or a thoracolumbar approach (T10–L2) and also (2) a right- or left-sided approach. For instance, the liver as well as the aorta and the inferior vena cava can be limiting factors in terms of the extent of retraction permitted to obtain a wider surgical corridor with a left-sided approach. Thus, although the location of the pathology is the critical determining factor, it is preferred to perform T4–T6 thoracotomies from the right side, since the descending aorta and aortic arch could make the surgical view narrower, whereas for T6–T11 thoracotomies, a left-sided approach is preferred to avoid the liver and the inferior vena cava, which may be difficult to repair in the event of inadvertent damage. Also, extravertebral tumor invasion is another important variable to be considered. In patients who have a history of previous thoracic operations, the contralateral approach should be selected, whenever feasible, to obviate the need for dissecting pleural adhesions and to lower the risks of postoperative air leaks and infectious complications. After selecting a thoracotomy approach, the patient is secured to the operating table with the use of tape in the lateral decubitus position, which allows for an orthogonal orientation of the spine.

Transthoracic Approach (T3-T11)

In terms of rib removal and incision placement, the following guidelines should be considered: (1) T3 and T4 lesions, fourth rib; (2) T5 and T6 lesions, fifth rib, (3) T7 and T8 lesions, one level above; and (4) T9–T12 lesions, two levels above. Of note, above T7, mobilization of the scapula is necessary to obtain a sufficient surgical corridor, so the patient's arm must be fully abducted and internally rotated. The skin incision should be made directly over the selected rib, extending from the lateral aspect of the rectus abdominis muscle to the lateral border of the paraspinal muscle, although a smaller incision with less anterior dissection can often be used successfully, and direct lateral minimally invasive options have been proposed. The latissimus dorsi muscle and the serratus anterior muscle should be dissected by cutting perpendicularly to the long axes and as caudally as possible to maximize the amount of muscle innervated. When stripping the muscles from the rib, staying in a subperiosteal plane is critical to avoid unnecessary blood loss and damage to the neurovascular bundle. Successful rib removal allows access to thoracic cavity and the targeted vertebra.

Corpectomy Technique

In order to safely perform a transthoracic corpectomy, we routinely follow these steps (Fig. 15.2) [59]: a rectangular cut into the anterior part of the

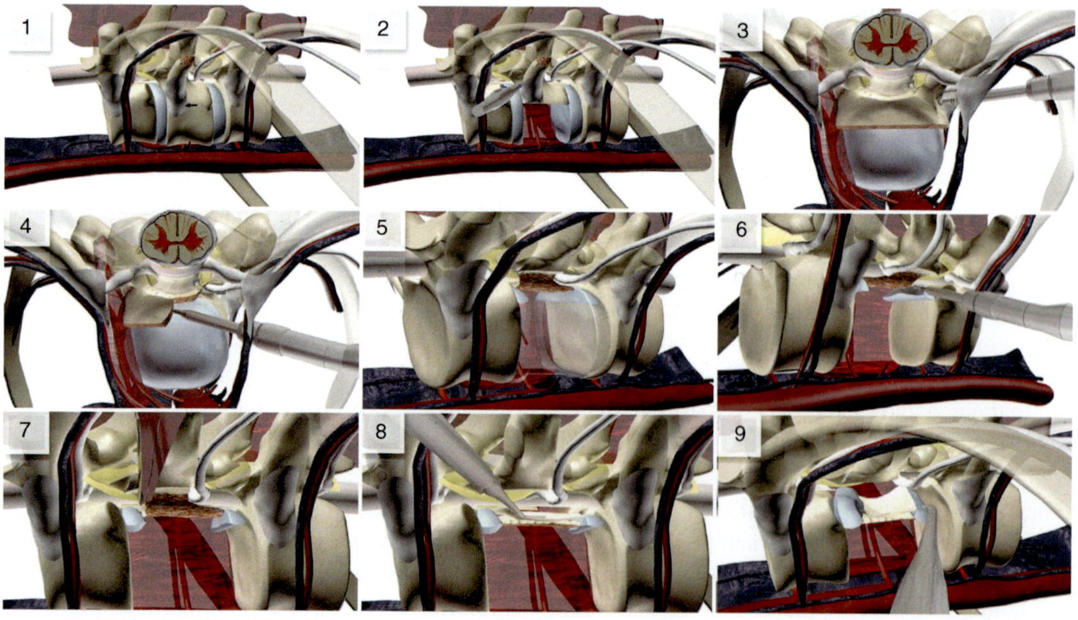

Fig. 15.2 Three-dimensional computer-assisted designs demonstrating each step of the nine-step transthoracic corpectomy technique (Reproduced with permission, Puvanesarajah et al., "Systematic Approach for Anterior Corpectomy through a Transthoracic Exposure," Turkish Neurosurgery, 26 (4): 646–652, 2016)

vertebral body is made; cauterize the soft tissue overlying the rib head, excise the muscular attachments, and then remove rib head to expose the ipsilateral pedicle; drill out the ipsilateral pedicle and vertebral body, leaving a shell of bone along the thecal sac; if required, the contralateral pedicle can be drilled out following removal of the ipsilateral pedicle and vertebral body, though this is challenging and often not required; remove the inferior and superior discs to expose the adjacent endplates; diamond-burr the superior endplate, starting from the junction with posterior longitudinal ligament (PLL); remove bone piece by piece from the rostral side to the caudal side, using a Kerrison punch; cautiously isolate the PLL from the thecal sac with the use of a nerve hook; excise any remnants of the ipsilateral (and contralateral pedicle if required) and PLL.

Thoracoabdominal Transdiaphragmatic Approach (T10–L2)

If access to upper lumbar vertebrae or lower thoracic vertebrae is needed (Fig. 15.3 and 15.4), lateral blunt dissection is performed to enter the retroperitoneal space while keeping the peritoneum intact. This allows for exposure of the diaphragm from both cavities. At this point, the ipsilateral lung may be deflated or can be simply retracted with a moist towel to deflect it out of the field and reduce the chance of postoperative atelectasis. In our practice, dual-lumen endotracheal tubes are rarely used unless the patient has a locally invasive lung malignancy requiring a lung lobectomy at the time of surgery. Then, the posterior portion of the diaphragm is detached. Special attention should be paid to the anatomy of the diaphragm since any incision through the diaphragm could potentially result in paralysis of the remnant of the muscle cuff. Identifying the attachment of the 11th and 12th ribs to the diaphragm and lateral and medial arcuate ligaments to the spine is important. By mobilizing the diaphragm, direct access to the thoracolumbar junction, especially the T12 and L1 vertebral bodies, can be obtained (Fig. 15.5) [60].

Reconstruction Techniques

The procedure is concluded with anterior reconstruction, using the aforementioned vertebral replacement devices or structural allograft. Anterior/lateral plating and screws and/or posterior instrumentation should be conducted in case of additional concern about spinal instability, based on the preoperative SINS and intraoperative findings.

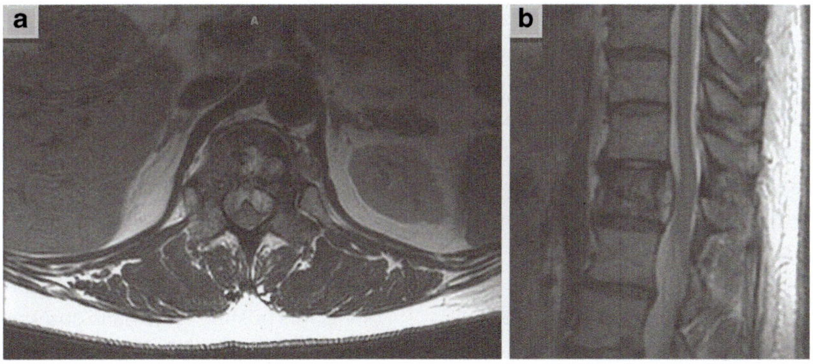

Fig. 15.3 (**a**) Axial and (**b**) sagittal preoperative images depicting a T12 metastatic lesion with involvement of the vertebral body, bilateral pedicles, and right rib head (Reproduced with permission, Puvanesarajah et al., "Systematic Approach for Anterior Corpectomy through a Transthoracic Exposure," Turkish Neurosurgery, 26 (4): 646–652, 2016)

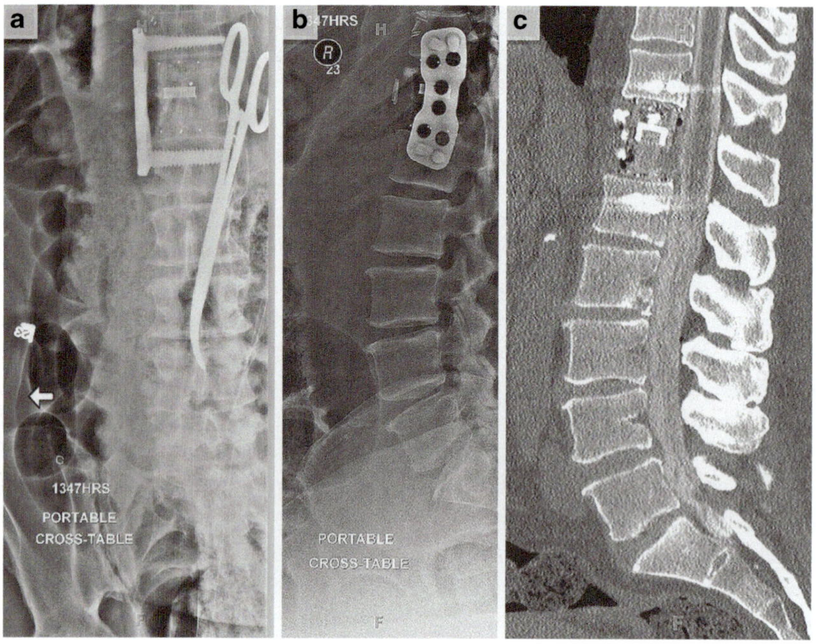

Fig. 15.4 Intraoperative (**a**) A–P and (**b**) lateral X-rays and postoperative (**c**) sagittal computed tomography myelogram demonstrating resection of the T12 mass and reconstruction with an expandable cage and lateral plate (Reproduced with permission, Puvanesarajah et al., "Systematic Approach for Anterior Corpectomy through a Transthoracic Exposure," Turkish Neurosurgery, 26 (4): 646–652, 2016)

Complications

Major complications from these approaches stem from damage to the critical structures including arteries, veins, thoracic duct, lungs, and all the visceral organs in the abdominal cavity. When sacrificing segmental arteries to maximize exposure of the targeted vertebra, one should note that the segmental arteries lie horizontally at the mid-body level and should be ligated between the anterior and posterior aspect of the vertebral body, which allows for collateral flow from other segments to prevent spinal cord ischemia.

Lumbar Approaches

Patient Positioning and Approaches

In an anterior retroperitoneal approach or a transperitoneal approach, the patient is placed in the supine position, angling the table underneath the sacral area between 0° and 40°. In a lateral flank retroperitoneal approach, the patient is secured on the operating table in the lateral decubitus position, with the approach side up. In lumbar approaches, a left-sided approach is preferred unless the pathology is predominantly located on the right side, due to limitations of surgical exposure and technical difficulties elicited by the liver and the inferior vena cava in comparison to the spleen and the aorta, respectively. A preoperative bowel preparation should also be considered. The lower leg remains straight and the upper leg is flexed to obtain relaxation of the ipsilateral psoas muscle. The arm on the operated side is placed across the chest in a sling. A lateral flank retroperitoneal approach can minimize the skin incision and the muscle exposure, particularly with some of the newer minimally invasive approaches, but L5 exposure is limited compared to anterior retroperitoneal and transperitoneal approaches, and access below L5 is impossible due to the location of the iliac crest. Therefore, the operative side and approach should be carefully chosen based on the location of the pathology.

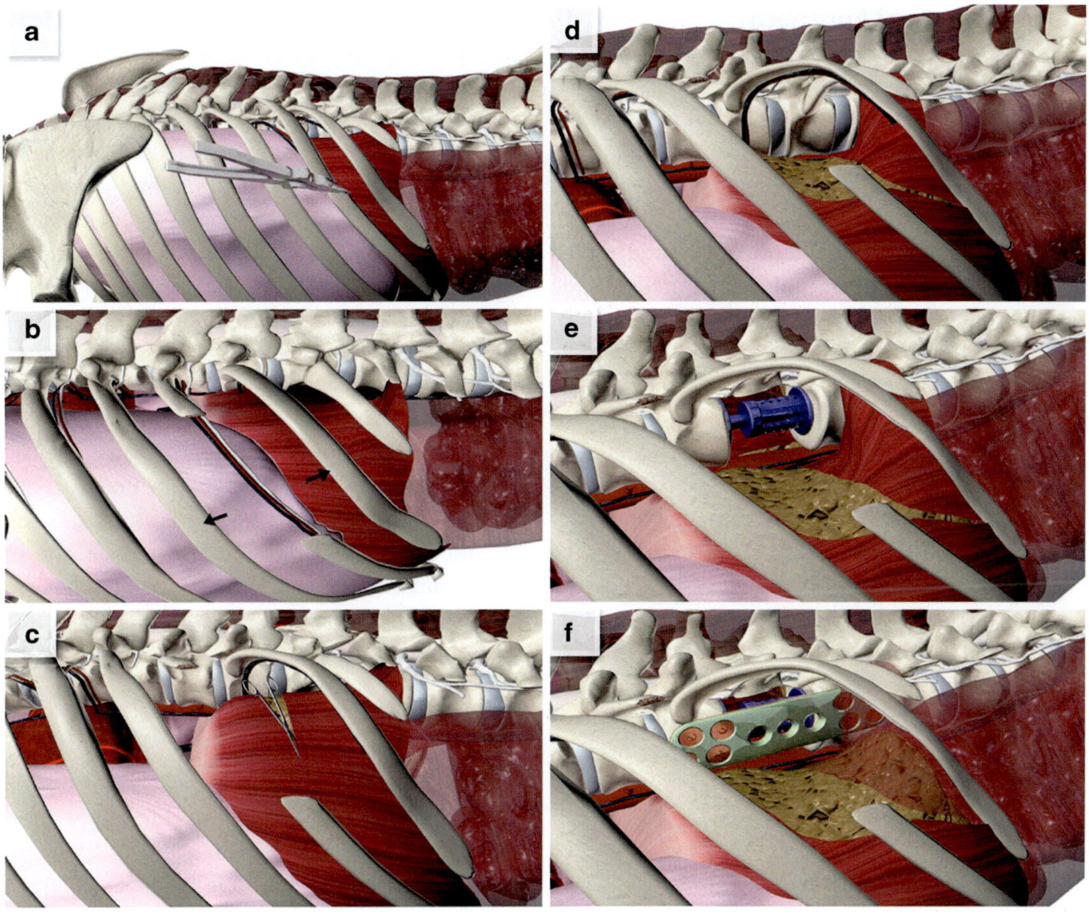

Fig. 15.5 Three-dimensional computer-assisted designs demonstrating key steps of the thoracoabdominal approach for the T12 mass. (**a**) Cutting of the rib. (**b**) Retraction of the ribs. (**c**) Cutting the diaphragm. (**d**) Retraction of the retroperitoneal fat. (**e**) Placement of an expandable cage. (**f**) Placement of lateral plate and screws (Reproduced with permission, Puvanesarajah et al., "Systematic Approach for Anterior Corpectomy through a Transthoracic Exposure," Turkish Neurosurgery, 26 (4): 646–652, 2016)

Anterior Retroperitoneal Approach

The lateral edge of the left rectus abdominis muscle is palpated approximately 5 cm lateral from the midline, and a paramedian skin incision is made. Then anterior rectus sheath is cut to expose the posterior rectus fascia, which is retracted to visualize the peritoneum. Once the peritoneum is well-mobilized and retracted, the left iliac fossa and the psoas muscle are identified. In this space, the ureter, the left iliac arteries and veins, and the aorta should be observed, which is of paramount importance in avoiding complications. Exposure of the lumbar spine is then accomplished by lateral dissection of the psoas muscle. When segmental arteries are identified, they should be ligated at the midpoint as discussed previously. If additional visualization of the upper lumbar spines is required, the skin incision can be extended rostral to the inferior part of the 10th–12th ribs, followed by careful mobilization of the kidney rostral and medial. Exposure of the lower lumbar spine requires mobilization of the great vessels often with sacrifice of the iliolumbar vein, while the working channel at the anterior lumbosacral junction is inferior to the crotch of the iliac vessels.

Transperitoneal Approach

This procedure is commonly performed in conjunction with a general surgery access surgeon. The same paramedian skin incision is made and the abdominal wall fascia is incised at the midline. The peritoneum is opened cautiously so that bowel is not damaged. The sigmoid, cecum, jejunum, and ileum are retracted rostrally, and the pelvic portion of the colon is retracted to the left, which allows for the clear visualization of the ureters. All of the prevertebral structures including the aorta, inferior vena cava, and the hypogastric nerve plexus are then identified. The hypogastric nerve plexus is generally located anterior to L5 and should be retracted to the left to expose the L5 vertebral body if necessary. Use of monopolar cauterization in this area should be minimized, given risk of injury to the hypogastric nerve plexus. Instead, bipolar electrocautery or vascular clips should be applied to control bleeding and control the middle sacral artery. After appropriate decompression, repositioning of the bowel loops is crucial to prevent bowel torsion and potential ischemia/herniation.

Lateral Flank Retroperitoneal Approach

The skin incision starts from the lateral edge of the posterior paraspinal muscles at the 12th rib. Depending on the region of interest, it can be above or below the 12th rib. For instance, if L1–L2 exposure is required, it should be made above the 12th rib, and excision of anterior two-thirds of the 12th rib should suffice in most cases. Next, the incision is extended to the intersection of the lateral border of the rectus abdominis muscle and the perpendicular bisector of the line segment between the umbilicus and the symphysis pubis. Then, external and internal oblique and transversus abdominis muscles are divided, which leads to visualization of the transversalis fascia. Since the transversalis fascia is fragile and in close proximity to the peritoneum, care should be taken not to inadvertently enter the abdominal cavity. Once the retroperitoneum is identified, the abdominal organs should be retracted medially and anteriorly, away from vertebral bodies to further visualize the targeted vertebrae and additional vital structures such as the ureters, the aorta, the common iliac vessels, and the genitofemoral nerve. After the psoas muscle is retracted, the segmental vessels are identified around the midpoint of the vertebral body. Again, ligation of segmental arteries must be performed at each level of interest. Lastly, in this approach, the plane between the aorta and the anterior longitudinal ligament can be easily established by blunt dissection in non-neoplastic cases, which could facilitate adequate decompression, but in cases with neoplastic pathology, this maneuver may result in uncontrollable blood loss. Thus, this part of the procedure should be performed with greatest care, or one should stay away from the great vessels and the region anterior to anterior longitudinal ligament if not required for the tumor resection. After decompression and reconstruction, the muscle and skin layers are reapproximated.

Reconstruction Techniques

As detailed previously, there are various options for reconstruction including structural bone grafts (often tricortical iliac crest, fibula, or femur), PEEK cages, titanium cages, PMMA, and lateral plates. The desired reconstruction technique should be selected carefully, depending on the surgical corridor available in each approach and biomechanical strength necessary for each case. Additional, one should consider that in a lateral flank retroperitoneal approach, it can be very challenging if not impossible to insert lateral instrumentation in the L5 vertebral body and given its shape, anterior reconstruction with a cage at L4 is possible, but supplemental posterior instrumentation should be strongly considered.

Complications

Injuries to the vasculature, ureters, lumbar plexus, and bowel may lead to major complications in all of the approaches. More specifically, vascular and bowel complications tend to occur in transperitoneal approaches, whereas ureteral injury and retrograde ejaculation induced by injury to the superior hypogastric plexus happen more frequently in retro- or extraperitoneal approaches.

Conclusions

Indications for resection and subsequent reconstruction of thoracolumbar spine tumors include intractable pain, impending Spine instability neoplastic score (SINS), progressive compression of the spinal cord by bony elements, and symptomatic compression of those neural structures by radio-resistant tumors. The predicted life expectancy of each patient (Tokuhashi score) should also be strongly considered when considering indications for surgery as well as reconstruction methods such as VBRs and bone graft options. Each surgical approach has its advantages and disadvantages and should be carefully tailored for each patient, with the deciding focus on the location of the pathology within the spinal column.

References

1. Gokaslan ZL. Spine surgery for cancer. Curr Opin Oncol. 1996;8(3):178–81.
2. Byrne TN. Spinal cord compression from epidural metastases. N Engl J Med. 1992;327(9):614–9.
3. Fourney DR, Gokaslan ZL. Spinal instability and deformity due to neoplastic conditions. Neurosurg Focus. 2003;14(1):e8
4. Fisher CG, Rhines LD, Bettegowda C, et al. Introduction to focus issue II in spine oncology: evidence-based medicine recommendations for spine oncology. Spine. 2016;41(Suppl 20):S159–s162.
5. Mobbs RJ, Coughlan M, Thompson R, Sutterlin CE, Phan K. The utility of 3D printing for surgical planning and patient-specific implant design for complex spinal pathologies: case report. J Neurosurg Spine. 2017;26(4):513–8.
6. Kim D, Lim JY, Shim KW, et al. Sacral reconstruction with a 3D-printed implant after hemisacrectomy in a patient with sacral osteosarcoma: 1-year follow-up result. Yonsei Med J. 2017;58(2):453–7.
7. Altaf F, Weber M, Dea N, et al. Evidence-based review and survey of expert opinion of reconstruction of metastatic spine tumors. Spine. 2016;41(Suppl 20):S254–s261.
8. Glennie RA, Rampersaud YR, Boriani S, et al. A systematic review with consensus expert opinion of best reconstructive techniques after osseous En bloc spinal column tumor resection. Spine. 2016;41(Suppl 20):S205–s211.
9. Wang Z, Wang J, Zhuang H, Wang P, Yuan Z. Stereotactic body radiation therapy induces fast tumor control and symptom relief in patients with iliac lymph node metastasis. Sci Rep. 2016;6:37987.
10. Verma V, Shostrom VK, Kumar SS, et al. Multi-institutional experience of stereotactic body radiotherapy for large (≥5 centimeters) non-small cell lung tumors. Cancer. 2017;123(4):688–96.
11. Thibault I, Whyne CM, Zhou S, et al. Volume of lytic vertebral body metastatic disease quantified using computed tomography-based image segmentation predicts fracture risk after spine stereotactic body radiation therapy. Int J Radiat Oncol Biol Phys. 2017;97(1):75–81.
12. Tanadini-Lang S, Rieber J, Filippi AR, et al. Nomogram based overall survival prediction in stereotactic body radiotherapy for oligo-metastatic lung disease. Radiother Oncol. 2017;123:182.
13. Chang JH, Shin JH, Yamada YJ, et al. Stereotactic body radiotherapy for spinal metastases: what are the risks and how do we minimize them? Spine. 2016;41(Suppl 20):S238–s245.
14. Zairi F, Arikat A, Allaoui M, Marinho P, Assaker R. Minimally invasive decompression and stabilization for the management of thoracolumbar spine metastasis. J Neurosurg Spine. 2012;17(1):19–23.
15. Di Martino A, Caldaria A, De Vivo V, Denaro V. Metastatic epidural spinal cord compression. Expert Rev Anticancer Ther. 2016:1–10.
16. Bakar D, Tanenbaum JE, Phan K, et al. Decompression surgery for spinal metastases: a systematic review. Neurosurg Focus. 2016;41(2):E2.
17. Fourney DR, Gokaslan ZL. Use of "MAPs" for determining the optimal surgical approach to metastatic disease of the thoracolumbar spine: anterior, posterior, or combined. Invited submission from the Joint Section Meeting on Disorders of the Spine and Peripheral Nerves, March 2004. J Neurosurg Spine. 2005;2(1):40–9.
18. Druschel C, Disch AC, Melcher I, et al. Surgical management of recurrent thoracolumbar spinal sarcoma with 4-level total en bloc spondylectomy: description of technique and report of two cases. Eur Spine J. 2012;21(1):1–9.
19. Aoude A, Fortin M, Aldebeyan S, et al. The revised Tokuhashi score; analysis of parameters and assessment of its accuracy in determining survival in patients afflicted with spinal metastasis. Eur Spine J. 2016.
20. Eap C, Tardieux E, Goasgen O, et al. Tokuhashi score and other prognostic factors in 260 patients with surgery for vertebral metastases. Orthop Traumatol Surg Res. 2015;101(4):483–8.
21. Tokuhashi Y, Matsuzaki H, Oda H, Oshima M, Ryu J. A revised scoring system for preoperative evaluation of metastatic spine tumor prognosis. Spine. 2005;30(19):2186–91.

22. Laufer I, Zuckerman SL, Bird JE, et al. Predicting neurologic recovery after surgery in patients with deficits secondary to MESCC: systematic review. Spine. 2016;41(Suppl 20):S224–s230.
23. Payer M, Sottas C. Mini-open anterior approach for corpectomy in the thoracolumbar spine. Surg Neurol. 2008;69(1):25–31; discussion 31-22.
24. Faciszewski T, Winter RB, Lonstein JE, Denis F, Johnson L. The surgical and medical perioperative complications of anterior spinal fusion surgery in the thoracic and lumbar spine in adults. A review of 1223 procedures. Spine. 1995;20(14):1592–9.
25. Perry TG, Mageswaran P, Colbrunn RW, Bonner TF, Francis T, McLain RF. Biomechanical evaluation of a simulated T-9 burst fracture of the thoracic spine with an intact rib cage. J Neurosurg Spine. 2014;21(3):481–8.
26. Mannen EM, Anderson JT, Arnold PM, Friis EA. Mechanical analysis of the human cadaveric thoracic spine with intact rib cage. J Biomech. 2015;48(10):2060–6.
27. Arana E, Kovacs FM, Royuela A, Asenjo B, Perez-Ramirez U, Zamora J. Spine instability neoplastic score: agreement across different medical and surgical specialties. Spine J. 2016;16(5):591–9.
28. Fourney DR, Frangou EM, Ryken TC, et al. Spinal instability neoplastic score: an analysis of reliability and validity from the spine oncology study group. J Clin Oncol. 2011;29(22):3072–7.
29. Versteeg AL, Verlaan JJ, Sahgal A, et al. The spinal instability neoplastic score: impact on oncologic decision-making. Spine. 2016;41(Suppl 20):S231–s237.
30. Ha KY, Kim YH, Ahn JH, Park HY. Factors affecting survival in patients undergoing palliative spine surgery for metastatic lung and hepatocellular cancer: dose the type of surgery influence the surgical results for metastatic spine disease? Clin Orthop Surg. 2015;7(3):344–50.
31. Zadnik PL, Goodwin CR, Karami KJ, et al. Outcomes following surgical intervention for impending and gross instability caused by multiple myeloma in the spinal column. J Neurosurg Spine. 2015;22(3):301–9.
32. Zadnik PL, Hwang L, Ju DG, et al. Prolonged survival following aggressive treatment for metastatic breast cancer in the spine. Clin Exp Metastasis. 2014;31(1):47–55.
33. Sahgal A, Atenafu EG, Chao S, et al. Vertebral compression fracture after spine stereotactic body radiotherapy: a multi-institutional analysis with a focus on radiation dose and the spinal instability neoplastic score. J Clin Oncol. 2013;31(27):3426–31.
34. Jawad MS, Fahim DK, Gerszten PC, et al. Vertebral compression fractures after stereotactic body radiation therapy: a large, multi-institutional, multinational evaluation. J Neurosurg Spine. 2016;24(6):928–36.
35. Cunha MVR, Al-Omair A, Atenafu EG, et al. Vertebral compression fracture (VCF) after spine stereotactic body radiation therapy (SBRT): analysis of predictive factors. Int J Radiat Oncol Biol Phys. 2012;84(3):e343–9.
36. Wilden JA, Moran SL, Dekutosky MB, Bishop AT, Shin AYS. Results of vascularized rib grafts in complex spinal reconstruction. J Bone Joint Surg Am. 2006;88-A(4):832–9.
37. Kaltoft B, Kruse A, Jensen LT, Elberg JJ. Reconstruction of the cervical spine with two osteocutaneous fibular flap after radiotherapy and resection of osteoclastoma: a case report. J Plast Reconstr Aesthet Surg. 2012;65(9):1262–4.
38. Elder BD, Ishida W, Goodwin CR, et al. Bone graft options for spinal fusion following resection of spinal column tumors: systematic review and meta-analysis. Neurosurg Focus. 2017;42(1):E16.
39. Miller DJ, Lang FF, Walsh GL, Abi-Said D, Wildrick DM, Gokaslan ZL. Coaxial double-lumen methylmethacrylate reconstruction in the anterior cervical and upper thoracic spine after tumor resection. J Neurosurg. 2000;92(2 Suppl):181–90.
40. Hayashi T, Lord EL, Suzuki A, et al. A comparison of commercially available demineralized bone matrices with and without human mesenchymal stem cells in a rodent spinal fusion model. J Neurosurg Spine. 2016;25(1):133–7.
41. Skovrlj B, Guzman JZ, Al Maaieh M, Cho SK, Iatridis JC, Qureshi SA. Cellular bone matrices: viable stem cell-containing bone graft substitutes. Spine J. 2014;14(11):2763–72.
42. McAnany SJ, Ahn J, Elboghdady IM, et al. Mesenchymal stem cell allograft as a fusion adjunct in one- and two-level anterior cervical discectomy and fusion: a matched cohort analysis. Spine J. 2016;16(2):163–7.
43. Zhou R, Huang Z, Liu X, et al. Kinematics and load-sharing of an anterior thoracolumbar spinal reconstruction construct with PEEK rods: an in vitro biomechanical study. Clin Biomech (Bristol, Avon). 2016;40:1–7.
44. Li Z-J, Wang Y, Xu G-J, Tian P. Is PEEK cage better than titanium cage in anterior cervical discectomy and fusion surgery? A meta-analysis. BMC Musculoskelet Disord. 2016;17(1):379.
45. Pekmezci M, Tang JA, Cheng L, et al. Comparison of expandable and fixed interbody cages in a human cadaver corpectomy model: fatigue characteristics. Clin Spine Surg. 2016;29(9):387–93.
46. Viswanathan A, Abd-El-Barr MM, Doppenberg E, et al. Initial experience with the use of an expandable titanium cage as a vertebral body replacement in patients with tumors of the spinal column: a report of 95 patients. Eur Spine J. 2012;21(1):84–92.
47. Ernstberger T, Kogel M, Konig F, Schultz W. Expandable vertebral body replacement in patients with thoracolumbar spine tumors. Arch Orthop Trauma Surg. 2005;125(10):660–9.
48. Disch AC, Schaser KD, Melcher I, Luzzati A, Feraboli F, Schmoelz W. En bloc spondylectomy reconstructions in a biomechanical in-vitro study. Eur Spine J. 2008;17(5):715–25.
49. Eleraky M, Papanastassiou I, Tran ND, Dakwar E, Vrionis FD. Comparison of polymethylmethacrylate

versus expandable cage in anterior vertebral column reconstruction after posterior extracavitary corpectomy in lumbar and thoraco-lumbar metastatic spine tumors. Eur Spine J. 2011;20(8):1363–70.
50. Viljoen SV, DeVries Watson NA, Grosland NM, Torner J, Dalm B, Hitchon PW. Biomechanical analysis of anterior versus posterior instrumentation following a thoracolumbar corpectomy: laboratory investigation. J Neurosurg Spine. 2014;21(4):577–81.
51. Liu X, Ma J, Park P, Huang X, Xie N, Ye X. Biomechanical comparison of multilevel lateral interbody fusion with and without supplementary instrumentation: a three-dimensional finite element study. BMC Musculoskelet Disord. 2017;18(1):63.
52. Sundaresan N, Shah J, Foley KM, Rosen G. An anterior surgical approach to the upper thoracic vertebrae. J Neurosurg. 1984;61(4):686–90.
53. Sar C, Hamzaoglu A, Talu U, Domanic U. An anterior approach to the cervicothoracic junction of the spine (modified osteotomy of manubrium sterni and clavicle). J Spinal Disord. 1999;12(2):102–6.
54. Darling GE, McBroom R, Perrin R. Modified anterior approach to the cervicothoracic junction. Spine. 1995;20(13):1519–21.
55. Lehman RM, Grunwerg B, Hall T. Anterior approach to the cervicothoracic junction: an anatomic dissection. J Spinal Disord. 1997;10(1):33–9.
56. Kraus DH, Huo J, Burt M. Surgical access to tumors of the cervicothoracic junction. Head Neck. 1995;17(2):131–6.
57. Cohen ZR, Fourney DR, Gokaslan ZL, Walsh GL, Rhines LD. Anterior stabilization of the upper thoracic spine via an "interaortocaval subinnominate window": case report and description of operative technique. J Spinal Disord Tech. 2004;17(6): 543–8.
58. York JE, Walsh GL, Lang FF, et al. Combined chest wall resection with vertebrectomy and spinal reconstruction for the treatment of Pancoast tumors. J Neurosurg. 1999;91(1 Suppl):74–80.
59. Puvanesarajah V, Lina IA, Liauw JA, et al. Systematic approach for anterior corpectomy through a transthoracic exposure. Turk Neurosurg. 2016;26(4):646–52.
60. Baaj AA, Papadimitriou K, Amin AG, Kretzer RM, Wolinsky J-P, Gokaslan ZL. Surgical anatomy of the diaphragm in the anterolateral approach to the spine: a cadaveric study. J Spinal Disord Tech. 2014;27(4):220–3.

16 Metastatic Disease of the Lumbar Spine

Scott E. Dart, Patrick Moody, and Joshua C. Patt

Introduction

Constantly evolving medical technology and treatments in the United States have prolonged the life expectancy of patients with cancer almost globally across the different diagnoses [1]. There has been a 20% increase in 5-year cancer survival rates over the past three decades [2]. In 2017, an estimated 1.7 million new cancer cases are expected to be diagnosed compared with only 600,000 cancer-related deaths. With the estimated number of cancer survivors expected to reach over twenty million by 2026 [3], the number of patients with metastatic disease is expected to increase accordingly. While once upon a time, cancer metastatic to bone was highly predictive of death, patients are now living longer with metastatic disease and how we treat them needs to change as well. Different cancer histologies have different predilection for skeletal metastasis with bone being behind only lung and liver when looking at overall incidence of metastases [4]. The vast majority, approximately 80%, of skeletal metastatic lesions come from breast, prostate, kidney, lung, and thyroid carcinomas [5]. Metastatic bone disease is economically burdensome to the healthcare system with surgical intervention often necessary for palliation. Despite an overall prevalence of 5.3% among US cancer diagnoses, metastatic bone disease contributes an estimated 17% to the national oncologic expense [6].

The spine is the most common site for skeletal metastases with autopsy studies suggesting upwards of a 70% prevalence at death although less than 14% had clinically apparent disease [7]. The thoracic spine is the most common spinal location for metastases and is proportional to its contribution to spinal bone volume. It also constitutes the highest probability of neurologic symptoms due to the small canal size, close proximity of the spinal cord, and predilection for kyphosis. A majority of the literature surrounding spinal metastasis is focused here due this higher incidence and morbidity, mostly related to spinal cord compression. The lumbar spine contributes 16–22% of spinal metastases [8] and is associated clinically with mechanical back pain because of its mobility and weight-bearing functions. Diagnosis is often delayed by several months in these patients as initial imaging can have low sensitivity and complaints can be dismissed as chronic low back pain unless there is a clear history of previous metastatic disease. Radicular symptoms often warrant earlier advanced imaging and, therefore, a more

S. E. Dart, MD · P. Moody, MD
Department of Orthopaedic Surgery, Carolinas Medical Center, Atrium Health, Charlotte, NC, USA
e-mail: scott.dart@carolinashealthcare.org; patrick.moody@carolinashealthcare.org

J. C. Patt, MD, MPH (✉)
Department of Orthopaedic Surgery, Carolinas Medical Center, Atrium Health, Charlotte, NC, USA

Levine Cancer Institute, Atrium Health, Charlotte, NC, USA
e-mail: joshua.patt@carolinashealthcare.org

R. A. W. Marco (ed.), *Metastatic Spine Disease*, https://doi.org/10.1007/978-3-319-76252-4_16

timely diagnosis from onset of initial symptoms. The predominant symptoms of patients presenting with lumbar metastatic disease are axial back pain and/or leg pain, and these patients less commonly present with significant neurologic deficits that can be seen with cord level disease.

Required workup of these patients is mostly reliant on previous workup and current diagnosis as someone with known metastatic disease will require less testing than a patient presenting without a known primary lesion. All patients will require a thoughtful and multidisciplinary team approach in order to develop an appropriate plan. Cauda equina and conus medullaris syndromes can present clearer surgical indications. However, instability, radiculopathy, and intractable pain are the more common reasons for surgical intervention in metastatic lumbar lesions. The mobility and the lordosis characteristics of the lumbar spine can present surgical challenges and decision-making that are unique compared to the thoracic or cervical spine, and, therefore, a comprehensive knowledge of lumbar spine anatomy plays a key role in successful treatment planning.

Anatomy

Multiple mechanisms have been proposed for the predilection of cancer metastasis to the vertebral column with the exact mechanism still unknown. Regardless of the cancer histology, the spine is the most common location of bony metastasis [9–11]. The leading theories involve arterial spread because of a predominance of hematopoietic bone marrow in vertebral bodies [12], venous reflux of the valveless Batson's plexus [13], and drop metastasis from shedding of cerebral or cerebellar tumors. The latter typically results in intradural metastases, which make up a minority of spinal metastases as extradural lesions account for upward of 95% of lesions [14]. As previously mentioned, the lumbar spine contributes 16–22% of spinal metastases [8], which closely corresponds to its overall volume of the bony spinal column.

The lumbar spine provides unique anatomical and biomechanical properties that differentiate it from other segments of the spine and can influence how metastatic disease presents and is treated. The vertebral bodies account for approximately 70% of the vertebral bony volume, and a corresponding percentage of metastatic lesions are found in these anterior elements [15]. The lumbar spine has a capacious spinal canal which contains the nerve roots for the majority of its course, as the conus medullaris ends at the L1 level in most of the population. With more room available to accommodate the neurologic elements and predominantly roots, as opposed to the more proximal spinal cord, catastrophic neurologic compression is less common than in the lumbar spine. The nerve roots of the cauda equina exit the spinal canal directly inferior to their corresponding vertebral pedicle. The lumbar nerve roots have a characteristic vertical course within the spinal canal, allowing central and paracentral disease to affect the traversing nerve roots, while any mass effect at or lateral to the pedicle will affect the exiting nerve root [16, 17].

The lumbar spine plays a key role in sagittal balance with an average of 60° of lordosis with majority of this occurring between L4 and S1 levels. The mobility of the lumbar spine is mostly in the sagittal plane with flexion and extension. There is a small amount of rotation in the caudal portions as the facet orientation progresses from a more sagittal to coronal orientation [18, 19]. Disruption of these anatomic relationships can affect spinal stability despite the intrinsic stability of the lumbar spine.

Clinical Presentation

Epidemiology studies suggest 70–85% of the population will experience low back pain at some point in their lives, and approximately 30% of the population at any time can be experiencing low back pain symptoms [20]. This creates a diagnostic trap for physicians when it comes to diagnosing lumbar spinal metastases. The most common and often initial symptom is back pain in up to 90% of patients with spinal metastatic disease [21]. Most patients will present with poorly characterized, nonmechanical axial back pain, and these vague symptoms are often treated conservatively without initial imaging studies unless certain "red flags" are uncovered. History of cancer and unexplained weight loss are the only two red flags that expedite the need for imaging according to the American College of Radiology Appropriateness Criteria [22]. More classically, we are taught to look for night pain and progressive or unrelenting pain as red flag symptoms. A delay in diagnosis of lumbar spinal metastasis is a common problem especially in the patient without a known history of cancer as their pain is often dismissed as the more common, benign degenerative etiology. A high index of suspicion and clinical intuition along with a detailed history of present illness and cancer risk factors is often necessary to ensure a timely diagnosis.

Pain often precedes neurologic symptoms by several months [5], but the appearance of neurologic symptoms is more commonly the impetus to order imaging studies. Most patients with neurologic symptoms will present with mild sensory deficits and some mild weakness mostly related to thoracic or upper lumbar lesions compressing on the spinal cord [23]. When focusing on the lumbar spine, a majority of neurologic symptoms present as radiculopathy, and this can be from direct compression by the tumor on the exiting nerve root or from mechanical collapse of the neural foramina due to a loss of structural integrity of the surrounding vertebrae. Unfortunately, this clinical presentation precisely mimics the most common lumbar diagnosis, radiculopathy, so it can be easily overlooked. An analogous entity to spinal cord compression of the thoracic or upper lumbar spine is central compression of the nerve roots in the lower lumbar spine causing cauda equina syndrome. Cauda equina syndrome from direct compression of metastatic tumor presents in a subacute fashion with sciatica, altered sensation in a saddle distribution, micturition dysfunction, and fecal dysfunction being the most prominent symptoms [24]. This incidence is not published in the literature with most case reports suggesting intradural spinal metastasis as the more common implicating lesion [25]. The much more common presentation for lumbar spinal metastasis is nonspecific axial back pain, as previously discussed, or symptomatic instability. Instability is defined by the Spine Oncology Study Group as pain, deformity, or neural compromise under physiologic loading [26], and this topic will be further explored in other areas of this book.

Imaging

The American College of Radiology appropriateness criteria suggests no imaging necessary for low back pain until at least 6 weeks of failed conservative treatment except in the presence of any red flags. If the patient has a history of cancer or unexplained weight loss, then this meets the criteria to proceed with imaging modalities as a red flag for malignancy [22]. A previous history of cancer has been shown to be the most reliable "red flag" [27]. The initial imaging of choice when malignancy is suspected is MRI with gadolinium contrast [22] as MRI has proven to be the best imaging modality for spinal tumors showing a 98.5% sensitivity and 98.9% specificity [28] with gadolinium enhancement allowing for better visualization of soft tissue involvement. It is recommended to obtain MRI imaging of the entire spine after diagnosis of a spinal metastatic lesion as there is a 15% incidence of noncontiguous lesions [29].

Standard radiographs have poor sensitivity for diagnosis of spinal malignancy. Studies suggest at least 30–50% involvement of trabecular bone is necessary before a lesion is reliably detectable on radiographs [30]. Pediculolysis, suggested by the "winking owl sign," is pathognomonic for a spinal tumor although is not always seen. Standard radiographs play a more important role in the monitoring of disease progression or spinal alignment over time. Standing or "upright" radiographs along with flexion-extension films play an important and more economic role in the assessment of spinal alignment and stability. These studies are helpful in patients with complaints consistent with spinal instability, as instability is a common indication for surgical intervention for lumbar spinal metastasis. Computed topography scans can be an important imaging modality in patients that are unable to obtain MRI imaging, or impending collapse is suspected. It can also be helpful for surgical planning and assessment of stability.

Workup

A multidisciplinary approach is always the best care strategy when considering surgical intervention for a patient with a metastatic spinal lesion. Patients can present in one of three scenarios: no previous diagnosis of cancer, history of cancer without known metastasis, or known metastatic disease. The first of these requires a more detailed workup to identify the primary tumor etiology. An initial workup consisting of thorough history and physical examination with CT scans of the chest, abdomen, and pelvis can complement routine and tumor-specific labs in diagnosis. This approach can yield the primary tumor source in approximately 85% of cases. Biopsy plays a complementary role in diagnosis as it has only shown to aid in an additional 8% of cases, whereas in isolation it can fail to identify the primary lesion in up to two-thirds of cases [31]. In the latter two patient presentations, a thorough understanding as to the extent of metastatic disease is important in determining prognosis. Incorporating medical oncology and radiation oncology specialists into decision-making early is important as treatment is evolving quickly in each of these fields. Each tumor histology typically responds differently to available non-operative treatments options and therefore is associated with different overall prognoses.

Multiple modalities exist to tailor treatment to each individual patient diagnosed with metastatic cancer of the lumbar spine. Such modalities range from nonoperative options like corticosteroids and radiotherapy to operative treatments that include kyphoplasty and the more invasive corpectomy. Each patient must be evaluated on an individual basis to determine the risks and benefits of treatment options and formulate an appropriate plan. Patient factors such as overall health, tumor histology, extent of metastasis, performance status, neurologic compromise, and expected survival must all be weighed [32]. Most important are the wishes of the patient and his or her family.

Treatment Strategy

Algorithms have been created to guide the care of patients with metastatic spinal disease. Two of the first published algorithms by Tokuhashi and Tomita helped physicians navigate patients down different treatment pathways based on factors such as tumor growth, metastatic site, and general condition of the patient [33, 34]. More recently, Laufer et al. described the NOMS system, which utilizes neurologic, oncologic, mechanical, and systemic criteria to drive decision-making for patients with spine metastasis [35]. In this method, neurologic assessment relies on the extent of epidural spinal cord compression. Oncologic assessment refers to the radiosensitivity of the metastatic subtype. Systemic assessment of the extent of disease burden relies on the staging process. And finally, mechanical assessment relates to intrinsic spinal stability, defined by the validated Spinal Instability Neoplastic Score, or SINS, laid out by the Spine Oncology Study Group [26, 36].

Using a systematic approach, multiple authors have created adaptations of similar algorithms designed to help walk the clinician through the clinical decision-making process from the perspective of the individual patient (see Fig. 16.1) [32, 37]. The National Comprehensive Cancer Network also has a dedicated metastatic spine tumor guideline [38]. Though they all differ slightly, each of these approaches seeks to ultimately help advise what treatment modality is most appropriate for a particular patient, whether nonoperative, operative, or both as we sometimes see in sequential treatment algorithms.

Nonoperative Treatment

Corticosteroids

Corticosteroids provide an anti-inflammatory effect to help alleviate pain and are frequently the first line of treatment for patients found to have spinal metastatic disease. Though their neurological benefit is typically only seen in the first 2 weeks of treatment, the effect can provide the sur-

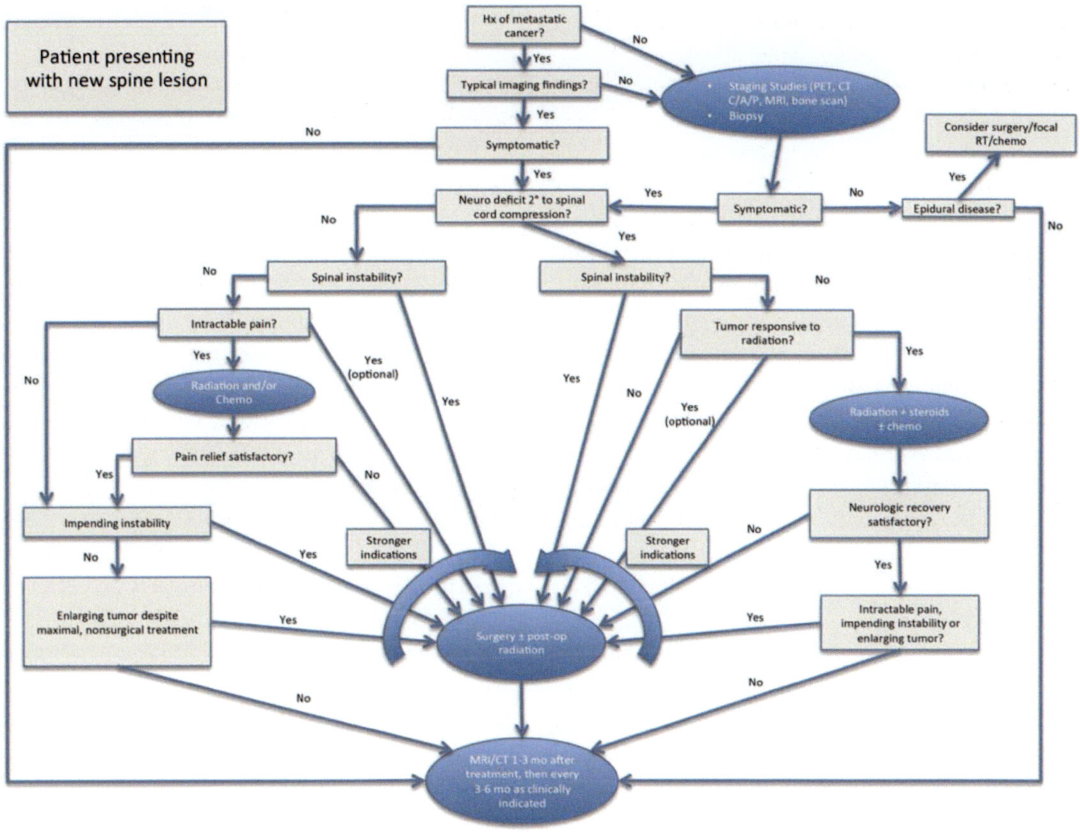

Fig. 16.1 Surgical algorithm for a patient diagnosed with spinal lumbar metastatic lesion (Adapted from Phelps K, Patt J. Diagnosis and management of patients with carcinoma metastatic to the spine. Current Orthopaedic Practice. 2014;25(6):525–533)

geon with time to establish a diagnosis and determine a plan. Corticosteroids are also known to have a tumoricidal effect on leukemias, lymphomas, myelomas, and occasionally breast cancer [39]. Optimum dosing has not yet been defined.

Chemotherapy

Although chemotherapy is a mainstay for treatment of metastatic disease, it is most commonly held as more of an adjuvant therapy in symptomatic spinal metastasis due to its delayed efficacy. The exception to this is if the histology has been determined to be highly chemosensitive, as in the case of lymphoma, neuroblastoma, and seminoma [7]. For patients with multilevel disease, especially those with noncontiguous areas of metastatic spread, or those who are not good surgical candidates due to other comorbidities, chemotherapy may be the best route. Although not directly cytotoxic, hormonal inhibition or blockade can be very helpful in both prostate and breast cancer as well as other gynecologic hormone-sensitive histologies [40]. Again, these modalities are not expected to have an acute effect on disease burden.

Radiotherapy

Most patients diagnosed with metastatic spinal disease will undergo radiation therapy at some point in their treatment. With goals that include pain control, prevention of local disease progression and pathologic fractures, and maintenance of neurologic function, radiation is usually offered

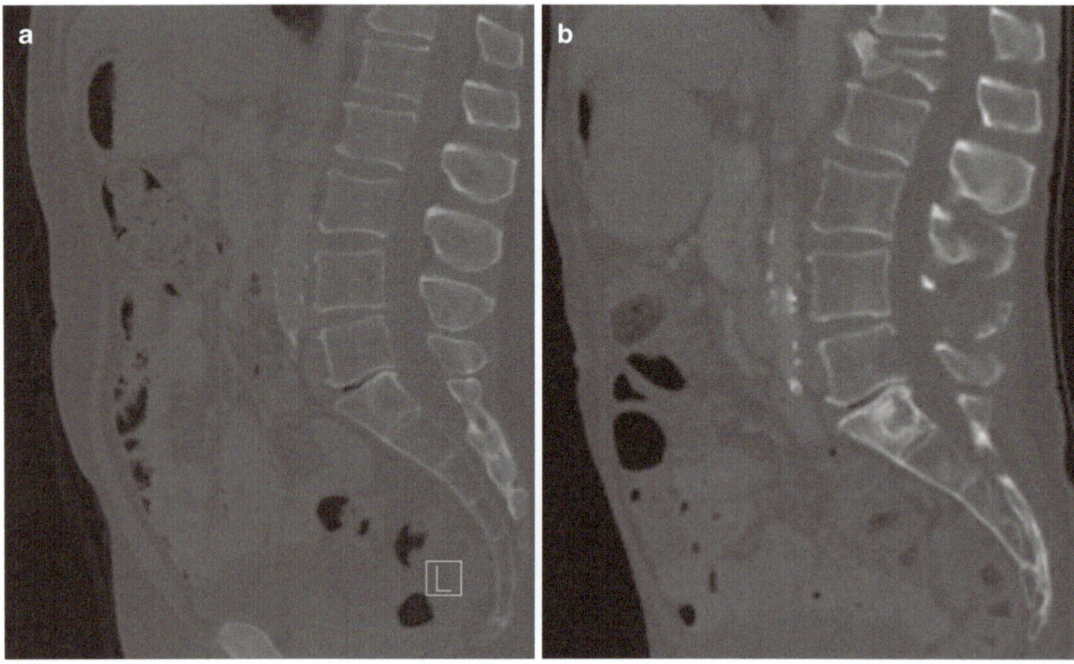

Fig. 16.2 (**a**) Sixty-three-year-old male with metastatic renal cell carcinoma lesion to S1. (**b**) The image to the left is 5 years after being treated successfully with palliative radiotherapy, 35 gray in five fractions. Notice that the patient was treated nonoperatively for multiple lumbar lesions

to those with at least 1 month of life remaining [41] (see Fig. 16.2). Some tumors are highly radiosensitive, including lymphoma, myeloma, and seminomas, so radiation is frequently first-line therapy in these diseases. Others including breast and prostate cancer have a more intermediate radiosensitivity, while radioresistance is common in most others such as renal cell and hepatocellular metastasis [7]. The efficacy of radiation therapy has been well established in patients found to have metastatic spinal cord compression where patients were found to have both significant pain relief and preservation or reestablishment of walking ability [29]. Tumor histology plays a major role in the expected results with external beam radiation.

The limiting factor in radiotherapy is typically the spinal cord, which can only safely tolerate between 3000 and 5000 centigray depending on the study. For this reason, conventional radiotherapy has reduced effects because it lacks precision. However, with the implementation of image-guided, intensity-modulated radiation therapy, or spinal radiosurgery, more effective doses can be safely delivered to spinal metastatic lesions without damaging the spinal cord or other nearby organs. However, these high doses of radiation can also contribute to pathologic fractures, so ongoing research will continue to seek the ideal radiation protocols [42].

Operative Treatment

When nonoperative measures alone will not suffice for metastatic disease of the lumbar spine, operative treatment must be considered. Widely held is the belief that those undergoing surgery for spinal metastases should have a life expectancy of at least 3 months beyond surgery and have the ability to withstand a major surgery. It is important to explain to the patient and their family that surgery will not cure them of their disease, but rather seeks to improve their pain and sometimes function in a palliative manner. Procedures range from percutaneous to invasive, based upon the indication. These indications include five main categories: neural compression, present or impending spinal instability, need for histologic diagnosis, local control, and intractable pain. Regarding diagnosis, surgery is performed when specimen is needed that cannot be obtained by another method, such as needle biopsy. The other indications will be discussed in more detail.

Neural Compression

The role of surgery must be considered carefully for patients with neural compromise. Recovery can be variable for those with deficits either at the cord or root level. However, if possible, acute changes in neurologic status in a patient with metastatic spinal disease should be addressed early, including the scenario of cauda equine syndrome. Those with metastatic spinal cord compression who have surgery within 48 h of symptom onset have been shown to have better neurologic outcomes [43]. An estimated 30% of patients found to have weakness will progress to paraplegia in 1 week [44]. Surgery can provide a more immediate form of intervention compared to other modalities.

In 2005, the work of Patchell et al. reported that decompression surgery and radiation were superior to radiation alone [45]. The study was stopped early because more surgical subjects regained or sustained the ability to walk for a longer period of time. Prior to this study, surgery had fallen out of favor when research showed no benefit for surgery with adjuvant radiation compared to radiotherapy alone for compressive spinal epidural metastasis [46]. However, the previous standard for decompression of metastatic spinal metastasis was a laminectomy. Given that most metastasis of the spine occurs in the vertebral body [47], laminectomies are inadequate for decompression and potentially destabilized the spine. The key element of the Patchell study was that surgery included "direct decompression" of the tumor on the spinal cord, in stark contrast to the old standard of laminectomy which sought to indirectly alleviate pressure on the spinal cord. The Patchell study has several limitations, and the findings cannot be routinely applied to patients with metastatic spinal cord compression. The limitations of the Patchell study are discussed in the chapter entitled "Metastatic Spine Disease: Critical Evaluation of the Current Literature."

Earlier research pointed toward the use of more effective surgical technique. In 1988, Kostuik et al. found anterior decompressions much more successful in neurologic return compared to posterior decompressions [47]. They recommended anterior decompression and stabilization with methyl methacrylate and internal fixation for one- to two-level disease or significant kyphosis. The work of Harrington released that same year also showed good results with anterior decompression and stabilization augmented by methyl methacrylate and anterior distraction rods [48]. He utilized an anterior approach that required detachment of the posterolateral corner of the diaphragm for the upper lumbar vertebrae, while below the diaphragm he used a retroperitoneal or intraperitoneal approach to access the remainder of the lumbar vertebrae. Once considered very risky because of the potential for vascular or superior hypogastric plexus damage, the designation and specialization of approach surgeons has made anterior approaches safer.

Posterior decompression still has a utility, especially for the 30% of patients whose metastases present posterior to the vertebral body. Though Harrington noted complications with the use of posterior stabilization, he did support its use when a lengthy anterior fixation was unable to achieve rigid stability, posterior instability developed due to facet joint destruction, or anterior or posterior lesions presented from L3 distally [48]. Many times, both anterior and posterior approaches are required to establish a circumferential spinal cord decompression. Such can be the case with three column involvement, multilevel vertebral body or epidural tumor, or major spinal deformity [49].

For most patients, it is now generally accepted that the location of the epidural compression should dictate the approach to decompression [37]. Yet in some patients, this is not always possible. Some patients who require vertebrectomy or circumferential decompression and fusion are poor candidates due to comorbidities such as poor pulmonary function, previous surgery, previous radiotherapy, or unresectable, anterior paraspinal tumor or scar. When an anterior approach could be difficult for these patients, circumferential decompression and spondylectomy can be accomplished via a single-stage posterolateral transpedicular approach. With this approach, the surgeon can perform a corpectomy while preserving the roots [49]. Among other options is the lateral transpsoas approach which provides great access to the lumbar spine though is limited by the pelvis in its exposure of L5. Also becoming popular is the concept of minimally invasive approaches. These include the Wiltse muscle-splitting approach, which gives direct access to the junction between the articular and transverse processes for dorsal decompression and partial vertebrectomy [50]. Reducing morbidity by minimally invasive surgery is important for cancer patients with significant comorbidities.

Instability

One of the main causes of neural compression in those with lumbar metastatic disease is spinal instability. Many classifications have been devised, but as mentioned earlier, the Spinal Instability Neoplastic Score presents a validated tool for mechanical assessment featured in the NOMS system of treatment strategy. This score takes into account both clinical signs and radiographic findings to predict instability [26]. Prior to the development of the SINS, physicians considered the work of Taneichi et al., who determined that 35–40% involvement of the vertebral body or 20–25% involvement with neural arch destruction were criteria for impending collapse of the thoracolumbar and lumbar spine, indicating surgical intervention [51].

The goal in treating spinal instability is rigid fixation, but the approach must take into account where decompression must occur, if necessary. Decompression, especially circumferential decompression, can destabilize the spine. Stabilization can have both anterior and posterior elements. Anteriorly, stabilization can be augmented with polymethylmethacrylate, allograft, and static or expandable cages, the latter of which can be metal or polyetheretherketone (PEEK). Posterior instrumentation options range from the more common pedicle screw to the use of hooks and tension bands. The use of fusion should be considered, but most cases do not require it given the limited life expectancy of the patient. Decortication is not generally recommended because it can weaken the bone and remove a barrier to tumor spread. Because both fusion and decortication are not always required, percutaneous screw fixation provides an excellent option for immediate stability while avoiding the morbidity of open procedures [52] (see Fig. 16.3). This is especially important for cancer patients with advanced disease who may not tolerate an extensive exposure and blood loss. Regardless of exposure, a long construct is usually needed. To create a durable construct, one must have good points of fixation. The advantage of posterior instrumentation of the lumbar spine is the ability to achieve fixation in the nearby sacrum as well as the pelvis. The use of sacral 2 alar-iliac screws is becoming more popular and provides another tool for rigid fixation [53].

Local Control

Most patients undergoing surgery for spinal metastatic disease will have intralesional tumor resection to provide neural decompression, stability, and gross total resection [7]. It is rare for patients to undergo en bloc resection, where the entire tumor is removed with margins, or even marginal resection. However, en bloc resection can be performed successfully in carefully selected patients with solitary metastasis and a long disease-free interval. These circumstances are considered in the algorithm of Tomita [33], and en bloc resections have had favorable outcomes [54] in those who could tolerate the morbidity of the surgery (see Fig. 16.4). Though outcomes may improve with en bloc resections in

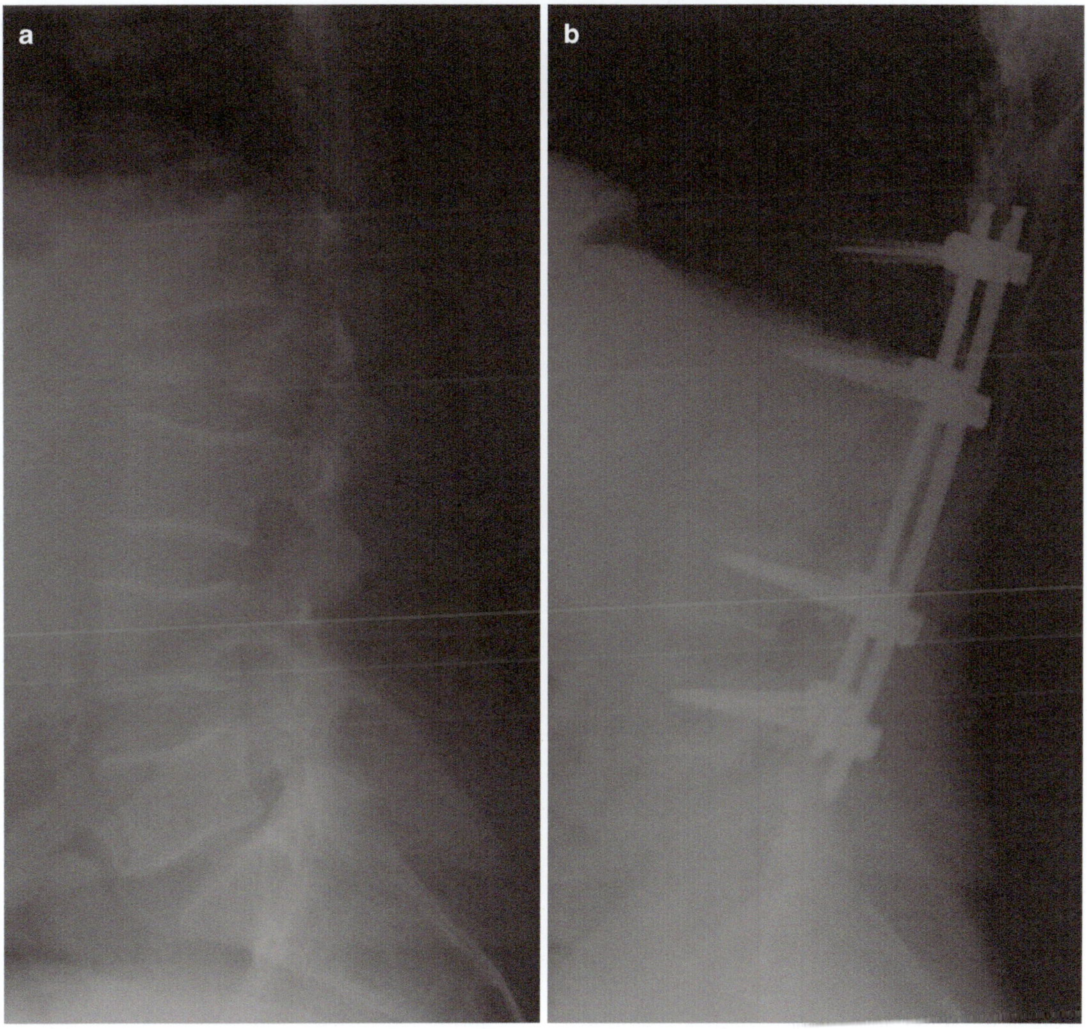

Fig. 16.3 (**a**) Pre- and (**b**) postoperative lateral lumbar radiographs of a 65-year-old gentleman with metastatic small cell carcinoma resulting in a pathologic L2 compression fracture. A posterior spinal instrumentation and fusion using percutaneous technique from T12 to L4 was performed

specified patients, no clear role exists for en bloc resection with most histologies.

Pain

Pain can have one or more of many origins in a patient with lumbar spine metastatic disease. As discussed earlier, neural compression and instability can generate tremendous pain. Painful pathologic fractures and microfractures in bone weakened by the metastatic lesion can also occur in this patient population. Vertebral compression fractures are the most common skeletal complication of metastatic cancer. Intractable pain, recalcitrant to radiation, chemotherapy, and bracing, is an indication for surgery. While decompression and instrumentation are options for neural compression and instability, vertebroplasty and kyphoplasty provide a treatment for pain resulting from pathologic fractures. Often used to treat osteoporotic vertebral compression fractures, these minimally invasive procedures involve the injection of cement into the vertebral

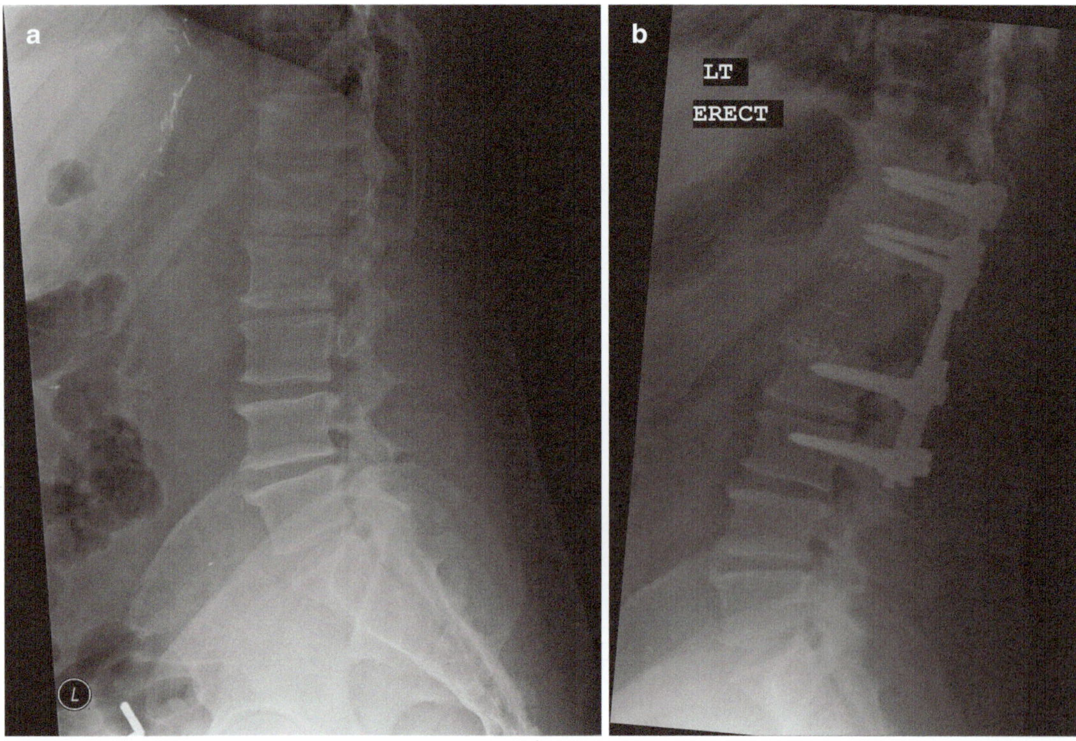

Fig. 16.4 (**a**) Pre- and (**b**) postoperative lateral radiographs of the thoracolumbar spine from a 62-year-old gentleman with stage IV colon cancer resulting in a pathologic fracture of L1 and epidural spinal cord compression. He would undergo en bloc resection of L1 with anterior inter- body fusion T12–L2, T12–L2 laminectomy for decompression, with posterior spinal instrumentation and fusion from T11 to L3

body to stabilize the fracture and attempt to restore alignment. They differ in that kyphoplasty involves the placement of a balloon that creates a cavity into which cement is slowly injected while vertebroplasty involves the direct injection of cement into the vertebral body. These procedures have been successful in treating vertebral compression fractures with short- and long-term pain relief [55].

Conclusion

In summary, lumbar spine metastatic disease presents a challenging problem for the patient and multidisciplinary treatment team. There are several aspects of the lumbar spine that differentiate it from the more cephalad levels of the spine. The most significant is that the lumbar roots are much more accommodating to compression than the thoracic spine that encased the spinal cord, and therefore, catastrophic neurologic injury is much less common. The other important aspect is that the naturally lordotic lumbar spine is intrinsically more stable than the thoracic or cervical levels, so again, it can more frequently be treated by nonoperative means or minimally invasive means.

Once the diagnosis is reached after a proper workup including imaging, a treatment plan should be devised with the aid of established algorithms to best fit the wishes of the patient and his or her family. This plan will include either nonoperative or operative treatment, for which there are many options due to the development of technology and novel approaches and techniques over the years. Although a cure is not the ultimate goal, treatment can lead to significant improvement in the quality of life for the patient.

References

1. Luksanapruksa P, et al. Perioperative complications of spinal metastases surgery. Clin Spine Surg. 2017;30(1):4–13.
2. American Cancer Society. Cancer Facts and Figures 2017. Atlanta: American Cancer Society; 2017.
3. Miller KD, et al. Cancer treatment and survivorship statistics, 2016. CA Cancer J Clin. 2016;66(4):271–89.
4. Disibio G, French SW. Metastatic patterns of cancers: results from a large autopsy study. Arch Pathol Lab Med. 2008;132(6):931–9.
5. Guillevin R, et al. Spine metastasis imaging: review of the literature. J Neuroradiol. 2007;34(5):311–21.
6. Schulman KL, Kohles J. Economic burden of metastatic bone disease in the U.S. Cancer. 2007;109(11):2334–42.
7. Rose PS, Buchowski JM. Metastatic disease in the thoracic and lumbar spine: evaluation and management. J Am Acad Orthop Surg. 2011;19(1):37–48.
8. Brihaye J, et al. The management of spinal epidural metastases. Adv Tech Stand Neurosurg. 1988;16:121–76.
9. Harrington K. Metastatic disease of the spine. In: Orthopaedic management of metastatic bone disease. St. Louis: Moshy Co.; 1988.
10. Bos GD, Edersold M, McLeod RA. Lesions of the spine. In: Sim FH, editor. Diagnosis and treatment of metastatic bone disease. New York: Raven Press; 1988.
11. Boland PJ, Lane JM, Sundaresan N. Metastatic disease of the spine. Clin Orthop Relat Res. 1982;169:95–102.
12. Arguello F, et al. Pathogenesis of vertebral metastasis and epidural spinal cord compression. Cancer. 1990;65(1):98–106.
13. Batson OV. The function of the vertebral veins and their role in the spread of metastases. Ann Surg. 1940;112(1):138–49
14. Jacobs WB, Perrin RG. Evaluation and treatment of spinal metastases: an overview. Neurosurg Focus. 2001;11(6):e10.
15. Bhatt AD, et al. Current and emerging concepts in non-invasive and minimally invasive management of spine metastasis. Cancer Treat Rev. 2013;39(2):142–52.
16. Weinstein PR. The application of anatomy and pathophysiology in the management of lumbar spine disease. Clin Neurosurg. 1980;27:517–40.
17. Crock HV. Normal and pathological anatomy of the lumbar spinal nerve root canals. J Bone Joint Surg Br. 1981;63B(4):487–90.
18. Schneck CD. The anatomy of lumbar spondylosis. Clin Orthop Relat Res. 1985;193:20–37.
19. Ebraheim NA, et al. Anatomic considerations of the lumbar isthmus. Spine (Phila Pa 1976). 1997;22(9):941–5.
20. Andersson GB. Epidemiological features of chronic low-back pain. Lancet. 1999;354(9178):581–5.
21. Gilbert RW, Kim JH, Posner JB. Epidural spinal cord compression from metastatic tumor: diagnosis and treatment. Ann Neurol. 1978;3(1):40–51.
22. Patel ND, et al. ACR appropriateness criteria low back pain. J Am Coll Radiol. 2016;13(9):1069–78.
23. White AP, et al. Metastatic disease of the spine. J Am Acad Orthop Surg. 2006;14(11):587–98.
24. Korse NS, et al. Cauda Equina syndrome: presentation, outcome, and predictors with focus on micturition, defecation, and sexual dysfunction. Eur Spine J. 2017;26(3):894–904.
25. Kotil K, Kilinc BM, Bilge T. Spinal metastasis of occult lung carcinoma causing cauda equina syndrome. J Clin Neurosci. 2007;14(4):372–5.
26. Fisher CG, et al. A novel classification system for spinal instability in neoplastic disease: an evidence-based approach and expert consensus from the Spine Oncology Study Group. Spine (Phila Pa 1976). 2010;35(22):E1221–9.
27. Henschke N, et al. Red flags to screen for malignancy in patients with low-back pain. Cochrane Database Syst Rev. 2013;(2):CD008686.
28. Buhmann Kirchhoff S, et al. Detection of osseous metastases of the spine: comparison of high resolution multi-detector-CT with MRI. Eur J Radiol. 2009;69(3):567–73.
29. Maranzano E, Latini P. Effectiveness of radiation therapy without surgery in metastatic spinal cord compression: final results from a prospective trial. Int J Radiat Oncol Biol Phys. 1995;32(4):959–67.
30. Edelstyn GA, Gillespie PJ, Grebbell FS. The radiological demonstration of osseous metastases. Experimental observations. Clin Radiol. 1967;18(2):158–62.
31. Rougraff BT, Kneisl JS, Simon MA. Skeletal metastases of unknown origin. A prospective study of a diagnostic strategy. J Bone Joint Surg Am. 1993;75(9):1276–81.
32. Phelps KP, Patt JC. Diagnosis and management of patients with carcinoma metastatic to the spine. Curr Orthop Pract. 2014;25(6):525–33.
33. Tomita K. Surgery strategy for spinal metastases. Spine (Phila Pa 1976). 2001;26(3):298–306.
34. Tokuhashi Y, et al. A revised scoring system for preoperative evaluation of metastatic spine tumor prognosis. Spine (Phila Pa 1976). 2005;30(19):2186–91.
35. Laufer I, et al. The NOMS framework: approach to the treatment of spinal metastatic tumors. Oncologist. 2013;18:744–51.
36. Fourney DR, et al. Spinal instability neoplastic score: an analysis of reliability and validity from the spine oncology study group. J Clin Oncol. 2011;29(22):3072–7.
37. Walker MP, et al. Metastatic disease of the spine: evaluation and treatment. Clin Orthop Relat Res. 2003;(415 Suppl):S165–75.
38. National Comprehensive Cancer Network: NCCN Guidelines—Metastatic Spine Tumors. https://www.nccn.org/professionals/physician_gls/pdf/cns.pdf. Retrieved April 30, 2017.

39. Cole JS, Patchell RA. Metastatic epidural spinal cord compression. Lancet Neurol. 2008;7(5):459–66.
40. Sciubba DM, et al. Diagnosis and management of metastatic spinal disease. J Neurosurg Spine. 2010;13:94–108.
41. Gerszten PC, Mendel E, Yamada Y. Radiotherapy and radiosurgery for metastatic spine disease: what are the options, indications, and outcomes? Spine (Phila Pa 1976). 2009;34(22 Suppl):S78–92.
42. Boyce-Fappiano D, et al. Analysis of the factors contributing to vertebral compression fractures after spine stereotactic radiosurgery. Int J Radiat Oncol Biol Phys. 2017;97(2):236–45.
43. Quraishi NA, et al. Effect of timing of surgery on neurological outcome and survival in metastatic spinal cord compression. Eur Spine J. 2013;22:1383–8.
44. Yalamanchili M, Lesser GJ. Malignant spinal cord compression. Curr Treat Options in Oncol. 2003;4:509–16.
45. Patchell RA, et al. Direct decompressive surgical resection in the treatment of spinal cord compression caused by metastatic cancer: a randomised trial. Lancet. 2005;366(9486):643–8.
46. Young RF, Post EM, King GA. Treatment of spinal epidural metastases. Randomized prospective comparison of laminectomy and radiotherapy. J Neurosurg. 1980;53:741–8.
47. Kostuik JP, et al. Spinal stabilization of vertebral column tumors. Spine (Phila Pa 1976). 1988;13(3):250–6.
48. Harrington KD. Anterior decompression and stabilization of the spine as a treatment for vertebral collapse and spinal cord compression from metastatic malignancy. Clin Orthop Relat Res. 1988;233:177–97.
49. Bilsky MH, et al. Single-stage posterolateral transpedicle approach for spondylectomy, epidural decompression, and circumferential fusion of spinal metastases. Spine (Phila Pa 1976). 2000;25(17):2240–9.
50. Zairi F, et al. Minimally invasive decompression and stabilization for the management of thoracolumbar spine metastasis. J Neurosurg Spine. 2012;17:19–23.
51. Taneichi H, et al. Risk factors and probability of vertebral body collapse in metastases of the thoracic and lumbar spine. Spine (Phila Pa 1976). 1997;22(3):239–45.
52. Lee Y, Kuper M. Percutaneous pedicle screw fixation in the lumbar spine. In: Wang JC, editor. Advanced reconstruction: spine. Rosemont: AAOS; 2011. p. 471–6.
53. Chang T, et al. Low profile pelvic fixation: anatomic parameters for sacral alar-iliac fixation versus traditional iliac fixation. Spine (Phila Pa 1976). 2009;34(5):436–40.
54. Yao KC, et al. En bloc spondylectomy for spinal metastases: a review of techniques. Neurosurg Focus. 2003;15(5):1–6.
55. Allen RT, Phillips FM. Kyphoplasty and vertebroplasty. In: Wang JC, editor. Advanced reconstruction: spine. Rosemont: AAOS; 2011. p. 651–60.

Vertebral Body Reconstruction in Metastatic Spine Disease

17

Zoe Zhang, Ahmed Mohyeldin, and Ehud Mendel

Introduction

The spine is the most common site of osseous metastases with 5–10% of cancer patients developing spinal metastases [1]. Of these, 60–80% are located in the thoracic region. Bone metastases disturb the activities of osteoclasts and osteoblasts, replacing the bone with tumor cells. Loss of bone can lead to the development of biological pain that is present regardless of body position, movement, and loading of the spine. When metastases result in pathologic fractures, patients report pain with movement and with loading the spine. In addition to pain, these fractures can also lead to instability, which in turn can cause neurologic deficits. This severely affects a patient's quality of life and can lead to joint contractures, muscle atrophy, pressure sores, pneumonia, and cardiovascular complications.

Z. Zhang, MD
Central Ohio Neurological Surgeons, Westerville, OH, USA
e-mail: zoe.z.zhang@gmail.com

A. Mohyeldin, MD, PhD
Department of Neurosurgery, Ohio State University Wexner Medical Center, Columbus, OH, USA
e-mail: Ahmed.mohyeldin@osumc.edu

E. Mendel, MD, MBA, FACS (✉)
Department of Neurosurgery, The Ohio State University—Wexner Medical Center, The James Cancer Hospital, Columbus, OH, USA
e-mail: Ehud.Mendel@osumc.edu

Surgical intervention in appropriately selected patients can dramatically impact quality of life. In addition, it can obtain tissue for diagnosis, decompress neural structures, and reconstruct stability and deformities. Unfortunately, surgery itself can cause instability via removal of affected vertebral bodies, pedicles, and facets. Denis' three-column model dictates that, in the thoracolumbar spine, two of the three columns must be maintained [2]. Thus, reconstruction is necessary to secure the spinal column from collapse and in turn damage to nerves and the spinal cord. Stabilization methods for vertebral reconstruction are ever improving with new materials and improved design. Though each year there are new products for clinical use or trial, the basic strategies remains the same: fixation and augmentation.

Fixation

Also known as instrumentation or implants, they come in a variety of sizes and shapes, i.e., screws, plates, rods, wires, hooks, and cages. All fixation devices are designed to stabilize the spinal column and they do so immediately upon placement. The goals of instrumentation are to (1) immobilize the weakened or destroyed spinal column until bony fusion occurs, (2) maintain the spinal canal from compression, (3) restore vertebral height and reestablish the alignment of the spine, and (4) allow early recovery and mobilization of patients.

R. A. W. Marco (ed.), *Metastatic Spine Disease*, https://doi.org/10.1007/978-3-319-76252-4_17

Implants made from prosthetic materials such as metal serve to form stiff constructs to maintain spinal stability. In the last two decades, a vast array of systems have been available: Harrington, Cotrel-Dubousset, Luque, Wisconsin Drummond, Vermont Internal Fixator, AO Fixateur Interne, Texas Scottish Rite, Isola, R-F, Edwards, anterior Moss-Miami and Z plate-anterior thoracolumbar construct system, Stryker, Medtronic, Globus, K2M, and Depuy Synthes to name a few. The choice of a particular instrumentation system depends on the purpose of surgery, the anatomic location, the degree of deformity, and the surgeon preference.

Anterior instrumentation with cage, plate or screw systems are preferred in the cervical spine. It is also a valuable technique in the thoracic and lumbar vertebral spine [3], however, with higher morbidity due to chest, abdominal, or retroperitoneal cavity exposure. Posterior instrumentation can be performed using pedicle screws, rods, or wire systems. Crosslinks may help to reinforce the stabilization [4]. Screws come in various different materials, sizes, and lengths. Titanium, cobalt chromium, and stainless steel are the most common alloys. Sizes and lengths depend on whether they are placed anteriorly or posteriorly. For reconstruction in metastatic patients, translaminar screws are rarely used as they are small but also because the lamina is usually removed during the decompression. Alloy wires are suitable to assist in binding the bony structures posteriorly especially in the cervical spine. There are multiple systems available including Wisconsin posterior wiring, Hartshill rectangles, and Luque wires. The wires resist tension loads by connecting to the spinous processes and lamina or sublaminarly. Similar to the wiring systems, hooks are also an option for posterior fixation by anchoring under the lamina.

Cages: The typical spinal cages are made from different materials and come in different shapes and sizes. They range from simple titanium non-expandable mesh cages to carbon fiber-reinforced polyetheretherketone (CFRP) cages [5]. They can also be expandable and have various endplate angulation capabilities [6, 7]. The advantage of using cages over a bone strut graft is the modular capability of these implants allows optimization of diameter and length for the reconstruction. The goal is to be compatible with the host tissue and act harmoniously with bone graft packing. Anterior column reconstruction with a cage is effective in preventing the progression of a kyphotic deformity.

Augmentation

In the reconstruction of the vertebral body, another strategy is filling or packing bony defects, which were caused by metastases or surgical removal.

Bone cement is a common material used with or without bio-properties of tissue compatibility and osteogenesis. They can be found in powder or liquid form. Chemically, their makeup can include calcium orthophosphate [8], Norian non-exothermic hydroxyapatite cement (Norian skeletal repair system), or polymethyl methacrylate. In addition, bone cements can be enhanced by adding other gradients such as nano-hydroxyapatite-coated bone collagen [9].

Bone cement is not only a replacement material but also reinforces strength. For example, after hardening, Norian non-exothermic hydroxyapatite cement had a compressive strength of 20–55 MPa. Though weaker than autogenous cortical bone (50–200 MPa), it was stronger than autogenous cancellous bone (2–20 MPa). Other allogeneic bone grafts have compressive strengths of 4–13 MPa. Bone cement can be injected into a vertebral body percutaneously [10, 11] or in an open fashion. It can also be used to augment screws when the bone is weak, injected into a screw tract or around a screw via a Jamshidi needle [12]. Cement can also serve as a substitute for a cage when placed from a posterior direction [13].

Bone grafts: Autologous bone collected from the iliac crest or fibula of patients are the traditional sources [14]. Ribs also can be collected when approaching the thoracic spine to decrease donor site morbidity. Bone from the vertebral body or lamina can also be collected during dissection or corpectomy for use; however, autografts as a whole are avoided due to possible inclusion of tumor cells.

Allogeneic bone grafts avoid the donor site morbidity and spread of tumor cells. There is also no limit to the amount or size of grafts. Bone products are supplied from a number of different companies, varing from demineralized cancellous bone matrix to cryopreserved viable cortical cancellous bone matrix. To fill the large gap of a corpectomy defect, however, larger sizes of bone are necessary, such as femoral strut allografts, fibular struts, or tricortical iliac crest grafts [15].

The materials mentioned above can be used independently or in combination to stabilize a spine weakened by metastatic disease in a circumferential reconstruction if required.

Surgical Selection

Though the basic reconstruction techniques for spinal metastasis are similar to the trauma or degenerative disorders, extra deliberation is needed in this patient population. Many of these patients do not have a long life expectancy and may have many medical comorbidities, which make surgery a dangerous endeavor and decrease postoperative fusion rates. Consideration of the patient's condition such as degree of tumor spread, speed of disease progression, prognosis, and surgical tolerance must be taken into account. The Tokuhashi index considers the patient's Karnofsky index, neurological status, metastatic type, and lesion resectability to help determine surgical candidacy [16]. The Tokuhashi score correlated well with life expectancy (0–4 < 3 months, 5–8 < 6 months, 9–12 > 6 months) and is also useful in determining the extent of spinal reconstruction as only patients with reasonable life expectancies should be candidates for aggressive reconstructive procedures [17]. The Tomita classification of metastatic stages based on tumor intracompartmental or extracompartmental invasion can also be used in surgical determination [18]. Despite this, recent advances in cancer immunotherapy, particularly clinical trials aimed at blockade of programmed death receptor 1 (PD-1), have dramatically extended survival outcomes in patients with non-small cell lung cancer, melanoma, and renal cell cancer [19]. Approximately one in four or one in five patients who historically had a dismal prognosis are now candidates for immunotherapy due to the molecular genetics of their tumor. These patients may now benefit from surgical intervention despite having a poor Tokuhashi score and considerable systemic disease burden on initial presentation. The ultimate treatment plan is optimally determined by a multidisciplinary team consisting of oncologists, radiation oncologists, radiologists, physiatrists, and spine surgeons with experience in treating patients with oncologic conditions.

Radiographic Studies

The initial study of choice to evaluate axial spine tumors includes plain radiographs which can localize lesions and are diagnostic in particular cases. However, they often require 30–60% loss of mineralization before osteolytic lesions can be detectable, making them unfortunately a poor screening test for neoplastic lesions. Plain film radiographs can identify kyphosis and scoliosis deformities in weight-bearing patients unlike magnetic resonance and computed tomography scans, which are imaged in the supine position, thus resulting in positional reduction of these deformities.

Advances in imaging have improved the sensitivity of detecting primary and secondary tumors of the spine. As a result the repertoire of imaging modalities at the disposal of the practicing clinician is constantly undergoing development to help improve diagnosis and resolve tumor burden from surrounding tissue. The most heavily used imaging techniques include magnetic resonance imaging (MRI), computed tomography (CT), myelogram, positron emission tomography (PET) bone scans, and angiography (Fig. 17.1).

CT and MRI scans have become the standard imaging modalities used to determine the location and extent of tumor burden. MRI provides powerful tissue resolution and can discriminate with the use of gadolinium, tumor from surrounding soft tissue anatomy. CT scans are often used in conjunction with MRI, and their utility is often used

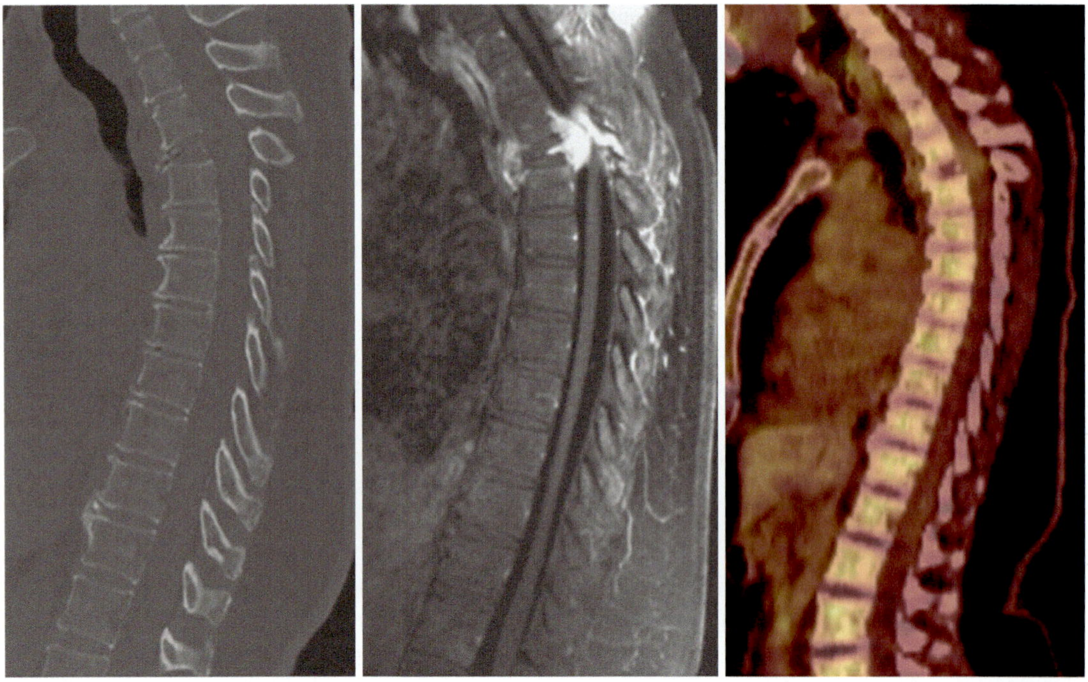

Fig. 17.1 From left to right, sagittal CT scan of the thoracic spine demonstrating a destructive lytic process at T3 with significant loss of height and a kyphotic deformity of the upper thoracic spine in a patient with metastatic disease. Middle panel demonstrates a T1 MRI with gadolinium in the same patient, demonstrating a large enhancing mass within the spinal canal, compressing the spinal cord. PET imaging of the same lesion reveals a likely high-grade malignancy with increased metabolic uptake of glucose

to assess the extent of bony destruction and quality of the surrounding bony architecture. Prior to MRI becoming widely available, CT myelography was the test of choice for assessing cord compression. This imaging modality is now often employed in scenarios where patients cannot obtain an MRI due to either metallic foreign objects or implanted medical devices. Bone scans, PET imaging, and angiography can collectively provide insightful information to supplement MRI and CT data. Bone scans which rely on a nuclear tracer, technetium-99m-methylenediphopshanate, allow for the identification of areas for bone growth or bone breakdown, thus making them highly sensitive but poorly specific for identifying neoplastic processes. PET imaging exploits cancer metabolism and the differential uptake of a glucose-labeled radiotracer by cancer cells. The technique has become popular because it allows for whole-body surveillance in a single study with reasonably accurate anatomical and functional information regarding a tumor. Angiography may often be used dually for diagnostic purposes and therapeutic intervention. It can aid in the diagnosis of a primary vascular lesions such as an aneurysmal bone cyst or a hemangioma. Alternatively it may be used to embolize highly vascular pathologies in the spine such as renal cell carcinoma, thyroid carcinoma, or melanoma while at the same time identifying primary segmental feeders to the tumor.

Preoperative Diagnosis

Ultimately prior to any surgical intervention and in the absence of a leading diagnosis of the lesion of interest, an accurate biopsy is essential to

Table 17.1 There are a number of approaches available depending on the surgical area of interest

	Anterior/lateral	Posterior	Comments
High cervical	Transoral, extraoral, far lateral	Midline	Anterior approaches in this area can lead to high morbidity rates
Cervical	Southwick Robinson	Midline	Anterior approach may be challenging above C3 (mandible) and below C7 (sternum)
Cervicothoracic	Trans-sternal, lateral extracavitary	Midline costotransversectomy	
Thoracic	Thoracotomy, lateral extracavitary	Costotransversectomy, transpedicular	
Thoracolumbar	Lateral extracavitary, retroperitoneal	Midline, posterolateral, transpedicular	Transpedicular becomes difficult at L1 and below as the nerve roots cannot be sacrificed for exposure
Lumbar	Retroperitoneal, transabdominal	Midline, posterolateral	At L5, retroperitoneal becomes less feasible due to the iliac crest and bifurcation of the great vessels

surgical planning and decision-making regarding management. Histopathological examination is most commonly achieved via CT-guided biopsy. This procedure has become safe, economical, and reasonably reliable as percutaneous CT-guided biopsy of spinal lesions is diagnostically accurate 93% of the time, with higher rates of success associated with high-grade lesions versus low-grade lesions. Once all of this data is acquired, the decision to manage and treat these patients is complex and relies on a multidisciplinary team that includes spine surgeons, oncologists, radiation oncologists, access surgeons, and neurovascular surgeons. Compelling arguments for surgery include palliation, decompression, and/or cure with some rare primary lesions; however all of this is factored in the context of the patient's overall survival, prognosis, and extent of disease burden making the decision to operate a very difficult one.

Presurgical Planning and Approach

After a tissue diagnosis is obtained, the decision to operate depends on several factors including tissue histology and grade, surgical accessibility, patient symptoms, and premorbid conditions. Each case must be evaluated on an individual basis. Some tumors' histology may predict a primarily nonoperative intervention such as chemotherapy and/or radiation therapy depending on the cancer's sensitivity to these agents, but patient symptoms or radiographic evidence of instability may dictate a need for operative intervention [20]. Based on anatomy, spinal alignment, and the need for deformity correction, the site of approach can be determined and the extent of surgery can be planned. Table 17.1 shows the approaches available in various areas of the spine. It is important to balance the goals of surgery with a patient's comorbidities to determine if they would do well with an approach. For example, if a patient with a previous transabdominal surgery presents with an L5 lesion compressing the thecal sac anteriorly, then an anterior approach may place the patient at an increased risk of surgery compared to a posterior approach due to previous scar tissue present in the abdominal cavity.

Positioning

Positioning of the patient changes with the approach. In a posterior cervical or upper thoracic surgery, consider fixating the patient's head in a Mayfield with the table moved as rostrally as possible to allow c-arm or X-ray to have access around the base of the bed. In the mid-thoracic to lumbar spines, it is reasonable to use a Jackson table or a table with bolsters to recreate the normal curvature of the spine to restore sagittal alignment.

Ultimately, since 85% of metastases occur in the thoracic spine, cooperation with thoracic, general, or vascular surgeons should be considered.

Reconstruction of the Vertebral Body

When a vertebral body is pathologically fractured or has the potential for instability and the patient's medical comorbidities preclude a major surgery, vertebroplasties and kyphoplasties should be considered to augment spine stability. These are procedures performed with either percutaneous injection of cement under radiographic guidance or in an open fashion. It can significantly decrease mechanical pain from fractures or instability and improve quality of life [21]. Kyphoplasties may be helpful in restoring some height loss [22]. Care must be taken in this patient population given the absence of a posterior wall and the risks of posterior cement migration and cord compression. If the patient's tumor is also a chemo-radiosensitive type, cement placement can stabilize a fracture, improving the patient's function and thus qualify the patient to begin systemic treatment.

In Fig. 17.2, a patient with metastatic colon cancer presented with a pathologic fracture associated with mechanical back pain and radiculopathy from nerve root compression. He had extensive metastatic disease including a previous colon resection and residual non-healing incision in his abdomen. A posterior laminectomy with removal of epidural tumor was performed for decompression of the thecal sac, and foraminotomies were performed for his radiculopathy. Posterior pedicle fixation for his mechanical pain was followed by intraoperative vertebroplasty of the pathologically fractured vertebral body.

Oftentimes, if there is cord compression ventrally, the most straightforward way to resect the body and the posterior longitudinal ligament is with a corpectomy. Reconstruction options include bone graft, cages, or methyl methacrylate. Surgical variations range from endoscopic transpedicular partial corpectomy followed with posterior instrumentation to multilevel corpectomy with circumferential stabilization [23, 24].

Technical Considerations

During surgery for these patients, the need for attention to detail and avoidance of complications is paramount for a quick recovery. The majority

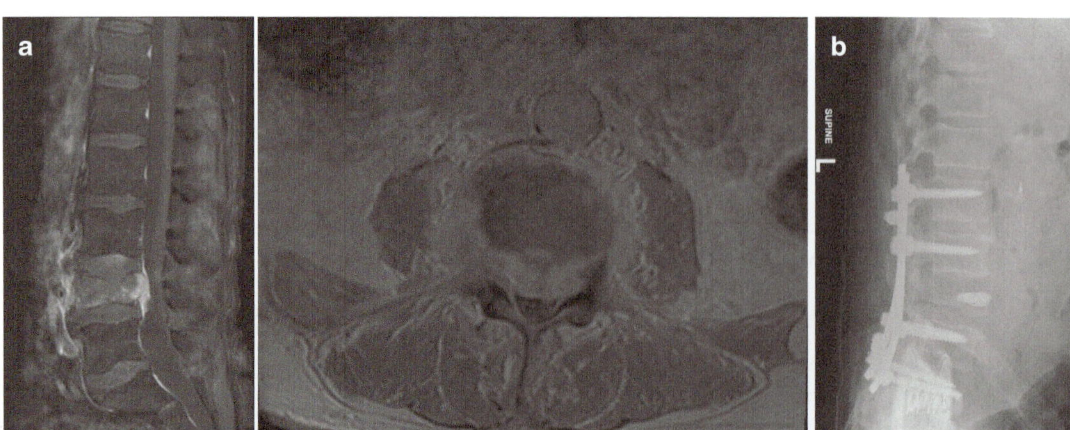

Fig. 17.2 (**a**) MRI post-contrast sagittal and axial views show metastatic colon cancer in L4 with a pathologic fracture and bilateral foraminal compression. (**b**) Postoperative lateral X-rays show a posterior construct with intraoperative cement injection

of these patients require a comprehensive chemotherapy and radiation regiment shortly after surgery.

Posterior pedicle screw placement is an essential step common to many reconstruction procedures. Longer and larger screws are optimal especially in a patient whose bone quality may be osteoporotic or riddled with small osseous metastases [25] (see Fig. 17.3).

The reconstruction of the vertebral body itself is the essential step for anterior weight bearing, deformity correction, and support for alignment correction from posteriorly. Use of a non-expandable cage can be challenging when positioning the cage. Distraction at the level may be necessary to allow the correctly sized cage to be placed, followed by compression. If too short a cage is placed, it can result in migration and neurological compression. An expandable cage can avoid some of these challenges. There are many shapes and sizes with height ranges to fit almost any corpectomy site. Unfortunately, given the expansion is performed by the surgeon's feel and experience, there is a higher risk of cage subsidence. The risk of this can be reduced with proper endplate preparation and a larger-diameter cage size to decrease the pressure placed on the endplates by the cage. Regardless of the expandability

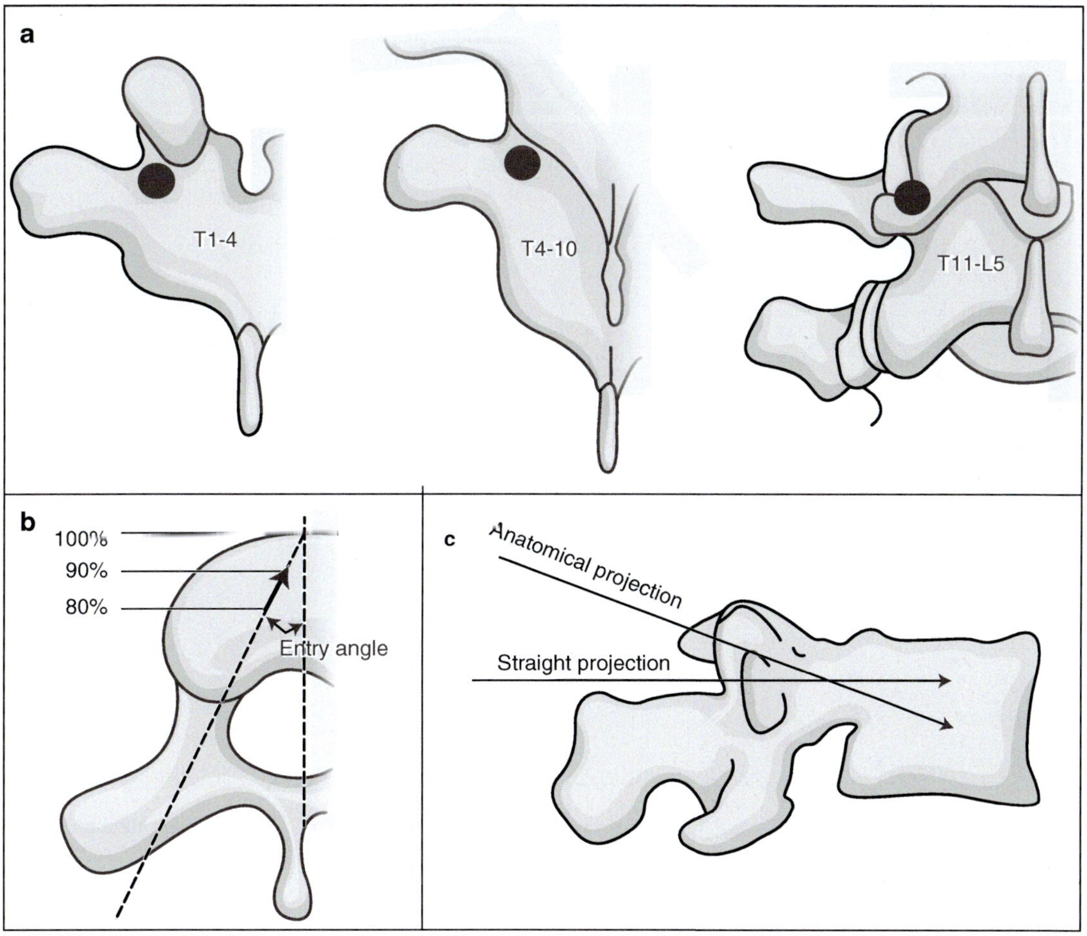

Fig. 17.3 Pedicle screw placement technique: (**a**) the entry points are noted by the black dots. They are usually at the intersection of the transverse process and facet joint, around 3–5 mm from the edge. (**b**) After penetrating the cortex, the medial angle is chosen with a goal of mid-vertebral body without entering the canal. Appropriate screw length should reach the anterior cortex when possible. (**c**) Both the straight and anatomical projections are acceptable. The anatomical projection allows for a longer screw; however, the straight projection allows for better insertional torque [26]

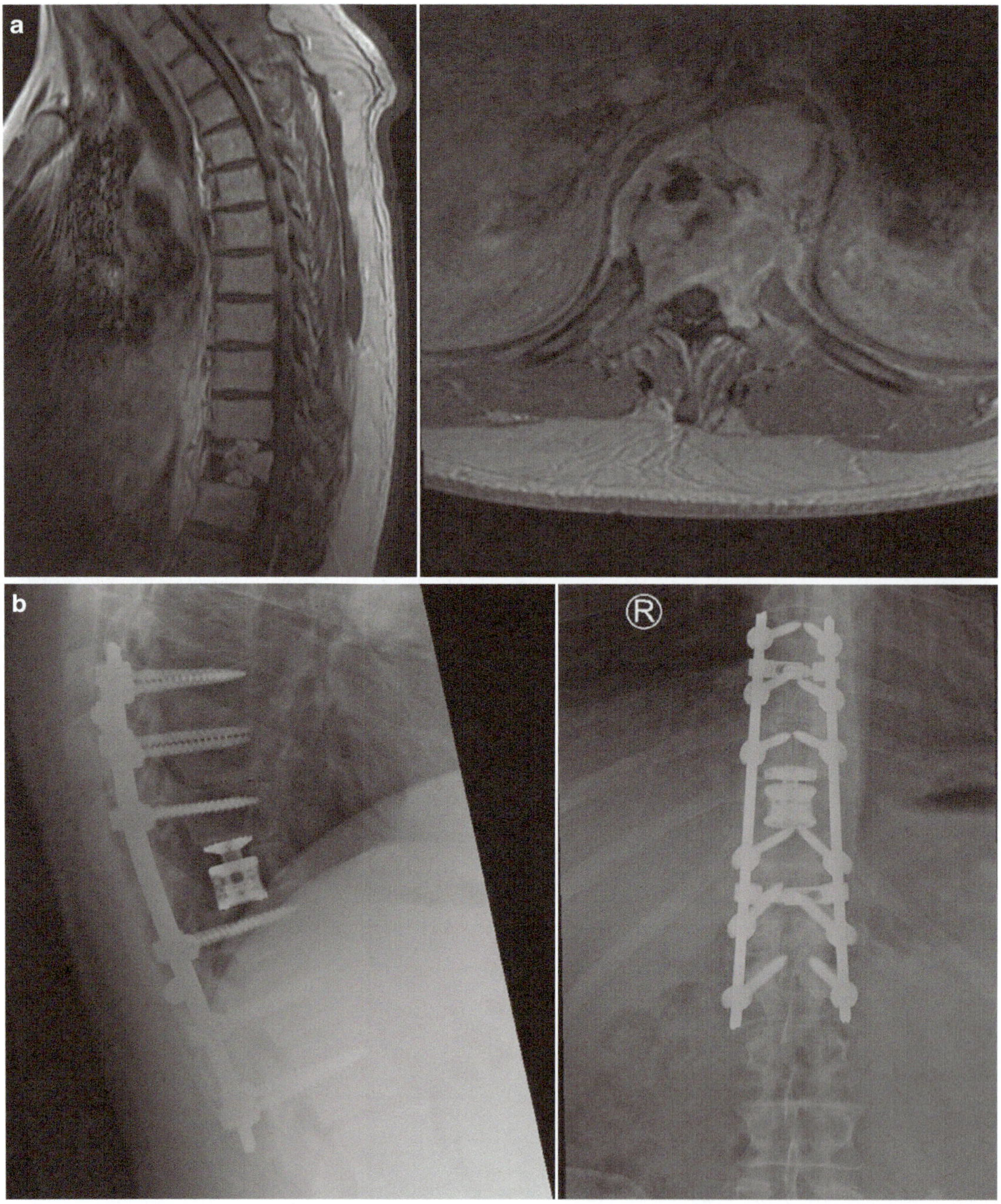

Fig. 17.4 (**a**) Post-contrast MRI sagittal and axial showing a T11 plasmacytoma with an unstable pathologic fracture. (**b**) Postoperative X-rays lateral and AP showing a posterior construct and cage placement through a costotransversectomy approach

of the cage, the angle of the endplates can be quite exacting (see Fig. 17.4).

With two or more levels, there is increased concern for sacrificing nerve roots and their concurrent segmental arteries in the watershed area of thoracic spine [27]. An anterior approach for completion of corpectomy and placement of a cage should be considered strongly in these situations.

If there is not a cage that fits the size and angle of the endplates or the height of the vertebral

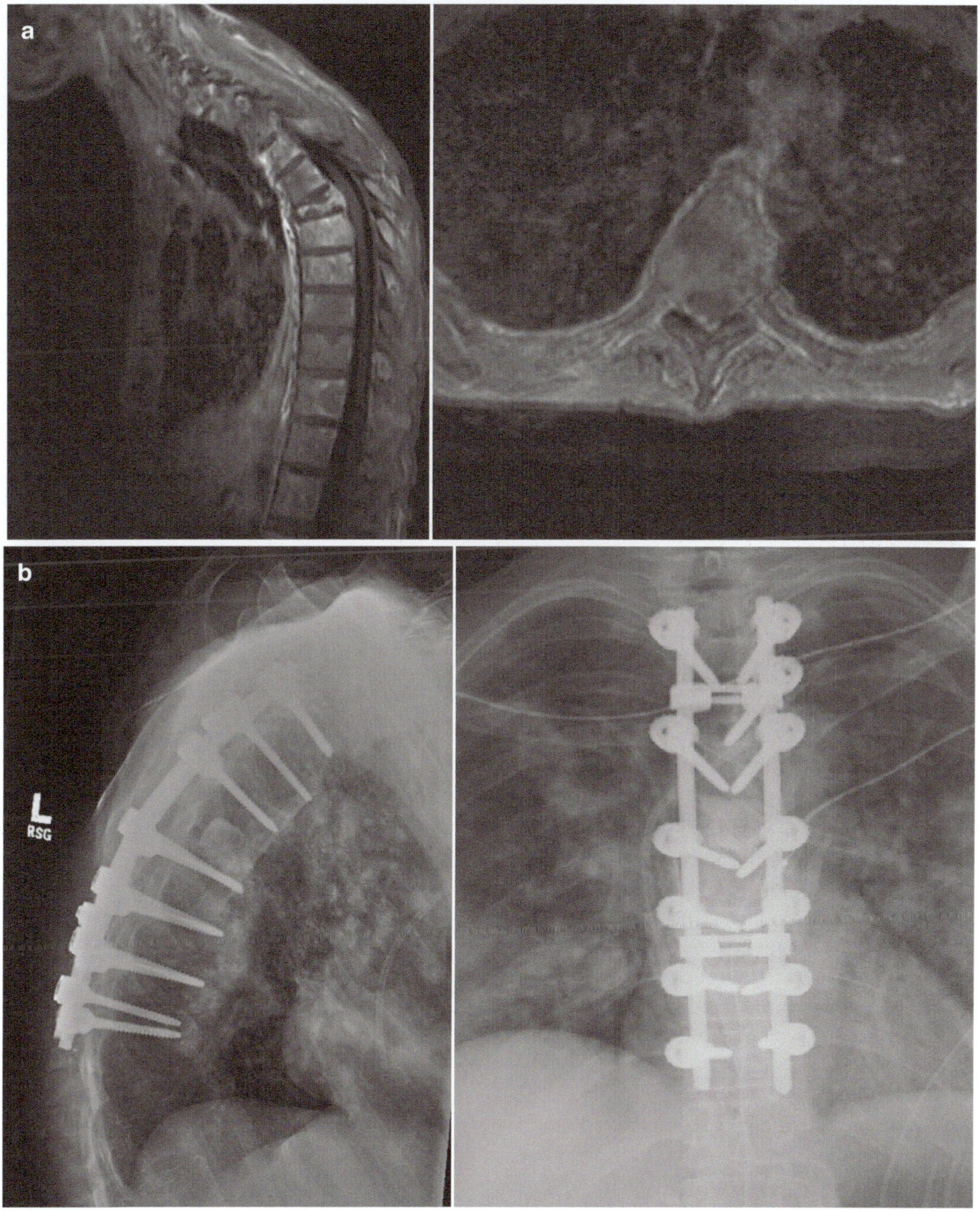

Fig. 17.5 (**a**) Post-contrast MRI sagittal and axial showing metastatic breast cancer to the thoracic spine with a pathologic fracture at T6 resulting in kyphosis. (**b**) Postoperative x-rays lateral and AP showing posterior instrumentation and methylmethacrylate artificial vertebra

body deficit well, methyl methacrylate can be considered. This can be placed into the defect, and as it hardens, irrigation can be used to reduce the effects of the exothermic reaction, and palpation is used to ensure it is not expanding and compressing any neurologic structures. The downside to methyl methacrylate is that an anterior fusion is unlikely to occur (see Fig. 17.5).

Fusion is difficult in this patient population given their medical comorbidities and their prognosis. As a result, careful decortication of the facets, lamina, transverse processes, etc. is critical.

The structural support of this reconstruction is a low-cost option that provides durable stability for most patients with metastatic spinal cord compression. Moreover, subsidence of the cement is less likely compared to cages due to the large surface area of the cement, which decreases the pressure on the adjacent vertebral endplates. The modulus of elasticity of the PMMA cement is closer to that of the adjacent vertebral bodies thereby further decreasing the likelihood of subsidence compared to an expandable, titanium cage. Many authors recommend stabilizing the cement with pins [28] or a chest tube [29] to decrease the likelihood of cement migration.

Discussion

The basics of reconstructing the metastatic spine are the same as for trauma and degenerative processes. However, there are more considerations required in treating the metastatic patient due to their bony disease, medical comorbidities, and life expectancy. Common challenges include severe deformity or instability, increased blood loss on a more fragile patient, previous radiation-induced scarring, and failure of fusion.

Autologous bone grafting, cell saver, and use of bioactive agents such as bone morphogenic protein are not commonly utilized in this patient population [30].

Conclusion

There are challenges associated with reconstructing the vertebral body in metastatic spine patients. Their fragility and prognosis make for difficult procedures even when they would usually be straightforward. The importance of preoperative planning and approach are stressed. Based on the extent of surgery, reconstruction includes augmentation, fixation, and placement of a cage or bone cement.

References

1. Perrin RG, Laxton AW. Metastatic spine disease: epidemiology, pathophysiology, and evaluation of patients. Neurosurg Clin N Am. 2004;15(4):365–73.
2. Denis F. Spinal instability as defined by the three-column spine concept in acute spinal trauma. Clin Orthop Relat Res. 1984;(189):65–76.
3. McDonough PW, Davis R, Tribus C, Zdeblick TA. The management of acute thoracolumbar burst fractures with anterior corpectomy and Z-plate fixation. Spine. 2004;29:1901–8.
4. Krag MH. Biomechanics of thoracolumbar spinal fixation. A review. Spine. 1991;(16):S84–99.
5. Heary RF, Parvathreddy NK, Qayumi ZS, Ali NS, Agarwal N. Suitability of carbon fiber-reinforced polyetheretherketone cages for use as anterior struts following corpectomy. J Neurosurg Spine. 2016;25(2):248–55.
6. Perrini P, Gambacciani C, Martini C, Montemurro N, Lepori P. Anterior cervical corpectomy for cervical spondylotic myelopathy: reconstruction with expandable cylindrical cage versus iliac crest autograft. A retrospective study. Clin Neurol Neurosurg. 2015;139:258–63.
7. Hunt T, Shen FH, Arlet V. Expandable cage placement via a posterolateral approach in lumbar spine reconstructions. J Neurosurg Spine. 2006;5:271–4.
8. Dorozhkin SV. Calcium orthophosphate-containing biocomposites and hybrid biomaterials for biomedical applications. J Funct Biomater. 2015;6:708–832.
9. Li T, Weng X, Bian Y, Zhou L, Cui F, Qiu Z. Influence of nano-HA coated bone collagen to acrylic (polymethylmethacrylate) bone cement on mechanical properties and bioactivity. PLoS One. 2015;10:e0129018.
10. Christodoulou A, Ploumis A, Terzidis I, Pournaras I. Vertebral body reconstruction with injectable hydroxyapatite cement for the management of unstable thoracolumbar burst fractures: a preliminary report. Acta Orthop Belg. 2005;71:597–603.
11. Cho DY, Lee WY, Sheu PC. Treatment of thoracolumbar burst fractures with polymethyl methacrylate vertebroplasty and short-segment pedicle screw fixation. Neurosurgery. 2003;53:1354–60.
12. Moussazadeh N, Rubin DG, McLaughlin L, Lis E, Bilsky MH, Laufer I. Short-segment percutaneous pedicle screw fixation with cement augmentation for tumor-induced spinal instability. Spine J. 2015;15(7):1609–17. https://doi.org/10.1016/j.spinee.2015.03.037.
13. Alleyne CH Jr, Rodts GE Jr, Haid RW. Corpectomy and stabilization with methylmethacrylate in patients with metastatic disease of the spine: a technical note. J Spinal Disord. 1995;8:439–43.
14. Schnee CL, Freese A, Weil RJ, Marcotte PJ. Analysis of harvest morbidity and radiographic outcome using autograft for anterior cervical fusion. Spine. 1997;22:2222–7.

15. Bridwell KH, Lenke LG, McEnery KW, Baldus C, Blanke K. Anterior fresh frozen structural allografts in the thoracic and lumbar spine. Do they work if combined with posterior fusion and instrumentation in adult patients with kyphosis or anterior column defects? Spine. 1995;(20):1410–8.
16. O'Toole DM, Golden AM. Evaluating cancer patients for rehabilitation potential. West J Med. 1991;155:384–7.
17. Tokuhashi Y, Matsuzaki H, Toriyama S, Kawano H, Ohsaka S. Scoring system for the preoperative evaluation of metastatic spine tumor prognosis. Spine (Phila Pa 1976). 1990;15:1110–3.
18. Aoude A, Amiot LP. A comparison of the modified Tokuhashi and Tomita scores in determining prognosis for patients afflicted with spinal metastasis. Can J Surg. 2014;57:188–93.
19. Topalian SL, Hodi FS, Brahmer JR, Gettinger SN, Smith DC, McDermott DF, et al. Safety, activity, and immune correlates of anti-PD-1 antibody in cancer. N Engl J Med. 2012;366(26):2443–54.
20. Bartels RH, van der Linden YM, van der Graaf WT. Spinal extradural metastasis: review of current treatment options. CA Cancer J Clin. 2008;58:245–59.
21. Xie P, Zhao Y, Li G. Efficacy of percutaneous vertebroplasty in patients with painful vertebral metastases: a retrospective study in 47 cases. Clin Neurol Neurosurg. 2015;138:157–61.
22. Garfin SR, Yuan HA, Reiley MA. New technologies in spine: kyphoplasty and vertebroplasty for the treatment of painful osteoporotic compression fractures. Spine. 2001;26:1511–5.
23. Archavlis E, Schwandt E, Kosterhon M, Gutenberg A, Ulrich P, Nimer A, et al. A modified microsurgical endoscopic assisted transpedicular corpectomy of the thoracic spine based on virtual 3D planning. World Neurosurg. 2016;91:424–33.
24. Venkatesh R, Tandon V, Patel N, Chhabra HS. Solitary plasmacytoma of L3 vertebral body treated by minimal access surgery: Common problem different solution! J Clin Orthop Trauma. 2015;6:259–64.
25. Cinotti G, Gumina S, Ripani M, Postacchini F. Pedicle instrumentation in the thoracic spine. A morphometric and cadaveric study for placement of screws. Spine. 1999;(24):114–9.
26. Benzel EC. Biomechanics of spine stabilization. New York: Thieme Medical Publishers; 2001.
27. Sugita S, Murakami H, Demura S, Kato S, Yoshioka K, Yokogawa N, et al. Repeated total en bloc spondylectomy for spinal metastases at different sites in one patient. Eur Spine J. 2015;24:2196–200.
28. Bilsky MH, Boland P, Lis E, Raizer JJ, Healey JH. Single-stage posterolateral transpedicle approach for spondylectomy, epidural decompression, and circumferential fusion of spinal metastases. Spine (Phila Pa 1976). 2000;25(17):2240–50.
29. Miller DJ, Lang FF, Walsh GL, Abi-Said D, Wildrick DM, Gokaslan ZL. Coaxial double-lumen methylmethacrylate reconstruction in the anterior cervical and upper thoracic spine after tumor resection. J Neurosurg Spine. 2000;92(2):181–90.
30. Thawani JP, Wang AC, Than KD, Lin CY, La Marca F, Park P. Bone morphogenetic proteins and cancer: review of the literature. Neurosurgery. 2010;66(2):233–46. ; discussion 246. https://doi.org/10.1227/01.NEU.0000363722.42097.C2.

Lumbosacral Metastatic Spine Disease

18

Andrew B. Kay and Rex A.W. Marco

Introduction

The treatment of metastatic disease to the lumbosacral region may require surgical resection, reconstruction, and fixation to adequately manage the disease. However, such aggressive measures are very challenging and not without considerable risks of causing serious morbidity owing in great part to the complex anatomy of the lumbosacral junction, particularly its unique biomechanical features. Two other important factors that may increase morbidity are the typically lengthy operative times and the significant blood loss that may occur.

The lumbosacral junction is a rare site of metastatic disease to the spine. Most commonly such metastases arise in the thoracic spine, followed by the lumbar and then the cervical spine [1]. The predominant primary malignancies are those of the breast, lung, kidney, thyroid, and prostate [2, 3]. Other common sources include lymphoma, myeloma, melanoma, and tumors of unknown origin. Typically the primary lesion spreads via hematogenous dissemination, although pelvic tumors may directly invade the lumbosacral region.

Lesions of the lumbosacral region typically reside in the anterior vertebral body but may also invade the lamina or pedicles [4]. Pain is the chief presenting symptom. Neurologic dysfunction, which is revealed by the development of bowel or bladder incontinence, sexual dysfunction, and lower extremity weakness, is less common in patients with lumbosacral lesions than in those with lesions in the thoracic region [5].

Covered in this chapter are the anatomic and biomechanical features of the lumbosacral junction that must be clearly understood when undertaking the surgical management of metastatic disease in this region. Also included is the authors' preferred technique for surgical resection, reconstruction, and fixation at this level.

Lumbopelvic Bony Anatomy and Biomechanics

The lumbosacral junction is a unique zone in the spine where the mobile lumbar spine connects (i.e., transitions into) to the relatively fixed sacrum and pelvis. Although it possesses a greater range of motion in the sagittal plane (flexion-extension) than at any thoracic or lumbar level, rotation and lateral bending are significantly reduced in the lumbosacral junction. This is the result of the region's need to support greater loads than more proximal regions of the spine.

The lumbosacral intervertebral disc is positioned at a steep angle respective to the horizontal plane due to the normal lordotic curvature in the

A. B. Kay, MD (✉) · R. A. W. Marco, MD
Department of Orthopaedic Surgery, Houston Methodist Hospital, Houston, TX, USA
e-mail: abkay@houstonmethodist.org

R. A. W. Marco (ed.), *Metastatic Spine Disease*, https://doi.org/10.1007/978-3-319-76252-4_18

lumbar spine and sacrum. For this reason, the lumbar spine has a tendency to slip forward relative to the sacrum. The coronally oriented facet joints at L5–S1, in conjunction with the musculature and ligamentous elements, resist this forward slip. In this way, body weight is transmitted through the sacroiliac joints and down into the hips and lower limbs. Because the sacrum is tilted forward, body weight is transmitted to the ventral aspect of the sacrum as a potentially rotatory force with the axis at S2. The dorsal ligaments, including the interosseous and dorsal sacroiliac ligaments, are the sturdiest stabilizers at the sacroiliac junction [6].

Neurovascular Anatomy

The lumbosacral region contains critical neurovascular and visceral structures that can complicate surgical treatment, especially if an anterior approach is utilized. In particular, the aorta commonly bifurcates at the caudal aspect of the L4 vertebra, just left of the midline, and thereby becomes the common iliac arteries, which run inferolateral to the medial surface of the psoas muscle before bifurcating into the internal and external iliac arteries anterior to the sacroiliac joints at the lumbosacral level. The common iliac veins likewise come together to form the inferior vena cava at the L4–L5 level. Additionally, the left and right ureters, which are loosely embedded in the retroperitoneal space, cross the common iliac arteries anteriorly at the level of the sacroiliac joint. Adding further complexity to the neurovascular anatomy of this region, sympathetic and parasympathetic nerve branches cross and descend into the superior hypogastric plexus in between the common iliac arteries, which then descend further to innervate pelvic structures. These autonomic fibers are important for coordinating anterograde ejaculation, as well erectile function. Injury to them could cause retrograde ejaculation in men [7].

From this it is clear that advances in surgical techniques, notwithstanding lumbopelvic fixation for any pathology, including degenerative disease, deformity, trauma, and oncologic disease, are a challenging proposition [8–17].

Surgical Indications and Preoperative Management

The primary goal of any surgery in the lumbosacral region is to reduce pain and neurologic dysfunction. Any surgical treatment should be highly individualized to the patient and generally follow the MOSS approach described earlier in this book. Surgery should only be undertaken after in-depth evaluation of the patient's medical and oncologic status, the presence and nature of any stenosis, and the functional stability of the region.

Preoperative planning should take into account the anatomic, biomechanical, and functional aspects of the lumbosacral region. Appropriate imaging should be done to reveal any underlying anomalous anatomy or some pathology that would require the surgical plan to be altered. Because significant blood loss is the norm in these procedures, the patient's hemoglobin level should be optimized preoperatively to minimize the threat of intraoperative hemodynamic instability. Angiographic embolization is worthwhile for vascular tumors such as renal and thyroid carcinomas. In this instance, large-bore intravenous catheters are necessary, and central venous access should be considered for the rapid administration of fluids and blood products as needed intraoperatively. Intra-arterial monitoring of blood pressure facilitates fluid management and intraoperative resuscitation.

Resection Considerations

Anterior Approach

Both anterior and posterior approaches have been used to resect metastatic vertebral body lesions, but the anterior approach is significantly more risky and is associated with increased morbidity. This is because it requires structural support and fixation with bone graft, cement, or cages with or without anterior instrumentation. The theoretic advantage of the anterior approach is that it provides more direct access to the vertebral body, but, as noted earlier, there is significant risk of injuring critical vascular, neurologic, and urologic structures. A further consideration is that it can be very difficult to safely prepare the caudal endplate at L4 for reconstruction because the great vessels commonly bifurcate at this level. While the L5–S1 disc is farther from this bifurcation, fixation at this level is challenging because of its significant lordosis. This lordosis can make it easy for a cage to be dislodged due to the shear forces between the anterior strut and the S1 endplate. Moreover, the inclined surface of the S1 body at this level makes it difficult to obtain adequate purchase for the fixation of anterior instrumentation.

In a systematic review of 40 studies meeting strict inclusion criteria, Wood et al. examined the incidence and consequences of vascular injury in patients who undergo anterior lumbosacral surgery. They found that although vascular injuries were rare (<5%), surgical exposure and intervention at L4–L5 appeared to be associated with a higher risk of injury than at L5–S1 owing to the close proximity of the bifurcation of the aorta and inferior vena cava at L4–L5. Nonetheless, these authors found that the consequences of vascular injuries were often minor, with only a small number of patients suffering devastating consequences such as fatal acidosis, compartment syndrome, massive blood loss, and pulmonary embolism [18]. A further complication, retrograde ejaculation, occurs in up to 7% of males in some studies [19, 20].

Posterior Approach

A posterior approach may also be used for the resection of metastatic disease of the lumbosacral vertebral bodies that avoids the morbidity associated with the anterior approach. Resections via a posterolateral approach also allow for adequate reconstruction of the vertebrectomy defect without the need for a separate anterior approach.

In 1999, Bilsky et al. published an article describing their technique for removing vertebral body tumors through an all-posterolateral transpedicular approach. In this article they also retrospectively reviewed the outcome in 25 of their cases treated using this technique. Of the 25 patients, 23 experienced significant pain relief, as well as stable or improved neurologic function. The authors concluded from their findings that their technique both effectively reduced patient symptoms and avoided the risks associated with an anterior approach [21].

Reconstruction and Stabilization

One particularly challenging aspect of lumbosacral resection, regardless of the approach used, is achieving adequate fixation in the sacrum where the bone density is typically poor [22]. Some of the materials and instrumentation used to achieve optimal fixation include the placement of tricortical screws to gain purchase into the sacral promontory, plus the use of bone cement, and expandable screws [23–25]. To achieve stabilization, surgeons have made use of S1 pedicle screws, sacral alar screws, intrasacral screws, iliosacral screws, Galveston rods, iliac screws (bolts), transiliac bars, and S2 alar iliac screws to create multiple proximal and distal fixation points and trajectories required [9–11, 26–29].

Incorporating the concept of a lumbosacral pivot point in the thinking underlying the reconstruction of lumbosacral tumors was introduced by McCord et al. These authors placed this point in the middle of the osteoligamentous column at L5–S1. They went on to find that stability was increased when constructs passed either more distal to the point or more anterior to this point ([30], Fig. 18.1). Cunningham et al. showed that iliac fixation decreased the likelihood of developing a sacral fracture below the S1 screw. In a similar vein, O'Brien et al. identified three zones of the sacropelvic region where fixation strength would be progressively increased ([31], Fig. 18.2). Lebwohl et al. and Tis et al. confirmed this concept in in vitro biomechanical studies of the strength and feasibility of different types of lumbopelvic fixation in calf spines. These authors found that only fixation distal to S1 reduced screw strain and peak failure significantly enough to improve stability [32, 33]. Iliac screws and S2

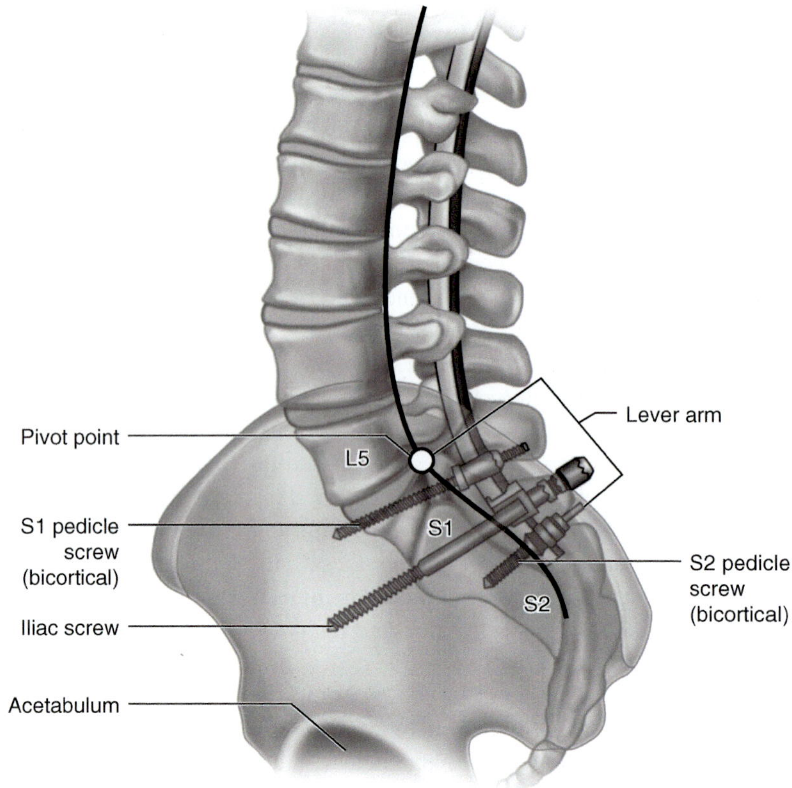

Fig. 18.1 The lumbosacral pivot point at the middle of the osteoligamentous column at L5–S1. McCord et al. found increasing stability with constructs passing more distal or anterior to the pivot point. Adapted from McCord D, Cunningham B, Shono Y, et al., Biomechanical Analysis of Lumbosacral Fixation. Spine. 1992 Jan 1;17

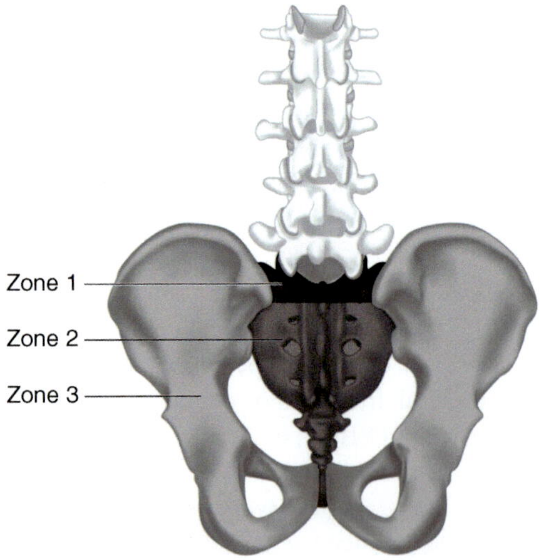

Fig. 18.2 Zones of sacropelvic fixation. Fixation strength has been shown to increase progressively by zone. Adapted from O'Brien M, Kuklo T, Lenke L. Sacropelvic Instrumentation: Anatomic and biomechanical zones of fixation. Semin Spine Surg. 2004 Jun 1;16(2):76–90. With permission from Elsevier

alar iliac screws both achieve fixation distal and anterior to the pivot point of McCord, as well as fixation through zones 2 and 3 described by O'Brien. These are some of the most popular techniques in current use.

There are drawbacks to iliac screws, however, that surgeons must bear in mind if using them. One is the need for a wider soft-tissue dissection, which may increase the likelihood of infection. A rate of infection of up to 4% over the course of 2 years was observed in a series of 81 patients in whom these screws were used [34]. The sciatic notch is also theoretically at risk when these screws are used, but no major case series has been done that has revealed an increased incidence of injury to the notch's contents (superior gluteal artery, sciatic nerve) [35].

Implant prominence and pain are the most common complications of these procedures, with screw removal necessary in up to 22% of patients by 2 years postoperatively [36, 37]. This problem might be avoided, however, if a portion of the iliac crest is resected to reduce bolt prominence. The S2 alar iliac (S2AI) technique might also be used to prevent this complication. In this technique the S2 ala is used as a starting point and projected into the ilium toward the anterior inferior iliac spine [38]. This technique also has the advantage of reducing implant prominence and connecting it directly to the longitudinal rod without the need for connectors [39]. It should be noted, however, that this technique is relatively new, and longer-term data are needed before we can fully understand how well it works and what the complication rate is.

Further aspects of these procedures that need to be considered are the biomechanical forces at the lumbosacral junction and the potential for rod fracture or other types of instrumentation failure [40]. To minimize such problems, Shen et al. developed a novel technique for lumbopelvic reconstruction that involves the use of four longitudinal rods that cross the lumbosacral junction and are anchored to the lumbar spine with pedicle screws ([26], Fig. 18.3). The rods are then coupled to a pair of Galveston-like screws starting in the posterior superior iliac spine and projecting toward the anterior inferior iliac spine. The rods are also coupled to a pair of more proximal iliac wing screws. Because this technique is relatively new, however, longer follow-up is needed before its place in lumbosacral surgery is clearly known. The authors did, however, convincingly demonstrate the feasibility of such a construct [26]. Kelly et al. studied a similar construct biomechanically and found that the four-rod technique was better than a two-rod technique at stabilizing the spine during flexion and extension and also during axial rotation through the addition of cross-links. The four-rod technique also significantly reduced L5-pelvic junction motion in flexion-extension, which could help improve fusion at this level [41].

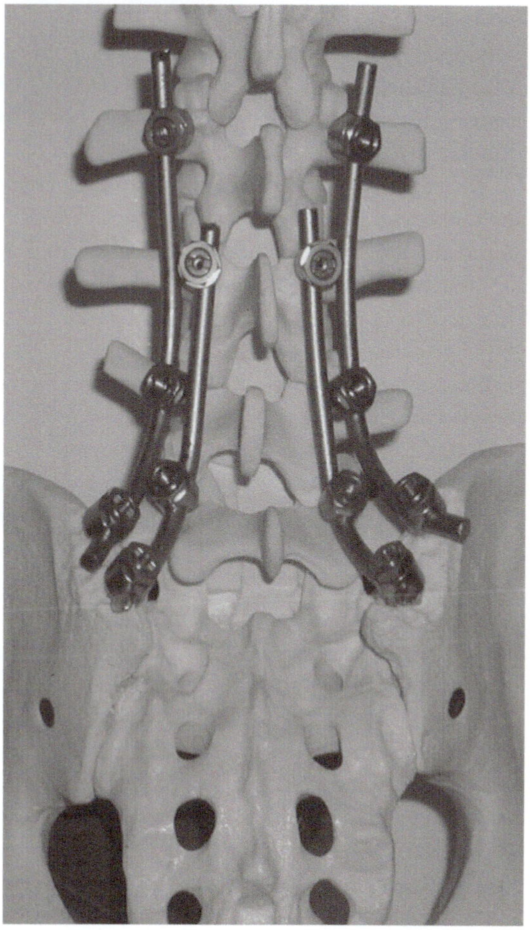

Fig. 18.3 Sawbones model depicting the four-rod technique for lumbopelvic fixation described by Shen et al. Adapted from Shen F, Harper M, Foster W, Marks I, Arlet V. A Novel "Four-Rod Technique" for Lumbo-Pelvic Reconstruction: Theory and Technical Considerations. Spine. 2006 May 20;31(12)

Authors' Preferred Technique for Resection and Reconstruction

Because of the challenges posed by lumbosacral resection, we often, at least initially, recommend nonoperative treatment. Our reason for this is that spines are often stable at this level and there is ample space in the spinal canal at L4–5 and L5–S1 to accommodate a metastatic tumor. If compression is significant, it can still be relieved nonoperatively by radiotherapy, if the tumor is radiosensitive. If surgery is indicated, we prefer posterior tumor resection, followed by the implantation of spinal instrumentation from L3 to the pelvis, possibly using two pelvic bolts on each side and four total rods, as described by Shen et al. [26].

To begin with, the patient is positioned prone on transverse gel rolls to maintain correct lumbar lordosis. We use a standard posterior, midline approach to the lumbar spine. We first place pedicle screws at L3, L4, and S1 and then place iliac bolts or screws. This is followed by the removal of the caudal two-thirds of the L4 lamina and the entire lamina of L5. The inferior articular facets of L4 and L5 are then completely removed, after which the L5 and S1 pedicles are skeletonized. This involves the removal of the medial and cephalad portions of the superior articular facets.

Next, the anterolateral epidural veins are dissected away from the shoulder of the L5 and S1 nerve roots, and bipolar cautery is used to coagulate these vessels. The careful dissection and coagulation of these vessels minimizes blood loss and facilitates dissection of the thecal sac away from the posterior longitudinal ligament. Discectomies at L4–L5 and L5–S1 are performed using a technique similar to that used for a standard transforaminal lumbar interbody fusion (TLIF). For this we use the down-biting or annulus-cutting curettes found in a typical pedicle subtraction osteotomy or TLIF instrument set [42]. A temporary rod is unilaterally connected to the instrumentation while the discectomies are performed. Preserving the anterior two-thirds to three-quarters of the annulus at L4–L5 and L5–S1 protects the iliac vessels.

Any readily removable tumor in the pedicle is removed with a pituitary rongeur. Preserving the medial wall of the pedicle protects the neural elements during this step. A transpedicular excision of the tumor is then performed anterior to the dura mater and nerve roots using reverse-angled curettes, cupped curettes, and up-biting pituitary ronguers in a manner similar to that used by Bilsky et al. (Fig. 18.4) [21]. This same technique is carried out on the contralateral pedicle.

All adhesions of the posterior longitudinal ligament (PLL) are gently dissected away from the thecal sac whenever possible, which facilitates tumor removal and local tumor control. Transecting the PLL across the midline at L4–L5 and L5–S1 also helps in completing dissection of the PLL from the neural elements. Occasionally, adhesions of the PLL to the neural elements prevent complete removal of this tumor barrier, and the potential risks of a durotomy or traction on the neural elements may preclude full dissection of the PLL from the dura. As much tumor is removed as is possible, while leaving the anterior cortex and anterior longitudinal ligament intact. Expeditious tumor removal is recommended for highly vascular tumors such as myeloma, thyroid carcinoma, and renal cell carcinoma. Preoperative embolization of lesions arising from thyroid and renal cell carcinoma can help decrease intraoperative blood loss.

Attention is then turned to reconstructing the anterior column. Our preferred technique is to use Steinmann pins and PMMA cement, which are relatively cost-effective materials compared with titanium mesh or expandable cages. For this procedure the Steinmann pins are cut and then bent at a 90° angle into an L shape. A right-angle clamp is used to penetrate the left L4 endplate just medial to the lateral edge of the dura and equidistant from the anterior and posterior aspects of the vertebral body. A needle driver is used to grasp the Steinmann pin along the long aspect of the shaft, with the short aspect turned inward along the clamp. This grasp allows for adequate control of the Steinmann pin as it is driven 1.5 cm into the L4 vertebral body. The long axis of the pin is then pushed anteriorly so that it parallels the anterior surface of the L5 vertebral body, and the leg of the pin is turned approximately 80° away from the thecal sac and L5 nerve roots. A second pin is placed within the S1 body.

A Toomey syringe with the sheath from a 16-gauge spinal needle added to its tip is used to inject cement into the corpectomy defect. The sheath extension needs to be cut to a length of 3–5 cm, which is best for facilitating cement placement. A small burr hole is also made at the

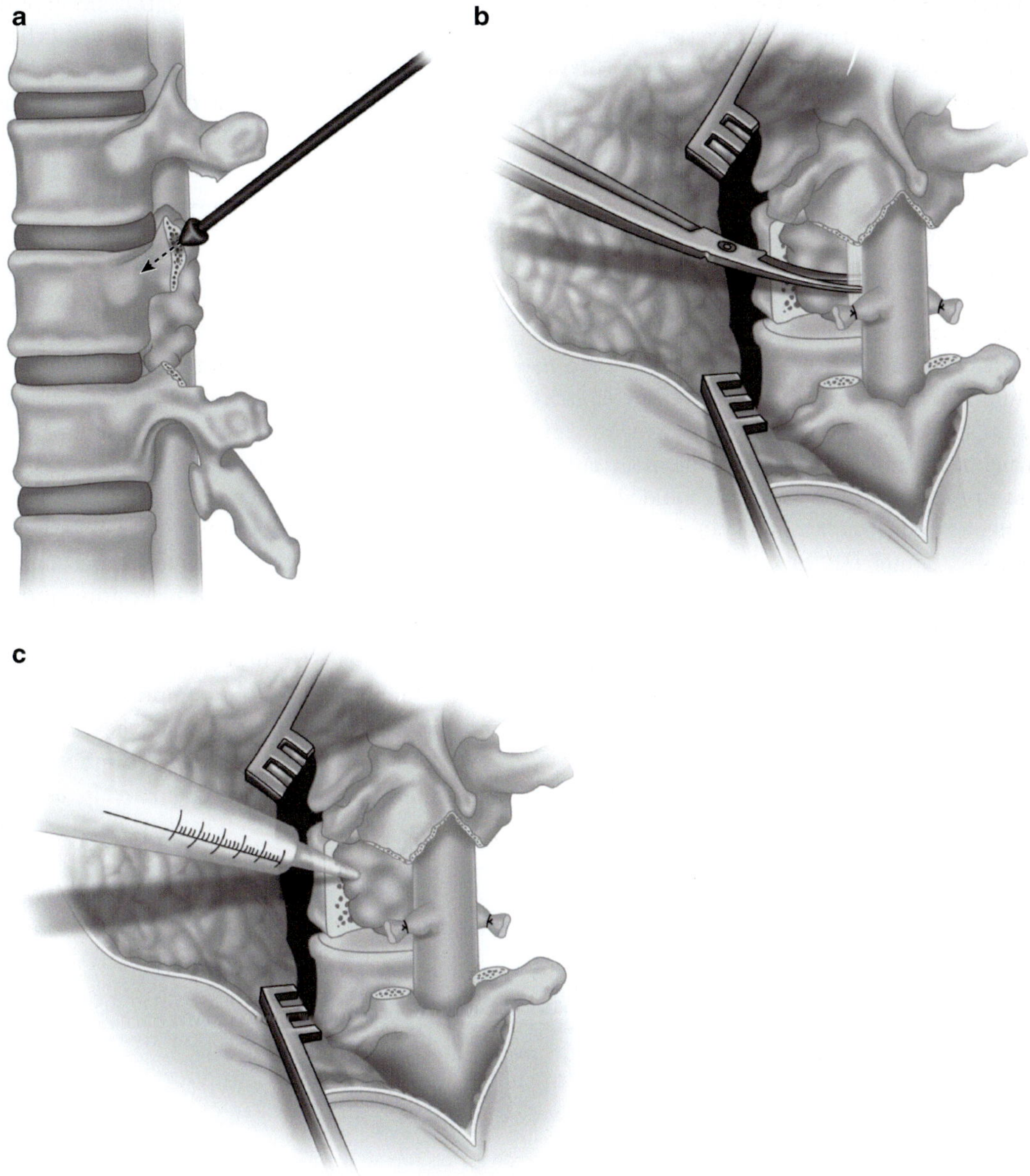

Fig. 18.4 Depiction of the transpedicular technique for vertebral body tumor excision as described by Bilsky et al. Pedicle resection and facet removal (**a**). After rhizotomy, the posterior longitudinal ligament is cut to secure the anterior margin (**b**). PMMA cement and pins are placed into vertebral body defect (**c**). Adapted from Bilsky M, Boland P, Lis E, Raizer J, Healey J. Single-stage Posterolateral Transpedicle Approach for Spondylectomy, Epidural Decompression, and Circumferential Fusion of Spinal Metastases. Spine. 2000 Sep 1;25(17)

40 cc mark on the syringe to enable air removal as the cement is injected.

Once the Toomey syringe had been modified as just described, the PMMA cement is mixed in a bowl with a tongue depressor or some other similar device and placed into the syringe. The plunger is then placed into the syringe and the tip with its sheath extension placed into the anterior-most aspect of the corpectomy defect (the floor of the tumor bed). The cement is injected going from anterior to posterior to fill the entire tumor bed. It is important that the tip of the syringe is kept at the anterior-most aspect of the tumor bed so that the defect is filled from the bottom up. Injection is halted once the cement touches the thecal sac. Penfield #3 instruments are used to mold the cement away from the neural elements after the sheen of the fresh cement disappears but before the cement cures completely.

Care is taken to ensure that there is no cement posterior to the L4 or S1 vertebral body or touching the L5 nerve root or thecal sac. We are vigilant about removing any excess cement as the posterior aspect of the cement is molded into an L5-like cement strut. Molding continues until the cement is completely cured and expands to fill the entire corpectomy and discectomy without compressing the neural elements (Fig. 18.5).

As a final step, rods are bent to match the patient's lumbar lordosis across the lumbosacral junction, with a slight kyphosis created where the rods enter the iliac bolts. These rods are placed into the previously inserted pedicle screws and iliac bolts, and compression across the rods at L4–L5 and L5–S1 further stabilizes the construct. The wound is copiously irrigated and closed over a drain in the usual manner.

Postoperative Care

Depending on the size of the resection and the nature of any intraoperative complications, patients may initially need to be cared for in an intensive care unit. Because of the potential for significant blood loss, ongoing assessment of the need for potential resuscitation is required. The administration of blood products may be called for. Wounds should be closely watched for the development of hematoma, seroma, or infection. Antibiotics should be continued until all drains have been removed. Venous thromboembolisms may be prevented by mechanical means such as sequential compression devices and early ambulation, as well as chemical anticoagulation. The use of chemical anticoagulation should be done very selectively as it is

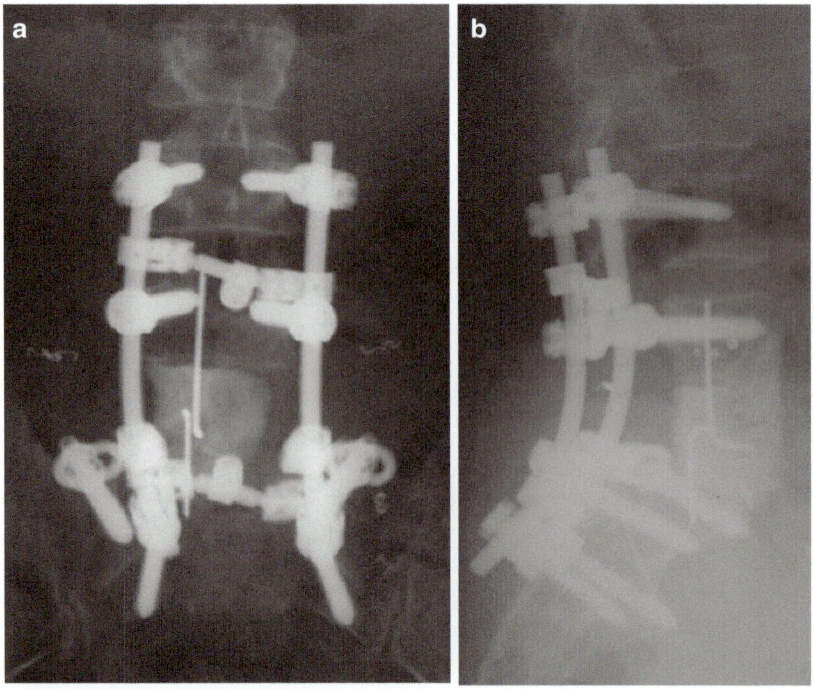

Fig. 18.5 L5 resection and reconstruction with PMMA cement and Steinmann pins through an all-posterior approach. Iliac fixation was not performed in this case

commonly associated with wound complications and hematoma formation. Supine positioning is avoided because of the direct pressure it places on the wound. Moreover, avoiding supine positioning may also decrease wound swelling, which may in turn decrease the incidence of wound complications.

The patient is typically mobilized as early as possible. Physical therapists and rehabilitation physicians are important members of the treatment team to help the patient regain independent mobility soon after surgery. Typically, patients are advised to refrain from bending, lifting, or twisting, at least early in the postoperative period.

References

1. Cummings BJ, Ian Hodson D, Bush RS. Chordoma: the results of megavoltage radiation therapy. Int J Radiat Oncol Biol Phys. 1983;9(5):633–42.
2. Raque GH, Vitaz TW, Shields CB. Treatment of neoplastic diseases of the sacrum. J Surg Oncol. 2001;76(4):301–7.
3. Wuisman P, Lieshout O, Sugihara S, van Dijk M. Total sacrectomy and reconstruction: oncologic and functional outcome. Clin Orthopaed Related Res. 2000;381:192–203.
4. Quraishi NA, Giannoulis KE, Manoharan SR, Edwards KL, Boszczyk BM. Surgical treatment of cauda equina compression as a result of metastatic tumours of the lumbo-sacral junction and sacrum. Eur Spine J. 2013;22(1):33–7.
5. Llauger J, Palmer J, Amores S, Bague S, Camins A. Primary tumors of the sacrum: diagnostic imaging. Am J Roentgenol. 2000;174(2):417–24.
6. Fourney DR, Gokaslan ZL. Complex lumbosacral resection and reconstruction procedure. In: Cancer in the spine: Humana Press; 2006. p. 265–77.
7. Gunterberg B, Romanus B, Stener B. Pelvic strength after major amputation of the sacrum: an experimental study. Acta Orthopaed Scand. 1976;47(6):635–42.
8. Chopin D. A new device for pelvic fixation for spinal surgery: the sacral block. Presented at the 8th International Congresson Cotrel-Dubousset instrumentation. Minneapolis, MN; 1991.
9. D'Ariano GD, Kostuik JP, Carbone JJ. Regional considerations in sacral and iliac fixation techniques. In: Spinal instrumentation. 2nd ed. Philadelphia, PA: Lippincott Williams Wilkins; 1999. p. 291–301.
10. Farcy JP, Rawlins BA, Glassman SD. Technique and results of fixation to the sacrum with iliosacral screws. Spine. 1992;17(6):S190–5.
11. Jackson RJ, Gokaslan ZL. Spinal-pelvic fixation in patients with lumbosacral neoplasms. J Neurosurg Spine. 2000;92(1):61–70.
12. Kuroki H, Tajima N, Kubo S. Instrument failure after total sacrectomy and reconstruction of the sacrum. Nishinihonsekituikenkyukaisi. 1998;24:209–12.
13. Gaines RW. The use of pedicle-screw internal fixation for the operative treatment of spinal disorders. J Bone Joint Surg Am. 2000;82(10):1458–76.
14. Miles WK, Chang DW, Kroll SS, Miller MJ, Langstein HN, Reece GP, Evans GR, Robb GL. Reconstruction of large sacral defects following total sacrectomy. Plast Reconstruct Surg. 2000;105(7):2387–94.
15. Pihlajamäki H, Myllynen P, Böstman O. Complications of transpedicular lumbosacral fixation for non-traumatic disorders. Bone Joint J. 1997;79(2):183–9.
16. Sar C, Eralp L. Surgical treatment of primary tumors of the sacrum. Arch Orthopaed Trauma Surg. 2002;122(3):148–55.
17. Zhang HY, Thongtrangan I, Balabhadra RS, Murovic JA, Kim DH. Surgical techniques for total sacrectomy and spinopelvic reconstruction. Neurosurg Focus. 2003;15(2):1–0.
18. Wood KB, DeVine J, Fischer D, Dettori JR, Janssen M. Vascular injury in elective anterior lumbosacral surgery. Spine. 2010;35(9S):S66–75.
19. Comer GC, Smith MW, Hurwitz EL, Mitsunaga KA, Kessler R, Carragee EJ. Retrograde ejaculation after anterior lumbar interbody fusion with and without bone morphogenetic protein-2 augmentation: a 10-year cohort controlled study. Spine J. 2012;12(10):881–90.
20. Sasso RC, Burkus JK, LeHuec JC. Retrograde ejaculation after anterior lumbar interbody fusion: transperitoneal versus retroperitoneal exposure. Spine. 2003;28(10):1023–6.
21. Bilsky MH, Boland P, Lis E, Raizer JJ, Healey JH. Single-stage posterolateral transpedicle approach for spondylectomy, epidural decompression, and circumferential fusion of spinal metastases. Spine. 2000;25(17):2240–50.
22. Jackson RP, McManus AC. The iliac buttress: a computed tomographic study of sacral anatomy. Spine. 1993;18(10):1318–28.
23. Renner SM, Lim TH, Kim WJ, Katolik L, An HS, Andersson GB. Augmentation of pedicle screw fixation strength using an injectable calcium phosphate cement as a function of injection timing and method. Spine. 2004;29(11):E212–6.
24. Turner AW, Gillies RM, Svehla MJ, Saito M, Walsh WR. Hydroxyapatite composite resin cement augmentation of pedicle screw fixation. Clin Orthopaed Related Res. 2003;406(1):253–61.
25. Cook SD, Barbera J, Rubi M, Salkeld SL, Whitecloud TS. Lumbosacral fixation using expandable pedicle screws: an alternative in reoperation and osteoporosis. Spine J. 2001;1(2):109–14.
26. Shen FH, Harper M, Foster WC, Marks I, Arlet V. A novel "four-rod technique" for lumbo-pelvic reconstruction: theory and technical considerations. Spine. 2006;31(12):1395–401.

27. Barber JW, Boden SD, Ganey T, Hutton WC. Biomechanical study of lumbar pedicle screws: does convergence affect axial pullout strength? Clin Spine Surg. 1998;11(3):215–20.
28. Boucher HH. A method of spinal fusion. Bone Joint J. 1959;41(2):248–59.
29. Kawahara N, Murakami H, Yoshida A, Sakamoto J, Oda J, Tomita K. Reconstruction after total sacrectomy using a new instrumentation technique: a biomechanical comparison. Spine. 2003;28(14):1567–72.
30. McCord DH, Cunningham BW, Shono Y, Myers JJ, McAfee PC. Biomechanical analysis of lumbosacral fixation. Spine. 1992;17:235–43.
31. O'Brien MF, Kuklo TR, Lenke LG. Sacropelvic instrumentation: anatomic and biomechanical zones of fixation. Semin Spine Surg. 2004;16(2):76–90.
32. Tis JE, Helgeson M, Lehman RA, Dmitriev AE. A biomechanical comparison of different types of lumbopelvic fixation. Spine. 2009;34(24):E866–72.
33. Lebwohl NH, Cunningham BW, Dmitriev A, Shimamoto N, Gooch L, Devlin V, Boachie-Adjei O, Wagner TA. Biomechanical comparison of lumbosacral fixation techniques in a calf spine model. Spine. 2002;27(21):2312–20.
34. Kuklo TR, Bridwell KH, Lewis SJ, Baldus C, Blanke K, Iffrig TM, Lenke LG. Minimum 2-year analysis of sacropelvic fixation and L5–S1 fusion using S1 and iliac screws. Spine. 2001;26(18):1976–83.
35. Kebaish KM. Sacropelvic fixation: techniques and complications. Spine. 2010;35(25):2245–51.
36. Emami A, Deviren V, Berven S, Smith JA, Hu SS, Bradford DS. Outcome and complications of long fusions to the sacrum in adult spine deformity: luque-galveston, combined iliac and sacral screws, and sacral fixation. Spine. 2002;27(7):776–86.
37. Tsuchiya K, Bridwell KH, Kuklo TR, Lenke LG, Baldus C. Minimum 5-year analysis of L5–S1 fusion using sacropelvic fixation (bilateral S1 and iliac screws) for spinal deformity. Spine. 2006;31(3):303–8.
38. O'Brien JR, Warren DY, Bhatnagar R, Sponseller P, Kebaish KM. An anatomic study of the S2 iliac technique for lumbopelvic screw placement. Spine. 2009;34(12):E439–42.
39. Chang TL, Sponseller PD, Kebaish KM, Fishman EK. Low profile pelvic fixation: anatomic parameters for sacral alar-iliac fixation versus traditional iliac fixation. Spine. 2009;34(5):436–40.
40. Stambough JL. Lumbosacral instrumented fusion: analysis of 124 consecutive cases. J Spinal Disord. 1999;12(1):1–9.
41. Kelly BP, Shen FH, Schwab JS, Arlet V, Diangelo DJ. Biomechanical testing of a novel four-rod technique for lumbo-pelvic reconstruction. Spine. 2008;33(13):E400–6.
42. Moskowitz A. Transforaminal lumbar interbody fusion. Orthoped Clin. 2002;33(2):359–66.

Sacral Metastases

19

A. Karim Ahmed, C. Rory Goodwin,
and Daniel M. Sciubba

Introduction

Tumors of the sacrum are relatively rare, comprising 1–7% of spine tumors [1]. Although the majority of metastatic spine lesions are in the thoracic spine, metastatic tumors of the sacrum are more common than primary tumors at that location and should be considered when malignancy is suspected. The neurologic functions, anatomy, and biomechanical properties of the sacral spine are unique, requiring special consideration in the management of sacral metastases. Adequate diagnosis, consisting of imaging and biopsy, guides the most appropriate management. Treatment options include adjuvant therapy, radiation, surgery, and cement augmentation. Clinical presentation, prognosis, tumor etiology, neurologic signs and symptoms, and spine stability dictate which combination of treatment options will best suit each individual patient.

A. K. Ahmed, BS · D. M. Sciubba, MD
Department of Neurosurgery, Johns Hopkins University School of Medicine, Baltimore, MD, USA
e-mail: aahmed33@jhmi.edu; dsciubb1@jhmi.edu

C. R. Goodwin, MD, PhD (✉)
Department of Neurosurgery, Duke University Medical Center, Durham, NC, USA
e-mail: crg30@duke.edu

Anatomy of the Sacrum

The sacrum plays a dynamic role that includes protecting the pelvic viscera, distributing the load from the cephalad spinal segments to the pelvis, and housing nerves with motor, sensory, and autonomic functions. As such, an overview of sacral anatomy is necessary in describing metastatic sacral lesions.

The bony sacrum is formed by five fused vertebrae, articulating superiorly with the fifth lumbar vertebra (via the L5–S1 disk and L5 inferior articulating process and S1 superior articulating process), inferiorly with the coccyx, and laterally with the ilium of the pelvic bone (via the sacroiliac joints). The sacral promontory forms an inflection point, anteriorly—influenced by the forward rotation of the pelvis. The lateral alae of the sacrum articulate with the ilium forming the bilateral sacroiliac joints—relatively immobile joints with less than 4° of rotation. The inferior aspect of the sacral canal forms a posterior opening, the sacral hiatus, terminating in the paired sacral cornua. The inferior apex of the sacrum articulates with the coccyx. The coccygeal cornua project superiorly to articulate with the sacral cornua. The sacral canal houses the sacral portion of the cauda equina, with nerve roots exiting through bilateral sacral foramina.

The sacrum serves as a point of attachment for numerous ligaments and muscles. Among other functions, tension from the sacrotuberous

R. A. W. Marco (ed.), *Metastatic Spine Disease*, https://doi.org/10.1007/978-3-319-76252-4_19

(attached to the ischial tuberosity) and sacrospinous (attached to the ischial spine) ligaments separates greater and lesser sciatic foramen and prevents the caudal sacrum from being lifted superiorly as a result of downward torque from the mass above. The interosseous and dorsal sacroiliac ligaments prevent forward rotation of the sacrum. The coccygeus muscle and levator ani, which contribute to the pelvic floor, and piriformis, which participates in lateral rotation of the hip, have key points of attachment on the sacrum.

The rectum, internal iliac arteries, uterus/ductus deferens, ureters, and bladder traverse the pelvic inlet and are essential landmarks due to their close proximity to the sacrum. The abdominal aorta usually gives rise to the common iliac arteries at the level of L4–5 disc. The median sacral artery branches from the posterior abdominal aorta as an unpaired vessel and anastomoses with the lateral sacral artery and supplies the lower lumbar vertebrae, sacrum, and coccyx. The lateral sacral arteries, arising from the posterior division of the internal iliac arteries, enter the anterior sacral foramina to supply blood to the bony sacrum and also the meninges. Lymphatic drainage is achieved through sacral lymph nodes and internal iliac lymph nodes—responsible for draining most of the viscera in the pelvic region.

The sacral portion of the cauda equina has a rich innervation, supplying roots to the sacral plexus (L4–S4), pelvic splanchnic nerves (S2–S4), and the coccygeal plexus (S4–Co). The largest nerve in the body, the sciatic nerve (L4–S3), bifurcates to form the tibial and common peroneal nerve—which branches further to form deep and superficial peroneal nerves. The tibial nerve participates in motor innervation to most of the muscles in the posterior thigh, all of the muscles in the posterior compartment of the leg, and all muscles in the sole of the foot. The common peroneal provides motor innervation to the remaining muscles in the posterior thigh, anterior and lateral compartments of the leg, and extensor digitorum brevis. The sciatic nerve carries cutaneous stimulation from the anterior, lateral, and dorsal portions of the foot and anterolateral portion of the leg.

The sacral plexus is additionally comprised of the pudendal nerve (S2–S4), the superior gluteal nerve (L4–S1), the inferior gluteal nerve (L5–S2), the nerve to obturator internus and superior gemellus (L5–S2), the nerve to quadratus femoris and inferior gemellus (L4–S1), the posterior cutaneous nerve of the thigh (S1, S3), the nerve to piriformis (S1, S2), the perforating cutaneous nerve (S2, S3), pelvic splanchnic nerves (S2–S4), and nerves to levator ani/coccygeus/external anal sphincter (S4). The coccygeal plexus (S4–Co) supplies the anococcygeal nerves.

Pelvic splanchnic nerves (S2–S4), which are preganglionic parasympathetic nerves, and sacral splanchnic nerves, from the sympathetic trunk, join the inferior hypogastric plexus. The inferior hypogastric plexus is responsible for autonomic control of the pelvic viscera, genital erection (male and female), and bowel/bladder function. Parts of the pelvic splanchnic nerves (S2–S4) travel superiorly to contribute parasympathetic innervation to the inferior mesenteric portion of the prevertebral plexus [1–10].

Clinical and Diagnostic Features

Sacral tumors comprise 1–7% of spine tumors [7]. Metastatic lesions of the spine are most commonly found in the thoracic spine, and the sacrum is a much more rare location for metastatic seeding [7, 8, 11]. Nonetheless, metastatic disease of the sacrum is still more common than primary tumors and should be considered when malignancy is suspected. The most common types of primary cancer that metastasize to the sacrum are myeloma, breast, lung, renal cell, thyroid, and prostate [11]. Metastatic lesions of the sacrum are less insidious in their growth than primary tumors, and 61% of cases have distant organ involvement at the time of diagnosis [8]. Metastases can occur through hematogenous spread, drop metastasis, or direct extension—as is seen in recurrent colorectal cancers [11–13]. Drop metastasis, or leptomeningeal spread, to the sacrum has been reported in patients with breast cancer, lung cancer, melanoma, leukemia, and malignant lymphoma [14]. However, due to the rich blood supply from the lateral sacral arteries, the majority of metastatic lesions to the sacrum are from hematogenous spread with osseous involvement.

Although the time to diagnosis of a metastatic sacral lesions is earlier than a primary sacral tumor, these tumors can grow substantially before becoming symptomatic. The large sacral canal provides significant room for metastatic lesions to grow without significant neurologic compromise. Moreover, bladder/bowel, epigastric, sacral plexus compression, and motor dysfunction do not become symptomatic until later in the disease course [11].

There is no unifying clinical presentation for sacral metastases. Pain is the most common initial symptom due largely to mass effect [15]. The dura, within the intervertebral foramen, can result in pain when stretched. Bone pain may also occur as a result of infiltration and possible fracture. Unilateral or bilateral radicular pain can occur with nerve root compression and is often multiradicular/nonspecific. Due to the innervation provided by the sacral plexus and sciatic nerve, radicular pain may present in the buttocks, perineum, genital region, posterior thigh, leg, and/or foot [16]. Radicular pain is worse at night, exacerbated by the Valsalva maneuver, and a positive straight leg test can indicate involvement of L5–S1 [10, 15]. When present, motor, bowel/bladder, and sexual dysfunction have been reported to follow sensory loss [17]. Constipation and/or urinary retention may also occur, due to presacral infiltration and mass effect on the bladder and/or rectum [16].

Imaging and Biopsy

Imaging is the mainstay for diagnosis of sacral lesions. Plain radiographs are commonly performed and frequently are the first-line imaging modality utilized; however, they have often been considered to have limited value in assessing sacral metastases [18]. Nonetheless, particular attention to the loss of one or more sacral arcuate lines, on plain radiographs, can provide meaningful insight into identifying metastatic lesions [19].

Magnetic resonance imaging (MRI) with and without gadolinium is unparalleled as a tool to identify sacral lesions, facilitating an accurate assessment of neurologic compromise, and vascularity. In addition, MRI can reveal infiltration into soft tissue structures, sacroiliac joints, and the epidural space [20, 21]. The hypo- and/or hyperintensity pattern on T1-weighted and T2-weighted sequences coupled with the enhancement pattern can provide meaningful insight into the diagnosis. When this is not possible, a computed tomography (CT) myelogram can be useful as a secondary option to assess compression of nerve roots. As an adjunct, CT plays its own pivotal role in determining osseous involvement, tumor calcification, and structural integrity and also providing clues to the diagnosis. For instance, metastatic prostate cancer has a characteristic blastic bony lesion pattern (hyperdense), whereas myeloma, thyroid, kidney, lung, and the majority of metastatic cancers have lytic bony lesion pattern (hypodense). Metastatic breast cancer can have a mixed blastic and lytic presentation. In this respect, CT can help guide treatment by providing information regarding both bony compression of neural elements and osseous integrity [21–23].

Nuclear bone scan/scintigraphy can be another imaging option for patients with a known cancer diagnosis and can demonstrate nuclear uptake in the presence of osseous metastases to the sacrum [22–25]. This imaging modality is often used in conjunction with other imaging modalities as part of a complete work-up. A more precise form of scintigraphy, single-photon emission computed tomography (SPECT), has been shown to increase the sensitivity and specificity to detect smaller lesions that may otherwise be undetectable on computed tomography (CT) or magnetic resonance imaging (MRI) [11, 21–26]. Positron emission tomography (PET), including ^{18}fluorodeoxyglucose (^{18}FDG) and ^{18}F-fluoride, is another imaging modality that can be crucial in staging metastatic disease throughout skeletal and soft tissue structures [27].

When a sacral lesion is detected, CT-guided biopsy should be utilized to determine the tumor pathology and grade prior to the initiation of any intervention and particularly in cases of an unknown cancer diagnosis [28]. Studies have demonstrated that a metastatic spine tumor pathology was diagnosed in 96% of cases when patients underwent CT-guided biopsy [29, 30]. CT-guided biopsy has several benefits, in comparison to fluoroscopy-guided biopsy, including easier identification of vertebral lesions and documented trajectory of the biopsy needle from the entry point, which may be crucial for appropriate treatment in cases where further surgical intervention is indicated (i.e., chordoma) [30].

A percutaneous CT-guided needle biopsy should be performed for sacral lesions when the diagnosis is not clear and when safe to do so. In cases where the needle biopsy is nondiagnostic or there are safety concerns, an open biopsy may be performed. However, in a situation where potential harm is limited, most commonly a nondiagnostic needle biopsy can be followed with repeat needle biopsy for adequate diagnosis prior to initiating a treatment plan [28–30].

Management of Sacral Metastasis

Diagnosis prior to treatment is imperative because the pathology of a sacral tumor can drastically alter management; contributing factors can include tumor vascularity, radiosensitivity, the presence of systemic metastases, and response to adjuvant therapy.

Metastatic lymphoma, seminoma, and myeloma to the spine are considered as highly radiosensitive tumors and respond well to radiation without the need for surgical intervention. Breast, prostate, ovarian, and neuroendocrine tumors are relatively radiosensitive. Colon, non-small cell lung carcinoma, hepatocellular, and previously treated thyroid tumors are moderately radioresistant, whereas metastatic renal cell carcinoma naïve to chemotherapy, melanoma, and some sarcomas are highly radioresistant [31–35]. Surgical decompression should be considered for relatively healthy patients with radioresistant tumors causing radiculopathy and/or pain. Conversely, neurologic symptoms and/or pain, in the absence of overt or impending instability, can be appropriately treated with radiation instead of surgery for radiosensitive tumors. Very radiosensitive metastatic lesions of the spine, such as lymphoma and myeloma, are commonly treated with corticosteroids and radiotherapy unless there are signs of physiologic instability.

Tumor-induced spinal instability, regardless of radiosensitivity or response to adjuvant chemotherapy, can be addressed by surgical stabilization [27, 33, 36–40] if the patient is well enough to undergo surgery. Instability can be defined in various ways but involves a loss of spinal integrity and/or range of motion, resulting in pain, deformity, or neurologic deficit [35, 41]. The Spinal Instability Neoplastic Score (SINS) takes various factors into consideration such as location, pain, lesion type, spine alignment, vertebral collapse, and involvement of spinal elements [41]. Sacral metastasis to a junction, such as L5–S1, is more likely to result in spinal instability, compared to a rigid location within S2–S5.

In the case presented (Fig. 19.1), a 32-year-old male experienced rapid and significant onset of pain due to multiple myeloma to the sacrum. The symptoms, lytic nature of the tumor, and involvement of the L5–S1 junction put this patient in a calculated SINS range of impending instability. This warranted further surgical consultation despite the radiosensitive nature of multiple myeloma (Fig. 19.2).

The risks and benefits of surgical intervention should be discussed with each patient as nonoperative treatment with corticosteroids and radiation therapy could provide equivalent intermediate and long-term functional outcomes for this patient who may be physiologically stable with modified weight bearing. A relatively healthy person with mechanical pain who prefers immediate weight bearing despite the inherent risks of surgery may choose to undergo spinal stabilization as in the illustrated case.

Highly vascularized tumors, such as metastatic renal cell carcinoma, should be embolized preoperatively to prevent excessive blood loss (Fig. 19.3) [11, 42]. However, surgery for metastatic lesions of the sacrum is generally for palliative treatment. Tumor staging and imaging play a key role in the overall management. Patients with

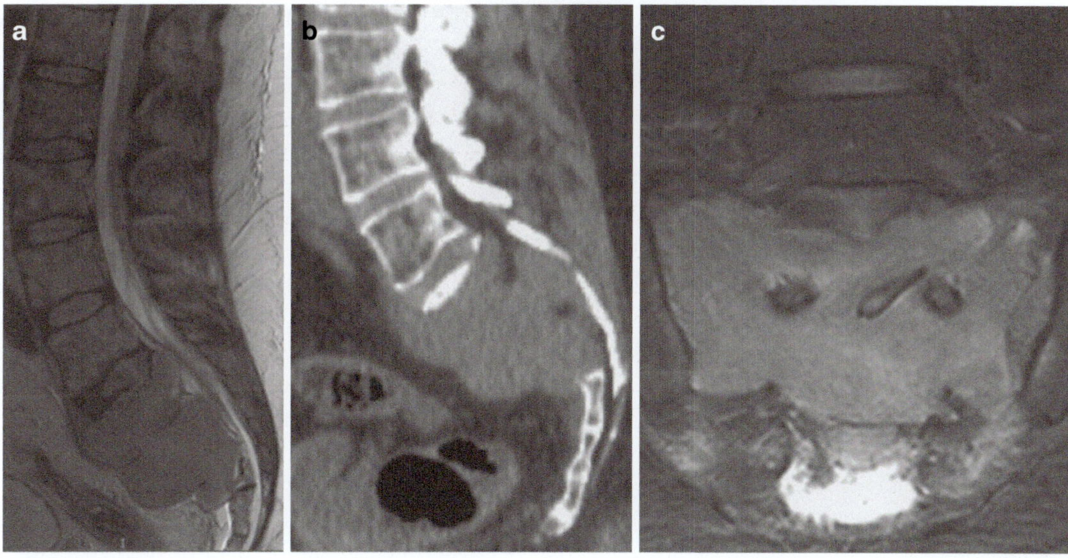

Fig. 19.1 A 32-year-old male with metastatic multiple myeloma of the sacrum; preoperative imaging. (**a**) Sagittal T2 MRI. (**b**) Sagittal CT with contrast. (**c**) Coronal T2 MRI

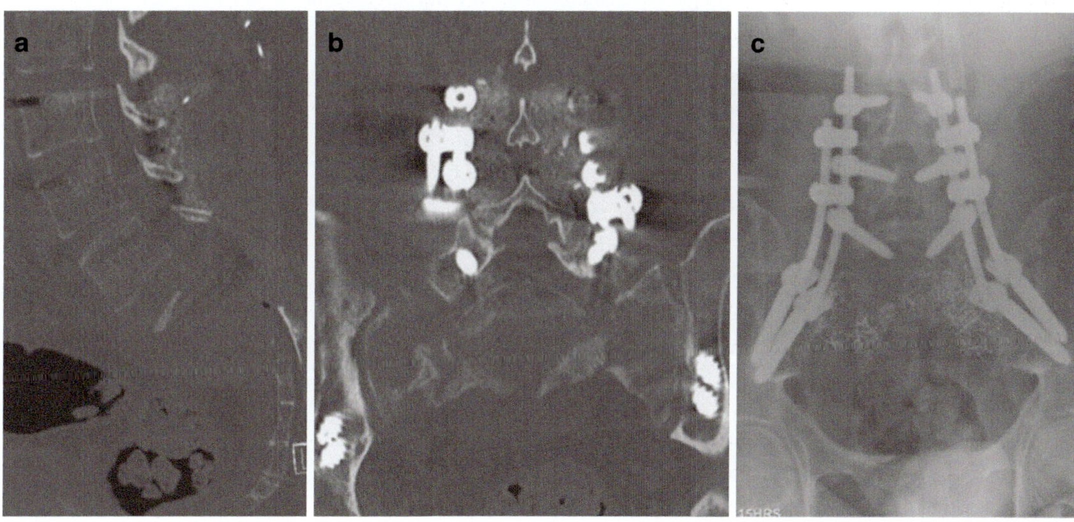

Fig. 19.2 A 32-year-old male with metastatic multiple myeloma of the sacrum; postoperative imaging of L3–S1 pelvic fixation with sacrectomy. (**a**) Sagittal T2 MRI. (**b**) Coronal T2 MRI. (**c**) Plain AP radiograph

a poor prognosis should preferably undergo interventions with limited morbidity and mortality (i.e., nonoperative treatment or minimally invasive procedures as opposed to traditional open surgery). Although there is no unanimously established time, patients with an estimated survival of less than 3 months are in general not considered appropriate surgical candidates in cases where surgical intervention for a sacral metastasis is warranted [27] (Fig. 19.4).

Because the aim of surgery is palliation, morbidity should be minimized with an emphasis on function. Nerve sparing, even with some adherent tumor, can drastically alter a patient's quality of life. There is a great variability, with regard to function, based on the sacral level and roots

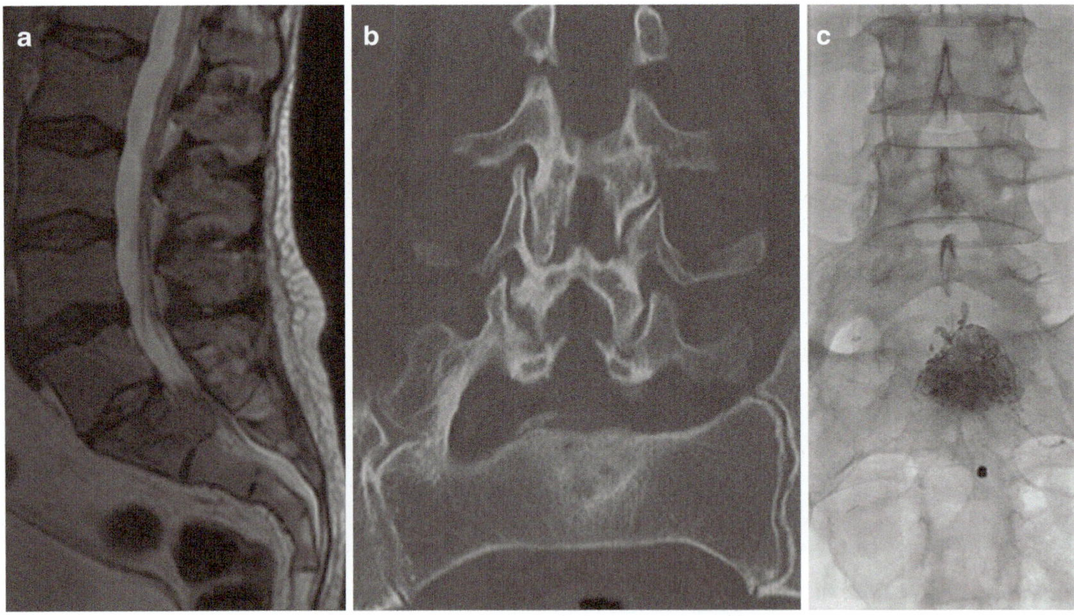

Fig. 19.3 A 49-year-old male with metastatic renal carcinoma of sacrum; preoperative imaging. (**a**) Sagittal T2 MRI. (**b**) Coronal CT without contrast. (**c**) Preoperative embolization of renal cell carcinoma via lateral sacral artery

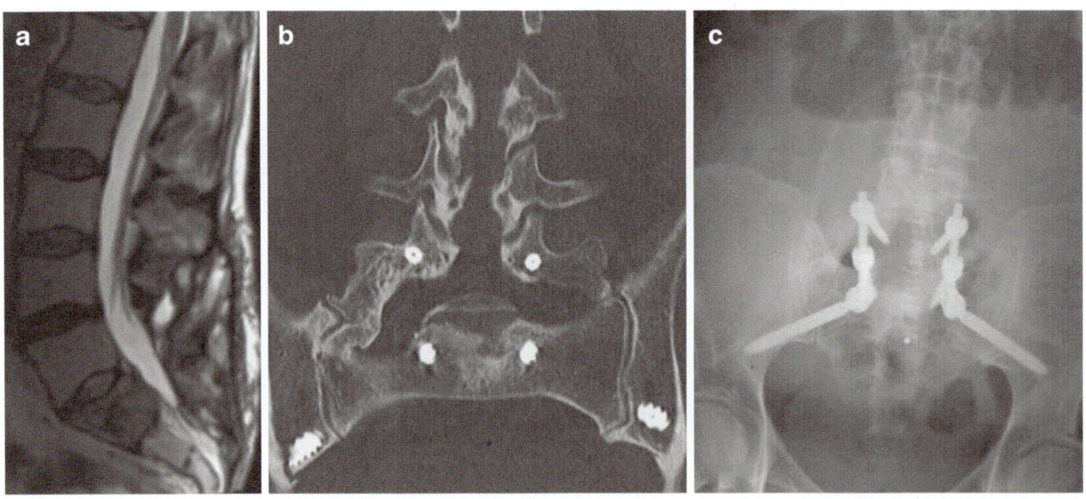

Fig. 19.4 A 49-year-old male with metastatic renal cell carcinoma of the sacrum; postoperative imaging of L5–S1 pelvic function. (**a**) Sagittal T2 MRI. (**b**) Coronal CT without contrast. (**c**) Plain AP radiograph

involved. Surgical lesioning of the L5 nerve root can result in impaired ankle dorsiflexion. Weakness in plantar flexion, and possible foot drop, may occur when the S1 root is sacrificed. However, patients can manage ambulating independently with an intact L4 and up—albeit with compensatory gait. Middle sacral amputation, including the S2 and S3 nerve roots, typically does not result in significant motor or gait disturbances. Unilateral lesioning of the S2 or S3 nerve roots generally results in preserved bowel/bladder and sexual function [11, 16], but several cases of eventual loss of sphincter and sexual function have been reported [43, 44]. Bilateral S2 or S3 lesioning leads to complete bowel/bladder incontinence, sexual dysfunction, and saddle anesthesia, with preserved motor and gait [11, 45]. Unilateral and bilateral lesioning of S4 and/or S5 in general do not lead to autonomic, bowel/bladder dysfunction or gait deviation. Hemisacrectomy with lesioning of the S1–5 roots may result in preserved sexual function and bowel/bladder function but results in unilateral motor and sensory deficits [16, 45].

In addition to the neural elements, sacral resection requires special attention to the adjacent structures. Tumors of direct extension, such as colorectal, may require a larger resection to remove a segment of the bowel. A sacroiliac resection can potentially cause iatrogenic injury to the lumbosacral trunk (L4 and L5 nerve roots) and may require complex lumbopelvic reconstruction with instrumentation to reestablish spinopelvic stability [11]. In terms of potential for vascular injury, a resection involving L5–S1 can cause damage to the common iliac artery. The internal iliac artery, lateral sacral artery, and median sacral artery are at risk in an upper sacral resection. Additionally, an osteotomy in the region of S2–S3 can cause damage to the superior gluteal vessels. Surgical resection of the lower sacrum, S3–S5, is relatively safe without significance of a risk of damage to a major vessel leading to hemorrhage [5].

In terms of timing and sequence of treatments that involve surgery, in certain cases, radiation is best performed after surgery instead of before, although this is pathology specific. For many solid tumors, decompressive surgery followed by postoperative radiotherapy may lead to better local control compared to surgery alone [11, 16, 32]. Radiation prior to surgery is associated with adverse outcomes including wound complication and failure of instrumentation [46]. High-dose hypofractionated stereotactic radiosurgery (SRS) to the spine has the added benefit of delivering radiation over a small area, which is particularly advantageous in treating sacral metastases because they are in close proximity to the pelvic viscera. This reduces the amount of time for radiation and reduces the side effects compared to conventional radiation therapy [11, 32]. CT myelography is ordered prior to SRS, especially for patients with instrumentation.

Similar to vertebroplasty, sacroplasty is gaining in popularity as a treatment for sacral fractures associated with metastases, where instability and neurologic dysfunction are absent [47]. This may be under CT or fluoroscopic guidance and has shown promising results in relieving pain associated with metastatic sacral fractures [48].

References

1. Feldenzer JA, McGauley JL, McGillicuddy JE. Sacral and presacral tumors: problems in diagnosis and management. Neurosurgery. 1989;25:884–91.
2. Bogduk N. Clinical anatomy of the lumbar spine and sacrum. 4th ed. Philadephia, PA: Elsevier; 2005. p. 59–76.
3. Wang T, Fielding LC, Parikh A, Kothari M, Alamin T. Sacral spinous processes; a morphologic classification and biomechanical characterization of strength. Spine J. 2015;15(12):2544–51.
4. Sae-Jung S, Khamanarong K, Woraputtaporn W, Amarttayakong P. Awareness of the median sacral artery during lumbosacral spinal surgery: an anatomic cadaveric study of its relationship to the lumbosacral spine. Eur Spine J. 2015;24(11):2520–4.
5. Zoccali C, Skoch J, Patel A, Walter CM, Maykowski P, Baaj AA. The surgical neurovascular anatomy relating to partial and complete sacral and sacroiliac resections: a cadaveric, anatomic study. Eur Spine J. 2015;24(5):1109–13.
6. Woon JT, Stringer MD. The anatomy of the sacrococcygeal corneal region and its clinical relevance. Anat Sci Int. 2014;89(4):207–14.
7. Gray H. Gray's anatomy: descriptive and applied. London, UK: Longmans; 1967. p. 286–547.
8. Rhee J, Kosztowski TA, Bydon M, Gokaslan ZL. Sacral tumors: regional challenges. In: Steinmets MP, Benzel EC, editors. Spine surgery: techniques, complications, avoidance, and management. 4th ed. Philadephia, PA: Elsevier; 2016. p. 1061–7.
9. Fourney DR, Gokaslan ZL. Surgical approaches for the resection of sacral tumors. In: Dickman CA, editor. Spinal cord and spinal column tumors: principles and practice. New York: Thieme; 2006. p. 632–6.
10. Payer M. Neurological manifestation of sacral tumors. Neurosurg Focus. 2003;1(2):1–6.
11. Quraishi NA, Giannoulis KE, Edwards KL, Boszczyk BM. Management of metastatic sacral tumours. Eur Spine J. 2012;21(10):1984–93.
12. Feiz-Erfan I, Fox BD, Nader R, Suki D, Chakrabarti I, Mendel E, Gokaslan ZL, Rao G, Rhines LD. Surgical treatment of sacral metastases: indications and results. J Neurosurg Spine. 2012;17:285–91.
13. Shah LM, Salsman KL. Imaging of spinal metastatic disease. Int J Surg Oncol. 2011;2011:1–12.

14. Fukushima T, Kasai Y, Kato K, Fujisawa K, Uchida A. Intradural squamous cell carcinoma of the sacrum. World J Oncol. 2009;7:16.
15. Pain GJ. Extremities and spine-evaluation and differential diagnosis. In: Omer G, Spinner M, Van Beek A, editors. Management of peripheral nerve problems. Philadelphia: WB Saunders; 1980. p. 169.
16. Sciubba DM, Petteys RJ, Garces-Ambrossi GL, Noggle JC, McGirt MJ, Wolinsky JP, Witham TF, Gokaslan ZL. Diagnosis and management of sacral tumors. J Neurosurg Spine. 2009;10:244–56.
17. Norstrom CW, Kernohan JW, Love JG. One hundred primary caudad tumors. JAMA. 1961;178:1071–7.
18. Diel J, Ortiz O, Losada RA, Price DB, Hayt MW, Katz DS. The sacrum: pathologic spectrum, multimodality imaging, and subspecialty approach. Radiographics. 2001;21(1):83–104.
19. Amorosa JK, Weintraub S, Amorosa LF, Safer JN, Rafii M. Sacral destruction: foraminal lines revisited. AJR. 1985;145(4):773–5.
20. Fourney DR, Gokaslan ZL. Sacral tumors: primary and metastatic. In: Dickman CA, Fehlings MG, Gokaslan ZL, editors. Spinal cord and spinal column tumors: principles and practice. New York: Thieme; 2006. p. 404–19.
21. Gerber S, Ollivier L, Leclere J, Vanel D, Missenard G, Brisse H, de Pinieux G, Neuenschwander S. Imaging of sacral tumours. Skelet Radiol. 2008;37(4): 277–89.
22. Algra PR, Bloem JL, Tissing H, FAlke TH, Arndt JW, Verteboom LJ. Detection of vertebral metastases: comparison between MR imaging and bone scintigraphy. Radiographics. 1991;11(2):219–32.
23. Galasko CS. Mechanisms of lytic and blastic metastatic disease of bone. Clin Orthop Relat Res. 1982;(169):20–7.
24. Horger M, Bares R. The role of sing-photon emission computed tomography/computed tomography in benign and malignant bone disease. Semin Nucl Med. 2006;36(4):286–94.
25. Savelli G, Chiti A, Grasselli G, Maccauro M, Rodai M, Bombardieri E. The role of bone SPECT study in diagnosis of single vertebral metastases. Anticancer Res. 2000;20:1115–20.
26. Bushnell DL, Kahn D, Huston B, Bevering CG. Utility of SPECT imaging for determination of vertebral metastases in patients with known primary tumors. Skelet Radiol. 1995;24:13–6.
27. Laufer I, Sciubba DM, Madera M, Bydon A, Witham TJ, Gokaslan ZL, Wolinsky JP. Surgical management of metastatic spinal tumors. Cancer Control. 2012;19(2):122–8.
28. Babu NV, Titus VT, Chittaranjan S, Abraham G, Prem H, Korula RJ. Computed tomographically guided biopsy of the spine. Spine. 1994;19:439–44.
29. Kattapuram SV, Khurana JS, Rosenthal DI. Percutaneous needle biopsy of the spine. Spine. 1992;17:561–4.
30. Lis E, Bilsky MH, Pisinski L, Boland P, Healey JH, O'Malley B, et al. Percutaneous CT-guided biopsy of osseous lesion of the spine in patients with known or suspected malignancy. AJNR Am J Neuroradiol. 2004;25:1583–8.
31. Talamo G, Dimaio C, Abbi KKS, Pandey MK, Malysz J, Creer MH, Zhu J, Mir MA, Varlotto JM. Current role of radiation therapy for multiple myeloma. Front Oncol. 2015;5(40):1–6.
32. Gerszten PC, Mendel E, Yamada Y. Radiotherapy and radiosurgery for metastatic spine disease: what are the options, indications, and outcomes? Spine. 2009;34:S78–92.
33. Laufer I, Rubin DG, Lis E, Cox BW, Stubblefield MD, Yamada Y, Bilsky MH. The NOMS framework: approach to the treatment of spinal metastatic tumors. Oncologist. 2013;18(6):744–51.
34. Maranzano E, Bellavita R, Rossi R, et al. Short-course versus split-course radiotherapy in metastatic spinal cord compression: results of a phase III, randomized, multicenter trial. J Clin Oncol. 2005;23:3358–65.
35. Fisher CG, DiPaola CP, Ryken TC, et al. A novel classification system for spinal instability in neoplastic disease: an evidence-based approach and expert consensus from the Spinal Oncology Study Group. Spine. 2010;35(2):E1221–9.
36. Bacci G, Savini R, Calderoni P, et al. Solitary plasmacytoma of the vertebral column: a report of 15 cases. Tumori. 1982;68(3):271–83.
37. Patchell RA, Ribbs PA, Regine WF, et al. Direct decompressive surgical resection in the treatment of spinal cord compression caused by metastatic cancer: a randomized trial. Lancet. 2005;366(9486):643–8.
38. Bilsky MH, Laufer I, Burch S. Shifting paradigms in the treatment of metastatic spine disease. Spine. 2009;34(22):S101–7.
39. Cybulski GR. Methods of surgical stabilization for metastatic disease of the spine. Neurosurgery. 1989;25:240–52.
40. Founrey DR, Gokaslan ZL. Spinal instability and deformity due to neoplastic conditions. Neurosurg Focus. 2003;14(1):E8.
41. Fourney DR, Frangou EM, Ryken TC, et al. Spinal instability neoplastic score: an analysis of reliability and validity from the spine oncology study group. J Clin Oncol. 2011;29(22):3072–7.
42. Langdon J, Way A, Heaton S, Bernard J, Molloy S. The management of spinal metastases from renal cell carcinoma. Ann R Coll Surg Engl. 2009;91(8):649–52.
43. Stener B, Gunterberg B. High amputation of the sacrum for extirpation of tumors. Principles and technique. Spine (Phila Pa 1976). 1978;3(4):351–66.
44. Althausen PL, Schneider PD, Bold RJ, Gupta MC, Goodnight JE, Khatri VP. Multimodality management of a giant cell tumor arising in the proximal sacrum: a case report. Spine. 2002;27(15):E361–5.
45. Biagini R, Ruggieri P, Mercuri M, et al. Neurologic deficit after resection of the sacrum. Chir Organi Mov. 1997;82(4):357–72.
46. Ghogawala Z, Mansfield FL, Borges LF. Spinal radiation before surgical decompression adversely affects

outcomes of surgery for symptomatic metastatic spinal cord compression. Spine. 2001;26(7):818–24.
47. Zhang J, Wu C, Gu Y, Li M. Percutaneous sacroplasty for sacral metastatic tumors under fluoroscopic guidance only. Korean J Radiol. 2008;9(6):572–6.
48. Whitlow CT, Mussat-Whitlow BJ, Mattern CWT, Baker MD, Morris PP. Sacroplasty versus vertebroplasty: comparable clinical outcomes for the treatment of fracture-related pain. AJNR Am J Neuroradiol. 2007;28:1266–70.

20 Radiation Therapy for Spinal Metastases

Waqar Haque and Bin S. Teh

Spinal metastatic disease is diagnosed in about 10% of cancer patients and 40% of patients who have metastatic disease [1–3]. The most common symptom associated with spinal disease is back pain, though spinal metastases can also cause sensory deficit, radicular pain, weakness, bowel/bladder dysfunction, and paralysis. Due to the potential for permanent neurologic damage, spinal cord compression due to metastases can be a medical emergency. Workup for patient's suspected of having spinal metastases includes complete neurologic exam including a digital rectal exam, assessment of pain, assessment of bladder/bowel function, and imaging of the entire spinal cord with magnetic resonance imaging (MRI). Treatment options include surgery, external beam radiation therapy, radionuclide treatment, chemotherapy, corticosteroids, pain medication including both nonsteroidal anti-inflammatory drugs (NSAIDs) and narcotics, kyphoplasty, and vertebroplasty. The present report will provide an overview of radiotherapy for spinal metastases, including radionuclide treatment and the two different methods of external beam radiation therapy (EBRT), conventional external beam radiation therapy (CEBRT), and spinal stereotactic body radiation therapy (SBRT).

Radionuclides are radioactive atoms that are injected intravenously to the bloodstream and are incorporated into the bone matrix. Radionuclides that have been demonstrated to improve pain in patients with skeletal metastases include the beta-emitters phosphorus-32, strontium-89, samarium-153, rhenium-186, and rhenium-188 and the alpha-particle emitter radium-223 [4]. Indications for radionuclide use include diffuse skeletal metastases visualized on nuclear medicine bone scan, painful skeletal metastases inadequately treated by analgesics, and patients with hormone-insensitive disease (for prostate cancer) [4]. Radionuclides are typically used in patients with osteoblastic metastatic disease, as in patients with prostate cancer or breast cancer, and can provide pain relief in 60–92% of patients for a median duration of 6 months [5, 6]. One randomized trial demonstrated that for patients with metastatic prostate cancer, equivalent palliation was achieved for patients treated with strontium-89 compared to EBRT, though patients receiving treatment with EBRT lived longer [7]. Radium-223 has been shown to improve overall survival and decrease risk of skeletal events in patients with castrate-resistant prostate cancer [8]. The most serious side effect associated with radionuclide treatment is myelosuppression, most commonly seen in the form of thrombocytopenia decreasing to 40–60% from baseline, while additional side effects include

W. Haque, MD, B. S. Teh, MD
Radiation Oncology Department,
Houston Methodist Hospital, Houston, TX, USA
e-mail: BTeh@houstonmethodist.org

R. A. W. Marco (ed.), *Metastatic Spine Disease*, https://doi.org/10.1007/978-3-319-76252-4_20

nausea, loose stools, hematuria, and heart palpitations [4].

EBRT is among the standard treatments for palliation for patients with spinal metastatic disease. In the following paragraphs, we will describe treatment with CEBRT, after which we will describe the more novel SBRT in greater detail. CEBRT can be offered to patients for management of pain, treatment of cord compression, or prevention of morbidity in bone metastases and can be offered definitively or postoperatively. Patients with spinal metastases should, if they meet the appropriate criteria listed in Table 20.1, receive surgery, followed by CEBRT.

In a randomized trial, patients with spinal cord compression were treated with direct decompressive surgery followed by either palliative radiation therapy to a dose of 30 gray (Gy) in 10 fractions or the same EBRT dose alone. There were statistically significant improvements for the surgical cohort in every endpoint: patients who regained ambulation (62% vs. 19%), duration of ambulatory status (122 days vs. 13 days), and overall survival (122 days vs. 100 days) [9].

Table 20.1 ASTRO criteria for patients considered for surgical management for spinal cord decompression followed by radiation therapy

Characteristic	Factors favoring surgical decompression plus postoperative CEBRT
Radiographic	1. Solitary site of tumor progression
	2. Absence of visceral of brain metastases
	3. Spinal instability
Patient	1. Age <65 years
	2. KPS ≥70
	3. Projected survival of >3 months
	4. Slow progression of neurologic symptoms
	5. Maintained ambulation
	6. Nonambulatory for <48 h
Tumor	1. Relatively radioresistant tumor histologic type (i.e., melanoma)
	2. Site of origin suggesting relatively indolent course (i.e., prostate, breast, kidney)
Treatment	1. Previous EBRT failed

From Lutz S, Berk L, Chang E et al. Palliative radiotherapy for bone metastases: an ASTRO evidence-based guideline. Int J Radiat Oncol Biol Phys. 2011;79:965–976. With permission from Elsevier

Multiple randomized trials have demonstrated that only 19–30% of patients with spinal cord compression regain ambulation following radiation therapy alone [10–12]. There are currently no published trials in the postoperative setting of CEBRT evaluating the use of single-fraction treatment (SFT), and the most commonly used postoperative fractionation scheme has been 30 Gy in 10 fractions.

CEBRT can also be used definitive for spinal metastases for patients that do not meet the aforementioned ASTRO criteria for surgical resection. The optimal fractionation scheme for CEBRT has been investigated in multiple randomized trials. The first such trial was the Radiation Therapy Oncology Group (RTOG) 74-02 that compared 40.5 Gy in 15 fractions to 20 Gy in 5 fractions for solitary metastases or 30 Gy in 10 fractions to 20 Gy, 25 Gy, or 15 Gy in 5 fractions for patients with multiple metastases and found that there was no difference in pain control (54% of patients achieved complete pain relief, and 90% achieved some level of pain relief), though reanalysis demonstrated that on multivariate analysis, a higher number of fractions were correlated with a greater likelihood of complete remission of pain [13, 14]. Since then, multiple randomized trials have demonstrated equivalency between SFT and multi-fraction treatment (MFT) in the setting of CEBRT for palliation of spinal metastases, with a complete or partial pain response rate of 53–88% [15–20]. The newly updated ASTRO guidelines regarding the use of radiation therapy for bone metastases state that a single 8 Gy fraction provides noninferior pain relief compared to MFT for patients with spinal metastasis and that this treatment is recommended for patients with a limited life expectancy due to its convenience [21].

Re-irradiation can also safely be administered using CEBRT for patients with recurrent spine pain after an initial course of EBRT, given that at least 1 month has elapsed since the completion of the initial course of treatment and that normal tissue dose constraints for the spinal cord can be adhered to [21]. A multicenter randomized trial demonstrated that re-treatment with either 8 Gy in a single fraction or 20 Gy in

5 fractions could safely be administered in patients receiving a prior course of spine RT, though only 28–32% of patients had a response to re-treatment [22]. The radiation oncologists were required to keep the biologically equivalent dose to the spinal cord ≤60 Gy. A meta-analysis of re-irradiation for bone metastases that included 36% of patients with spinal disease confirmed that re-irradiation can be safely delivered in this patient population and reported a 58% response rates in all sites, with no cases of radiation myelopathy reported [23]. Healthy patients who have recurrent spinal cord compression despite previous radiation therapy may benefit from surgery followed by radiation therapy rather than re-irradiation alone. Patients who are candidates for re-irradiation are thus evaluated by a multidisciplinary team to determine whether re-irradiation or surgery is preferred. It should be noted that re-irradiation further disrupts the surrounding soft tissue, thus potentially increasing the likelihood of wound complications in the event that surgery is later indicated.

CEBRT is typically administered with the use of a linear accelerator using photons. The field arrangement varies by disease site. The entire vertebral body, transverse processes, spinous process, and spinal cord are included within the treatment volume. In the cervical spine, the optimal beam arrangement is two opposed lateral beams in order to spare toxicity associated with dose delivery to the esophagus. For lesions in the thoracic spine, a single posterior-anterior (PA) beam can be used, which allows sparing of the anterior mediastinal organs, or an anterior-posterior (AP)/PA beam arrangement. Lesions in the lumbar spine are typically treated using an AP/PA beam arrangement. One vertebral body above the lesion and one vertebral body below the lesion are included within the treatment field to provide treatment to any microscopic metastatic disease. A computed tomography (CT) simulation is typically performed prior to treatment for assistance with treatment planning, a process in which a patient lays down on the treatment table and is immobilized using an indexable vacuum bag device, though in emergent situations patients can be placed on the treatment table of the linear accelerator and a clinical treatment can be performed without three-dimensional planning. On the day of the treatment, the patient is lined up by marks made during the CT simulation, and a kilovoltage (kV) image is taken prior to treatment to ensure an accurate setup. Pretreatment images can be taken every five treatments to ensure the patient is being set up in the correct position.

The most concerning side effect in any instance of spinal irradiation is radiation myelopathy. The Quantitative Analysis of Normal Tissue Effects in the Clinic (QUANTEC) reports that the risk of radiation myelopathy with a maximum cord dose of 50 Gy is 0.2%, with a 6% chance of myelopathy when the spinal cord dose is treated with 60 Gy and a 50% chance of myelopathy with a spinal cord dose of 69 Gy [24]. Due to the catastrophic consequences associated with myelopathy, radiation oncologists make every attempt to prevent this outcome, and the recommended maximum spinal cord dose is typically 45 Gy. Additional side effects can include dysphagia, odynophagia, fatigue, skin irritation, radiation fibrosis, nerve damage, fracture, or lymphedema.

Advances in radiation therapy technology including the use of image fusion, development of more rigid immobilization devices, computerized treatment planning, image-guided treatment, intensity-modulated radiation therapy, and sub-millimeter treatment accuracy have allowed radiation oncologists to offer a more conformal, higher-dose, lower fraction EBRT technique called SBRT [25]. Based on technology developed for intracranial stereotactic radiosurgery (SRS) [26], SBRT is a radiation technique that employs significantly higher doses delivered in one or a few fractions to a conformal target volume with steep dose falloff. Data suggests that the higher, ablative doses employed in SBRT may provide a therapeutic advantage when compared to treatment with CEBRT [27, 28]. Indeed, the inadequate response rates offered by CEBRT lead to the experimentation with and use of SBRT for treatment of spinal metastases.

Table 20.2 ASTRO inclusion and exclusion criteria for patients suitable for spine SBRT

Characteristic	Inclusion	Exclusion
Radiographic	1. Spinal or paraspinal metastasis by MRI 2. No more than two consecutive or three noncontiguous spine segments involved	1. Spinal MRI cannot be completed 2. Epidural compression of spinal cord or cauda equina 3. Spinal canal compromise >25% 4. Unstable spine requiring surgical stabilization 5. Tumor location within 5 mm of spinal cord or cauda equina
Patient	1. Age ≥18 years 2. KPS of ≥40–50 3. Medical inoperable (or patient refused surgery)	1. Active connective tissue disease 2. Worsening or progressive neurologic deficit 3. Inability to lie flat on table for SBRT 4. Patient in hospice or with <3-month life expectancy
Tumor	1. Histologic proof of malignancy 2. Biopsy of spine lesion if first suspected metastasis 3. Oligometastatic or bone-only metastatic disease	1. Radiosensitive histology such as multiple myeloma 2. Extraspinal disease not eligible for further treatment
Previous treatment	1. Previous EBRT <45 Gy total dose 2. Failure of previous surgery to that spinal level 3. Presence of gross residual disease after surgery	1. Previous SBRT to the same level 2. Systemic radionuclide delivery within 30 days of SBRT 3. EBRT within 90 days before SBRT 4. Chemotherapy within 30 days of SBRT

From Rades D, Fehlauer F, Stalpers LJ et al. A prospective evaluation of two radiotherapy schedules with 10 versus 20 fractions for the treatment of metastatic spinal cord compression: final results of a multicenter study. Cancer. 2004;101:2687–2692. With permission from Elsevier

The indications for spine SBRT were initially described by Lutz et al. in the ASTRO guidelines regarding palliative radiation therapy for bone metastases and are included below in Table 20.2 [12].

The largest experience for SBRT in spinal metastases comes from the University of Pittsburgh, where in a single-institution prospective nonrandomized cohort they describe treated 500 cases of spinal metastases with a single fraction of SBRT or spinal stereotactic radiosurgery (SSRS) to a mean dose of 20 Gy [29]. Long-term local control was achieved in 90% of patients, and 86% of patients reported improvement in pain (Fig. 20.1).

Furthermore, unlike CEBRT, SSRS has been shown to directly decrease epidural spinal cord compression. In a phase II study from Henry Ford Hospital, 62 patients with metastatic epidural cord compression, including patients with relatively radioresistant histologies such as renal cell carcinoma, were treated with SSRS to a median dose of 16 Gy [30]. Investigators reported both a mean reduction in the volume of epidural tumor of 65 ± 14% and improvement in thecal sac patency from 55 ± 4% to 76 ± −3% ($p < 0.001$) within 2 months of treatment. Furthermore, among patients presented with neurologic deficit, 74% (20/27) of patients had improved or stable neurologic function, and among patients presenting with intact neurologic function, 94% (33/35) of patients continued to have an intact neurologic exam after treatment, demonstrating the efficacy of SSRS in patients with epidural spinal cord compression. In addition to single-fraction delivery, spine SBRT can be delivered in multiple fractions. In a phase I/II trial from MD Anderson, authors describe treating patients in 3 fractions to a dose of 27–30 Gy, resulting in 54% of patients reporting no pain at 6 months and 81% local control at 1 year [31]. Spine SBRT can safely be administered in patients who have previously

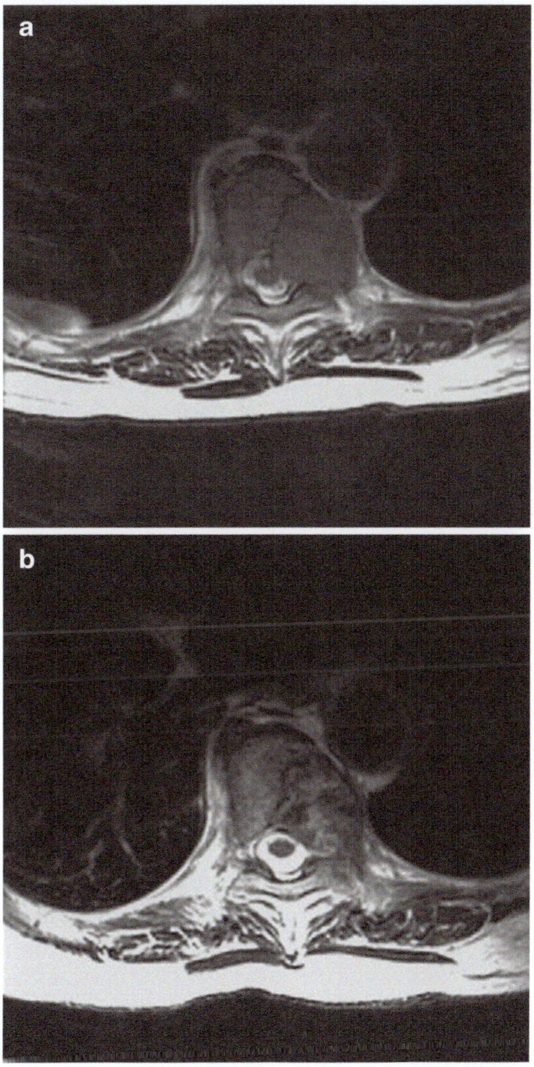

Fig. 20.1 Patient with colorectal cancer metastasis demonstrated regression of epidural and paraspinal component of tumor 8 weeks after 21 Gy delivered in a single fraction. (**a**) Pretreatment. (**b**) Three months posttreatment. From Yamada Y, Bilsky MH, Lovelock M et al. High-dose, single-fraction image-guided intensity-modulated radiotherapy for metastatic spinal lesion. Int J Radiat Oncol Biol Phys. 2008;71:484–490. With permission from Elsevier

received radiation therapy. In a study from the University of Toronto, investigators treated patients who had previously received radiation for spinal metastases with re-irradiation to a dose of 24 Gy in 3 fractions and reported a 1-year local control rate of 96% with no radiation-induced myelopathy [32].

The optimal dose for SSRS is currently an active question. There may be a dose-response relationship, though the evidence for this is largely circumstantial. In a phase I trial from Henry Ford, there was a non-statistically significant trend to increased pain relief when the SSRS dose was increased from 10 to 20 Gy in 2 Gy increments, with 80% of patients reporting pain relief with doses ≥16 Gy, very similar to the 86% of patients with pain relief in the study from the University of Pittsburgh [29, 33, 34]. Indeed, in a single-institution report from the University of Florida, only 43% of patients reported pain relief when treated with an SSRS dose of 15 Gy [35]. Consequently, in a multi-institution phase I/II trial to assess the safety of feasibility of SSRS for spine metastases, RTOG 0631, the investigators opted to require a dose of either 16 or 18 Gy in a single fraction to be delivered to the tumor [36].

SSRS and spine SBRT can also be delivered to spinal metastatic disease postoperatively. Consensus recommendations state that optimal patients for postoperative SBRT are patients with a radioresistant primary, patients with only one to two levels of adjacent disease, and those with previous radiation therapy [37]. Though the optimal dose for postoperative spinal SBRT is currently under investigation, the available data suggest that high-dose single or multi-fraction SBRT provides superior local control to low-dose fractionated SBRT. In a retrospective review from Memorial Sloan Kettering, 186 patients with epidural spinal cord compression were treated with surgical decompression followed by postoperative radiation with SSRS to 24 Gy, high-dose hypofractionated SBRT to 24–30 Gy in 3 fractions, or low-dose hypofractionated SBRT to 18–36 Gy in 5–6 fractions. Local progression was 4.1% for the high-dose SBRT arm, while it was 22.6% for the low-dose SBRT arm [38]. A second retrospective review reporting on outcomes for patients with spinal metastases treated postoperatively with SBRT from the University of Toronto confirmed superior local control for patients treated with high-dose SBRT (18–26 Gy in 1 or 2 fractions) when compared to patients treated with low-dose SBRT (18–40 Gy in 3–5 fractions) [39].

The high doses used in SBRT treatment to eradicate tumor along with the steep dose gradients required to respect the tolerance dose for the adjacent organs at risk (OAR) necessitate a high degree of accuracy while delivering SBRT treatment. The accuracy of the treatment delivered should be within 1–2 mm, as a shift of 2–3 mm can significantly increase the dose delivered to the spinal cord [40, 41]. The initial step in ensuring accuracy during treatment delivery begins during the CT simulation process, which is a necessary prerequisite to begin treatment planning for spinal SBRT. The patient undergoes a CT scan with the goal of obtaining a three-dimensional map of the patient's internal anatomy while being placed in an immobilization device in an effort to place the patient in a fixed, reproducible position during treatment delivery. The most commonly used device to place the patient in a reproducible position with minimal motion is the noninvasive near-rigid stereotactic body frame, which minimizes intrafractional patient motion [42] (Fig. 20.2).

As displayed in Fig. 20.2, the commercially available BodyFIX® system (Medical Intelligence; Schwabmuenchen, Germany) contains a sealed whole-body vacuum cushion, a clear plastic foil wrap, and a carbon fiber base. The system also includes a dual vacuum system, one of which creates a vacuum seal with a uniform pressure that covers the patient and the other one removes the air from the cushion device so it conforms to the unique anatomy of the patient. The BodyFIX® system is typically used for immobilization when SBRT is delivered using a conventional linear accelerator, whereas treatment with the CyberKnife® (Accuray; CA, USA) device does not require a stringent immobilization due to its ability to conduct real-time intrafractional image guidance.

Delineation of the target volume typically requires image fusion between a pre- and post-contrast T1 and T2 multiplanar MRI to the CT obtained during the simulation, as the MRI is more sensitive at displaying the gross disease and subclinical disease spread [43, 44]. The International Spine Radiosurgery Consortium has created guidelines regarding the delineation of the target for spine SBRT [45]. The gross tumor volume (GTV) is the gross disease within the vertebra, the paraspinal component of the disease, and the disease within the epidural space. The clinical target volume (CTV) includes any abnormal marrow signal and an expansion into the normal bony space to ensure treatment of subclinical disease. The International Spine Radiosurgery Consortium recommends using a Weinstein-Boriani-Biagini system to divide the vertebra into six anatomic

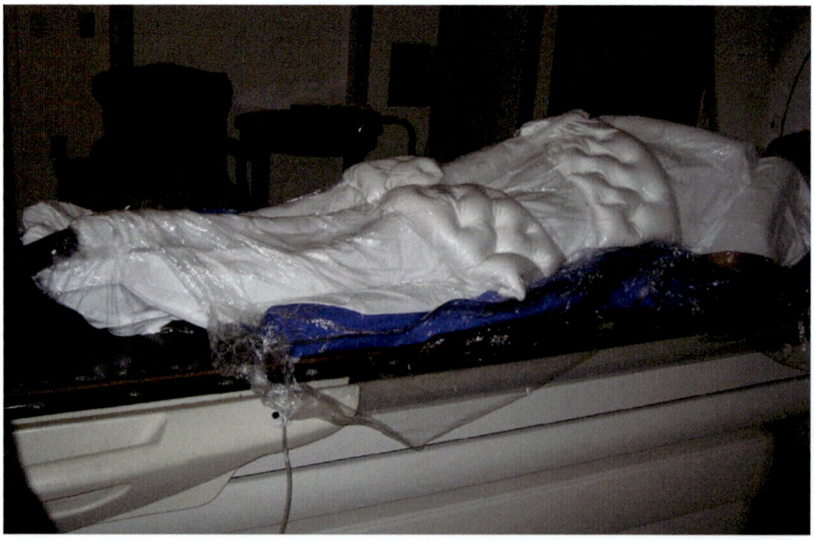

Fig. 20.2 BodyFIX® system (Medical Intelligence; Schwabmuenchen, Germany). From Lo SS, Sahgal A, Teh BS, Gerszten PC, Chang EL. Stereotactic Body Radiation Therapy for Spinal Metastases. London, UK: Future Medicine; 2014

compartments to select the adjacent normal bony spaces for inclusion of contouring within the CTV [45, 46]. The planning treatment volume (PTV) describes a margin placed around the CTV to ensure the target receives adequate dose while accounting for uncertainty with the patient setup. The PTV margin is recommended to be ≤3 mm and should be carved out of the spinal cord or cauda equina. Since dose to the PTV must oftentimes be carved around the OAR, specifically the spinal cord, the sculpting of the dose around these structures is best achieved using inversely planned treatment algorithms including intensity-modulated radiation therapy (IMRT) and volumetric-modulated arc therapy (VMAT), with VMAT adding the possible advantage of decreased treatment time which may increase patient comfort and decrease the likelihood of patient movement during treatment [47, 48] (Fig. 20.3).

Spinal SBRT can be delivered using either a conventional linear accelerator or the CyberKnife® system. Available data suggest either treatment platform provides similar clinical outcomes. Image-guided radiotherapy (IGRT) is essential to ensuring accurate patient setup prior to the delivery of each fraction of treatment. On a conventional linear accelerator, the patient is initially placed within the immobilization device on the treatment couch based on in-room lasers and marks created during the CT simulation. Subsequently to initial patient placement, images of the patient are taken using imaging systems either mounted on the gantry such as volumetric cone-beam CT or planar kV X-rays, a mobile CT scanner on rails, or stereoscopic kV X-ray sources on the floor of the treatment room with detector panels placed in the ceiling (ExacTrac®, Brainlab). The patient images taken before treatment are compared to the images obtained at the time of CT simulation to ensure that the patient's positioning is accurate. The CyberKnife® device is a robotic radiosurgery system that is able to deliver radiation treatment while using orthogonal X-rays to provide intrafraction imaging of the patient and provides intrafraction image guidance that achieves submillimeter accuracy [48–51]. During treatment, orthogonal X-rays are taken every 30–60 s and registered to the images obtained during the CT simulation process, and any changes required are delivered to the robot which is able to adjust the beam to accurately treat the updated target position without requiring repositioning of the patient.

Possible toxicities following spinal SBRT include radiation myelopathy, radiculopathy, plexopathy, vertebral compression fracture, and pain flare. Due to the devastating consequences of radiation-induced myelopathy, it is necessary that dose tolerances for the spinal cord be respected. The multi-institutional RTOG 0631 required a minimum of 3 mm distance between the tumor and the spinal cord [36]. The dose constraint for the spinal cord in this trial was a maximum cord dose of 14 Gy to <0.03 cc of the spinal cord, and that <10% of the cross-sectional area of the cord, defined as the cord at 6 mm above and below the SSRS target volume, received <10 Gy. Additional spinal cord dose constraints for hypofractionated SBRT with or without prior radiation therapy are recorded in consensus guidelines for spinal SBRT [37].

While there are several potential advantages to SBRT for spinal metastasis including rapid and durable pain control, decreased volume of bone marrow in the volume of treatment, and possible decompression due to epidural compression, there are also disadvantages such as the potential for catastrophic events and increased cost [50]. Whether or not SBRT can offer superior palliation and local control than CEBRT is currently an active research question [52]. We await the results of RTOG 0631 which is a phase II/III trial, which has completed the phase II portion demonstrating the feasibility and safety of SSRS in a multi-institutional setting, and is now comparing the efficacy of SSRS of 16–18 Gy to a single fraction of CEBRT to 8 Gy [36]. In the future, we anticipate that spine SBRT may be the standard of care for patients with inoperable spinal metastatic disease and that it will be incorporated into treatment paradigms for minimally invasive or noninvasive treatment for patients with spinal cord compression [52–55].

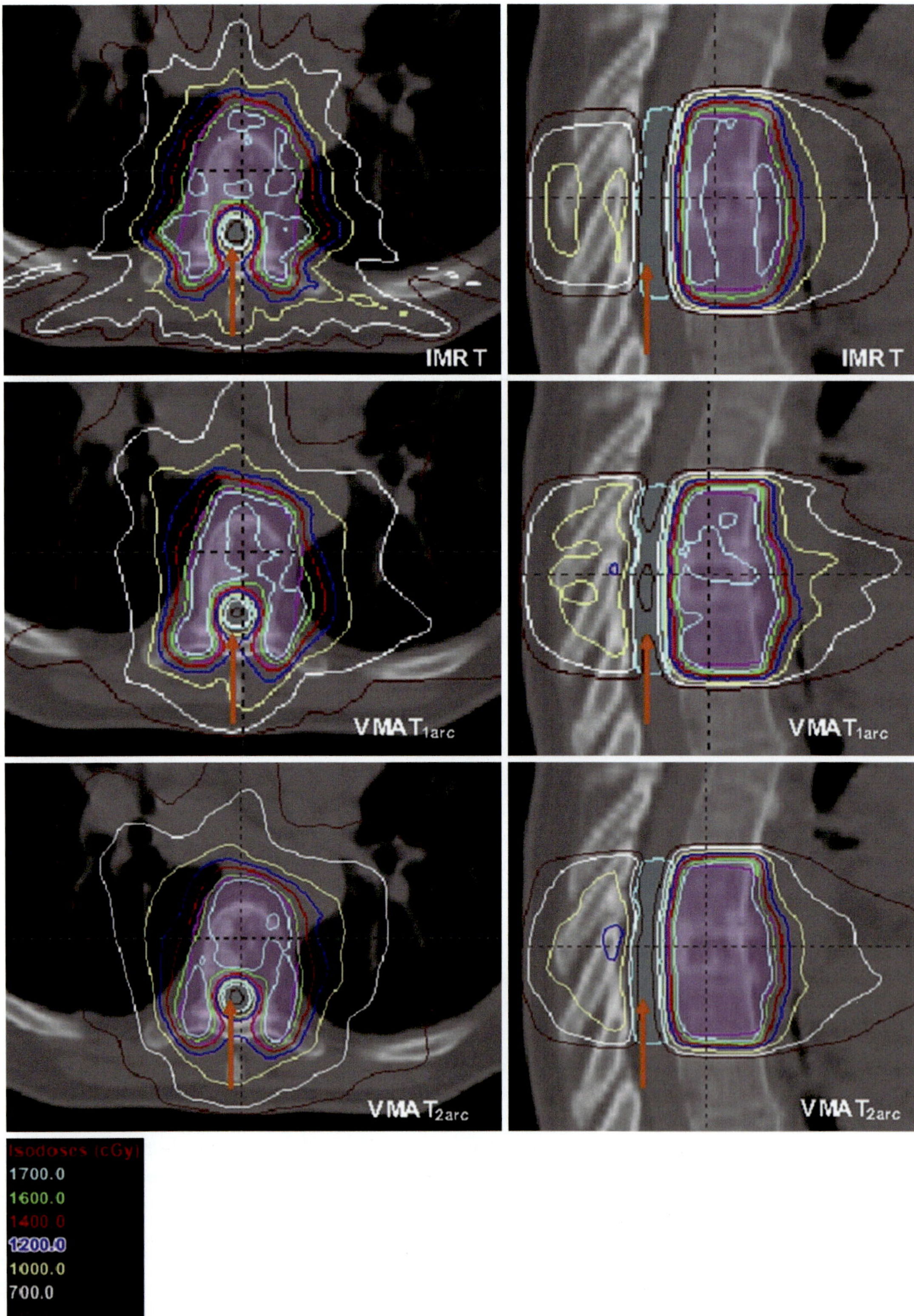

Fig. 20.3 Image displaying the ability of IMRT and VMAT to sculpt dose around the spinal cord. From Wu QJ, Yoo S, Kirkpatrick JP et al. Volumetric arc intensity-modulated therapy for spine body radiotherapy comparison with static intensity-modulated treatment. Int J Radiat Oncol Biol Phys 2009;75:1596–1604. With permission from Elsevier

References

1. Fornasier VL, Horne JG. Metastases to the vertebral column. Cancer. 1975;36(2):590–4.
2. Grant R, Papadopoulos SM, Greenberg HS. Metastatic epidural spinal cord compression. Neurol Clin. 1991; 9(4):825–41.
3. Hatrick NC, Lucas JD, Timothy AR, et al. The surgical treatment of metastatic disease of the spine. Radiother Oncol. 2000;56(3):335–9.
4. Tomblyn M. The role of bone-seeking radionuclides in the palliative treatment of patients with painful osteoblastic skeletal metastases. Cancer Control. 2012; 19:137–44.
5. Fuster D, Herranz D, Vidal-Sicart S, et al. Usefulness of strontium-89 for bone pain palliation in metastatic breast cancer patient. Nucl Med Commun. 2000; 21:623–6.
6. Gunawardana DH, Lichtenstein M, Better N, et al. Results of strontium-89 therapy in patients with prostate cancer resistant to chemotherapy. Clin Nucl Med. 2004;29:81–5.
7. Oosterhof GO, Roberts JT, de Reijke TM, et al. Strontium(89) chloride versus palliative local field radiotherapy in patients with hormonal escaped prostate cancer: a phase III sstudy of the European Organisation for Research and Treatment of Cancer, Genitourinary Group. Eur Urol. 2003;44:519–26.
8. Parker C, Nilsson S, Heinrich D, et al. Alpha Emitter Radium-223 and survival in metastatic prostate cancer. N Engl J Med. 2013;369:213–23.
9. Patchell RA, Tibbs PA, Regine WF, et al. Direct decompressive surgical resection in the treatment of spinal cord compression caused by metastatic cancer: a randomized trial. Lancet. 2005;366:643–8.
10. Maranzano E, Bellavita R, Rossi R, et al. Short-course versus split-course radiotherapy in metastatic spinal cord compression: results of a phase III, randomized, multicenter trial. J Clin Oncol. 2005;23:3358–65.
11. Maranzano E, Trippa F, Casale M, et al. 8Gy single-dose radiotherapy is effective in metastatic spinal cord compression: results of a phase III randomized multicenter Italian trial. Radiother Oncol. 2009;93: 174–9.
12. Rades D, Fehlauer F, Stalpers LJ, et al. A prospective evaluation of two radiotherapy schedules with 10 versus 20 fractions for the treatment of metastatic spinal cord compression: finals results of a multicenter study. Cancer. 2004;101:2687–92.
13. Tong D, Gillick L. The palliation of symptomatic osseous metastases final results of the study by the radiation therapy group. Cancer. 1982;50:893–9.
14. Blitzer PH. Reanalysis of the RTOG study of the palliation of symptomatic osseous metastasis. Cancer. 1985;55:1468–72.
15. Steenland E, Leer JW, van Houwelingen H, et al. The effect of a single fraction compared to multiple fractions on painful bone metastases: a global analysis of the Dutch Bone Metastasis Study. Radiother Oncol. 1999;52:101–9.
16. 8 Gy single fraction radiotherapy for the treatment of metastatic skeletal pain: randomized comparison with a multifraction schedule over 12 months of followup. Bone Pain Trial Working Party. Radiother Oncol. 1999;52:111–121.
17. Meeuse JJ, van der Linden YM, van Tienhoven G, et al. Efficacy of radiotherapy for painful bone metastases during the last 12 weeks of life: results from the Dutch Bone Metastasis Study. Cancer. 2010;116:2716–25.
18. Majumder D, Chatterjee D, Bandyopadhyay A, et al. Single fraction versus multiple fraction radiotherapy for palliation of painful vertebral bone metastases: a prospective study. Indian J Palliat Care. 2012;18:202–6.
19. Howell DD, James JL, Hartsell WF, et al. Single-fraction radiotherapy versus multifraction radiotherapy for palliation of painful vertebral bone metastases-equivalent efficacy, less toxicity, more convenient: a subset analysis of Radiation Therapy Oncology Group trial 97-14. Cancer. 2013;119:888–96.
20. Gutierrez Bayard L, Salas Buzon Mdel C, Angulo Pain E, et al. Radiation therapy for the management of painful bone metastases: results from a randomized trial. Rep Pract Oncol Radiot. 2014;19:405–11.
21. Lutz S, Balbone T, Jones J, et al. Palliative radiation therapy for bone metastases: update of an ASTRO evidence-based guideline. Pract Radiat Oncol. 2017;7(1): 4–12.
22. Chow E, van der Linden Y, Roos D, et al. Single versus multiple fractions of repeat radiation for painful bone metastases: a randomized, controlled, non-inferiority trial. Lancet Oncol. 2014;15:164–71.
23. Huisman M, van den Bosch MA, Wijlemans JW, et al. Effectiveness of reirradiation for painful bone metastases: a systematic review and meta-analysis. Int J Radiat Oncol Biol Phys. 2012;84:8–14.
24. Marks LB, Yorke ED, Jackson A, et al. Use of normal tissue complication probably models in the clinic. Int J Radiat Oncol Biol Phys. 2010;76:S10–9.
25. Sahgal A, Roberge D, Schellenberg D, et al. The Canadian Association of Radiation Oncology Scope of Practice guidelines for lung, liver and spine stereotactic body radiotherapy. Clin Onco (R Coll Radiol). 2012;24:629–39.
26. Leksell L. The stereotaxic method and radiosurgery of the brain. Acta Chir Scand. 1951;102:316–9.
27. Flickinger JC, Kondziolka D, Lunsford LD. Radiobiological analysis of tissue responses following radiosurgery. Technol Cancer Res Treat. 2003;2: 87–92.
28. Jhaveri PM, Teh BS, Paulino AC, et al. A dose-response relationship for time to bone pain resolution after stereotactic body radiotherapy (SBRT) for renal cell carcinoma (RCC) bony metastases. Acta Oncol. 2012;51:584–8.
29. Gerszten PC, Burton SA, Ozhasoglu C, et al. Radiosurgery for spinal metastases: clinical experience in 500 cases from a single institution. Spine (Phila Pa 1976). 2007;32(2):193–9.
30. Ryu S, Rock J, Jain R, et al. Radiosurgical decompression of metastatic epidural spine metastasis. Cancer. 2010;116:2250–7.

31. Wang XS, Rhines LD, Shiu AS, et al. Stereotactic body radiation therapy for management of spinal metastases in patients without spinal cord compression: a phase 1–2 trial. Lancet Oncol. 2012;13:395–402.
32. Ryu S, Jin JJ, Jin RY, Rock J, Ajlouni M, Movsas B, Kim JH. Partial volume tolerance of spinal cord and complication of single dose radiosurgery. Cancer. 2007;109:628–36.
33. Sahgal A, Ames C, Chou D, et al. Stereotactic body radiotherapy is effective salvage therapy for patients with prior radiation of spinal metastases. Int J Radiat Oncol Biol Phys. 2009;74:723–31.
34. Ryu S, Jin R, Jin JJ, Qing C, Rock J, Anderson J, Movsas B. Pain control by image-guided radiosurgery for solitary spinal metastasis. J Pain Sympt Manage. 2008;35:292–8.
35. Amdur RJ, Bennett J, Olivier K, et al. A prospective, phase II study demonstrating the potential value and limitation of radiosurgery for spine metastases. Am J Clin Oncol. 2009;32(5):515–20.
36. Ryu S, Pugh SL, Gerszten PC, et al. RTOG 0631 phase 2/3 study of image guided stereotactic radiosurgery for localized (1-3) spinal metastases: phase 2 results. Pract Radiat Oncol. 2014;4:76–81.
37. Redmond KJ, Lo SS, Soltys SG, et al. Consensus guidelines for postoperative stereotactic body radiation therapy for spinal metastases: results of an international survey. J Neurosurg Spine. 2016;26(3): 299–306.
38. Laufer I, Iorgulescu JB, Chapman T, et al. Local disease control for spinal metastases following "separation surgery" and adjuvant hypofractionated or high-dose single-fraction stereotactic radiosurgery: outcome analysis in 186 patients. J Neurosurg Spine. 2014;18:207–14.
39. Al-Omair A, Masucci L, Masson-Cote L, et al. Surgical resection of epidural disease improves local control following postoperative spine stereotactic body radiotherapy. Neuro-Oncology. 2013;15:1413–9.
40. Lo SS, Sahgal A, Wang JZ, et al. Stereotactic body radiation therapy for spinal metastases. Disc Med. 2010;9:289–96.
41. Chang EL, Shiu AS, Lii MF, et al. Phase I clinical evaluation of near-simultaneous computed tomographic image-guided stereotactic body ariotherapy for spinal metastases. Int J Radiat Oncol Biol Phys. 2004; 59:1288–94.
42. Guckenberger M, Meyer J, Wilbert J, et al. Precision of image-guided radiotherapy (IGRT) in six degrees of freedom and limitations in clinical practice. Strahlenther Onkol. 2007;183:307–13.
43. Lo SS, Sahgal A, Teh BS, Gerszten PC, Chang EL. Stereotactic body radiation therapy for spinal metastases. London, UK: Future Medicine; 2014.
44. Dahele M, Zindler JD, Sanchez E, et al. Imaging for stereotactic spine radiotherapy: clinical considerations. Int J Radiat Oncol Biol Phys. 2011;81:321–30.
45. Cox BW, Spratt DE, Lovelock M, et al. International spine radiosurgery consortium consensus guidelines for target volume definition in spinal stereotactic radiosurgery. Int J Radiat Oncol Biol Phys. 2012; 83:e597–605.
46. Boriani S, Weinstein JN, Biagini R. Primary bone tumors of the spine. Terminology and surgical staging. Spine. 1997;22:1036–44.
47. Yin FF, Ryu S, Ajlouni M, et al. A technique of intensity-modulated radiosurgery (IMRS) for spinal tumors. Med Phys. 2002;29:2815–22.
48. Wu QJ, Yoo S, Kirkpatrick JP, et al. Volumetric arc intensity-modulated therapy for spine body radiotherapy comparison with static intensity-modulated treatment. Int J Radiat Oncol Biol Phys. 2009; 75:1596–604.
49. Kilby W, Dooley JR, Kuduvalli G, et al. The CyberKnife robotic radiosurgery system in 2010. Technol Cancer Res Treat. 2010;9:433–52.
50. Ho AK, Fu D, Cotrutz C, et al. A study of the accuracy of cyberknife spinal radiosurgery using skeletal structure tracking. Neurosurgery. 2007;60:147–56.
51. Fürweger C, Drexler C, Kufeld M, et al. Patient motion and targeting accuracy in robotic spinal radiosurgery: 260 single-fraction fiducial-free cases. Int J Radiat Oncol Biol Phys. 2010;78:937–45.
52. Haley ML, Gerszten PC, Heron DE, et al. Efficacy and cost–effectiveness analysis of external beam and stereotactic body radiation therapy in the treatment of spine metastases: a matched-pair analysis. J Neurosurg Spine. 2011;14:537–42.
53. Tatsui CE, Stafford RJ, Li J, et al. Utilization of laser interstitial thermotherapy guided by real-time thermal MRI as an alternative to separation surgery in the management of spinal metastasis. J Neurosurg Spine. 2015;23:400–11.
54. Massicotte E, Foote M, Reddy R, Sahgal A. Minimal access spine surgery (MASS) for decompression and stabilization performed as an out-patient procedure for metastatic spinal tumours followed by spine stereotactic body radiotherapy (SBRT): first report of technique and preliminary outcomes. Technol Cancer Res Treat. 2012;11:15–25.
55. Gerszten PC, Monaco EA 3rd. Complete percutaneous treatment of vertebral body tumors causing spinal canal compromise using a transpedicular cavitation, cement augmentation, and radiosurgical technique. Neurosurg Focus. 2009;27:E9.

Reconstructive Flap Coverage

21

Dmitry Zavlin and Michael J. Klebuc

Background

Flap reconstruction plays an important role in the management of metastatic spine disease. Flaps can be employed prophylactically to significantly decrease the rates of wound healing complications and instrumentation exposure associated with metastatic tumor extirpation [1]. Their ability to obliterate dead space, enhance local perfusion, and facilitate collagen deposition apportions flap reconstruction with a pivotal role along with thorough debridement and antimicrobial therapy in the management of complex postoperative wounds. A regional approach based on location, size, blood supply, and donor site morbidity can be utilized to facilitate flap selection and enhance the potential for successful wound healing [2, 3].

The spinal column is the most frequent site of bony metastasis for solid tumors, and individuals who fail to respond to nonoperative therapy often experience progressive recalcitrant pain, weakness, pathologic fractures, and incontinence. Surgical intervention has the potential to significantly enhance quality of life in this patient population; however, major complications can be encountered in up to 52% of individuals undergoing resection of spinal metastasis [4]. Tumor extirpation is often extensive, producing complex soft tissue defects and bony instability requiring the use of internal fixation. Patients are frequently elderly with multiple comorbidities and have often undergone previous radiation and chemotherapy causing various degrees of immunosuppression and malnutrition [5]. In many ways, this creates a perfect storm for the development of wound healing complications that can yield significant consequences. Wound breakdown with associated hardware exposure and infection creates a risk for meningitis and sepsis [6]. Treatment frequently requires serial debridement, lengthy intravenous antibiotic therapy, and prolonged hospitalization and is associated with an increased risk of readmission. If removal of instrumentation is necessary, then spinal instability with progressive loss of neurologic function is a considerable risk [3, 7]. If the full health-related quality of life benefits stemming from the surgical treatment of spinal metastasis are to be realized, then uncomplicated wound healing is paramount. In the presence of postoperative wound healing complications, the plastic surgeon's role in the multidisciplinary team becomes even more pivotal if favorable outcomes are to be realized [8].

D. Zavlin, MD
Institute for Reconstructive Surgery, Houston Methodist Hospital, Houston, TX, USA
e-mail: dzavlin@houstonmethodist.org

M. J. Klebuc, MD (✉)
Institute for Reconstructive Surgery, Houston Methodist Hospital, Weill Cornell Medical College, Houston, TX, USA
e-mail: mklebuc@houstonmethodist.org

R. A. W. Marco (ed.), *Metastatic Spine Disease*, https://doi.org/10.1007/978-3-319-76252-4_21

The provision of stable, well-vascularized soft tissue coverage and prevention of wound healing complications are the principal roles of plastic and reconstructive surgery in the multidisciplinary management of the patient with metastatic spine disease. Flap coverage, timing of surgical intervention, physiologic optimization, and wound healing strategies are all employed to this end.

Principles of Flap Coverage

Superficial wounds with limited contamination can be successfully managed with local skin and muscle-sparing fasciocutaneous flaps. However, these types of defects are rare in this patient population with most individuals demonstrating deep, spatially complex wounds with associated hardware often in the presence of bacterial colonization and/or infection.

In this type of hostile wound environment, muscle and/or myocutaneous flap coverage have proved superior outcomes to local skin and/or fasciocutaneous flaps for obtaining stable soft tissue coverage. Muscle flaps are pliable, can effectively obliterating dead space, and can aid in preventing seroma formation. They demonstrate superior blood flow and improved wound oxygenation as compared to skin and fasciocutaneous flap. This enhanced perfusion accelerates leukocyte activity and antibiotic delivery producing more rapid bacterial elimination while enhancing collagen deposition [9]. The posterior thorax possesses a series of muscles that can be utilized for flap coverage (i.e., trapezius, latissimus dorsi, paraspinous, and gluteus). A regional approach is employed in flap selection giving careful consideration to the muscles arch of rotation, bulk, and the functional deficit produced by its utilization. In patients with previous radiation, it is important that the muscle segment employed in the reconstruction has not been subjected to radiation and that the wound is covered with well-vascularized, non-radiated tissue. The flap pedicle should be outside the zone of injury, and one must give careful consideration to old incisions and a history of previous spinal exposures that may produce vascular pedicle injury. Deep wounds will often require a two-flap reconstruction with one flap dedicated to obliteration of dead space, while the other provides skin coverage. Fasciocutaneous flaps often suffice for the more superficial portion of the reconstruction. However, it is critically important to provide complete coverage of any spinal instrumentation with well-vascularized soft tissue. If this goal has been achieved, then the development of limited regions of superficial wound separation can usually be managed with local wound care avoiding return trips to the operating room as hardware exposure becomes unlikely.

Surgical Timing and Risk Factors for Wound Complications

There are a series of preoperative risk factors that are predictive for the development of complex, postoperative spine wounds and infections. A series of studies have identified the presence of spinal instrumentation, previous spinal surgery, spinal malignancy, preoperative radiation, and chemotherapy along with advanced age as primary concerns. A multitude of comorbid factors has also been acknowledged to have a detrimental effect on wound healing including diabetes, hypertension/coronary artery disease, chronic obstructive pulmonary disease, morbid obesity, paralysis, tobacco, and chronic steroid use [6, 10]. In this "high-risk" patient population, several studies have demonstrated a significant reduction in postoperative wound healing complications with the use of prophylactic muscle flaps [1]. Garvey et al. reported on the use of "preemptive" muscle flap coverage in 52 high-risk patients undergoing immediate soft tissue reconstruction following spinal neoplasm resection [11]. They identified a 12% major complication rate that compared favorably to the 38% complication rate they had witnessed in an earlier study prior to adopting prophylactic soft tissue reconstruction. None of the patients required hardware removal, and all went on to achieve a healed wound. Similarly, Spector et al. describe their experience with the use of prophylactic muscle flaps in 96 patients [12]. There was a 0 and 6.8% rate of wound healing complications in the increased risk and high-risk group, respectively. This compared favorably to historical controls where wound healing complications are encountered in nearly 30% of patients. The value of prophylactic flap coverage in high-risk patients is also demonstrated by Dumanian and associates who encountered no wound healing complications in patients treated with immediate flap coverage verses a rate of 26% in the delayed coverage group [13]. It is apparent that immediate soft tissue reconstruction at the time of tumor excision has the potential to facilitate uncomplicated wound healing and has become an integral part of our surgical approach to the patient with metastatic spine disease.

Strategies for Delayed Management of Complex Spine Wounds

In addition to prophylactic soft tissue coverage, muscle flaps in particular can play a central role in management of complex postoperative wounds. Infection and hardware exposure frequently necessitate a return to the operating room. The wound is explored, soft tissue is sent for culture, and broad-spectrum empiric intravenous antibiotics are initiated. Meticulous debridement is then performed removing all devitalized tissue. This is usually best performed as a collaborative effort between the plastic surgeon and spine surgeon. Hydrosurgery systems, for example, Versajet (Smith & Nephew Plc, London, UK), can be utilized to perform a precise, layered removal of tissue, and pulse lavage with a povidone-iodine is used to treat exposed hardware taking advantage of its detergent effect [14]. In the absence of a cerebrospinal fluid leak, temporary wound coverage is achieved with either an antibiotic bead pouch [15, 16] or negative pressure wound therapy. Antibiotic beads fashioned from polymethylmethacrylate containing vancomycin, tobramycin, and/or voriconazole have the potential to produce high local antimicrobial concentrations, up to 100 times MIC with limited systemic absorption (Fig. 21.1). This can prove valuable in reducing bacterial colonization and

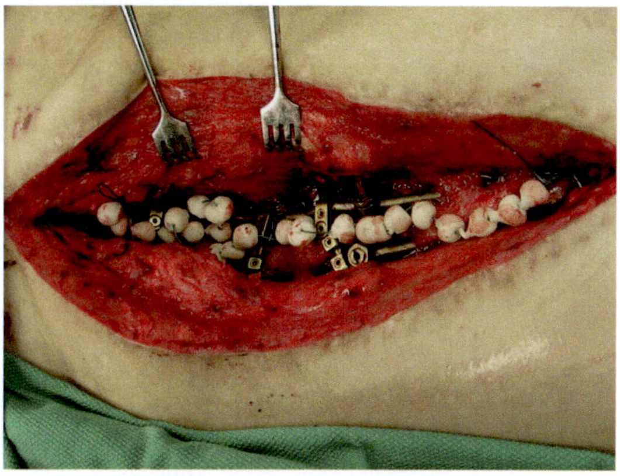

Fig. 21.1 Antibiotic bead placement prior to definite reconstruction

preparing the wound for closure [17]. Alternately, negative pressure wound therapy (NPWT) can provide an effective means of covering the wound between debridements. NPWT removes excess fluid from the wound, reduces edema, and enhances local blood flow stimulating formation of granulation tissue [18].

Regional Approach to Flap Selection

Posterior spine wounds can be stratified into zones in an effort to facilitate the flap selection process, with the upper third ranging from C1 to T7, the middle third spanning T7–L1, and the lower third extending from L1 to S5. Flap choices can also be categorized as primary, secondary, and tertiary options based on the frequency of their utilization. Table 21.1 and Figs. 21.2, 21.3, and 21.4 provide a broad overview of reconstructive management options for spinal defects based on their location.

Upper third defects (C1–T7) are most frequently managed with the trapezius flap [19]. The inferior portion of the muscle is perfused by the descending branch of the transverse cervical artery and can be used as a rotation, advancement, or turnover flap. During the standard, vertical flap elevation, the dissection is terminated at the level of the scapular spine to maintain muscular attachments that prevent shoulder

Table 21.1 Overview of flap techniques for various spinal defects

Spinal region	Primary options	Secondary options	Tertiary options
C1–T7	• Trapezius • Latissimus dorsi • Combined muscle flap with fasciocutaneous advancement flap for deep wounds	• Parascapular fasciocutaneous flap • Freestyle perforator flaps, keystone flaps	• Free flaps
T7–L1	• Latissimus dorsi rotation-advancement or v-y • Reverse latissimus dorsi • Paraspinous muscle flap • Combined paraspinous and latissimus dorsi muscle flaps ± fasciocutaneous advancement for deep wounds	• Intercostal neurovascular flap • Freestyle perforator flaps, keystone flaps	• Pedicled omental flap • Free flaps ± A-V loop
L1–S5	• Reverse latissimus dorsi • Paraspinous muscle flap (turnover or bipedicle) • Superior gluteal artery perforator (SGAP) flap	• Posterior thigh flap • Lumbar artery perforator flap • Composite latissimus dorsi and segmental gluteus maximus myocutaneous flap • Segmental gluteus maximus myocutaneous flap • Freestyle perforator flaps, keystone flaps	• Pedicled omental flap • Free flaps ± A-V loop • Transabdominal VRAM

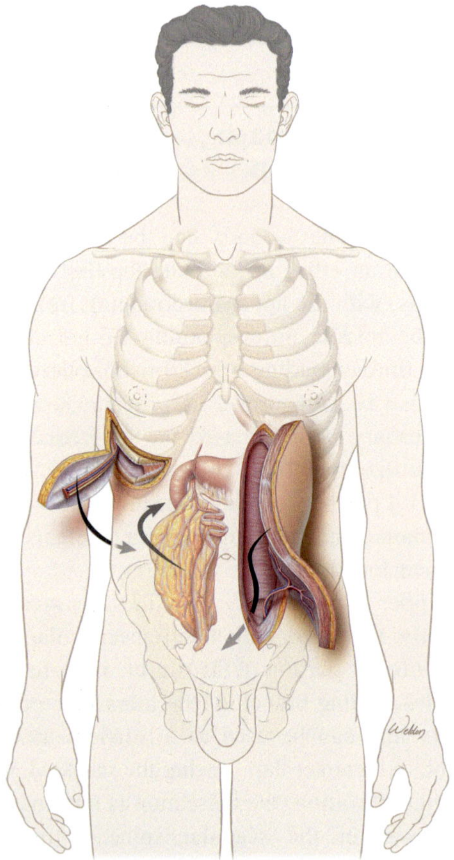

Fig. 21.2 Delineation of muscular and musculocutaneous flaps. Anterior trunk view

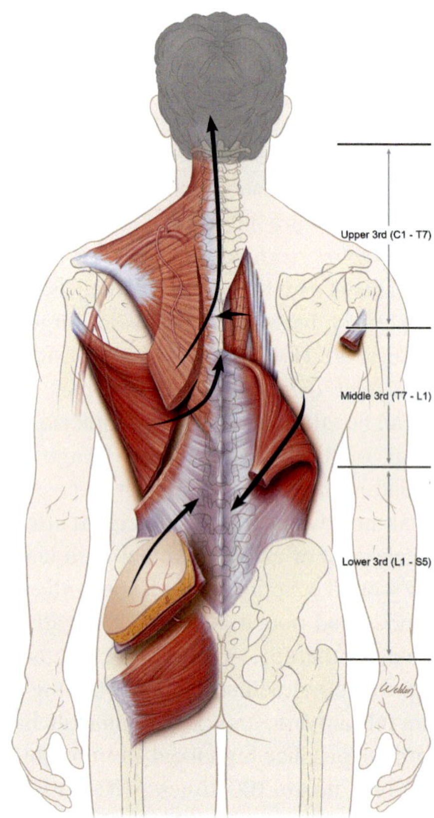

Fig. 21.3 Delineation of muscular and musculocutaneous flaps. Posterior trunk view

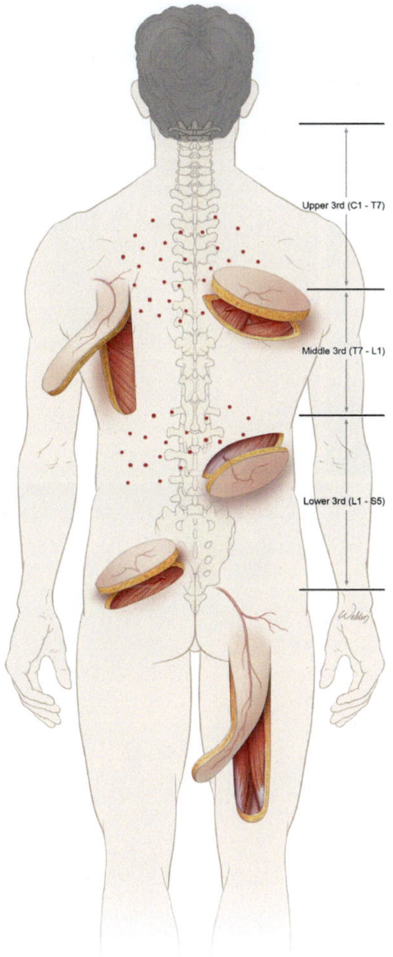

Fig. 21.4 Delineation of fasciocutaneous flaps. Posterior trunk view

droop. The mobilized muscle segment will reliably reach the cervical spine and skull base; however, the muscle flap dissection can be extended proximally to further enhance its reach. A skin island can be incorporated into the flap design; however, it should be situated directly over the muscle with limited extension past its borders to maximize reliability. The defects produced by extirpation of metastatic spine defects are typically deep and spatially complex. The trapezius is often utilized to obliterate dead space, while skin coverage is achieved with a second flap (fasciocutaneous advancement flaps, latissimus dorsi myocutaneous flap, parascapular flap, freestyle perforator flap) [3]. The latissimus dorsi rotation-advancement flap is another primary option in proximal third defects with the humeral insertion of the muscle frequently released to extend its reach (Fig. 21.5) [20].

Less spatially complex wounds can be managed with parascapular fasciocutaneous flaps designed around the circumflex scapular artery [21]. Additionally, there are clusters of cutaneous perforators in the thoracic and lumbar region that can be utilized in local flap design [22, 23]. In the thoracic region, a high density of perforators is present in a zone 10 cm from the midline and 0–15 cm from C7. In the lumbar region, two clusters of perforators are situated within 10–20 cm of the coccyx and 10 cm from the midline. A "freestyle" skin or fasciocutaneous flap can be designed around one or more cutaneous perforators with the flap usually being oriented perpendicular to the midline to maximize perforasome vascular connections. Similarly, these cutaneous perforators can be incorporated into a modified V-Y advancement or "keystone" flap to cover more superficial defects in all three zones [24].

Free flap reconstruction can also be employed in proximal third defects; however, they are considered tertiary options with the exception of free fibula bone flaps [25, 26] that can be effectively utilized to achieve bony union in a previously radiated field.

In middle third defects, the (reverse) latissimus dorsi and paraspinous muscle flaps are the most frequently utilized (Figs. 21.6 and 21.7) [20, 27, 28]. The latissimus dorsi muscle/myocutaneous flap provides a versatile treatment option in this zone and can be employed as a muscular rotation-advancement flap or reversed turnover flap to manage dead space. Blood supply to the reverse latissimus dorsi flap emanates from three large vascular pedicles branching off of the 9th, 10th, and 11th intercostal arteries that are situated approximately 5 cm lateral to the midline. During flap elevation the thoracodorsal vessels are temporarily occluded with bulldog clamps to verify adequate retrograde perfusion prior to ligation. Incorporation of a cutaneous island or mobilizing the flap as a musculocutaneous V-Y advancement allows provision of well-vascularized cutaneous coverage. A two-flap strategy is effective and frequently employed in this zone. Paraspinous muscle flaps are utilized to obliterate dead space, and cutaneous

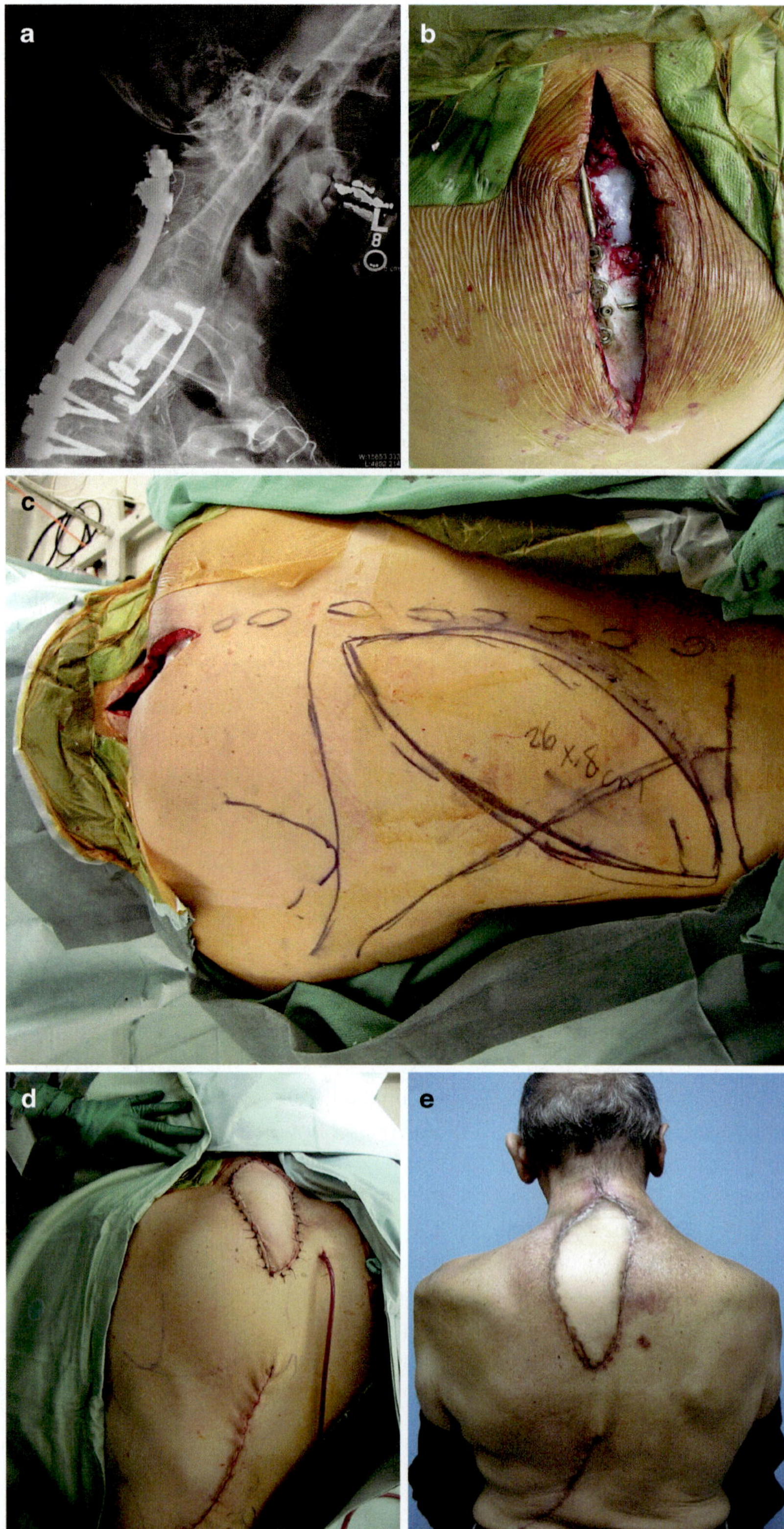

Fig. 21.5 Latissimus dorsi flap. (**a**) Radiograph of spinal instrumentation following excision of cervical spine metastasis and postoperative radiation. (**b**) Complex posterior, cervical wound following hardware revision. (**c**) Surgical plan for latissimus dorsi myocutaneous flap. (**d**) Initial flap inset. (**e**) Three-month postoperative follow-up

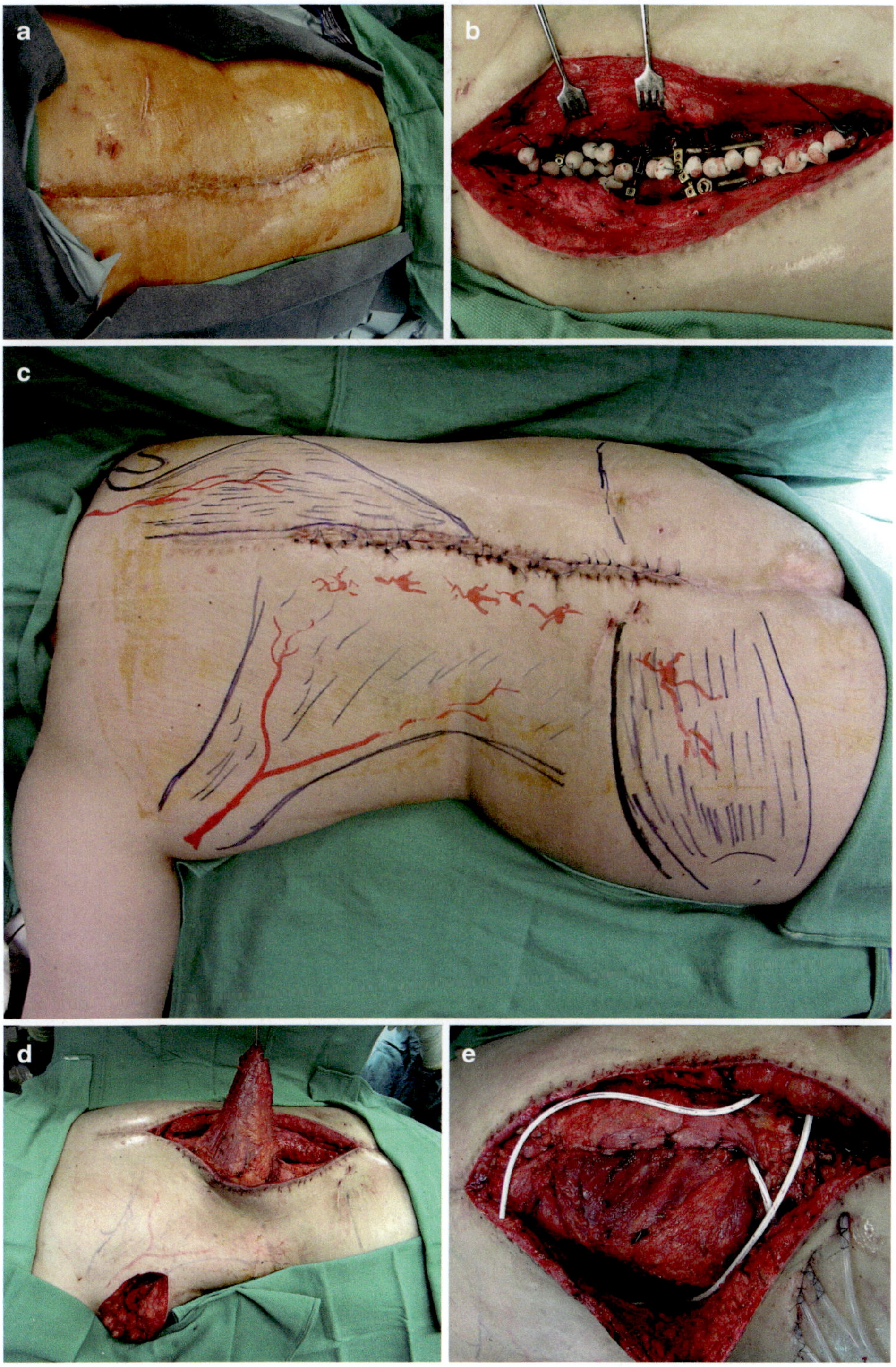

Fig. 21.6 Reverse latissimus dorsi flap with paraspinous flap. (**a**) Draining sinus tract after resection of metastatic renal cell carcinoma to the spine and hardware stabilization. (**b**) Debridement and antibiotic bead placement for treatment of methicillin-sensitive staphylococcus aureus (MSSA) colonization. (**c**) Planning for muscle flap coverage. (**d**) Elevation of reverse latissimus dorsi muscle flap. (**e**) Obliteration of dead space and complete hardware coverage with left reverse latissimus dorsi muscle flap and right paraspinous muscle flap

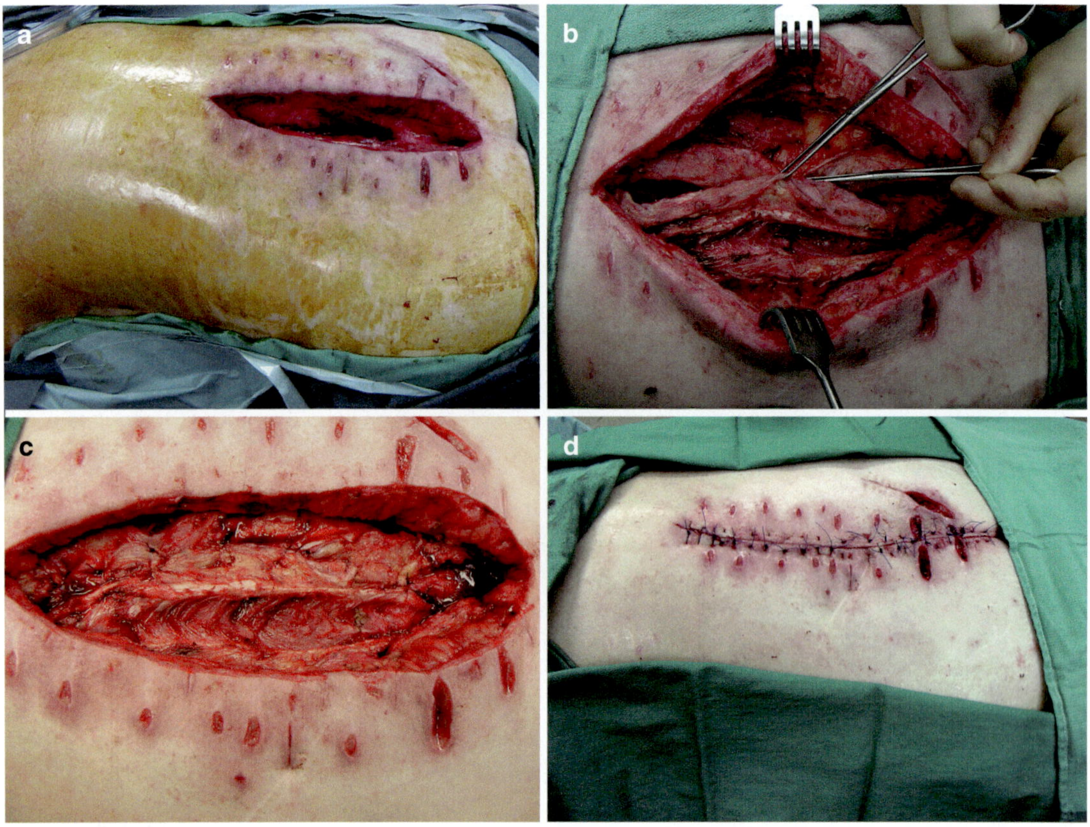

Fig. 21.7 Bilateral paraspinous flap (**a**) complex back wound (middle third) following serial debridement. (**b**) Mobilization of bilateral paraspinous muscle flaps. (**c**) Obliteration of dead space and full muscle coverage of vertebrae. (**d**) Bilateral fasciocutaneous advancement flaps for skin coverage

coverage is provided with a latissimus dorsi myocutaneous flap. If adequate skin laxity is present in this region, then either the latissimus dorsi muscle flap or the paraspinous muscle flap can be utilized to manage dead space and bilateral fasciocutaneous advancement flaps can provide skin coverage. Additional fasciocutaneous flap mobility can be achieved by carrying the dissection past the musculocutaneous perforators. The fascia lateral to the perforators is then incised vertically allowing greater movement toward the midline.

Secondary flap options in this zone include freestyle perforator [29] and keystone flaps. Intermittently, one will encounter a situation where the primary flap options have been previously utilized "burned bridges" and the posterior thoracic region demonstrates extensive scarring. In this event, the intercostal neurovascular flap has the ability to import well-vascularized, sensate tissue from an adjacent region and can provide an elegant solution to a complex problem [30, 31]. The flap is designed around the 9th, 10th, or 11th posterior intercostal arteries, and incorporation of the lateral cutaneous branch at the midaxillary line permits inclusion of a sizeable skin island. Segmental resection of the cephalic rib enhances the arch of rotation allowing the flap to reach the mid-thoracic region.

Although seldom employed the omental flap remains an important salvage option and can function well in individuals with large, complex wounds where reconstructive options have been limited by prior surgery [32, 33]. The omentum has a large surface area (~25 × 30 cm) and a dense lymphatic network providing immunologic privilege and good functionality in previously contaminated wounds. The flap can be designed on either the right or left gastroepiploic arteries, and its reach can be further enhanced by the release of its internal vascular arcade. It can be harvest laparoscopically or with an open laparotomy. Regardless, its use will require an intraoperative position change and creation of a tunnel in the posterolateral abdominal wall with the associated risk of hernia formation. Skin graft coverage will be required if inadequate laxity is present adjacent to the defect to achieve primary skin approximation. Free tissue transfer provides an additional tertiary reconstructive option in the mid-thoracic region. Although representing the first choice in the reconstructive elevator in many regions of the body, free flap utility is reduced in the posterior thorax. The presence of a large number of reliable local flap options, potential for postoperative flap compression (difficult positioning) and lack of recipient vessels, accounts for the infrequent use. When free flap reconstruction is mandated, the dorsal branch of the fourth lumbar artery and vein can provide reasonable recipient vessels. The vessel can usually be identified at the lateral border of the sacrospinalis muscle in a line perpendicular to the cephalic segment of the fourth lumbar vertebrae. The superior gluteal artery and vein can also be utilized with more inferiorly located defects. The use of arteriovenous loops fashioned from the saphenous or cephalic veins can greatly enhance the reach and flexibility of free flap reconstruction in both the middle and lower thirds of the posterior thorax. The thoracodorsal, circumflex scapular, and superior gluteal vessels can all be utilized in this regard.

Lower third defects (L1–S5) frequently can be closed with the reverse latissimus dorsi flap alone or in combination with paraspinous muscle flaps [20, 34]. The paraspinous muscle can be utilized as a turnover flap or the medial row of intercostal perforators can be ligated and the muscles advanced as bipedicled flaps [28] perfused by the lateral row of segmental intercostal perforators. The superior gluteal artery perforator flap (SGAP) has great utility in this region and in our practice has largely superseded the gluteus maximus flap [35, 36]. The muscle-sparing flap design is particularly appealing in ambulatory patients, although utilization of the proximal portion of the gluteus maximus muscle appears to have little negative impact on mobility. A large fasciocutaneous island can be designed around one or two perforators radiating from the superior gluteal artery. The perforator's muscular branches are ligated and divided, and the intramuscular space is opened parallel to the gluteus muscle fibers obviating the need for transection. Releasing the perforators creates significant mobility and allows the flap to be advanced medially to provide a tension free closure in the sacral region. The donor site is then closed in a V-Y fashion without the need for skin grafting. Alternately, the skin island can be extended laterally, and the flap transposed allowing it to reach the T12–L1 region. The lumbar artery perforator flap also has significant utility in this region [22]. The flap is fasciocutaneous in nature and is most frequently perfused by terminal branches of the lumbar arteries at the L3 and L4 level. The dominant perforator has an average diameter of 2.8 mm and can usually be identified entering the subcutaneous tissue 6–7 cm for the midline. The perforator runs in the interval between the erector spinae and the quadratus lumborum. Release of this space and division of side branches will enhance pedicle length and allow for an increased arch of rotation with less risk of pedicle torsion. Additionally, there is a rich network of vascular communications between the thoracodorsal perforators that penetrate the latissimus dorsi muscle and the superior gluteal artery and vein. These vascular connections permit elevation of large composite (latissimus dorsi-gluteus maximus) myocutaneous advancement flaps [37, 38]. The flap is elevated beneath the latissimus dorsi muscle and the thoracolumbar fascia, and the dissection is extended laterally to enhance mobility. A lateral relaxing incision and skin grafting of the acquired defect may be necessary to achieve the desired advancement.

In addition, the posterior thigh flap is another reliable option for lower third defects and can provide well-vascularized, sensate skin coverage in the sacral region [39]. The posterior thigh flap is an axial patterned, fasciocutaneous flap, which is centered on the descending branch of the inferior gluteal artery with a large skin island measuring up to 34 × 15 cm. The flap design includes the posterior femoral cutaneous nerve providing an opportunity for a sensate reconstruction. Similar to middle third defects, pedicled omental flaps and free tissue transfers also play an ancillary role in this zone.

The transabdominal, vertical rectus abdominis myocutaneous flap (VRAM) is a seldom, utilized yet important option for soft tissue coverage in the sacral region (Fig. 21.8) [40]. Sacrectomy for the treatment of bony malignancies in this region is often associated with ligation of the internal iliac vessels interrupting the blood supply to many regional flaps. The external iliac artery is

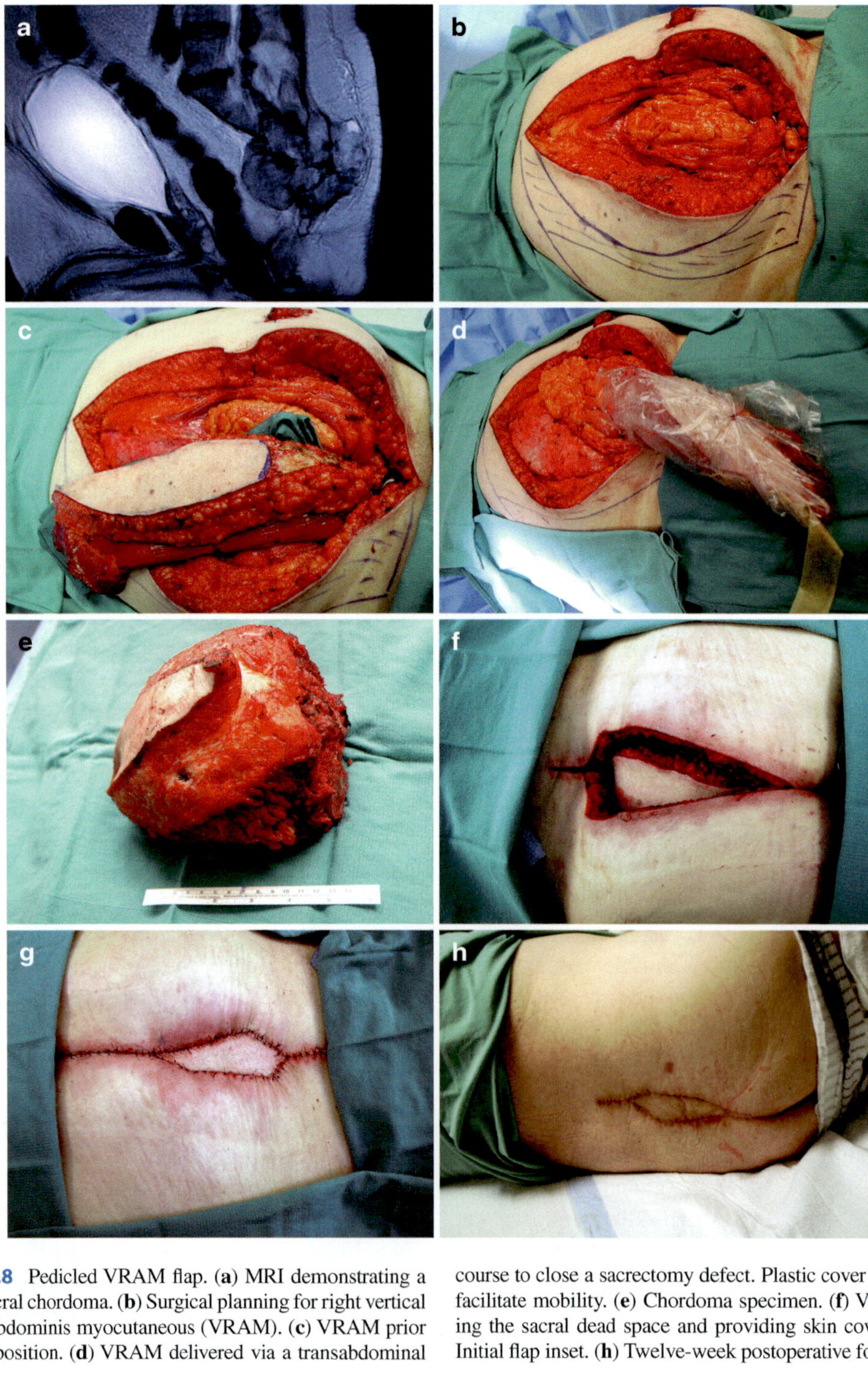

Fig. 21.8 Pedicled VRAM flap. (**a**) MRI demonstrating a large sacral chordoma. (**b**) Surgical planning for right vertical rectus abdominis myocutaneous (VRAM). (**c**) VRAM prior to transposition. (**d**) VRAM delivered via a transabdominal course to close a sacrectomy defect. Plastic cover utilized to facilitate mobility. (**e**) Chordoma specimen. (**f**) VRAM filling the sacral dead space and providing skin coverage. (**g**) Initial flap inset. (**h**) Twelve-week postoperative follow-up

usually unaffected during sacrectomy, and the rectus abdominis muscle with an overlying, longitudinally oriented skin island based on the deep inferior epigastric can provide reliable coverage while obliterating pelvic dead space. The mobilized flap is secured to a sterile plastic bag to facilitate the transabdominal (intraperitoneal) delivery into the pelvis. As with many of the flap reconstructions in this region, pressure reduction and postoperative positioning are critically important to achieving a successful outcome.

Air-fluidized beds, e.g., Clinitron (Hill-Rom, Chicago, IL), can produce a resting surface with pressures lower than end capillary pressure. This allows flap perfusion even with the patient in the recumbent position and removes the need for frequent turning and position changes. A series of other conservative interventions can be employed in an effort to minimize postoperative wound healing complications. These include active nutritional support with monitoring of prealbumin levels, liberal utilization of closed suction drains to prevent seroma formation, and the use of temporary diverting colostomies in the management of complex sacral-perineal wounds. Application of cyanoacrylate tissue adhesive can also prove effective in achieving a watertight seal and protecting the suture line during the initial weeks of wound healing.

Summary

Flap reconstruction plays an important role in the management of metastatic spine disease. Flaps can be employed prophylactically to significantly decrease the rates of wound healing complications and hardware exposure associated with metastatic tumor extirpation. They also play a pivotal role along with thorough debridement and antimicrobial therapy in the management of complex postoperative wounds. A regional approach based on location, size, and blood supply can be employed to facilitate flap selection and enhance the potential for successful wound healing. Further classification divides reconstructive techniques into primary, secondary, and tertiary approaches depending on their frequency and their complexity.

References

1. Glassman SD, Dimar JR, Puno RM, Johnson JR. Salvage of instrumental lumbar fusions complicated by surgical wound infection. Spine. 1996;21(18):2163–9.
2. Behr B, Wagner JM, Wallner C, Harati K, Lehnhardt M, Daigeler A. Reconstructive options for oncologic posterior trunk defects: a review. Front Oncol. 2016;6:51.
3. Chieng LO, Hubbard Z, Salgado CJ, Levi AD, Chim H. Reconstruction of open wounds as a complication of spinal surgery with flaps: a systematic review. Neurosurg Focus. 2015;39(4):E17.
4. Dunning EC, Butler JS, Morris S. Complications in the management of metastatic spinal disease. World J Orthop. 2012;3(8):114–21.
5. Mericli AF, Tarola NA, Moore JH Jr, Copit SE, Fox JW, Tuma GA. Paraspinous muscle flap reconstruction of complex midline back wounds: risk factors and postreconstruction complications. Ann Plast Surg. 2010;65(2):219–24.
6. Chaudhary SB, Vives MJ, Basra SK, Reiter MF. Postoperative spinal wound infections and postprocedural diskitis. J Spinal Cord Med. 2007;30(5):441–51.
7. Hochberg J, Ardenghy M, Yuen J, Gonzalez-Cruz R, Miura Y, Conrado RM, et al. Muscle and musculocutaneous flap coverage of exposed spinal fusion devices. Plast Reconstr Surg. 1998;102(2):385–9; discussion 90–2.
8. Epstein NE. When does a spinal surgeon need a plastic surgeon? Surg Neurol Int. 2013;4(Suppl 5):S299–300.
9. Calderon W, Chang N, Mathes SJ. Comparison of the effect of bacterial inoculation in musculocutaneous and fasciocutaneous flaps. Plast Reconstr Surg. 1986;77(5):785–94.
10. Chang DW, Friel MT, Youssef AA. Reconstructive strategies in soft tissue reconstruction after resection of spinal neoplasms. Spine. 2007;32(10):1101–6.
11. Garvey PB, Rhines LD, Dong W, Chang DW. Immediate soft-tissue reconstruction for complex defects of the spine following surgery for spinal neoplasms. Plast Reconstr Surg. 2010;125(5):1460–6.
12. Cohen LE, Fullerton N, Mundy LR, Weinstein AL, Fu KM, Ketner JJ, et al. Optimizing successful outcomes in complex spine reconstruction using local muscle flaps. Plast Reconstr Surg. 2016;137(1):295–301.
13. Dumanian GA, Ondra SL, Liu J, Schafer MF, Chao JD. Muscle flap salvage of spine wounds with soft tissue defects or infection. Spine. 2003;28(11):1203–11.
14. Chang FY, Chang MC, Wang ST, Yu WK, Liu CL, Chen TH. Can povidone-iodine solution be used safely in a spinal surgery? Eur Spine J. 2006;15(6):1005–14.
15. Chen JF, Lee ST. Antibiotic-polymethylmethacrylate strut: an option for treating cervical pyogenic spondylitis. Case report. J Neurosurg Spine. 2006;5(1):90–5.

16. Lee BJ, Lee SR, Kim ST, Kim TH, Lee SH. Spinal epidural abscess with pyogenic arthritis of facet joint treated with antibiotic-bone cement beads—a case report. Asian Spine J. 2007;1(1):61–4.
17. Khan NR, Thompson CJ, DeCuypere M, Angotti JM, Kalobwe E, Muhlbauer MS, et al. A meta-analysis of spinal surgical site infection and vancomycin powder. J Neurosurg Spine. 2014;21(6):974–83.
18. Adogwa O, Fatemi P, Perez E, Moreno J, Gazcon GC, Gokaslan ZL, et al. Negative pressure wound therapy reduces incidence of postoperative wound infection and dehiscence after long-segment thoracolumbar spinal fusion: a single institutional experience. Spine J. 2014;14(12):2911–7.
19. Mathes SJ, Nahai F. Trapezius flap. In: Reconstructive surgery: principles, anatomy & technique, vol. 1. New York: Churchill Livingston Inc.; 1997. p. 651–78.
20. Mathes SJ, Nahai F. Latissimus dorsi flap. In: Reconstructive surgery: principles, anatomy & technique, vol. 1. New York: Churchill Livingston Inc.; 1997. p. 565–616.
21. Mathes SJ, Nahai F. Scapular flap. In: Reconstructive surgery: principles, anatomy & technique, vol. 1. New York: Churchill Livingston Inc.; 1997. p. 617–42.
22. Hamdi M, Craggs B, Brussaard C, Seidenstueker K, Hendrickx B, Zeltzer A. Lumbar artery perforator flap: an anatomical study using multidetector computed tomographic scan and surgical pearls for breast reconstruction. Plast Reconstr Surg. 2016;138(2):343–52.
23. Aho JM, Laungani AT, Herbig KS, Wong C, Kirchoff RW, Saint-Cyr M. Lumbar and thoracic perforators: vascular anatomy and clinical implications. Plast Reconstr Surg. 2014;134(4):635e–45e.
24. Behan FC. The keystone design perforator island flap in reconstructive surgery. ANZ J Surg. 2003;73(3):112–20.
25. Moran SL, Bakri K, Mardini S, Shin AY, Bishop AT. The use of vascularized fibular grafts for the reconstruction of spinal and sacral defects. Microsurgery. 2009;29(5):393–400.
26. Saltzman BM, Levy DM, Vakhshori V, DeWald CJ. Free vascularized fibular strut autografts to the lumbar spine in complex revision surgery: a report of two cases. Korean J Spine. 2015;12(3):185–9.
27. Saint-Cyr M, Nikolis A, Moumdjian R, Frenette G, Ciaburro H, Harris PG, et al. Paraspinous muscle flaps for the treatment and prevention of cerebrospinal fluid fistulas in neurosurgery. Spine. 2003;28(5):E86–92.
28. Wilhelmi BJ, Snyder N, Colquhoun T, Hadjipavlou A, Phillips LG. Bipedicle paraspinous muscle flaps for spinal wound closure: an anatomic and clinical study. Plast Reconstr Surg. 2000;106(6):1305–11.
29. Lecours C, Saint-Cyr M, Wong C, Bernier C, Mailhot E, Tardif M, et al. Freestyle pedicle perforator flaps: clinical results and vascular anatomy. Plast Reconstr Surg. 2010;126(5):1589–603.
30. Mathes SJ, Nahai F. Intercostal flap. In: Reconstructive surgery: principles, anatomy & technique, vol. 1. New York: Churchill Livingston Inc.; 1997. p. 537–64.
31. Wong MC, Allison K, Yap LH, Peart F. The pedicled intercostal neurovascular island skin flap for lumbosacral trunk reconstruction. Br J Plast Surg. 2004;57(6):520–4.
32. Mathes SJ, Nahai F. Omental flap. In: Reconstructive surgery: principles, anatomy & technique, vol. 2. New York: Churchill Livingston Inc.; 1997. p. 1141–60.
33. O'Shaughnessy BA, Dumanian GA, Liu JC, Ganju A, Ondra SL. Pedicled omental flaps as an adjunct in the closure of complex spinal wounds. Spine. 2007;32(26):3074–80.
34. Mericli AF, Mirzabeigi MN, Moore JH Jr, Fox JW, Copit SE, Tuma GA. Reconstruction of complex posterior cervical spine wounds using the paraspinous muscle flap. Plast Reconstr Surg. 2011;128(1):148–53.
35. Verpaele AM, Blondeel PN, Van Landuyt K, Tonnard PL, Decordier B, Monstrey SJ, et al. The superior gluteal artery perforator flap: an additional tool in the treatment of sacral pressure sores. Br J Plast Surg. 1999;52(5):385–91.
36. Blondeel PN, Van Landuyt K, Hamdi M, Monstrey SJ. Soft tissue reconstruction with the superior gluteal artery perforator flap. Clin Plast Surg. 2003;30(3):371–82.
37. Strauch B. Bilateral interconnected latissimus dorsi-gluteus maximus musculocutaneous flaps for closure of large lumbosacral meningomyelocele defects. In: Grabb's encyclopedia of flaps. 3rd ed. Philadelphia: Lippincott Williams & Wilkins; 2009. p. 1318–21.
38. Mathes SJ, Nahai F. Gluteus maximus—gluteal thigh flap. In: Reconstructive surgery: principles, anatomy & technique, vol. 1. New York: Churchill Livingston Inc.; 1997. p. 501–36.
39. Friedman JD, Reece GR, Eldor L. The utility of the posterior thigh flap for complex pelvic and perineal reconstruction. Plast Reconstr Surg. 2010;126(1):146–55.
40. Miles WK, Chang DW, Kroll SS, Miller MJ, Langstein HN, Reece GP, et al. Reconstruction of large sacral defects following total sacrectomy. Plast Reconstr Surg. 2000;105(7):2387–94.

Complications

22

Hannah Morehouse and Adedayo O. Ashana

Introduction

Complications related to the treatment of metastatic spine disease are often associated with inaccurate preoperative assessment and diagnosis. This leads to inappropriate medical or surgical treatments, further increasing complication rates. Obtaining a careful history and physical examination is the first step in approaching these patients, and other coexisting premorbid conditions may be discovered during this process intervention [1]. Radiological and laboratory studies serve important roles in establishing diagnosis and staging. However, a biopsy is necessary for making a definitive diagnosis. Exact techniques of the biopsy and the definitive treatment should be tailored to the nature and location of the lesion and the patient's general condition. A multidisciplinary team consisting of surgical, medical, and radiation oncologists, combined with experienced radiologists and pathologists, helps optimize patient care. When indicated, the goals of operative intervention of spinal metastatic tumors are pain control, maintenance or improvement of neurological function, maintenance of spinal stability, and the attainment of normal coronal and sagittal alignment. Attention to details and appropriate goal-oriented intervention should help decrease the incidence of complications related to spinal surgery. The complications of the treatment of metastatic spine disease and ways to anticipate and treat them are discussed in this chapter.

H. Morehouse, MD
Department of Orthopedic Surgery, Houston Methodist Hospital, Houston, TX, USA
e-mail: hmorehouse@houstonmethodist.org

A. O. Ashana, MD (✉)
Department of Orthopedic Spine Surgery, OSS Health, York, PA

Preoperative Planning

Many complications could be obviated by a careful initial evaluation. The history is often helpful in separating neoplastic processes from other causes of back pain. Pain associated with tumors is characteristically persistent, progressive, worse at night, and present at rest. The age of the patient helps narrow the differential diagnosis. A previous history of cancer increases the likelihood that the lesion is a metastatic deposit.

The physical examination should include a general survey, which may detect primary tumors from breast, prostate, lung, rectum, or thyroid. Elderly patients with new onset persistent back pain should have a thorough evaluation to rule out tumors or infections. Certain physical exam findings can help detect tumors early in disease onset and can improve survival rates. A careful neurological examination is mandatory to detect early signs of spinal cord compression. Signs and

R. A. W. Marco (ed.), *Metastatic Spine Disease*, https://doi.org/10.1007/978-3-319-76252-4_22

symptoms of spinal cord compression include persistent back pain, difficulty maintaining balance, wide-based gait, fatigue after a short walk, bowel or bladder incontinence, paresthesias, and weakness of the extremities. Early diagnosis of spinal cord compression and the commencement of appropriate treatment may prevent irreversible neurological deficits and deformity.

A thorough panel of laboratory studies may help diagnose inflammatory versus neoplastic disorders and may assist with diagnosis of primary tumor. Further metastatic studies, such as mammography and chest or abdominal computed tomography (CT), should be obtained in accordance with the suspected primary carcinoma. Although metastatic lesions are the most common tumors of the spine, primary tumors, including benign and malignant bone tumors, intraspinal tumors, and cysts, should be considered in the differential diagnosis. Metabolic disorders such as osteoporosis and Paget's disease should also be considered in the differential diagnosis and may mimic metastatic tumors. Spinal infections should be ruled out, particularly in the immunocompromised patients. Occasionally, an infection and tumor may exist in the same individual [2].

Imaging studies are essential in further diagnosis and treatment of metastatic spine tumors. Plain radiographs are used initially to evaluate the level of the lesion, the local anatomy, and the overall alignment. CT helps further define the bony architecture and integrity, whereas magnetic resonance imaging (MRI) provides additional information on soft tissue and neural involvement. MRI is indispensible when differentiating malignant spinal tumors from infections and benign compression fractures [3–6]. Vertebral osteomyelitis usually involves the disc space and adjacent vertebral body end plates, whereas spinal tumors usually do not involve the disc space. Malignant compression fractures of the spine, as compared to benign compression fractures, are more likely to demonstrate bony destruction, involvement of the pedicle, and a soft tissue epidural component.

Preoperative angiography is invaluable for tumors with hypervascularity, especially metastatic renal cell carcinoma. Preoperative embolization has been shown to be effective in reducing perioperative blood loss and decreasing operative time without significantly increasing complication rates [7, 8]. Angiography also identifies the feeding artery to the spinal cord, which may be involved by tumor. Additionally, if the tumor is close to a major artery, angiography will help define this relationship and its clinical significance.

Biopsy

A biopsy of the lesion is often essential before rendering definitive treatment. Biopsy can be deferred if the patient has known metastatic disease with characteristic radiographic findings. Careful planning and execution of the biopsy decreases the likelihood of adverse effects on the prognosis and treatment options. Image-guided large-bore core needle biopsies are usually diagnostic when evaluated by an experienced pathologist [9] and minimize soft tissue contamination and hematoma formation compared to open biopsy. Open biopsies are performed if the needle biopsy is nondiagnostic or if the patient has spinal cord compression that requires emergent decompression. Patients with a solitary lesion and high-grade spinal cord compression may benefit from an emergent needle or open biopsy to determine the histology of the tumor. A patient with a diagnosis of lymphoma, myeloma, or carcinoma is usually treated with corticosteroids combined with radiation therapy. A patient with a biopsy consistent with a primary malignant bone tumor may be a candidate for an en bloc resection. An emergent decompression with minimal contamination of the soft tissues and minimal destabilization of the facets can be performed if indicated. The definitive palliative procedure can be performed at the time of an open biopsy if the frozen section analysis is diagnostic of metastatic disease and the patient would benefit from surgical intervention. Proceeding with a definitive procedure is not prudent if equivocal frozen section analysis results are rendered or if the diagnosis is consistent with a primary bone tumor. In this situation, it may be ideal to await final histologic results, further staging studies, and multidisciplinary planning prior to performing the definitive procedure. Sending tissue for cultures and sensitivities for bacteria, fungus, and mycobacterium is also recommended, particularly if biopsy is nondiagnostic on frozen section analysis.

Needle biopsies for the cervical, thoracic, lumbar, and sacral spine are usually performed under ultrasound, MR imaging, endoscopic, fluoroscopic, or CT guidance [10–18]. Following biopsy, the patient should be closely monitored for bleeding complications. Complications associated with needle biopsies include neural injury, paraspinal hematoma, infection, pneumothorax, meningitis, tumor spread, and death [12–14, 16, 17]. CT guidance has a very low complication rate with a high accuracy rate and relatively low cost (vs. MRI) [13].

Open biopsies are uncommonly performed, unless done at the time of definitive fixation due to an emergent condition. Historically, there was a perceived danger with percutaneous biopsies in the thoracic spine, and more open or mini-open techniques were employed, but this has become less applicable with newer imaging techniques [17]. If the definitive procedure is not performed at the time of the biopsy, meticulous hemostasis should be obtained before skin closure to minimize risk of hematoma formation.

Surgical Decision-Making and Approach

Metastatic lesions are medically managed concurrently with surgical evaluation. Once the primary tumor is diagnosed, each tumor must be approached individually. Each intervention, be it radiotherapy, chemotherapy, kyphoplasty, or surgery, carries its own complication risks. Overall, direct surgical decompression demonstrates improved outcomes versus radiotherapy alone when applied to the appropriate patient (e.g., not for radiosensitive tumors) [19].

Before performing a specific procedure, indications for surgery must be defined and applied to the patient. The surgical indications and considerations for metastatic tumors include the presence of significant neurological deficits, deformity, failure of nonoperative treatment, medical status, and oncological prognosis of the patient.

There are several scoring systems to evaluate metastatic spine tumor prognosis [20]. Tokuhashi et al. outlined a scoring system comprised of six key parameters, to include general condition, number of extraspinal bone metastases, number of metastases in the vertebral body, presence or absence of metastases to major internal organs, site of the primary lesion, and severity of the palsy, which closely correlates with survival period [21, 22]. Tomita et al. also evaluated a new scoring system based on three factors: grade of malignancy, visceral metastases, and bone metastases [23–25]. Each system attempts to correlate patient's overall disease burden with survivability. Logically, a higher level of comorbidities also increases the risks associated with surgical intervention. Murakami et al. evaluated an aging population (>70 years old), which overall takes into account a greater number of medical comorbidities, but surprisingly did not recommend avoiding radical procedures (i.e., total en bloc spondylectomy) merely based on age [25]. Boriani et al.'s system does not take into account multilevel disease, since it is aimed at primary bone tumors [26]. However, it can provide guidance for surgical treatment based on tumor location within individual spinal levels. These scoring systems can be applied to guide treatment decisions regarding patient feasibility for operative versus nonoperative care. As a traditional guideline, patients with a likelihood of survival <3 months are treated with nonoperative supportive care, while patients with better physical health and higher longevity are more appropriate surgical candidates [27].

The surgical approach depends on the type and location of the tumor. Most metastatic tumors in the spinal column are present in the vertebral body, and therefore an anterior or lateral approach is frequently used to perform corpectomy. Regardless of approach, the PLL provides a clear barrier for metastatic spine disease. En bloc resection is advocated in select patients since it would obviate the need for radiotherapy [20, 24, 28]. Spinal reconstruction includes assuring that the neural elements are patent, the spine is properly aligned, the anterior column is supported, and the posterior column is stabilized. Since these surgeries are primarily palliative, preventing pseudarthrosis and allowing for high fusion rates are relatively less important. Dorsal augmentation with instrumentation is considered to maximize the rigidity of the surgical construct. Thorough familiarity of surgical anatomy and surgical approaches to the cervical, thoracic, and lumbar spine is important to prevent intraoperative complications.

Positioning

Avoidance of abnormal pressure on the eyes can prevent corneal abrasions and blindness. Constant attention by the surgeon and the anesthesiologist helps minimize ocular pressure. Foam headrests with open areas over the eyes and Mayfield tongs or headrests all work to minimize direct pressure on the eyes.

Many complications can be avoided by certain positioning techniques. Avoiding shoulder abduction beyond 80° minimizes the likelihood of brachial plexus traction injuries. Avoiding direct pressure on the ulnar nerves decreases the likelihood of ulnar nerve neuropraxia. Minimizing external pressure on the abdomen increases blood flow through the inferior vena cava, which likely decreases blood flow through the epidural venous system resulting in decreased blood loss, increased visibility during excision of the tumor, and decreased perioperative time. An axillary roll is utilized in the lateral decubitus position to prevent brachial plexopathy of the down arm. Proper padding of the greater trochanters and knees helps prevent pressure ulcers in these regions. Protection of the fibular head can prevent peroneal nerve injuries.

Appropriate Level and Side

Intraoperative examination and radiographs facilitate identification of the appropriate spinal level. The level of the clavicle and mandible relative to the cervical level is readily visible on a lateral radiograph. Certain anterior structures help delineate the cervical level: the hyoid bone at C3, the thyroid cartilage overlying C4 and C5, and the cricoid cartilage over C6. Following a ventral approach, a spinal needle placed within the disc helps confirm the appropriate level. A bayonet bend at the end of the needle helps prevent posterior over penetration of the needle into the spinal canal.

Palpation of the last rib and counting the ribs from within the thoracic cavity help identify the appropriate thoracic level during ventral thoracic approaches. Lateral radiographs and palpation of the L1 transverse process and the last rib help identify the thoracolumbar junction during dorsal approaches. Palpation of the iliac crest in comparison to the corresponding lumbar level combined with an intraoperative radiograph and palpation of the sacrum help identify the target site in the lumbar spine [29]. Ultimately, a soft tissue mass, tumor, and local bone destruction and collapse usually will confirm the appropriate level.

Complications

Neurological Complications

Although the goal of surgery in metastatic spine disease is to improve neurologic function, patients with advanced neurological deficits preoperatively may develop worsening of their symptoms postoperatively. Rates of neurological deficits have been reported as high as 5.6% in the lumbar spine and even higher in the cervical spine. Excessive cervical manipulation during intubation should be avoided in patients with cervical spine tumors. Careful removal of tumor, bone, and disc material in the lateral corner near the uncovertebral joint may help avoid the nerve root. Cautious use of a diamond burr along the posterior longitudinal ligament (PLL) may also facilitate tumor removal. Removing the PLL can help overall prognosis by removing microscopic tumor deposits and may decrease local recurrence. Dorsolateral decompressions consist of a laminectomy at the involved level and the bone overlying the rostral and caudal disc spaces adjacent to the involved level.

Inadvertent penetration of the spinal canal can occur at any point in the surgery and can lead to a range of minor to catastrophic neurologic complications. Radiological studies can assist in determining areas of weak bone, wide interlaminar spaces, and other defects. The utilization of broad elevators over large interlaminar spaces or posterior arch deficiency is preferred over sharp-pointed instruments, which can pass through the defects. Gentle subperiosteal dissection of the soft tissue at levels of the spinal cord compression is recommended to minimize motion and pressure during exposure of the dorsal elements.

The depth and placement of anterior grafts, cages, or cement should be assessed intraoperatively with lateral radiographs. If neurologic deficits are discovered postoperatively, an accessory lateral radiograph or CT myelogram should be obtained to check the position of the ventral interbody strut. If hematoma or bone graft malalignment is suspected, immediate surgical exploration is warranted.

Iatrogenic nerve injuries are rare, but most commonly occur due to a space-occupying lesion, such as a hematoma or compression by instrumentation. Neuromonitoring has helped to mitigate the risks of neurologic deficits in spine surgery and can provide reassurance of preserved neurologic status, particularly in metastatic spine disease where blood loss and tumor infiltration can disrupt visualization of anatomy [30, 31]. Recording both SSEP's and tceMEP's is used by some center to monitor different spinal cord tracts; EMG monitoring can provide additional information about nerve root function [30–32]. Additional monitoring modalities can be utilized if further information is required based on location of the operative field and structures at risk.

Injury to the sympathetic chain can result in a Horner's syndrome. The cervical sympathetic chain lies on the ventral surface of the longus colli muscles just dorsal to the carotid sheath [33]. Subperiosteal dissection helps prevent damage to these nerves. Horner's syndrome is usually temporary but was found to be permanent in less than 1% of patients in one study [34]. In rare instances, it may be the presenting symptom for a metastatic lesion in the spine and should be evaluated closely preoperatively [35]. The lumbar sympathetic chain lies medial of the psoas muscle. Transection of this structure usually causes a vasodilation of the vessels in the ipsilateral extremity.

Dural Tears

Incidental dural tears or durotomies occur with approximately a 3.1% overall incidence but vary depending on surgical procedure. A higher incidence is noted in patients undergoing revision surgery or with prior irradiation [36–38]. Dural tears have an incidence of 1.0% in the cervical spine but can range anywhere from 1 to 16% in lumbar spine surgeries [36, 39, 40]. Perforations of the dura mater can subsequently lead to cerebrospinal fluid leakage, neurological impairment, pseudomeningocele formation, CSF fistula, meningitis, and/or wound healing problems. The dura mater is at highest risk during manipulation of the dural sac to free adhesions, although may also be torn during excision of the ligamentum flavum. Dural tears are usually closed primarily while avoiding constriction of the spinal cord or cauda equina. A watertight repair is essential to avoid future complications and must be balanced with desire to avoid compression at the level of repair. Postoperative spinal fluid leaks and pseudomeningoceles are paradoxically more likely to occur with small perforations. Preoperative radiation therapy increases the incidence of wound dehiscence and spinal fluid leakage. If prompt improvement is not observed with minor bedside procedures, the surgeon is encouraged to explore the wound and repair the dural leak.

There is no consensus on postoperative management of dural tears, leaving the ultimate decision based upon strength of the repair to the surgeon. Some surgeons recommend bed rest, positioning determined by location to minimize pressure on the tear (e.g., flat for lumbar tears vs. seated for cervical). Other studies have also reported good results without bed rest [41]. Symptoms of a dural tear may persist for a few days postoperatively regardless of repair, but patients should be reassured that dural tears do not usually cause long-term sequelae [39–41].

Complications Associated with Spinal Instrumentation

Complications related to posterior spinal instrumentation include neural element encroachment, pedicle screw failure, hardware prominence, and junctional kyphosis. Erosion of visceral or vascular structures, penetration of the spinal canal, and interbody instrumentation dislodgment can occur with ventral spinal instrumentation. The goal of instrumentation is to provide sufficient spinal stability to allow early mobilization and maintain spinal alignment since most surgery for metastatic spine disease is palliative [20]. Patients with prolonged life expectancies will benefit from instrumentation for increased likelihood of fusion.

Visceral Injury

Esophageal perforation can occur during anterior cervical spine procedures. A nasogastric tube helps to identify the esophagus during surgery. If injury is suspected to the esophagus, an intraoperative consultation with a head and neck or general surgeon is recommended to primarily repair the injury [42]. If not recognized, an esophageal perforation can present as an abscess, tracheoesophageal fistula, or mediastinitis, which would necessitate aggressive treatment including intravenous antibiotics, incision, and drainage as well as repair by an appropriate surgeon.

Injury to the lung can occur, particularly during exposure of the rib or costovertebral junction during anterior or posterolateral spinal procedures. Careful subperiosteal dissection of the ribs can usually expose the ribs without violating the parietal pleura. Holding ventilation and using a double-lumen endotracheal tube during transthoracic approaches before entering the pleura can decrease risk of injury to the lung during anterior procedures. A tube thoracostomy should be placed after anterior and lateral approaches.

The rectum is at risk during sacral procedures and coccygectomies. Transection of the anococcygeal ligaments allows for careful separation of the rectum from the sacrum. A rectal tube can also help identify the rectum to avoid damaging it during surgery.

Pulmonary Complications

Pulmonary complications commonly occur after reconstructive spinal procedures in patients with cancer. Atelectasis, pneumonia, pneumothorax, and aspiration are most frequently encountered. However, other concerning complications include pulmonary edema, acute respiratory distress syndrome, and transfusion-related acute lung injury [43]. Multiple techniques are utilized to prevent atelectasis, including expansion of the lung before extubation, deep breathing, coughing, and early mobilization. Pneumonia should be treated aggressively with pulmonary toilet, early mobilization, antibiotics, and possibly bronchoscopy. A small apical pneumothorax is common following chest tube removal but usually resolves without treatment. However, a large, persistent, or symptomatic pneumothorax may require placement of a tube thoracostomy. Aspiration risk in these patients increases with lower mobility and nausea and vomiting. This can be prevented with elevation of the head of the bed, aggressive control of nausea and vomiting, minimizing sedation, and consideration of nasogastric suction.

Genitourinary Complications

Ureteral injuries typically occur during retroperitoneal dissections around the bifurcation of the common iliac vessels. Identification, mobilization, and protection of the ureter during these approaches decrease the likelihood of ureteral injury. Placement of retrograde ureteral stents may facilitate identification and protection of the ureter in patients undergoing anterior surgery to remove lumbosacral and sacral tumors with large, anterior soft tissue masses. Retrograde ejaculation can also occur if the superior hypogastric sympathetic plexus is injured during dissection on the ventral portion of the upper sacrum [44]. Bowel, bladder, and sexual dysfunction are relatively common occurrences after a total sacrectomy due to proximity to visceral structures.

Dysphagia and Hoarseness

Dysphagia after anterior cervical surgery is relatively common and may be caused by hemorrhage, edema, denervation, or infection. Smoking and revision surgery are risk factors for persistent dysphagia postoperatively [45]. A hematoma is an emergent problem that can cause airway obstruction or spinal cord compression. Risk of hematoma can be decreased with meticulous hemostasis, especially identification and ligation of the superior or inferior thyroid artery, placement of a drain, and elevation of the head in the immediate postoperative period. Airway obstruction after extubation can occur in the postoperative period and necessitates close monitoring. Prolonged retraction of the soft tissues can result in retropharyngeal edema. Postoperative intubation and corticosteroids are considered until the edema decreases, although steroid use is controversial due to limited evidence proving efficacy and increased rates of poor wound healing [46, 47].

If persistent dysphagia is present, a barium swallow or an endoscopy should be considered. Minor hoarseness or sore throat after a ventral cervical approach is usually caused by edema or endotracheal intubation. Occasionally, laryngeal nerve palsy causes hoarseness [48]. The external branch of the superior laryngeal nerve travels along with the superior thyroid artery to innervate the cricothyroid muscle. Damage to this nerve may result in hoarseness but often produces symptoms such as easy fatiguing of the voice. The left recurrent laryngeal nerve is protected in the left tracheoesophageal groove, whereas the right recurrent laryngeal nerve is vulnerable as it passes from subclavian artery to the right tracheoesophageal groove. If hoarseness persists for more than 6 weeks following anterior cervical surgery, laryngoscopy can be done to evaluate the vocal cord and laryngeal muscles. Treatment of inferior laryngeal nerve palsy includes observation to allow for spontaneous recovery of function [49]. Further treatment or surgery by an otolaryngologist may be necessary in persistent cases.

Ileus/Gastrointestinal

Gastrointestinal complications are a risk with any spine surgery but particularly with anterior approaches to the thoracic and lumbar spine. Perforation is a rare complication, but repair by a qualified surgeon is recommended. Postoperative ileus can occur after spinal procedures, particularly following ventral procedures at the thoracolumbar, lumbar, or sacral levels. Ileus is often treated with nasogastric tube suction, intravenous fluids, and delayed oral intake until intestinal function returns [50]. Ogilvie's syndrome, or acute colonic pseudo-obstruction, is a severe complication that can be deadly if it remains untreated. Treatment depends on patient's clinical condition and whether or not they have perforated but may require surgical intervention versus monitoring [51, 52].

Vascular

Vascular injury is a potentially life-threatening complication in spine surgery [53]. The common carotid artery, the vertebral artery, and the internal jugular vein can be injured during anterior cervical approaches. The vertebral arteries and veins are usually located within the transverse foramen of C2–C6. The vertebral veins are usually located medial to the arteries and are injured more frequently than the vertebral arteries. Hemostasis is usually managed with gentle packing with thrombotic agents. Persistent hemorrhage may require further decompression and exposure of the vessels followed by bipolar electrocautery, repair, or ligation of the vessel. Ligation of the vertebral artery is associated with an increased risk of neurological deficit; thus, repair is preferred if possible [54]. The dominance of the artery should enter this decision-making process and can be assessed with preoperative CT angiography if operating close to the artery. The smaller of the two ventral arteries, if sacrificed, poses less of a neurological risk than the sacrifice of the larger artery.

The vertebral artery emerges from the foramen of C2 and then courses medially on the superior portion of C1 within the vertebral artery groove. The distance from the midline of C1 to the medial aspect of the groove ranges from 12 to 23 mm on the dorsal aspect of the ring and from 8–13 mm on the rostral aspect of the ring in adult vertebrae [42, 55, 56]. Dorsal dissection on the C1 ring should remain within 12 mm lateral of midline, and deep dissection on the rostral aspect of the ring should remain within 8 mm of midline to minimize risk of injury to the vertebral artery.

Thoracic and lumbar procedures can have catastrophic vascular complications. The arch of the aorta with its innominate, left common carotid, and left subclavian artery branches, as well as the right and left brachiocephalic veins, are at risk of injury during exposures of tumors involving C7–T3 through low cervical or median sternotomy approaches [57]. The descending aorta is at risk for injury during left-sided ventral approaches from T4 to L4 and the inferior vena cava is at risk for injury during procedures involving L1–L4 [58, 59]. Protection of the aorta, inferior vena cava, azygos, and hemiazygos veins with a malleable retractor helps prevent injuries to these structures. Ligation of the segmental vessels, followed by gentle dissection off the vertebral body, helps identify the plane between the anterior longitudinal ligament and the larger vessels. Careful utilization of curettes and pituitary rongeurs combined with protection of the vessels with a laparotomy pad or malleable retractors helps prevent injuries to the large vessels. Identification and ligation of the iliolumbar vein aids visualization of the lower lumbar spine and increases the mobility of the common iliac vein. Ligation or mobilization of the internal iliac vessels and its branches helps decrease blood loss during total and partial sacrectomies. When attempting complex surgical approaches for spine tumors, having a vascular surgeon involved in the case can significantly decrease EBL, total incision time, and length of stay [60].

The radicular artery of Adamkiewicz contributes to the anterior spinal artery and provides the main blood supply to the lower spinal cord. It usually originates from a segmental artery on the left side and accompanies the ventral root of T9, T10, or T11 but can originate anywhere from T5 to L5 [61]. Ligation of segmental vessels over the midportion of the vertebral body may help minimize risk of injury to the artery of Adamkiewicz. Dissection or electrocautery near the foramen and disarticulation of the costotransverse and costovertebral joints can injure the artery or important collateral vessels. Paraplegia resulting from segmental vessel ligation is rare if vessel ligation is unilateral and normotensive anesthesia is utilized [1].

Injury to the aorta, azygos, inferior vena cava, and iliac vessels can also occur during dorsal approaches to the spine. Most injuries occur during the discectomy but can be limited by strict attention to the depth of penetration of rongeurs and curettes. Late hemorrhage owing to erosion, leakage, or false aneurysm formation of the vessel is possible but thought to be related to prominent metal implants.

Thoracic Duct Injury

The thoracic duct is at risk for injury during ventral approaches to the spine [62, 63]. The cisterna chyli is the beginning of the thoracic duct and usually lies on the surface of the second lumbar vertebra between the right crus and the aorta. The thoracic duct remains between the aorta and the azygos vein in the lower thoracic spine and then crosses over to the left side at about T5. The thoracic duct ascends into the neck as high as C6 before it descends to empty near the internal jugular and subclavian vein junction. If damaged, the thoracic duct should be doubly ligated proximally and distally to prevent chylothorax. Tube thoracostomy drainage, intravenous hyperalimentation, and no oral intake are instituted for persistent leaks [63]. Exploration and thoracic duct ligation may be required if nonoperative measures fail.

Thromboembolic Disease

Patients with metastatic disease of the spine are at higher baseline risk for thromboembolic disease due to the thrombotic nature of cancer. However, the efficacy and safety of prophylactic anticoagulation is disputed. Postoperative fatal pulmonary embolism is rare [64, 65]. The complications associated with pharmacologic anticoagulation include wound hematoma, deep wound infection, upper gastrointestinal bleeding, cauda equina syndrome secondary to epidural hematoma, and paraplegia secondary to epidural formation and are concerning enough to hold anticoagulation. Patients who develop pulmonary emboli or significant deep venous thromboses may benefit from placement of a vena cava filter preferentially to anticoagulation. There is no known safe timing for prophylactic pharmacologic anticoagulation. These patients should be encouraged to ambulate and have compression boots and stockings placed postoperatively.

Infection

Spinal procedures for metastatic disease are associated with higher wound infection rates as compared to other spine surgeries. Additionally, surgical site infection was shown to have a negative impact on survival, triggering greater cause for concern [66–68]. Weinstein et al. reported a 20% incidence of wound infections with metastatic cancer in the spine compared to 0.4–3.2% infection rates after laminectomies, fusion with and without instrumentation [69]. The incidence of wound infection is 2.5 times greater with dorsal procedures compared to anterior. Early cellulitis may be treated with antibiotics, but exploration is indicated for persistent signs of infection. Purulent drainage warrants exploration, irrigation, and debridement. Instrumentation should be left in place unless the infection persists despite proper irrigation and debridement. Typically, the wound is closed over drains but occasionally must be left open with wound vac placement with delayed primary or secondary closure. Broad spectrum antibiotics should continue until sensitivity results allow tailoring. IV antibiotics are generally continued for 6 weeks.

Wound Complications

Radiation therapy, chemotherapy, preoperative embolization, poor nutrition, and immobility contribute to increased wound complications in cancer patients. Anterior decompressive procedures through a thoracotomy, thoracolumbar, or retroperitoneal approach may decrease the incidence of wound complications [70, 71] compared to dorsal procedures using a midline incision.

Known risk factors include albumin <3.5, lymphocyte count <1000 mm^3, and preoperative corticosteroid administration [72]. The incidence of wound complications is significantly higher in patients who received preoperative radiation therapy within a week of the operation compared to patients that had surgery several weeks after radiation therapy [73].

Minimizing pressure on the wound helps prevent wound complications. Early mobilization, logrolling, and specialized mattresses diminish pressure and length of time lying on the wound. Local flaps utilizing the latissimus or trapezius muscle may prevent or treat wound complications associated with prominent or exposed hardware [9, 73]. Revision cases may benefit from the expertise of a plastic surgeon to assist in decreasing postoperative wound complications [72].

Radiation-Associated

Radiation therapy is an effective adjuvant treatment modality to treat symptomatic metastatic carcinoma of the spine and to decrease the rate of local recurrence. Radiation therapy before surgical intervention for spinal cord compression is associated with a higher wound complication rate compared to patients that receive radiation therapy after surgical decompression [70]. However, new techniques using radiosurgery and high-dose, hypofractionated, image-guided radiation techniques may change this basic principle [74]. Judicious use of local flaps and the utilization of low-profile instrumentation may decrease wound complications. If postoperative radiation therapy is planned, a delay of at least 2–4 weeks may decrease the incidence of wound complications.

Complications Associated with Corticosteroid Utilization

Corticosteroids are frequently administered to patients with spinal cord compression. There are similar neurological outcomes using high-dose and moderate-dose dexamethasone, while fewer complications occur with moderate doses [75]. Steroids are also given after initiation of radiation treatment but should be given with H2-receptor antagonists to prevent steroid-associated stress ulcers [76]. Steroids can also cause psychiatric disturbances and can be treated with neuroleptics [77]. Patients on chronic corticosteroid therapy have weakened immune systems and are more susceptible to opportunistic infections.

Deformity

Patients with tumors involving the vertebral body have increased risk of developing a kyphotic deformity. If nonoperative treatment is indicated, the use of a molded thoracolumbar spinal orthosis may prevent collapse of the vertebral body during radiation therapy. A laminectomy alone is reserved for patients with lesions that only involve the dorsal elements. If a laminectomy was performed in a patient with ventral column involvement, there would be an increased likelihood of pathological fracture of the vertebral body and subsequent kyphotic deformity. These patients would benefit from more robust instrumentation to decrease risk of postoperative deformity [78].

Fluid and Electrolyte Imbalance

Fluid and electrolyte status is critical to monitor during and after large spine surgeries. Although seemingly minor, fluid and electrolyte imbalance can lead to pulmonary congestion, dehydration, and cardiac arrhythmia. Patients with diffuse spinal metastases may develop hypercalcemia with associated complications such as nausea, vomiting, abdominal pain, or cardiac symptoms. Early mobilization, hydration, and utilization of bisphosphonates may prevent or treat hypercalcemia.

Conclusion

Potential sources of complications exist at each step along the process for evaluation and treatment of metastatic spine disease. Decreasing complication risk begins with proper initial preoperative workup of each patient, including identifying appropriate surgical candidates and obtaining a histologic diagnosis, and continues with meticulous surgical technique and postoperative care.

References

1. Wise JJ, Fischgrund JS, Herkowitz HN, Montgomery D, Kurz LT. Complication, survival rates, and risk factors of surgery for metastatic disease of the spine. Spine. 1999;24(18):1943–51.
2. Eismont FJ, Green BA, Brown MD, Ghandur-Mnaymneh L. Coexistent infection and tumor of the spine. A report of three cases. J Bone Joint Surg Am. 1987;69:452–8.
3. An HS, Vaccaro AR, Dolinskas CA, Cotler JM, Balderston RA, Bauerle WB. Differentiation between spinal tumors and infections with magnetic resonance imaging. Spine. 1991;16:S334–8.
4. An HS, Andreshak TG, Nguyen C, Williams A, Daniels D. Can we distinguish between benign versus malignant compression fractures of the spine by magnetic resonance imaging? Spine. 1995;20:1776–82.
5. Wang B, Fintelmann FJ, Kamath RS, Kattapuram SV, Rosenthal DI. Limited magnetic resonance imaging of the lumbar spine has high sensitivity for detection of acute fractures, infection, and malignancy. Skelet Radiol. 2016;45(12):1687–93.
6. Kato S, Hozumi T, Yamakawa K, Saito M, Goto T, Kondo T. META: an MRI-based scoring system differentiating metastatic from osteoporotic vertebral fractures. Spine J. 2015;15(7):1563–70.

7. Awad AW, Almefty KK, Ducruet AF, Turner JD, Theodore N, McDougall CG, et al. The efficacy and risks of preoperative embolization of spinal tumors. J Neurointervent Surg. 2016;8:859–64.
8. Olerud C, Jonsson H Jr, Lofberg AM, Lorelius LE, Sjostrom L. Embolization of spinal metastases reduces perioperative blood loss. 21 patients operated on for renal cell carcinoma. Acta Orthop Scand. 1993; 64:9–12.
9. Ayala AG, Raymond AK, Ro JY, Carrasco CH, Fanning CV, Murray JA. Needle biopsy of primary bone lesions. M.D. Anderson experience. Pathol Annu. 1989;24:219–51.
10. Davis TM. Spinal biopsy techniques. In: McGraw JK, editor. Interventional radiology of the spine. Totowa, NJ: Humana Press; 2004. p. 181–96.
11. Kang M, Gupta S, Khandelwal N, Shankar S, Gulati M, Suri S. CT-guided fine-needle aspiration biopsy of spinal lesions. Acta Radiol. 1999;40:474–8.
12. Rajeswaran G, Malik Q, Saifuddin A. Image-guided percutaneous spinal biopsy. Skelet Radiol. 2013; 42(1):3–18.
13. Tehranzadeh J, Tao C, Browning CA. Percutaneous needle biopsy of the spine. Acta Radiol. 2007; 48(8):860–8.
14. Rimondi E, Staals EL, Errani C, Bianchi G, Vasadei R, Alberghini M, et al. Percutaneous CT-guided biopsy of the spine: results of 430 biopsies. Eur Spine J. 2008;17(7):975–81.
15. Gupta RK, Gupta S, Tandon P, Chhabra DK. Ultrasound-guided needle biopsy of lytic lesions of the cervical spine. J Clin Ultrasound. 1993;21(3): 194–7.
16. Mankin HJ, Mankin CJ, Simon MA. The hazards of the biopsy, revisited. Members of the Musculoskeletal Tumor Society. J Bone Joint Surg Am. 1996;78: 656–63.
17. Clamp JA, Bayley EJ, Ebrahimi FV, Quraishi NA, Boszczyk BM. Safety of fluoroscopy guided percutaneous access to the thoracic spine. Eur Spine J. 2012;21:207–11.
18. McLain RF. Spinal cord decompression: an endoscopically assisted approach for metastatic tumors. Spinal Cord. 2001;39:482–7.
19. Patchell RA, Tibbs PA, Regine WF, Payne R, Saris S, Kryscio RJ, et al. Direct decompressive surgical resection in the treatment of spinal cord compression caused by metastatic cancer: a randomised trial. Lancet. 2005;366:643–8.
20. Rose PS, Buchowski JM. Metastatic disease in the thoracic and lumbar spine: evaluation and management. J Am Acad Orthop Surg. 2011;19:37–48.
21. Tokuhashi Y, Matsuzaki H, Oda H, Oshima M, Ryu J. A revised scoring system for preoperative evaluation of metastatic spine tumor prognosis. Spine. 2005;30(19):2186–91.
22. Tokuhashi Y, Matsuzaki H, Toryama S, Kawano H, Ohsaka S. Scoring system for the preoperative evaluation of metastatic spine tumor prognosis. Spine. 1990;15(11):1110–3.
23. Tomita K, Kawahara N, Baba H, Tsuchiya H, Fujita T, Toribatake Y. Total en bloc spondylectomy: a new surgical technique for primary malignant vertebral tumors. Spine. 1997;22(3):324–33.
24. Tomita K, Kawahara N, Kobayashi T, Yoshida A, Murakami H, Akamaru T. Surgical strategy for spinal metastases. Spine. 2001;26(3):298–306.
25. Murakami H, Kawahara N, Demura S, Kato S, Yoshioka K, Sasagawa T, Tomita K. Perioperative complications and prognosis for elderly patients with spinal metastases treated by surgical strategy. Orthopedics. 2010;33(3). https://doi.org/10.3928/01477447-20100129-10.
26. Boriani S, Weinstein JN, Biagini R. Primary bone tumors of the spine. Terminology and surgical staging. Spine. 1997;22(9):1036–44.
27. Verlaan JJ, Choi D, Versteeg A, Albert T, Arts M, Balabaud L, et al. Characteristics of patients who survived <3 months or >2 years after surgery for spinal metastases: can we avoid inappropriate patient selection? J Clin Oncol. 2016;34(25):3054–61.
28. Yao KC, Boriani S, Gokaslan ZL, Sundaresan N. En bloc spondylectomy for spinal metastases: a review of techniques. Neurosurg Focus. 2003;15(5):E6.
29. Ebraheim NA, Inzerillo C, Zu R. Are anatomic landmarks reliable in determination of fusion level in posterolateral lumbar fusion? Spine. 1999;24:973–4.
30. Devlin VJ, Schwartz DM. Intraoperative neurophysiologic monitoring during spinal surgery. J Am Acad Orthop Surg. 2007;15(9):549–60.
31. Avila EK, Elder JB, Singh P, Chen X, Bilsky MH. Intraoperative neurophysiologic monitoring and neurologic outcomes in patients with epidural spine tumors. Clin Neurol Neurosurg. 2013;115:2147–52.
32. Ney JP, van der Goes DN, Nuwer MR. Does intraoperative neurophysiologic monitoring matter in noncomplex spine surgeries? Neurology. 2015;85:2151–8.
33. Civelek E, Karasu A, Cansever T, Hepgul K, Kiris T, Sabanci A, et al. Surgical anatomy of the cervical sympathetic trunk during anterolateral approach to the cervical spine. Eur Spine J. 2008;17:991–5.
34. Flynn TB. Neurologic complications of anterior cervical interbody fusion. Spine. 1982;7(6):536–9.
35. Zhao CQ, Jiang SD, Jiang LS, Dai LY. Horner syndrome due to a solitary osteochondroma of C7. A case report and review of the literature. Spine. 2007; 32(16):E471–4.
36. Cammisa FP, Girardi FP, Sangani PK, Parvataneni HK, Cadag S, Sandhu HS. Incidental durotomy in spine surgery. Spine. 2000;25(20):2663–7.
37. O'Neill KR, Neuman BJ, Peters C, Riew KD. Risk factors for dural tears in the cervical spine. Spine. 2014;39(17):E1015–20.
38. Espiritu MR, Rhyne A, Darden BV. Dural tears in spine surgery. J Am Acad Orthop Surg. 2010;18:537–45.
39. Hannallah D, Lee J, Khan M, Donaldson WF, Kang JD. Cerebrospinal fluid leaks following cervical spine surgery. J Bone Joint Surg Am. 2008;90(5):1101.
40. Wang JC, Bohlman HH, Riew KD. Dural tears secondary to operations on the lumbar spine. Management and

results after a two-year-minimum follow-up of eighty-eight patients. J Bone Joint Surg Am. 1998;80:1728–32.
41. Hodges SD, Humphreys SC, Eck JC, Covington LA. Management of incidental durotomy without mandatory bed rest: a retrospective review of 20 cases. Spine (Phila Pa 1976). 1999;24(19):2062–4.
42. Grabowski G, Cornett CA, Kang JD. Esophageal and vertebral artery injuries during complex cervical spine surgery—avoidance and management. Orthop Clin North Am. 2012;43(1):63–74.
43. Swann MC, Hoes KS, Aoun SG, McDonagh DL. Postoperative complications of spine surgery. Best Pract Res Clin Anaesthesiol. 2016;30:103–20.
44. Lindley EM, McBeth ZL, Henry SE, Cooley R, Burger EL, Cain CM, Patel VV. Retrograde ejaculation after anterior lumbar spine surgery. Spine. 2012; 37(20):1785–9.
45. Olsson EC, Jobson M, Lim MR. Risk factors for persistent dysphagia after anterior cervical spine surgery. Orthopedics. 2015;38(4):e319–23.
46. Joaquim AF, Murar J, Savage JW, Patel AA. Dysphagia after anterior cervical spine surgery: a systematic review of potential preventative measures. Spine J. 2014;14(9):2246–60.
47. Siasios I, Fountas K, Dimopoulos V, Pollina J. The role of steroid administration in the management of dysphagia in anterior cervical procedures. Neurosurg Rev. 2018;41(1):47–53.
48. Tan TP, Govindarajulu AP, Massicotte EM, Venkatraghavan L. Vocal cord palsy after anterior cervical spine surgery: a qualitative systematic review. Spine J. 2014;14(7):1332–42.
49. Jung A, Schramm J, Lehnerdt K, Herberhold C. Recurrent laryngeal nerve palsy during anterior cervical spine surgery: a prospective study. J Neurosurg Spine. 2005;2(2):123–7.
50. Doorly MG, Senagore AJ. Pathogenesis and clinical and economic consequences of postoperative ileus. Surg Clin N Am. 2012;92:259–72.
51. Feldman RA, Karl RC. Diagnosis and treatment of Ogilvie's syndrome after lumbar spinal surgery. Report of three cases. J Neurosurg. 1992;76: 1012–6.
52. Fineberg SJ, Nadyala SV, Kurd MF, Marquez-Lara A, Noureldin M, Sankaranarayanan S, et al. Incidence and risk factors for postoperative ileus following anterior, posterior, and circumferential lumbar fusion. Spine J. 2014;14(8):1680–5.
53. Hans SS, Shepard AD, Reddy P, Rama K, Romano W. Iatrogenic arterial injuries of spine and orthopedic operations. J Vasc Surg. 2011;53:407–13.
54. Lunardini DJ, Eskander MS, Even JL, Dunlap JT, Chen AF, Lee JY, et al. Vertebral artery injuries in cervical spine surgery. Spine J. 2014;14(8):1520–5.
55. Schroeder GD, Hsu WK. Vertebral artery injuries in cervical spine surgery. Surg Neurol Int. 2013;4(Suppl 5): S362–7.
56. Heary RF, Albert TJ, Ludwig SC, Vaccaro AR, Wolansky LJ, Leddy TP, et al. Surgical anatomy of the vertebral arteries. Spine. 1996;18:2074–80.
57. Sundaresan N, Shah J, Foley KM, Rosen G. An anterior surgical approach to the upper thoracic vertebrae. J Neurosurg. 1984;61:686–90.
58. Hamdan AD, Malek JY, Schermerhorn ML, Aulivola B, Blattman SB, Pomposelli FB. Vascular injury during anterior exposure of the spine. J Vasc Surg. 2008; 48(3):650–4.
59. Baker JK, Reardon PR, Reardon MJ, Heggeness MH. Vascular injury in anterior lumbar surgery. Spine. 1993;18:2227–30.
60. Zahradnik V, Lubelski D, Abdullah KG, Kelso R, Mroz T, Kashyap VS. Vascular injuries during anterior exposure of the thoracolumbar spine. Ann Vasc Surg. 2013;27(3):306–13.
61. Alleyne CH, Cawley CM, Shengelaia GG, Barrow DL. Microsurgical anatomy of the artery of Adamkiewicz and its segmental artery. J Neurosurg. 1998;89(5):791–5.
62. Verhoeven W, Low CO, See HF, Chacha PB, Tan NC. Massive chylothorax after anterior fusion of the thoracic spine. Ann Acad Med Singap. 1996;25(2): 286–8.
63. Colletta AJ, Mayer PJ. Chylothorax: an unusual complication of anterior thoracic interbody spinal fusion. Spine. 1982;7:46–9.
64. Cheng JS, Arnold PM, Anderson PA, Fischer D, Dettori JR. Anticoagulation risk in spine surgery. Spine. 2010;35(9):S117–24.
65. Schulte LM, O'Brien JR, Bean MC, Pierce TP, Yu WD, Meals C. Deep vein thrombosis and pulmonary embolism after spine surgery: incidence and patient risk factors. Am J Orthop. 2013;42(6):267–70.
66. Atkinson RA, Davies B, Jones A, van Popta D, Ousey K, Stephenson J. Survival of patients undergoing surgery for metastatic spinal tumours and the impact of surgical site infection. J Hosp Infect. 2016;94:80–5.
67. Demura S, Kawahara N, Murakami H, Nambu K, Kato S, Yoshioka K, et al. Surgical site infection in spinal metastasis: risk factors and countermeasures. Spine. 2009;34:635–9.
68. Omeis IA, Dhir M, Sciubba DM, Gottfried ON, McGirt MJ, Attenollo FJ, et al. Postoperative surgical site infections in patients undergoing spinal tumor surgery: incidence and risk factors. Spine (Phila Pa 1976). 2011;36:1410–9.
69. Weinstein MA, MCCabe JP, Cammisa FP Jr. Postoperative spinal wound infection: a review of 2,391 consecutive index procedures. J Spinal Disord. 2000;13:422–6.
70. Ghogawala Z, Mansfield FL, Borges LF. Spinal radiation before surgical decompression adversely affects outcomes of surgery for asymptomatic metastatic spinal cord compression. Spine. 2001;26:818–24.
71. McPhee IB, Williams RP, Swanson CE. Factors influencing wound healing after surgery for metastatic disease of the spine. Spine. 1998;23:726–32.
72. Mesfin A, Sciubba DM, Dea N, Nater A, Bird JE, Quraishi NA, et al. Changing the adverse event profile in metastatic spine surgery: evidence-based approach to target wound complications and instrumentation failure. Spine. 2016;41(20):S262–70.

73. Itshayek E, Yamada J, Bilsky M, Schmidt M, Shaffrey C, Gerszten P, et al. Timing of surgery and radiotherapy in the management of metastatic spine disease: a systematic review. Int J Oncol. 2010;36: 533–44.
74. Gerszten PC, Mendel E, Yamada Y. Radiotherapy and radiosurgery for metastatic spine disease: what are the options, indications and outcomes? Spine. 2009;34(225):S78–92.
75. Heimdal K, Hirschberg H, Slettebo H, Watne K, Nome O. High incidence of serious side effects of high-dose dexamethasone treatment in patients with epidural spinal cord compression. J Neuro-Oncol. 1992;12:141–4.
76. Barletta JF, Bruno JJ, Buckley MS, Cook DJ. Stress ulcer prophylaxis. Crit Care Med. 2016;44(7):1395–405.
77. Kenna HA, Poon AW, de los Angeles CP, Koran LM. Psychiatric complications of treatment with corticosteroids: review with case report. Psychiatry Clin Neurosci. 2011;65(6):549–60.
78. Kim HJ, Buchowski JM, Moussallem CD, Rose PS. Modern techniques in the treatment of patients with metastatic spine disease. J Bone Joint Surg Am. 2012;94:944–51.

Percutaneous Thermal Ablation of Spine Metastasis

23

Alexander Theologis, Jack W. Jennings, and Jacob M. Buchowski

Background

Approximately 1.7 million people were diagnosed with a new malignancy in 2016 in the United States [1]. The number of new cancer diagnoses is anticipated to rise to 22 million within the next two decades [1]. Within their lifetime, 30–70% of these individuals will develop an osseous metastasis [2, 3]. The most common osseous metastatic site is the spinal column due to its rich blood supply, vascular red marrow, and valveless vertebral venous plexuses that communicate with deep thoracic and pelvic veins [2, 4]. As patients with spinal metastasis have varied clinical presentations, their management requires a multidisciplinary approach commonly comprised of radiation and medical oncologists, interventional radiologists, neurosurgeons, and orthopedic surgeons.

The goal of treatment for patients with spinal metastases is primarily palliative. Systemic therapies, including chemotherapy, hormonal therapy [5–7], radiopharmaceuticals [8–10], and bisphosphonates [11–15], are reserved for asymptomatic spinal lesions with the intent to control tumor locally and prevent pain, fracture, and spinal cord compression [2]. While these interventions are effective at decreasing skeletally related events, many patients will eventually develop symptoms that can be a source of significant physical and psychological morbidity [2, 16–19]. Painful and unstable spine metastatic lesions, as determined by the spinal instability neoplasm score [20, 21], with or without a neurologic deficit are most often treated with surgical stabilization. Standard fractionated radiation therapy (i.e., external beam radiation therapy [EBRT] and more recently stereotactic body radiation therapy [SBRT]) is the mainstay for treatment for painful osseous metastases and metastatic spinal disease without mechanical instability or neurologic symptoms [19, 22–38]. Conventional radiation therapy has several limitations with many patients having incomplete pain relief [37]. In a meta-analysis of randomized palliative radiotherapy trials for painful bone metastases, Chow et al. reported an overall response rate of 60% and a complete response rate of only 23% [37]. A study of patients with spinal metastases treated with

A. Theologis, MD
Department of Orthopaedic Surgery, University of California—San Francisco (UCSF), San Francisco, CA, USA
e-mail: Alekos.Theologis@ucsf.edu

J. W. Jennings, MD, PhD
Department of Radiology, Mallinckrodt Institute of Radiology, Washington University School of Medicine, Barnes-Jewish Hospital, St. Louis, MO, USA
e-mail: jackwjennings@wustl.edu

J. M. Buchowski, MD, MS (✉)
Department of Orthopaedic Surgery, BJC Institute of Health, Washington University in St. Louis—School of Medicine, St. Louis, MO, USA
e-mail: buchowskij@wustl.edu

R. A. W. Marco (ed.), *Metastatic Spine Disease*, https://doi.org/10.1007/978-3-319-76252-4_23

radiation therapy also found that average visual analog pain scores decreased by only 1.1 points after 30 days of radiation therapy (pre-radiation 5.7; postradiation 4.6) [26]. This partial pain relief may not be evident for nearly a month [26, 38, 39] and may not last for an appreciable amount of time [26, 39–41]. In a study of 320 patients who underwent radiation therapy and survived >52 weeks, 49% reported pain progression [40, 41]. Re-treatment of spinal metastases with radiation has also been demonstrated to only be 40% effective and may not be possible due to the risk of radiation myelopathy [41, 42]. However, recent data on SBRT have demonstrated it to be an effective method to achieve local control in recurrent spinal metastases [23, 24, 43, 44]. In a cohort of 54 patients with recurrent spinal metastases treated with SBRT, Chang et al. reported radiographic control rates of 96% at 6 months, 81% at 12 months, and 79% at 24 months [43]. Importantly, there were also no associated cases of radiation myelopathy [43]. In addition to SBRT, alternative approaches that provide adequate and lasting pain relief for symptomatic spinal metastases have been developed. Two of these modalities, which have proven particularly effective, are radiofrequency ablation (RFA) and cryoablation.

This chapter will discuss the current indications for RFA and cryoablation in the treatment of spinal metastases and how each technique is performed. Moreover, we present the most current evidence regarding each modality's efficacy in the treatment of patients with spinal metastases and the importance of supplemental cement augmentation for treatment and prevention of pathologic fractures. An examination of RFA and cryoablations' limitations and risk profiles will also be provided.

Fundamental Concepts

Radiofrequency ablation and cryoablation are percutaneous, minimally invasive, image-guided techniques that rely upon the production of extreme temperatures to induce cell death. Radiofrequency ablation uses an electrode to create thermal energy and extremely high temperatures (>50 °C), which results in coagulative necrosis of tissue [45]. Conversely, cryoablation induces cell apoptosis by creating and thawing an exceedingly cold environment (< negative 40 °C) [46–48]. The utility of these modalities for tumor ablation was first recognized in the successful treatment of primary and metastatic visceral tumors (i.e., hepatic, renal, pulmonary) [49–51]. More recently, they each have been found to significantly decrease pain and provide local control of bone tumors [16, 42, 45, 48, 52–65]. For example, in 2002 Callstrom et al. first demonstrated that RFA-treated osteolytic metastases resulted in significant decreases in pain, opiate usage, and functional disability within 4 weeks of the treatment [55]. Callstrom et al. reported very similar findings for osteolytic metastases treated with cryoablation [59]. Given these promising original reports and the advancements of technology, indications for RFA and cryoablation have since expanded to the treatment of metastatic spinal disease.

Current Indications and Pre-procedural Planning

In spinal metastatic disease, RFA and cryoablation are reserved for patients with mechanically stable spines without neurologic deficits and in whom radiation therapy is contraindicated, persistent pain or radiographic tumor progression has been documented despite radiation therapy, or combination ablation and radiation therapy are planned for radiation-resistant tumors [66].

There are several factors involved in the decision to utilize RFA or cryoablation. These include bone quality, tumor location, and tumor size, all of which are determined from pre-procedural computed tomography (CT) and/or magnetic resonance imaging (MRI). In regard to bone quality, purely osteolytic lesions and mixed metastases (i.e., lytic and blastic) are most frequently targeted with RFA, while entirely osteoblastic metastases are better treated with cryoablation, as sclerotic bone hampers the ability of RFA probes to produce cytotoxic temperatures secondary to imped-

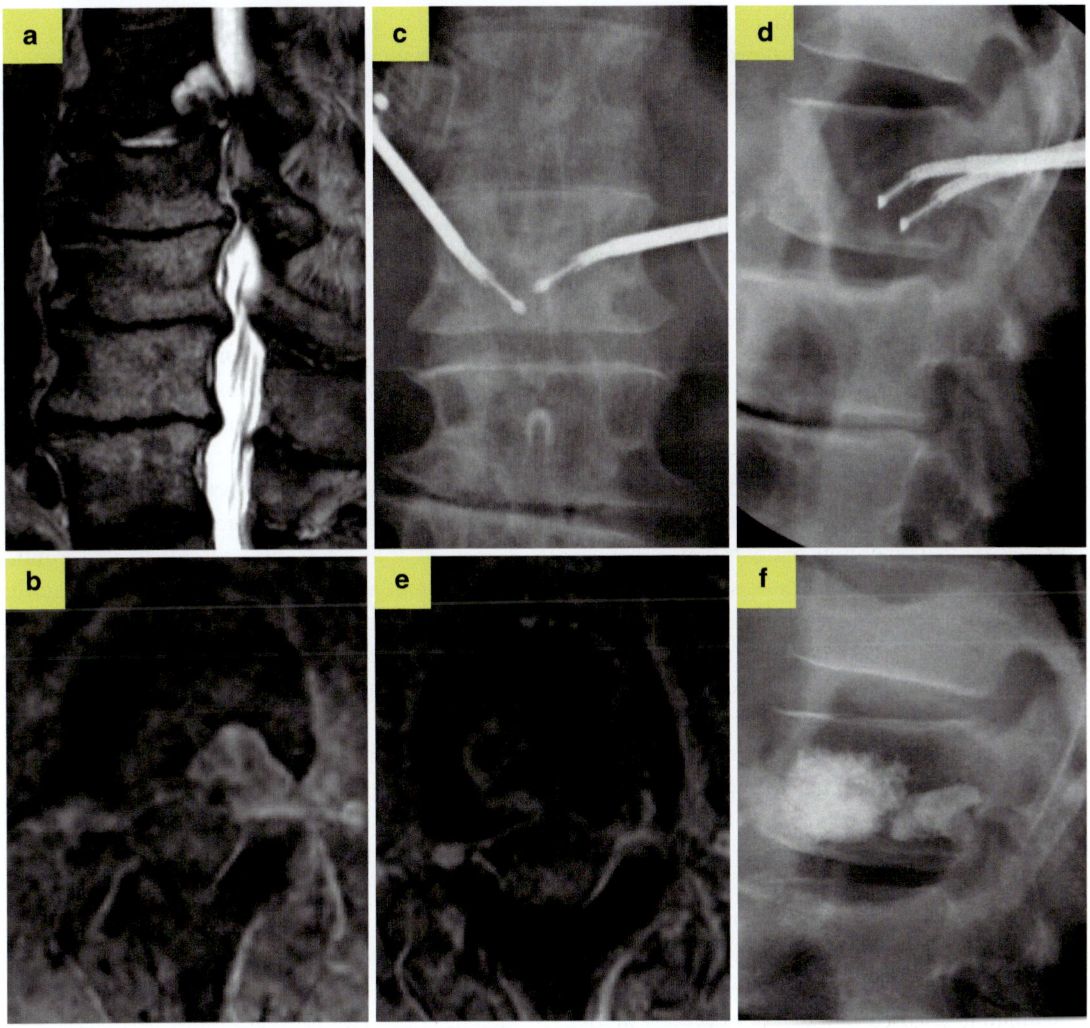

Fig. 23.1 A 78-year-old male with metastatic squamous cell carcinoma to the posteriolateral aspect of the L2 vertebral body (**a**, **b**). The tumor occupied more than 50% of the body's posterior wall. As such, the patient underwent radiofrequency ablation (RFA) via bilateral transpedicular approaches (**c**, **d**) and cement augmentation (**f**) to prevent pathologic fracture. Note that 2 months after RFA, there was no enhancement of the lesion on MRI with contrast (**e**)

ance [66]. Tumor location is also an important factor in choosing which ablation technique to employ. Lesions that have an extra-osseous soft tissue component are primarily managed with cryoablation, as CT can better detect ablation edges produced by cryoablation than by RFA [66]. Tumors contained within the osseous borders of the vertebra (i.e., body, pedicles, lamina) may be treated with either RFA or cryoablation. Anterior and posterolateral vertebral body lesions can be accessed from a transpedicular approach with straight probes [66]. However, tumors in the central-posterior aspect of the vertebral body cannot be accessed with traditional straight probes, and newer articulating probes are required [3] (Fig. 23.1). In addition to difficult access, posteriorly based lesions within 1 cm of the spinal canal or with posterior cortical bone destruction were originally deemed unsafe to treat with ablation because of concern for neurologic injury [3, 45]. In a porcine model, Nour et al. reported immediate post-ablation radiculopathy and paraplegia when RFAs were performed in the pedicle and posterior body, respectively [67]. As extensive neurologic injury has been determined to occur quickly at ≥45 °C [68–71], the use of more modern, bipolar electrode probes combined with thermal protection and thermal monitoring has made ablation of posterior lesions possible [2, 3, 41, 42, 45, 72]. Dupuy et al. first reported on four patients with tumors located adjacent to the spinal canal who were treated with internally cooled RFA probes [70]. The highest temperature observed in the epidural space was 44 °C, and no patients had a new neurologic deficit [70]. In a separate study in which ten patients with spinal metastases within 1 cm of the spinal canal were treated with RFA and spinal canal temperature was recorded, Nakatsuka et al. noted that one patient had transient neurologic injury after spinal canal temperature rose to 48 °C [73]. All other nine patients had spinal canal temperatures <45 °C, and none suffered new neurologic symptoms [73]. Multiple additional studies have since demonstrated that posterior vertebral body lesions can be safely ablated [2, 3, 41, 42, 45, 72] (Fig. 23.1). As such, recommendations from 2015 from the Metastatic Spine Disease Multidisciplinary Working Group state that "ablation is not contraindicated when the posterior vertebral body cortex is eroded by tumor; however, ablation cannot be performed safely when epidural tumor abuts or surrounds the spinal cord" [2].

Size of a tumor is also important to assess on pre-procedural imaging. Small tumors that are confined to one half of the vertebral body are adequately accessed through a unilateral transpedicular approach. This is in contrast to larger tumors that occupy a portion of both vertebral body's hemispheres, which are best addressed through both pedicles. Bilateral transpedicular approaches are often also required when the tumor involves >50% of the posterior wall [3] (Fig. 23.1). If pedicle sizes are too small to use for access to the vertebral body, as may be the case in the thoracic spine, a para-pedicular approach may be used.

Procedural Technique

Interventional radiologists perform the majority of ablations with image guidance in outpatient operating suites. While most of these procedures can be performed with conscious sedation and local anesthetic, conversion to general anesthesia may be required especially in cases in which neuromonitoring is necessary. After induction of anesthesia, patients are placed prone onto a radiolucent table associated with an imaging-guidance system (i.e., fluoroscopy, CT, MRI). For cases that are deemed to have the potential to risk neurologic structures, neuromonitoring may be used [66, 74]. An advantage of CT during cryoablation is that it allows for visualization of the frozen tissue as a low-attenuation lesion (Fig. 23.2). This is particularly important because it provides the opportunity to confirm that the entire tumor volume has been ablated.

Under image guidance, a trajectory to the region of interest is first established. An introducer cannula is then placed over the appropriate trajectory into the vertebral body via a transpedicular approach, which provides the working access through which the ablation probe is placed. Intraosseous placement can be accomplished with navigating osteotomes and/or bone biopsy needles [41]. When performing RFA and cryoablation, a variety of probes can be used. For cryoablation, the probes vary in length, diameter, and ice ball size that are available from Endocare (Perc-15, Perc-17, and Perc-24; Healthtronics/Endocare Incorporated, Irvine, California) and Galil (BTG) (IceRod, IceSeed; Arden Hills, MN) [48, 57, 63]. The probes should be placed 2 cm apart and approximately 1 cm from the lesion's periphery [48]. To freeze the tissue, probes deliver argon gas that can reach −140 °C as a result of gas expansion during the transition from the probes' insulated shafts to uninsulated tips [46–48]. Following a period of freezing, the tissue may be thawed passively or actively by instillation of helium gas [46–48]. To optimize cell death, a minimum of two 10-min freeze cycles with an intervening 5- to 10-min thaw cycle is advised and commonly used [46–48, 61, 62, 64]. Tissue injury is complete between −20 °C and −40 °C, which is reported to be approximately 3–5 mm deep to the visible edge of the "ice ball," which represents 0 °C [65]. For RFA, probes differ based on their modularity and type of radiofrequency (i.e., straight v. articulating; monopolar

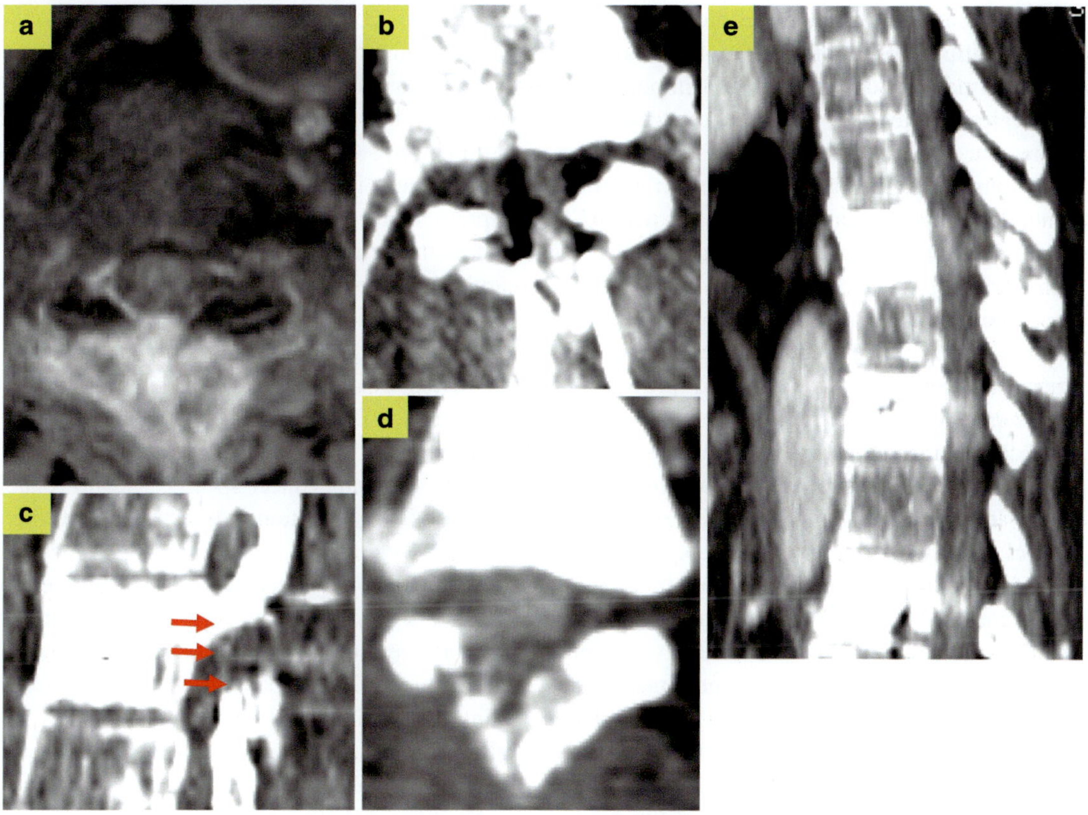

Fig. 23.2 A 58-year-old male with a history of metastatic renal cell carcinoma to T9. After undergoing a previously successful RFA with vertebral augmentation for a vertebral body metastatic lesion, he represented with a symptomatic lesion of the posterior elements (**a**). He underwent a cryoablation (**b**, **c**)—note the low-attenuation ice ball extending into the spinal canal (**c**, red arrows). Given the proximity of the lesion to the spinal canal, CO_2 was used in the epidural space for cord protection (**b**). No neurologic deficit occurred. Nineteen months post-cryoablation, there was no progression of disease at T9 (**d**) and no tumor within the canal (**e**)

v. bipolar). Modern RFA probes contain two thermocouples that allow for real-time monitoring of temperatures at the periphery of the ablation zone at a certain distance (i.e., 10–15 mm) from an ablation zone's center [41]. The zone of ablation is important to know because it will dictate how many ablations are required to cover an entire tumor and it defines the safe working distance between the probe and vital neurovascular structures.

When addressing a tumor in close proximity to the spinal canal or neural foramen with RFA and cryoablation, thermal protection is required. Thermal protection techniques involve placing an 18-gauge needle coaxial to a thermocouple within the epidural space or neural foramen. When temperatures exceed 45 °C during RFA or fall below 10 °C during cryoablation, CO_2 is injected for neural insulation, and 5% dextrose water is instilled [3, 41, 66, 75] (Fig. 23.2). Normal saline is not used as the coolant in RFA due to its ionic content as it can create a plasma field resulting in larger ablation zones than intended.

In addition to avoiding injury, pain relief is an important goal. As such, metastases involving contiguous vertebrae should be ablated during the same procedural setting. Furthermore, the entire volume of the lesion should be ablated. This may be accomplished by aiming to ablate marrow enhancement or T2-hyperintensity on MRI, osteolysis on CT, and/or increased FDG uptake on PET-CT [41]. An additional 3-mm rim around the lesion's periphery should also be targeted to account for microscopic tumor spread [41]. Multiple overlapping ablations should also be performed, which is particularly important for larger lesions [3]. As cryoablation technology allows for multiple probes to be used simultaneously, large tumors may be ablated in a shorter amount of time with cryoablation than with RFA, which requires multiple, sequential passes of the same probe.

After ablation has been performed, cement augmentation of the tumor is recommended to treat pathologic fractures and to prevent the development of future compression fractures (Fig. 23.1). In a case report, Wallace et al. presented a 46-year-old woman with a painful metastatic leiomyosarcoma located in the posterior aspect of L4 who sustained a vertebral compression fracture 4 months after RFA treatment without cement augmentation at the same time [76]. In a retrospective review of consecutive patients who underwent RFA of spinal metastases, 60% of the patients (three out of five) who did not receive vertebral cement augmentation sustained a compression fracture within 12 months of the treatment [41]. Furthermore, 50% of tumors not augmented with cement went on to fracture within 3 months of RFA treatment in a large multicenter retrospective analysis [45]. No report has documented vertebral fracture after cryoablation used in isolation. Nevertheless, the use of vertebral cement augmentation has been endorsed for cryoablation of larger lesions (>50%) [63]. While the need for cement augmentation of larger tumors is intuitive, its necessity for smaller tumors is not known. As instillation of cement is associated with rare but potentially serious complications (i.e. pulmonary embolism, spinal cord thermal necrosis, extravasation), careful consideration is required when deciding to use cement augmentation after ablation of smaller lesions.

Effectiveness of Treatment

Current literature has consistently demonstrated that RFA and cryoablation provide meaningful improvements in pain and quality of life for patients with spinal metastatic disease [41, 42, 45, 52, 54, 72, 77, 78]. In a retrospective review of 41 patients with unresectable primary ($n = 2$) or secondary tumors ($n = 39$) of the thoracolumbar spine that were unresponsive to chemo- and radiotherapy, Gevargez et al. reported a 36% improvement in pain at 6 weeks and 50% pain improvement at 6 months after RFA [54]. Functional activity scores also improved significantly at 6 weeks (8%) and at 6 months (10%) [54]. Furthermore, 85% were free of tumor progression [54]. In a multicenter, prospective clinical series of 50 patients with vertebral body metastases, Bagla et al. found significant improvements in average scores for pain, disability (ODI), and cancer-specific health-related quality of life (Functional Assessment of Cancer Therapy-General 7; Functional Assessment of Cancer Therapy Quality-of-Life Measurement in Patients with Bone Pain) from baseline to all post-intervention time intervals [79] Greenwood et al. found 62% of patients had a decrease in pain medication and 81% of patients had improvement in functional activity 1 month after RFA combined with radiation therapy for spinal metastases [42]. In another study of metastatic spinal disease treated with RFA, Grönemeyer et al. reported reduced pain in 90% of patients with an average relative pain reduction of 74.4% [77]. Disability related to back pain decreased on average by 27%, and general health significantly increased in 50% of patients [77]. Postoperatively, there was no further tumor growth on MRI [77]. In a large multicenter retrospective study of 128 metastatic spinal lesions treated with bipolar RFA, Anchala et al. noted significant improvements in visual analog pain scores (VAS) at 1 week (average 1.73), 1 month (average 2.25), and 6 months (average 1.73) post-procedure compared to pre-procedural scores (average 7.51) [45]. At the largest institution in this study, 54% of patients reported a reduction in pain medication usage [45]. Investigations solely evaluating posterior vertebral body lesions have also demonstrated promising results [3, 72, 73]. Of 12 patients with spinal tumors treated with RFA and vertebroplasty, all had decrease in pain medication usage and significant improvements in VAS pain scores (pre-procedure, 17.33 ± 2.46; 1 week post-procedure, 9.25 ± 4.81; 3 months post-procedure, 7.00 ± 5.26) [72]. In a separate study of 47 metastatic posterior vertebral body spinal tumors treated with RFA, Hillen et al. also found 50% of patients had decrease in pain medication usage and the entire cohort had significant improvements in VAS scores at 1 week (average 2.82) and 1 month (average 3.30) post-procedure compared to pre-op (average 7.82) [3]. There were no permanent neurologic injuries [3]. Similar findings were also reported by Wallace et al. for spinal metastases treated with a combination of RFA and vertebral cement augmentation [41].

Documented efficacy and safety of cryoablation for spinal metastases is less robust than RFA. In a case report, de Freitas et al. presented a 55-year-old woman with stage IV non-small cell lung cancer metastatic to the body of T9 and S2 that was treated with cryoablation [60]. There were no complications associated with the ablation, and after the procedure, the patient required no further pain medications and reported no pain [60]. Masala et al. presented a retrospective analysis of 23 patients with single vertebral metastases treated with cryoablation and vertebroplasty and found a significant improvement in VAS pain scores (baseline, 8.6 ± 1.1; 1 week, 2.9 ± 1.2; 1 month, 2.5 ± 1.0; 6 months, 2.1 ± 1.1) and Oswestry Disability Index scores (baseline, 60.65 ± 8.36; 3 months, 25.60 ± 4.35; 6 months, 22.43 ± 4.12) [63]. In a separate analysis of recurrent sacrococcygeal tumors (5 chordoma, 1 myxopapillary ependymoma) treated with cryoablation, Kurup et al. reported complete pain relief in one patient and good pain relief (VAS 6 to 2) in another patient for whom palliation of pain was the surgical indication [64]. Of the four other tumors that were treated for local control, all had no evidence of recurrence at 15 months follow-up [64]. The largest series of spinal metastases treated with cryoablation was performed by Tomasian et al. [56]. In their series of 14 patients with 31 spinal metastases (lumbar, 14; thoracic, 8; sacrum, 6; coccyx, 2; cervical, 1; vertebral body, 12; pedicle, 5; lamina, 5; spinous process, 2), there were significant decreases in pain scores and median analgesic usage 1 week, 1 month, and 3 months after the procedure [56]. Additionally, local tumor control was achieved in 96.7% of tumors at a median follow-up of 10 months [56]. While these studies specifically report upon cryoablation for spinal metastases, other investigations of cryoablation for musculoskeletal tumors include scattered cases of spinal tumors that also had successful outcomes [57–59, 61, 62].

Risks and Limitations

Radiofrequency ablation and cryoablation are relatively safe. However, they are not without risks and complications. While the aforementioned studies demonstrate outstanding improvements in pain and local tumor control, the response rates are not always complete. Furthermore, as discussed previously, ablations of tumors located adjacent to the spinal cord and nerve roots risk neurologic injury. Although thermal protection techniques minimize the risk of neurologic injury, they do not entirely prevent them. In the aforementioned analysis by Gevargez et al. of 41 patients with spinal tumors treated with RFA, two patients suffered RFA-associated complications [54]. One patient reported a new monoradiculopathy that was successfully treated with an intraforaminal corticosteroid injection [54]. A second patient had pain from an incomplete thermally induced paraplegia that was relieved within 12 h by an intraspinal corticosteroid injection [54]. In the study of 26 patients with posterior vertebral body metastases, Hillen et al. noted four patients had new post-procedure radiculopathies after RFA of tumors that extended into the pedicles [3]. All were successfully treated with corticosteroid injections, and there were no permanent neurologic deficits [3]. Tomasian et al. also reported two patients who developed transient post-procedural unilateral lower extremity radiculopathies and weakness after cryoablation that were resolved with transforaminal nerve root blocks [56]. Of note, nerve roots are more vulnerable to potential thermal injury with cryoablation than with RFA due to greater sensitivity to cold [56, 80] (we have added a new reference to confirm this statement).

Other potential risks are injury to segmental arteries during para-pedicular approaches, infection, hemorrhage, skin burns, post-RFA ablation syndrome, and cryoshock [48, 53]. Post-RFA ablation syndrome is characterized by low-grade fever ≤100 °F/37.8 °C, myalgia, and malaise that can last persistently for 1 week after the procedure [53]. Cryoshock is most commonly seen after hepatic cryoablations (approximately 1%) and results in release of various cytokines that precipitate severe coagulopathy, diffuse intravascular coagulopathy, and multi-organ failure [48]. Approximately one third of patients who experience it pass away; the overall death rate from all causes is nearly 1.5% [48]. While this phenomenon has never been reported in relation to musculoskeletal cryoablation, it is an important entity of which to be aware, as it can be life threatening. Patients should be counseled accordingly.

In conclusion, radiofrequency and cryoablation are important tools in the armamentarium of physicians involved in the treatment of patients with spinal metastases. Ideal candidates for RFA or cryoablation are those patients with mechanically stable spines without neurologic deficits and in whom radiation therapy is contraindicated, persistent pain or radiographic tumor progression has been documented despite radiation therapy, or combination ablation and radiation therapy are planned for radiation-resistant tumors [66]. Cryoablation is often favored for sclerotic lesions and those with paraspinal soft tissue components, while RFA can be used for entirely osteolytic and mixed lesions and preferred in lesions with posterior central vertebral body involvement with added benefit of articulating RFA probes. Both techniques can provide meaningful improvements in pain and provide local tumor control. To achieve the most desirable outcomes, pre-procedural planning with an emphasis on analysis of tumor size, location, and quality is a prerequisite. Additionally, vertebral body cement augmentation is important for pathologic fracture stabilization and should be performed after ablation so as to prevent pathologic fractures. Furthermore, a fundamental understanding of spinal anatomy and a firm working knowledge of ablation principles and technologies are needed to perform these techniques safely.

References

1. National Cancer Institute. Cancer statistics. National Institutes of Health; 2016.
2. Wallace A, Robinson C, Meyer J, Tran N, Gangi A, Callstrom M, et al. The metastatic spine disease multidisciplinary working group algorithms. Oncologist. 2015;20(10):1205–15.
3. Hillen T, Anchala P, Friedman M, Jennings J. Treatment of metastatic posterior vertebral body osseous tumors by using a targeted bipolar radiofrequency ablation device: technical note. Radiology. 2014;273(1):261–7.
4. Wiltse L, Fonseca A, Amster J, Dimartino P, Ravessoud F. Relationship of the dura, Hofmann's ligaments, Batson's plexus, and a fibrovascular membrane lying on the posterior surface of the vertebral bodies and attaching to the deep layer of the posterior longitudinal ligament. An anatomical, radiologic, and clin. Spine (Phila Pa 1976). 1993;18(8):1030–43.
5. Stopeck A, Lipton A, Body J, Steger G, Tonkin K, de Boer R, et al. Denosumab compared with zoledronic acid for the treatment of bone metastases in patients with advanced breast cancer: a randomized, double-blind study. J Clin Oncol. 2010;28(35):5132–9.
6. Fizazi K, Carducci M, Smith M, Damião R, Brown J, Karsh L, et al. Denosumab versus zoledronic acid for treatment of bone metastases in men with castration-resistant prostate cancer: a randomised, double-blind study. Lancet. 2011;377(9768):813–22.
7. Henry D, Costa L, Goldwasser F, Hirsh V, Hungria V, Prausova J, et al. Randomized, double-blind study of denosumab versus zoledronic acid in the treatment of bone metastases in patients with advanced cancer (excluding breast and prostate cancer) or multiple myeloma. J Clin Oncol. 2011;29(9):1125–32.
8. Harrison M, Wong T, Armstrong A, George D. Radium-223 chloride: a potential new treatment for castration-resistant prostate cancer patients with metastatic bone disease. Cancer Manag Res. 2013;5:1–14.
9. Quilty P, Kirk D, Bolger J, Dearnaley D, Lewington V, Mason M, et al. A comparison of the palliative effects of strontium-89 and external beam radiotherapy in metastatic prostate cancer. Radiother Oncol. 1994;31(1):33–40.
10. Serafini A, Houston S, Resche I, Quick D, Grund F, Ell P, et al. Palliation of pain associated with metastatic bone cancer using samarium-153 lexidronam: a double-blind placebo-controlled clinical trial. J Clin Oncol. 1998;16(4):1574–81.
11. Wong M, Stockler M, Pavlakis N. Bisphosphonates and other bone agents for breast cancer. Cochrane Database Syst Rev. 2012;2:CD003474.

12. Yuen K, Shelley M, Sze W, Wilt T, Mason M. Bisphosphonates for advanced prostate cancer. Cochrane Database Syst Rev. 2006;4:CD006250.
13. Lopez-Olivo M, Shah N, Pratt G, Risser J, Symanski E, Suarez-Almazor M. Bisphosphonates in the treatment of patients with lung cancer and metastatic bone disease: a systematic review and meta-analysis. Support Care Cancer. 2012;20(11):2985–98.
14. Hortobagyi G, Theriault R, Porter L, Blayney D, Lipton A, Sinoff C, et al. Efficacy of pamidronate in reducing skeletal complications in patients with breast cancer and lytic bone metastases. Protocol 19 Aredia Breast Cancer Study Group. N Engl J Med. 1996;335(24):1785–91.
15. Conte P, Latreille J, Mauriac L, Calabresi F, Santos R, Campos D, et al. Efficacy of pamidronate in reducing skeletal complications in patients with breast cancer and lytic bone metastases. Protocol 19 Aredia Breast Cancer Study Group. J Clin Oncol. 1996;14(9):2552–9.
16. Goetz M, Callstrom M, Charboneau J, Farrell M, Maus T, Welch T, et al. Percutaneous image-guided radiofrequency ablation of painful metastases involving bone: a multicenter study. J Clin Oncol. 2004;22(2):300–6.
17. Massie M, Holland J. The cancer patient with pain: psychiatric complications and their management. J Pain Symptom Manag. 1992;7(2):99–109.
18. Spiegel D, Sands S, Koopman C. Pain and depression in patients with cancer. Cancer. 1994;74(9):2570–8.
19. Kim J, Losina E, Bono C, Schoenfeld A, Collins J, Katz J, et al. Clinical outcome of metastatic spinal cord compression treated with surgical excision ± radiation versus radiation therapy alone: a systematic review of literature. Spine (Phila Pa 1976). 2012;37(1):78–84.
20. Fisher C, DiPaola C, Ryken T, Bilsky M, Shaffrey C, Berven S, et al. A novel classification system for spinal instability in neoplastic disease: an evidence based approach and expert consensus from the Spine Oncology Study Group. Spine (Phila Pa 1976). 2010;35(22):E1221–9.
21. Fourney D, Frangou E, Ryken T, Dipaola C, Shaffrey C, Berven S, et al. Spinal instability neoplastic score: an analysis of reliability and validity from the spine oncology study group. J Clin Oncol. 2011;29(22):3072–7.
22. Gerszten P, Burton S, Ozhasoglu C, Welch W. Radiosurgery for spinal metastases: clinical experience in 500 cases from a single institution. Spine (Phila Pa 1976). 2007;32(2):193–9.
23. Choi C, Adler J, Gibbs I, Chang S, Jackson P, Minn A, et al. Stereotactic radiosurgery for treatment of spinal metastases recurring in close proximity to previously irradiated spinal cord. Int J Radiat Oncol Biol Phys. 2010;78(2):499–506.
24. Ahmed K, Stauder M, Miller R, Bauer H, Rose P, Olivier K, et al. Stereotactic body radiation therapy in spinal metastases. Int J Radiat Oncol Biol Phys. 2012;82(5):e803–9.
25. Ryu S, Yoon H, Stessin A, Gutman F, Rosiello A, Davis R. Contemporary treatment with radiosurgery for spine metastasis and spinal cord compression in 2015. Radiat Oncol J. 2015;33(1):1–11.
26. Valesin Filho E, de Abreu L, Lima G, de Cubero D, Ueno F, Figueiredo G, et al. Pain and quality of life in patients undergoing radiotherapy for spinal metastatic disease treatment. Int Arch Med. 2013; 6(1):6.
27. Tong D, Gillick L, Hendrickson F. The palliation of symptomatic osseous metastases; final results of the study by the radiation therapy oncology group. Cancer. 1982;50(5):893–9.
28. Madsen E. Painful bone metastasis: efficacy of radiotherapy assessed by the patients: a randomized trial comparing 4 Gy X 6 versus 10 Gy X 2. Int J Radiat Oncol Biol Phys. 1983;9(12):1775–9.
29. Blitzer P. Reanalysis of the RTOG study of the palliation of symptomatic osseous metastasis. Cancer. 1985;55(7):1468–72.
30. Price P, Hoskin P, Easton D, Austin D, Palmer S, Yarnold J. Prospective randomised trial of single and multifraction radiotherapy schedules in the treatment of painful bony metastases. Radiother Oncol. 1986;6(4):247–55.
31. Arcangeli G, Micheli A, Giannarelli D, La Pasta O, Tollis A, Vitullo A, et al. The responsiveness of bone metastases to radiotherapy: the effect of site, histology and radiation dose on pain relief. Radiother Oncol. 1989;14(2):95–101.
32. Cole D. A randomized trial of a single treatment versus conventional fractionation in the palliative radiotherapy of painful bone metastases. Clin Oncol (R Coll Radiol). 1989;1(2):59–62.
33. Poulter C, Cosmatos D, Rubin P, Urtasun R, Cooper J, Kuske R, et al. A report of RTOG 8206: a phase III study of whether the addition of single dose hemibody irradiation to standard fractionated local field irradiation is more effective than local field irradiation alone in the treatment of symptomatic osseous metastases. Int J Radiat Oncol Biol Phys. 1992;23(1):207–14.
34. Arcangeli G, Giovinazzo G, Saracino B, D'Angelo L, Giannarelli D, Micheli A. Radiation therapy in the management of symptomatic bone metastases: the effect of total dose and histology on pain relief and response duration. Int J Radiat Oncol Biol Phys. 1998;42(5):1119–26.
35. Ratanatharathorn V, Powers W, Moss W, Perez C. Bone metastasis: review and critical analysis of random allocation trials of local field treatment. Int J Radiat Oncol Biol Phys. 1999;44(1):1–18.
36. Chow E, Harris K, Fan G, Tsao M, Sze W. Palliative radiotherapy trials for bone metastases: a systematic review. J Clin Oncol. 2007;25(11):1423–36.
37. Chow E, Zeng L, Salvo N, Dennis K, Tsao M, Lutz S. Update on the systematic review of palliative radiotherapy trials for bone metastases. Clin Oncol (R Coll Radiol). 2012;24(2):112–24.
38. Agarawal J, Swangsilpa T, van der Linden Y, Rades D, Jeremic B, Hoskin P. The role of external beam

radiotherapy in the management of bone metastases. Clin Oncol (R Coll Radiol). 2006;18(10):747–60.
39. Lo S, Sahgal A, Hartsell W, Lutz S, Kardamakis D, van der Linden Y, et al. No the treatment of bone metastasis with highly conformal radiation therapy: a brave new world or a costly mistake? Clin Oncol (R Coll Radiol). 2009;21(9):662–4.
40. Van der Linden Y, Steenland E, van Houwelingen H, Post W, Oei B, Marijnen C, et al. Patients with a favourable prognosis are equally palliated with single and multiple fraction radiotherapy: results on survival in the Dutch Bone Metastasis Study. Radiother Oncol. 2006;78(3):245–53.
41. Wallace A, Greenwood T, Jennings J. Radiofrequency ablation and vertebral augmentation for palliation of painful spinal metastases. J Neuro-Oncol. 2015;124(1):111–8.
42. Greenwood T, Wallace A, Friedman M, Hillen T, Robinson C, Jennings J. Combined ablation and radiation therapy of spinal metastases: a novel multimodality treatment approach. Pain Physician. 2015;18(6):573–81.
43. Chang U, Cho W, Kim M, Cho C, Lee D, Rhee C. Local tumor control after retreatment of spinal metastasis using stereotactic body radiotherapy; comparison with initial treatment group. Acta Oncol. 2012;51(5):589–95.
44. Masucci G, Yu E, Ma L, Chang E, Letourneau D, Lo S, et al. Stereotactic body radiotherapy is an effective treatment in reirradiating spinal metastases: current status and practical considerations for safe practice. Expert Rev Anticancer Ther. 2011;11(12):1923–33.
45. Anchala P, Irving W, Hillen T, Friedman M, Georgy B, Coldwell D, et al. Treatment of metastatic spinal lesions with a navigational bipolar radiofrequency ablation device: a multicenter retrospective study. Pain Physician. 2014;17(4):317–27.
46. Theodorescu D. Cancer cryotherapy: evolution and biology. Rev Urol. 2004;6(Suppl 4):S9–S19.
47. Gage A, Baust J. Cryosurgery for tumors. J Am Coll Surg. 2007;205(2):342–56.
48. Ullrick S, Hebert J, Davis K. Cryoablation in the musculoskeletal system. Curr Probl Diagn Radiol. 2008;37(1):39–48.
49. McGhana J, Dodd G 3rd. Radiofrequency ablation of the liver: current status. AJR Am J Roentgenol. 2001;176(1):3–16.
50. Hoffmann R, Jakobs T, Trumm C, Helmberger T, Reiser M. RFA of renal cell carcinoma in a solitary kidney. Abdom Imaging. 2008;33(2):230–6.
51. Brace C. Radiofrequency and microwave ablation of the liver, lung, kidney, and bone: what are the differences? Curr Probl Diagn Radiol. 2009;38(3):135–43.
52. Lane M, Le H, Lee S, Young C, Heran M, Badii M, et al. Combination radiofrequency ablation and cementoplasty for palliative treatment of painful neoplastic bone metastasis: experience with 53 treated lesions in 36 patients. Skelet Radiol. 2011;40(1):25–32.
53. Thanos L, Mylona S, Galani P, Tzavoulis D, Kalioras V, Tanteles S, et al. Radiofrequency ablation of osseous metastases for the palliation of pain. Skelet Radiol. 2008;37(3):189–94.
54. Gevargez A, Groenemeyer D. Image-guided radiofrequency ablation (RFA) of spinal tumors. Eur J Radiol. 2008;65(2):246–52.
55. Callstrom M, Charboneau J, Goetz M, Rubin J, Wong G, Sloan J, et al. Painful metastases involving bone: feasibility of percutaneous CT- and US-guided radiofrequency ablation. Radiology. 2002;224(1):87–97.
56. Tomasian A, Wallace A, Northrup B, Hillen T, Jennings J. Spine cryoablation: pain palliation and local tumor control for vertebral metastases. AJNR Am J Neuroradiol. 2016;37(1):189–95.
57. Prologo J, Passalacqua M, Patel I, Bohnert N, Corn D. Image-guided cryoablation for the treatment of painful musculoskeletal metastatic disease: a single-center experience. Skelet Radiol. 2014;43(11):1551–9.
58. Thacker P, Callstrom M, Curry T, Mandrekar J, Atwell T, Goetz M, et al. Palliation of painful metastatic disease involving bone with imaging-guided treatment: comparison of patients' immediate response to radiofrequency ablation and cryoablation. AJR Am J Roentgenol. 2011;197(2):510–5.
59. Callstrom M, Atwell T, Charboneau J, Farrell M, Goetz M, Rubin J, et al. Painful metastases involving bone: percutaneous image-guided cryoablation—prospective trial interim analysis. Radiology. 2006;241(2):572–80.
60. De Freitas R, de Menezes M, Cerri G, Gangi A. Sclerotic vertebral metastases: pain palliation using percutaneous image-guided cryoablation. Cardiovasc Interv Radiol. 2011;34(Suppl 2):S294–9.
61. Callstrom M, Dupuy D, Solomon S, Beres R, Littrup P, Davis K, et al. Percutaneous image-guided cryoablation of painful metastases involving bone: multicenter trial. Cancer. 2013;119(5):1033–41.
62. McMenomy B, Kurup A, Johnson G, Carter R, McWilliams R, Markovic S, et al. Percutaneous cryoablation of musculoskeletal oligometastatic disease for complete remission. J Vasc Interv Radiol. 2013;24(2):207–13.
63. Masala S, Chiocchi M, Taglieri A, Bindi A, Nezzo M, De Vivo D, et al. Combined use of percutaneous cryoablation and vertebroplasty with 3D rotational angiograph in treatment of single vertebral metastasis: comparison with vertebroplasty. Neuroradiology. 2013;55(2):193–200.
64. Kurup A, Woodrum D, Morris J, Atwell T, Schmit G, Welch T, et al. Cryoablation of recurrent sacrococcygeal tumors. J Vasc Interv Radiol. 2012;23(8):1070–5.
65. Rodriguez Castañeda W, Callstrom M. Effective pain palliation and prevention of fracture for axial-loading skeletal metastases using combined cryoablation and cementoplasty. Tech Vasc Interv Radiol. 2011;14(3):160–9.
66. Wallace A, Greenwood T, Jennings J. Use of imaging in the management of metastatic spine disease with percutaneous ablation and vertebral augmentation. AJR Am J Roentgenol. 2015;205(2):434–41.

67. Nour S, Aschoff A, Mitchell I, Emancipator S, Duerk J, Lewin J. MR imaging-guided radio-frequency thermal ablation of the lumbar vertebrae in porcine models. Radiology. 2002;224(2):452–62.
68. Froese G, Das R, Dunscombe P. The sensitivity of the thoracolumbar spinal cord of the mouse to hyperthermia. Radiat Res. 1991;125(2):173–80.
69. Letcher F, Goldring S. The effect of radiofrequency current and heat on peripheral nerve action potential in the cat. J Neurosurg. 1968;29(1):42–7.
70. Dupuy D, Hong R, Oliver B, Goldberg S. Radiofrequency ablation of spinal tumors: temperature distribution in the spinal canal. AJR Am J Roentgenol. 2000;175(5):1263–6.
71. Yamane T, Tateishi A, Cho S, Manabe S, Yamanashi M, Dezawa A, et al. The effects of hyperthermia on the spinal cord. Spine (Phila Pa 1976). 1992;17(11):1386–91.
72. Van der Linden E, Kroft L, Dijkstra P. Treatment of vertebral tumor with posterior wall defect using image-guided radiofrequency ablation combined with vertebroplasty: preliminary results in 12 patients. J Vasc Interv Radiol. 2007;18(6):741–7.
73. Nakatsuka A, Yamakado K, Takaki H, Uraki J, Makita M, Oshima F, et al. Percutaneous radiofrequency ablation of painful spinal tumors adjacent to the spinal cord with real-time monitoring of spinal canal temperature: a prospective study. Cardiovasc Interv Radiol. 2009;32(1):70–5.
74. Kurup A, Morris J, Boon A, Strommen J, Schmit G, Atwell T, et al. Motor evoked potential monitoring during cryoablation of musculoskeletal tumors. J Vasc Interv Radiol. 2014;25(11):1657–64.
75. Rybak L, Gangi A, Buy X, La Rocca Vieira R, Wittig J. Thermal ablation of spinal osteoid osteomas close to neural elements: technical considerations. AJR Am J Roentgenol. 2010;195(4):W293–8.
76. Wallace A, Vyhmeister R, Hsi A, Robinson C, Chang R, Jennings J. Delayed vertebral body collapse after stereotactic radiosurgery and radiofrequency ablation: case report with histopathologic-MRI correlation. Interv Neuroradiol. 2015;21(6):742–9.
77. Grönemeyer D, Schirp S, Gevargez A. Image-guided radiofrequency ablation of spinal tumors: preliminary experience with an expandable array electrode. Cancer J. 2002;8(1):33–9.
78. Ha K, Kim Y, Yoo T. Intraoperative radiofrequency ablation for metastatic spine disease: report of 4 cases and review. Eur J Orthop Surg Traumatol. 2013;23(Suppl 2):S129–34.
79. Bagla S, Sayed D, Smirniotopoulos J, Brower J, Neal RJ, Dick B, et al. Multicenter prospective clinical series evaluating radiofrequency ablation in the treatment of painful spine metastases. Cardiovasc Interv Radiol. 2016;39(9):1289–97.
80. Zwart J, Sand T, Unsgaard G. Warm and cold sensory thresholds in patients with unilateral sciatica: C fibers are more severely affected than A-delta fibers. Acta Neurol Scand. 1998;97(1):41–5.

24 Minimally Invasive Spine Surgery for Metastatic Spine Disease

Joseph H. Schwab

Introduction

Cancer is expected to eclipse cardiovascular disease as the number one cause of death in the United States. One out of every two men and one out of every three women will develop cancer in their lifetime. Lung, breast, and prostate cancers are common cancers that spread to the bone. These cancers are responsible for over 200,000 deaths each year in the United States [1]. It is estimated that nearly 80% of patients who died from cancer will have metastatic disease in their spine. A number of these patients will have pathologic fractures and neurologic compromise from spinal cord compression. Unfortunately, metastatic disease is not curable, and the treatment of spinal metastases can be associated with significant morbidity, which must be considered given the limited life expectancy of many of these patients. Efforts to limit the morbidity associated with treatment are gaining traction. The use of less invasive operative techniques such as percutaneous screws and percutaneous cement augmentation combined with improvements in adjuvant therapy offers the promise of less morbidity. Less morbidity translates to more rapid recovery which is essential for all patients but particularly for patient who only have several months to live.

J. H. Schwab, MD, MS
Harvard Medical School, Massachusetts General Hospital, Boston, MA, USA
e-mail: JHSCHWAB@mgh.harvard.edu; JHSCHWAB@partners.org

Survival

Fifty percent of the patients who undergo surgery for spinal metastases will not survive over 1 year [2, 3]. Patients with lung carcinoma metastatic to the spine have a median survival of approximately 3 months after surgery [4]. Most clinicians would agree that a patient should not spend his final days recovering from surgery. In other words, the benefits of surgery ought to be considered in the context of the recovery required after surgery. If recovery from the morbidity of surgery will outlast the expected survival of the patient, then one should consider whether or not surgery is warranted. Less invasive operative techniques may help tip the scale toward considering surgery if the morbidity is decreased. However, one must be able to predict survival accurately in order to gauge whether or not the morbidity of surgery, even with less invasive techniques, is warranted. However, the ability of clinicians to predict survival in patients with bone metastases is about as good as the flip of a coin [5]. One should not rely on their ability to predict survival in these patients but rather utilize various predictive scoring systems currently available. The most accurate scoring system

R. A. W. Marco (ed.), *Metastatic Spine Disease*, https://doi.org/10.1007/978-3-319-76252-4_24

available utilizes a nomogram to provide the probability of survival at 3, 6, and 12 months [6]. The nomogram utilizes parameters well established to be important in predicting survival such as the histology of the primary tumor, number of bony metastases, and number of visceral metastases among others. Unlike other systems, however, the nomogram provides the user to ascribe a probability that the patient will survive. This of course does not allow the clinician to make a judgment. However, it does provide useful information that can be incorporated into making a clinical judgment. Being able to predict survival with some accuracy may influence decisions such as whether or not to operate and whether or not to utilize less invasive techniques.

Quality of Life

Since metastatic disease is not curable, the primary goal of surgery is to maintain or improve quality of life. The first question is whether or not surgery improved the quality of life for these patients. A large prospective cohort of over 900 patients revealed that indeed quality-of-life edge measured by the EQ-5D is improved after surgery [2]. Patients who had a better quality of life prior to surgery naturally had a better quality of life after surgery. Furthermore, patients who had a better performance status prior to surgery also seemed to do better after surgery. Quality of life like survival seems to be on a spectrum. While all of these patients are stage IV, they are at different points in their cancer development. Patients who are earlier in their metastatic phase will do better in terms of quality of life and survival than those later in their metastatic phase. The improvement seen in quality of life seems to be durable for those patients who survive [7]. Naturally, there comes a time when quality of life begins to decline for all of these patients as they approach death. Common sense would lead us to think that being readmitted to the hospital would not be a positive influence on quality of life. One recent study revealed a readmission rate of 57%. Twenty-seven percent of the readmissions were for surgical complications. Another one third of the patients were readmitted for disease progression, and the remaining third were admitted for medical reasons [8]. Clearly, avoiding readmission should be a priority in terms of maintaining quality of life not to mention overall costs. The question is whether or not minimally invasive approaches provide the same improvements in quality of life with less morbidity. While we don't know the answer to this question based on the literature, there have been studies that show that minimally invasive surgery is comparable with regard to outcomes such as performance status and pain improvements. The less invasive group had shorter hospital stays by nearly 50%. Unfortunately, the study did not evaluate readmission rate between the two groups [9].

Adjuvant Therapy

Spinal cord compression from metastatic disease is one of the primary indications for surgical intervention. Improvements in adjuvant therapies such as stereotactic radiosurgery have allowed less aggressive operative approaches to take hold. Stereotactic radiosurgery is a form of high-precision radiation therapy which allows high biologically effective doses of radiation to be delivered very near the spinal cord. This form of radiation relies on several key improvements in the delivery of radiation therapy. One improvement involves the use of real-time axial imaging such as in suite CT scanning. Another improvement has been with the methods by which radiation is delivered. Rather than using large beams of radiation, many centers are using beams of radiation with the size of a no. 2 pencil. The radiation within each of these beams of radiation can be modulated in order to optimize the dose of radiation to the tumor while minimizing the dose to normal tissues. Patients are often held in place with formfitting molds that minimize their movement in order to protect normal structures. These methods have allowed radiation oncologist to increase the dose of radiation used all the while protecting the spinal cord. The spinal cord does not tolerate doses of radiation over 55 gray. With the methods described above, higher biologically effective doses of radiation can be delivered to the tumor while ensuring that lower doses are delivered to normal structures such as the spinal cord. However, even with these advances in radiation delivery, some separation between the tumor and the spinal cord may be beneficial. Reconstitution of the thecal sac is usually all that is necessary for radiation oncologist to then safely deliver radiation to the remaining tumor. The concept of separation surgery implies the reconstitution of the thecal sac which can then be followed by stereotactic radiation therapy. This method of treatment has shown to be quite effective in controlling these tumors locally [10]. Separation surgery has also allowed the utilization of less invasive operative techniques since a gross debulking of the tumor is no longer necessary. Some centers use stereotactic radiotherapy without separation surgery to decompress the thecal sac in patients with high-grade spinal cord compression [11]. Studies comparing the outcomes of separation surgery to decompressive stereotactic radiotherapy may help delineate which patients would benefit from these interventions.

Other adjuvant therapies are also gaining acceptance in the management of spinal metastases. As with radiation, one of the key aspects of these adjuvants is safety. Most of these ablative techniques are quite effective at destroying tumor cells. However, they can also cause damage to neurologic structures, and so the penumbra associated with these techniques must be assessable in order for them to be used safely.

One well-known method of killing tumor cells is to freeze them. The original techniques involved the use of liquid nitrogen in open surgery [12]; however, less invasive methods of using cryosurgery have evolved. These methods generally use argon gas. The argon gas is injected with a percutaneous metal catheter. As the argon gas exits the catheter, the gas expands. Rapid expansion of argon gas leads to rapid cooling, and an ice ball forms [13, 14]. The ice ball forms crystals within the tumor cells. Three freeze-thaw cycles are generally used to lyse the cells. Cell lysis is accomplished through complex mechanisms including destruction of the cell membrane. One advantage of percutaneous cryoablation is that the ice ball can be seen with computed tomography. This is particularly true in soft tissues and is less true in the bone. Visualization of the ice ball provides some measure of safety when one is utilizing this technique around the spinal cord. However, using this technique around the epidural space is potentially dangerous, and spinal cord injury can occur. Some centers have gained expertise using this technique and will actually inject air or other barriers between the tumor and the spinal cord to allow safer application of cryosurgery. They generally use neuro-monitoring under general anesthesia for these techniques [13].

Microwave ablation and radiofrequency ablation are excellent techniques for destroying tumor cells. However, their safety has not been fully established in the spine since the heat zone can be difficult to assess [15–17]. For that reason one must use caution around neurologic structures.

One newer technique utilizes intraoperative magnetic resonance imaging to assess increases in heat which provides a measure of safety. The authors describe SLITT or spinal laser interstitial thermotherapy. Although this technique is time-consuming and technically demanding, the results have been reported to be excellent in small series with regard to tumor ablation and safety [18].

Vertebral Augmentation with Cement

Vertebral augmentation with cement is commonly utilized for the treatment of pathologic fractures in the spine. Only one study achieves Level 1 evidence. However, there have been multiple studies examining the outcomes of the use of cement augmentation either in the form of vertebroplasty or kyphoplasty. A recent synopsis of the published literature included the use of vertebroplasty in 2545 patients and kyphoplasty in 1690 patients. The synopsis of the literature found that within 48 h of augmentation either with kyphoplasty or vertebroplasty, patient's pain scores were significantly improved. In addition, the use of opioids was also significantly decreased. Furthermore, disability as measured by patient report outcomes was also significantly improved [19]. In the single prospective randomized study examining kyphoplasty versus usual care, kyphoplasty was superior with regard to improvements in pain, disability, and quality of life. The primary outcome measure was assessed at 1 month; however, the results appeared to be durable up to 1 year [20]. In addition, the safety profile of vertebral augmentation appears to be excellent. Cement leakage does occur and is usually asymptomatic although there are some case reports of neurologic complaints due to cement leakage [19].

Posterior Percutaneous Stabilization

Symptomatic pathologic vertebral compression fractures are typically not treated with surgical stabilization. Radiation therapy alone is often sufficient to improve pain. However, as mentioned cement augmentation has been shown to be an effective means to rapidly improve pain in many of these patients with symptomatic pathologic compression fractures. There are circumstances where patients have symptomatic pathologic compression fractures that have not responded to radiation therapy and in whom cement augmentation is considered high risk. For instance, in cases where no posterior wall exists in the vertebral body, some interventionalists find the use of cement augmentation to be potentially unsafe. In addition, there are circumstances, such as in multiple myeloma, where little to no bone and no trabecular bone remain for cement to interdigitate, thus making cement augmentation less attractive. In these cases, when stabilization is indicated, percutaneous pedicle screw placement may play a role. Small studies have shown improvements in function after minimally invasive stabilization with pedicle screws [21]. The use of percutaneous pedicle screws has gained acceptance, and the technique is well established now. Still, percutaneous pedicle screw placement in the treatment of spinal metastases is most often utilized in conjunction with a form of spinal decompression. The main reason for this is that cement augmentation techniques have improved such that stabilization with cement is often sufficient and pedicle screw placement is not needed as a stand-alone procedure.

Minimally Invasive Decompression

Minimally invasive techniques have improved over time largely based on the experiences in degenerative spinal conditions. However, the techniques utilized in degenerative conditions of the spine can be extrapolated into treatment of spinal metastases. The advances in minimally invasive techniques have occurred simultaneously with advances in adjuvant therapies as I described above. The principal change in the operative techniques utilized for the management of spinal metastases includes the use of separation surgery. Since separation surgery lends itself well to minimally invasive techniques, there has been a dovetail effect.

An important caveat to the use of minimally invasive techniques to achieve spinal decompression involves the treatment of historically vascular tumors including renal cell carcinoma, thyroid carcinoma, and hepatocellular carcinoma. While all tumors can have a robust blood supply, these three tumors generally present a larger problem with bleeding than others. Another tumor that can be quite difficult to manage from a hemostasis perspective is myeloma. The principal difference between myeloma and the three tumors that have been mentioned is that myeloma tends not to have large vascular inflow and instead bleeds from smaller vessels. The reason that it is important is that myeloma tends not to respond as well to preoperative embolization. If one is considering a minimally invasive technique, then preoperative embolization should certainly be considered for these tumors. Some would argue that minimally invasive techniques are not indicated in these tumors owing to the robust blood supply. Clearly though, one must be prepared for bleeding, and if bleeding is too robust to complete a minimally invasive technique, then one must be prepared for an open decompression. If embolization is planned, then the embolization should occur as close to the time of surgery as possible to maximize the effectiveness of the embolization [22].

The technique utilized for minimally invasive decompression depends upon the comfort of the surgeon. There are various retractors that have been designed to assist with lateral approaches utilizing a minimally invasive technique. Furthermore, there are several retractor systems that can assist in posterior and posterior lateral approaches. Some surgeons continue to favor using tubular retractor systems which offer simplicity and versatility, but there are many different options available depending upon the surgeon's comfort level. In some instances it is necessary to utilize two approaches in order to provide circumferential decompression of the spinal cord. Again, the goal of the surgery must be kept in mind. In most cases separation surgery is the goal in which case the position of the tumor dictates the best approach. For instance, if the tumor is principally dorsal to the spinal cord, then a dorsal approach makes the most sense obviously. For 360° compression, one must utilize either a longer midline approach or more than one incision. It is generally my preference to approach the spine through a posterolateral approach. If only one half of the spinal cord is being compressed laterally, I often utilize a paraspinal incision to affect a costotransversectomy approach. However, if both sides of the spinal cord need to be addressed, I will either perform a longer midline incision which allows me to approach the spinal cord from both sides, or I will use two paraspinal incisions.

Case Example No. 1

A 55-year-old female with history of metastatic breast carcinoma presents with severe thoracolumbar pain and right thigh pain. She was diagnosed with breast cancer 5 years earlier, and she has received chemotherapy as well as radiation therapy to her upper lumbar spine. She has known lung metastasis and several other bony metastases in her spine that are not symptomatic. The pain is severe but she still manages to work part time and tries to remain active. Her hemoglobin is 12 and her white blood cell count is 10. She has numbness over her right thigh and significant pain and tenderness to the midline of her upper lumbar spine. We utilized a nomogram to help understand her probability of survival. Her probability of surviving to 3 months was over 90%, and her probability of surviving to 1 year was 73% [3]. Given her relatively good survival probability, it was determined that she was a good surgical candidate if her goals were aligned with what surgery could offer. She has a pathologic fracture in her lumbar spine that would likely be amenable to cement augmentation (Fig. 24.1). However, she also has

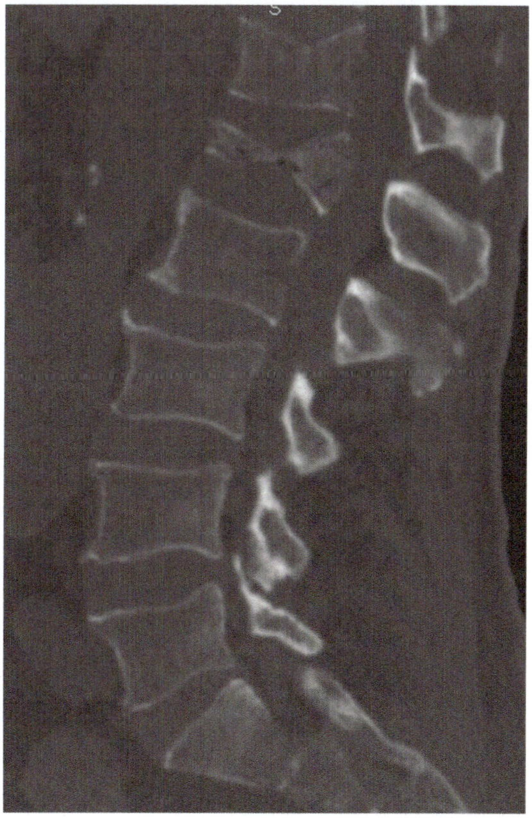

Fig. 24.1 This sagittal computed tomographic image demonstrates the pathologic fracture in the first lumbar vertebrae

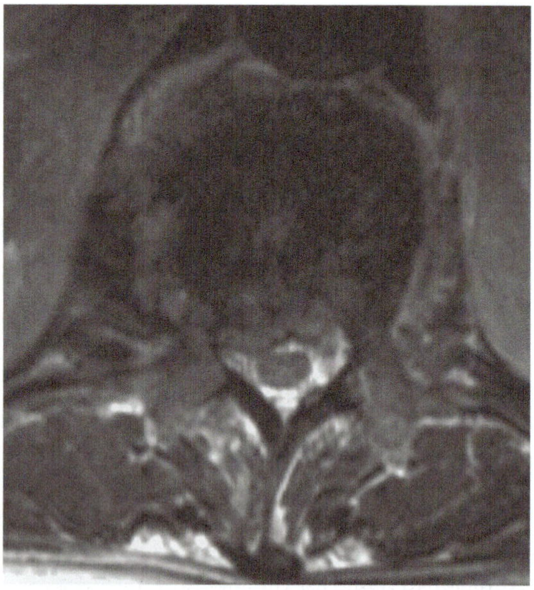

Fig. 24.2 This is an axial T2-weighted image of the first lumbar vertebrae demonstrating the epidural spinal cord compression. The spinal cord is not displaced but it is touching the tumor. It was decided that there was not enough space to safely deliver stereotactic radiation therapy

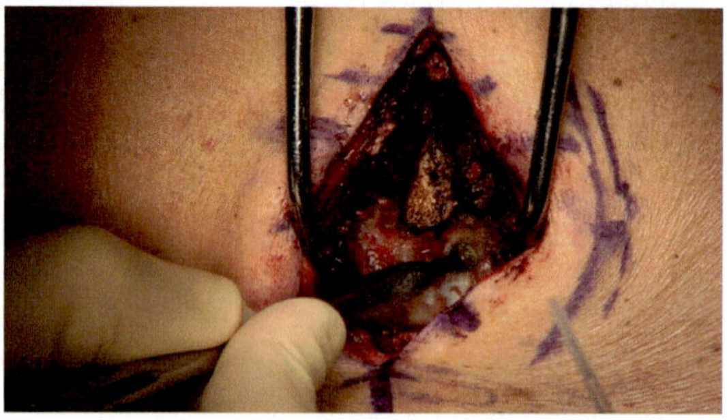

Fig. 24.3 This is an intraoperative photograph demonstrating a mini-open incision over the first lumbar vertebrae. A high-speed Burr is being utilized (Legend, Medtronic, Minneapolis, MN) to remove the posterior elements

epidural spinal cord compression (Fig. 24.2). She has already received radiation to this region. Stereotactic radiosurgery was considered, but our multidisciplinary team did not believe that there was enough clearance between the tumor and the spinal cord. For that reason, we elected to perform separation surgery. A mini-open incision was used in the midline to facilitate access to both sides of the spinal cord (Fig. 24.3). We decided to stabilize her spine with percutaneous pedicle screws; however, kyphoplasty may have also been adequate (Fig. 24.4a–c).

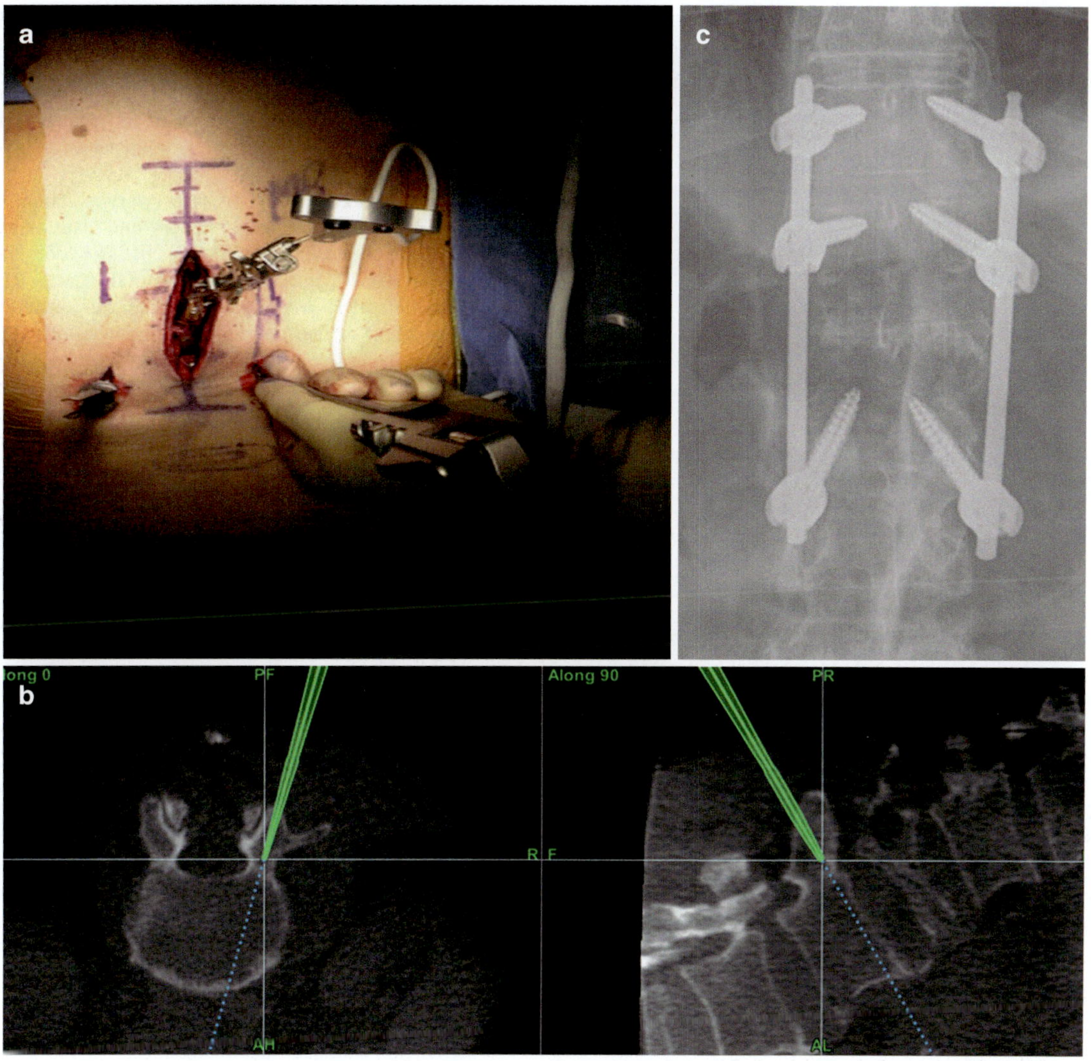

Fig. 24.4 (**a**–**c**) Panel (**a**) is an intraoperative image showing the navigation instruments (Stryker, Kalamazoo, MI) relative to the mini-open incision. Panel (**b**) reveals the navigation display utilized to insert the pedicle screws, and panel (**c**) shows the screws and rods after they have been secured into position

References

1. American Cancer Society 2013 [Internet]; 2013 [cited November 4]. www.cancer.org.
2. Choi D, Fox Z, Albert T, Arts M, Balabaud L, Bunger C, et al. Prediction of quality of life and survival after surgery for symptomatic spinal metastases: a multicenter cohort study to determine suitability for surgical treatment. Neurosurgery. 2015;77(5):698–708.
3. Paulino Pereira NR, Janssen SJ, van Dijk E, Harris MB, Hornicek FJ, Ferrone ML, et al. Development of a prognostic survival algorithm for patients with metastatic spine disease. J Bone Joint Surg Am. 2016;98(21):1767–76.
4. Goodwin CR, Khattab MH, Sankey EW, Elder BD, Kosztowski TA, Sarabia-Estrada R, et al. Factors associated with life expectancy in patients with metastatic spine disease from adenocarcinoma of the lung. Global Spine J. 2015;5(5):417–24.
5. Nathan SS, Healey JH, Mellano D, Hoang B, Lewis I, Morris CD, et al. Survival in patients operated on for pathologic fracture: implications for end-of-life orthopedic care. J Clin Oncol. 2005;23(25):6072–82.
6. Paulino Pereira NR, Mclaughlin L, Janssen SJ, van Dijk CN, Bramer JAM, Laufer I, et al. The SORG nomogram accurately predicts 3- and 12-months survival for operable spine metastatic disease: external validation. J Surg Oncol. 2017;115(8):1019–27.
7. Choi D, Fox Z, Albert T, Arts M, Balabaud L, Bunger C, et al. Rapid improvements in pain and quality of life are sustained after surgery for spinal metastases in a large prospective cohort. Br J Neurosurg. 2016;30(3):337–44.
8. Abu-Bonsrah N, Goodwin CR, De la Garza-Ramos R, Sankey EW, Liu A, Kosztowski T, et al. Readmissions after surgical resection of metastatic tumors of the spine at a single institution. World Neurosurg. 2017;101:701.e1.
9. Hansen-Algenstaedt N, Kwan MK, Algenstaedt P, Chiu CK, Viezens L, Chan TS, et al. Comparison between minimally invasive surgery and conventional open surgery for patients with spinal metastasis: a prospective propensity score-matched study. Spine (Phila Pa 1976). 2017;42(10):789–97.
10. Laufer I, Iorgulescu JB, Chapman T, Lis E, Shi W, Zhang Z, et al. Local disease control for spinal metastases following "separation surgery" and adjuvant hypofractionated or high-dose single-fraction stereotactic radiosurgery: outcome analysis in 186 patients. J Neurosurg Spine. 2013;18(3):207–14.
11. Ryu S, Rock J, Jain R, Lu M, Anderson J, Jin JY, Rosenblum M, Movsas B, Kim JH. Radiosurgical decompression of metastatic epidural compression. Cancer. 2010;116(9):2250–7.
12. Marcove RC, Miller TR. Treatment of primary and metastatic bone tumors by cryosurgery. JAMA. 1969;207(10):1890–4.
13. Rose PS, Morris JM. Cryosurgery/cryoablation in musculoskeletal neoplasms: history and state of the art. Curr Rev Musculoskelet Med. 2015;8(4):353–60.
14. McMenomy BP, Kurup AN, Johnson GB, Carter RE, McWilliams RR, Markovic SN, et al. Percutaneous cryoablation of musculoskeletal oligometastatic disease for complete remission. J Vasc Interv Radiol. 2013;24(2):207–13.
15. Ha KY, Kim YH, Yoo TW. Intraoperative radiofrequency ablation for metastatic spine disease: report of 4 cases and review. Eur J Orthop Surg Traumatol. 2013;23(Suppl 2):S129–34.
16. Adachi A, Kaminou T, Ogawa T, Kawai T, Takaki Y, Sugiura K, et al. Heat distribution in the spinal canal during radiofrequency ablation for vertebral lesions: study in swine. Radiology. 2008;247(2):374–80.
17. Simon CJ, Dupuy DE. Image-guided ablative techniques in pelvic malignancies: radiofrequency ablation, cryoablation, microwave ablation. Surg Oncol Clin N Am. 2005;14(2):419–31.
18. Tatsui CE, Nascimento CNG, Suki D, Amini B, Li J, Ghia AJ, et al. Image guidance based on MRI for spinal interstitial laser thermotherapy: technical aspects and accuracy. J Neurosurg Spine. 2017;26(5): 605–12.
19. Health Quality Ontario. Vertebral augmentation involving vertebroplasty or kyphoplasty for cancer-related vertebral compression fractures: a systematic review. Ont Health Technol Assess Ser. 2016;16(11):1–202.
20. Berenson J, Pflugmacher R, Jarzem P, Zonder J, Schechtman K, Tillman JB, et al. Balloon kyphoplasty versus non-surgical fracture management for treatment of painful vertebral body compression fractures in patients with cancer: a multicentre, randomised controlled trial. Lancet Oncol. 2011;12(3):225–35.
21. Schwab JH, Gasbarrini A, Cappuccio M, Boriani L, De Iure F, Colangeli S, et al. Minimally invasive posterior stabilization improved ambulation and pain scores in patients with plasmacytomas and/or metastases of the spine. Int J Surg Oncol. 2011;2011:239230.
22. Hong CG, Cho JH, Suh DC, Hwang CJ, Lee DH, Lee CS. Preoperative embolization in patients with metastatic spinal cord compression: mandatory or optional? World J Surg Oncol. 2017;15(1):3.

Index

R. A. W. Marco (ed.), *Metastatic Spine Disease*, https://doi.org/10.1007/978-3-319-76252-4